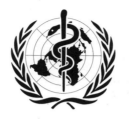

WORLD HEALTH ORGANIZATION

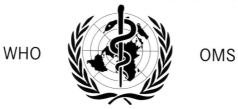

WHO   OMS

International Agency for Research on Cancer

WORLD CANCER REPORT

Edited by

Bernard W. Stewart
Paul Kleihues

IARCPress
Lyon 2003

Published by IARC*Press*, International Agency for Research on Cancer,
150 cours Albert Thomas, F-69372 Lyon, France

For bibliographic citations, please use the following format:
Stewart B. W. and Kleihues P. (Eds): World Cancer Report. IARC*Press*. Lyon 2003.

IARC Library Cataloguing in Publication Data
World Cancer Report/editors, B. W. Stewart, P. Kleihues

1. Neoplasms - epidemiology 2. Neoplasms - etiology 3. Neoplasms - prevention & control 4. Neoplasms - therapy 5. World Health I. Stewart B.W., II. Kleihues P., III. Title

ISBN 92 832 0411 5   (NLM Classification W 1)

WORLD CANCER REPORT

Editors	Bernard W. Stewart, Ph.D.
	Paul Kleihues, M.D.
Coordinating editor	Heidi Mattock, Ph.D.
Layout	Pascale Dia
	Catrin Goebels
	Sibylle Söring
Illustrations	Catrin Goebels
	Felix Krönert
	Georges Mollon
Printed by	Darantiere
	21801 Quetigny, France
Publisher	IARC*Press*
	International Agency for
	Research on Cancer (IARC)
	World Health Organization (WHO)
	69372 Lyon, France
	www.iarc.fr/press

CONTENTS

FOREWORD

The global burden of cancer continues to increase. In the year 2000, 5.3 million men and 4.7 million women developed a malignant tumour and 6.2 million died from the disease. Given the current trends in smoking prevalence and the adoption of unhealthy lifestyles, the number of new cases is expected to grow by 50% over the next 20 years to reach 15 million by 2020. Worldwide, twelve per cent of people die from cancer and in industrialised countries more than one in four will die from the disease. Each of us will experience grief and pain as a result of cancer, as a patient, a family member or a friend.

In developed countries, the overall cancer mortality is more than twice as high as in developing countries. The main reasons for the greater cancer burden of affluent societies are the earlier onset of the tobacco epidemic, the earlier exposure to occupational carcinogens and the Western diet and lifestyle. In developing countries, up to one quarter of malignancies are caused by infectious agents, including the hepatitis (HBV and HCV), and human papillomaviruses (HPV). HBV vaccination has already been shown to prevent liver cancer in high-incidence countries and it is likely that HPV vaccination will become a reality within the next 3-5 years. Today, more than 80% of women dying from cervical cancer live in developing countries. Successful prevention of HPV infection would make an immense contribution to women's health.

Tobacco consumption remains the most important avoidable cancer risk. During the twentieth century, approximately 100 million people died worldwide from tobacco-associated diseases. Half of all regular smokers are killed by the habit and one quarter will die prematurely before the age of 70. The World Health Organization and its member states will soon adopt the Framework Convention on Tobacco Control, a major step towards reducing the enormous morbidity and mortality associated with tobacco consumption.

During the past decade, research into the causes of human cancer, the molecular basis of malignant transformation and gene-environment interactions that contribute to individual cancer risks has made significant progress. Insight into cellular signalling pathways has led to the development of new anticancer drugs that are more specific and carry a lesser burden for the patient.

It is possible to prevent at least one-third of the cases that occur every year throughout the world through better use of existing knowledge. Where sufficient resources are available, current knowledge also allows the early detection and effective treatment of a further one-third of cases. Pain relief and palliative care can improve the quality of life of cancer patients and their families, even in very low resource settings.

My colleagues at the International Agency for Research on Cancer in Lyon and more than 50 contributors from all over the world have compiled a summary of the current understanding of cancer causes, cancer development, prevention and treatment. Together with the recently published WHO guidelines for national cancer control programmes, it will provide a scientific basis for public health action and assist us in our goal to reduce the morbidity and mortality from cancer and to improve the quality of life of cancer patients and their families, everywhere in the world.

Gro Harlem Brundtland, M.D.
Director-General,
World Health Organization

1

The global burden of cancer

Cancer is a major disease burden worldwide but there are marked geographical variations in incidence overall and at specific organ sites. Reliable estimation of the number of new cases (incidence) and death from the disease (mortality) requires population-based cancer registration. Compilation of worldwide age-standardized cancer rates allows the identification of countries and regions where particular tumour types are most prevalent. Such differences usually reflect exposure to distinct causative environmental factors. In addition to providing data on the distribution and the causation of neoplastic disease, descriptive epidemiology provides the basis for prevention, health service planning and resource allocation.

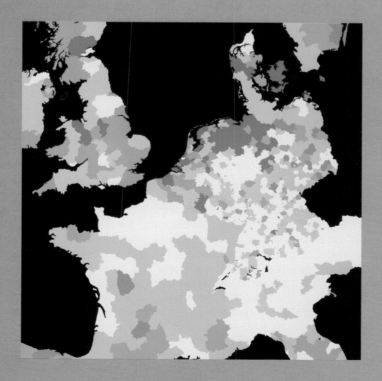

THE GLOBAL BURDEN OF CANCER

SUMMARY

> Worldwide, approximately 10 million people are diagnosed with cancer annually and more than 6 million die of the disease every year; currently, over 22 million people in the world are cancer patients.

> All communities are burdened with cancer, but there are marked regional differences. The total cancer burden is highest in affluent societies, mainly due to a high incidence of tumours associated with smoking and Western lifestyle, i.e. tumours of the lung, colorectum, breast and prostate.

> In developing countries, up to 25% of tumours are associated with chronic infections, e.g. hepatitis B virus (liver cancer), human papillomaviruses (cervical cancer), and *Helicobacter pylori* (stomach cancer).

> Differences in the regional distribution of cancer and its outcome, as documented by a worldwide network of population-based cancer registries, help to identify causative factors and those influencing survival.

> In some Western countries, cancer mortality rates have recently started to decline, due to a reduction in smoking prevalence, improved early detection and advances in cancer therapy.

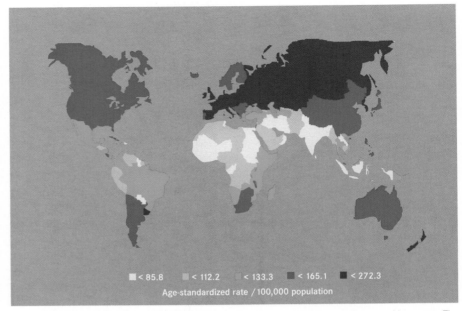

< 85.8   < 112.2   < 133.3   < 165.1   < 272.3
Age-standardized rate / 100,000 population

Fig. 1.1 Mortality rates in men for all cancer sites combined, excluding non-melanoma skin cancer. The highest rates are recorded in affluent countries.

Cancer afflicts all communities. Worldwide, the burden of disease impinges on the lives of tens of millions annually. Based on the most recent incidence and mortality data available, there were 10.1 million new cases, 6.2 million deaths and 22.4 million persons living with cancer in the year 2000 [1]. This represents an increase of around 19% in incidence and 18% in mortality since 1990.

Cancer involves a pathological breakdown in the processes which control cell proliferation, differentiation and death of particular cells. Most commonly, the malignant cells which form a tumour arise from epithelial tissue (i.e. tissue which has a secretory or lining function) and are termed "carcinoma". In many organs (breast, lung, bowel, etc.), most cancers are carcinomas. While having certain characteristics in common, different types of cancer have very different causes and show widely differing response to treatment. The biological basis of malignant transformation, the influence of environmental factors and options for prevention, screening and treatment are addressed in this Report. This chapter delineates the burden of cancer in numerical terms by reference to incidence, mortality and prevalence (Box: *Terms used in cancer epidemiology*, p18) on the basis of data generated through cancer registries and vital statistics systems (death registration).

The major cancer types

In terms of incidence, the most common cancers worldwide (excluding non-melanoma skin cancers) (Fig. 1.2) are lung (12.3% of all cancers), breast (10.4%) and colorectum (9.4%). For any disease, the relationship of incidence to mortality is an indication of prognosis, similar incidence and mortality rates being indicative of an essentially fatal condition. Thus, lung cancer accounts for most deaths from cancer in the world (1.1 million annually), since it is almost invariably associated with poor prognosis. On the other hand, appropriate intervention is often effective in avoiding a fatal outcome following diagnosis of breast cancer. Hence this particular cancer, which ranks second in terms of incidence, is not among the top three causes of death from cancer, which are respectively cancers of the lung (17.8% of all cancer deaths), stomach (10.4%) and liver (8.8%).

The most conspicuous feature of the distribution of cancer between the sexes is

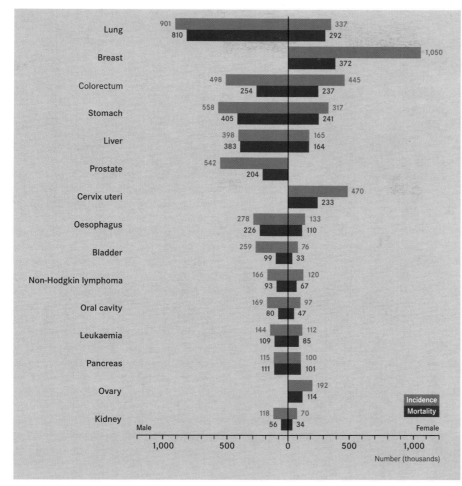

Cancer	Male Incidence	Male Mortality	Female Incidence	Female Mortality
Lung	901	810	337	292
Breast			1,050	372
Colorectum	498	254	445	237
Stomach	558	405	317	241
Liver	398	383	165	164
Prostate	542	204		
Cervix uteri			470	233
Oesophagus	278	226	133	110
Bladder	259	99	76	33
Non-Hodgkin lymphoma	166	93	120	67
Oral cavity	169	80	97	47
Leukaemia	144	109	112	85
Pancreas	115	111	100	101
Ovary			192	114
Kidney	118	56	70	34

Incidence
Mortality

Male Female

Number (thousands)

Fig. 1.2 Incidence and mortality of the most common cancers worldwide.

the male predominance of lung cancer (Fig. 1.2). Stomach, oesophageal and bladder cancer are also much more common in males. For the most part, differences in distribution between the sexes are attributable to differences in exposure to causative agents rather than to variations in susceptibility. For other tumour types, including cancers of the colorectum and pancreas, there is little difference in the sex distribution. Generally speaking, the relationship of incidence to mortality is not affected by sex. Thus, for example, the prognosis following diagnosis of liver or pancreatic cancer is dismal for both males and females. Many other tumour types are more responsive to therapy, so that cancers of breast, prostate and uter-ine cervix, for example, are the cause of death in only a minority of patients diagnosed.

The burden of cancer is distributed unequally between the developing and developed world, with particular cancer types exhibiting different patterns of distribution (Fig. 1.7). All of Europe, Japan, Australia, New Zealand and North America are classified here as more developed regions, whilst Africa, Latin America and the Caribbean, Asia (excluding Japan), Micronesia, Polynesia and Melanesia are classified as developing or less developed regions.

As discussed in later chapters, many differences in the distribution of cancer between regions are explicable with refer-ence to etiological factors. For example, populations in developing countries are vulnerable to cancers in which infectious agents (and associated non-malignant diseases) play a significant role [2] (*Chronic infections*, p56). These include cancers of the stomach, uterine cervix, liver and possibly oesophagus. Conversely, there are other cancers – exemplified by cancers of the colorectum and prostate – where the burden of disease falls disproportionately on the developed world. These observations seem to be largely attributable to differences in lifestyle, with dietary factors believed to be of major significance.

Monitoring

The extent of variation in the impact of cancer between different regions of the world has been studied for more than 50 years. Data permitting such comparisons come from cancer registries and from local and national health statistics, with respect to deaths from cancer. The completeness and accuracy of data accumulated by cancer registries has progressively increased, as has the proportion of the

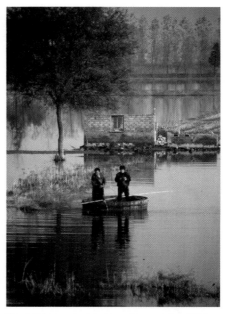

Fig. 1.3 In some regions, such as parts of China, flood waters can become sources of chronic *Schistosoma* infection which may cause bladder cancer.

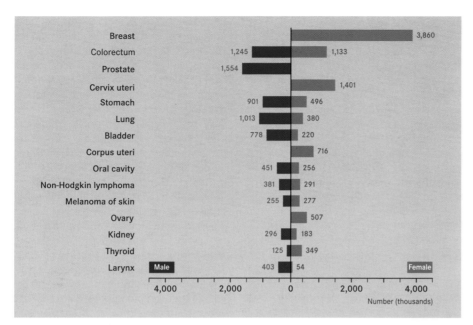

Fig. 1.4 The most prevalent cancers worldwide in 2000, expressed as thousands of persons diagnosed with cancer within the previous five years.

world's population included in such databases.

The International Agency for Research on Cancer has played a primary role in the establishment of cancer registries, the accreditation of data collection procedures and the integration and reporting of findings [3]. An aspect of this work has been publication of the volumes *Cancer Incidence in Five Continents* and such data are currently available via the Internet [4].

Incidence data are available from cancer registries. For this Report, incidence rates for a country were obtained whenever possible from cancer registries serving the whole population, or a representative sample of it. The number of cancer registries has increased steadily over the years. Registries cover entire national populations, selected regions or sub-samples of selected regions. Registries also provide statistics on cancer survival. With data on incidence and on survival, the prevalence of cancer (number of persons living with cancer that was diagnosed within the preceding five years) can be estimated. Mortality data by cause are available for many countries because of

registration of vital events (birth and death), although the degree of detail and quality of the data (both in terms of the accuracy of the recorded cause of death and the completeness of registration) vary considerably.

The most recent national mortality data from the WHO mortality data bank were used to obtain information on cancer deaths. For some countries a correction factor was applied to account for known and quantified under-reporting of mortality.

In the absence of either of these data sources, an estimate of cancer incidence was built up from available information on the relative frequency of different cancers (by age-group and sex), applied to an overall "all sites" incidence figure for the corresponding area. These "all sites" figures were derived from such data as could be found for the corresponding geographic area.

For some countries, data on mortality could be found, but nothing on incidence. In this case, incidence was estimated using sets of regression models which, for a given area, cancer, sex and age group, predict incidence from mortality, based on

cancer registry data from the same area. Conversely, incidence rates were available for some countries where there were no data on mortality. For these countries, information on cancer survival was used to obtain estimates of mortality. Prevalence was estimated from incidence and survival. Three sources of data on population-based survival were used: the *Cancer Survival in Developing Countries* project by IARC [5], which provides cancer survival data for populations of China, the Philippines, Thailand, India and Cuba for all of the sites considered; the SEER programme covering 10% of the US population [6] and the *EUROCARE II* project providing figures from several European cancer registries [7]. Estimates of the population of countries (by age and sex) for the year 2000 were taken from the 1998 UN population projections [8].

By these methods, comprehensive databases have been generated including information on the incidence, mortality, prevalence and age distribution of cancer for many countries and in some cases for local areas (or sub-populations) within countries. Additional information and the methods used to produce estimates of incidence, mortality, and prevalence are summarized elsewhere [9, 10]. Only a partial overview of the total available data is presented here.

Regional distribution of cancer

The incidence of cancer for 12 broad "regions" is shown in Figure 1.8. Even when considered in relation to such broad geographical areas, marked differences are apparent in terms of the sites of the most common tumours in a region, and the ranking of those cancer sites. Equally important, some similarities are evident.

The validity of contrasting cancer incidence in more and less developed countries (Fig. 1.7) is supported, at least in part, by the similar patterns of cancer incidence recorded for North America, Northern Europe, Western Europe and Oceania (predominantly Australia and New Zealand). In all these regions the predominant cancers are those of colorectum, lung, breast and prostate, the only deviation from this pattern being the emergence of melanoma as a major cancer in Australia and New Zealand. Both Central and Southern Europe differ marginally from this pattern as a result of the relatively high incidence of stomach cancer. Bladder cancer occupies the fifth or sixth position in all these regions (except Oceania).

East Asia, which includes Japan and regions of China, comprises nations and communities divided between the "more developed" and "less developed" categories. Accordingly, the distribution of cancer is evocative of that in more developed regions with regard to lung, colorectal and breast cancer, but different insofar as cancers of the stomach, oesophagus and liver are of major concern. In the less developed world, there is no single grouping of cancers constituting a clear pattern; rather particular patterns are specific to broad regions.

Breast cancer is of importance to communities in both more and less developed countries. In contrast, cervical cancer is a particularly serious problem for much of the developing world including South Central Asia, sub-Saharan Africa and South America. Otherwise, there are cancers that are of singular significance to certain regions. Thus cancer of the oral cavity ranks high in South Central Asia, liver cancer is of particular relevance to sub-Saharan Africa and parts of Asia, while bladder cancer is a major problem for Northern Africa and Western Asia.

Possibilities for cancer prevention and treatment

As previously indicated, the overview of cancer in the world presented here represents a superficial examination of the comprehensive data that are available concerning the distribution of cancer. Despite the limitations of the present assessment, certain principles are clearly evident. The burden of cancer in the world varies according to the community. The extent of variation when subcontinental regions are compared is equally apparent at a national level and may be clear even at the local district level. As this Report describes, variation in cancer incidence is primarily explicable in terms of, and indicative of, the influence of particular risk factors. Many established risk factors operate as causes of disease, for which the relevant biological mechanisms are

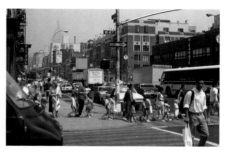
Fig. 1.5 Traffic emissions and other sources of atmospheric, soil and water pollution may account for as many as 4% of all cancers.

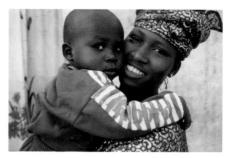
Fig. 1.6 A young mother from Senegal holding her son wearing a sweatshirt with cigarette industry logo.

being progressively clarified. For the most part, understanding the causes of cancer

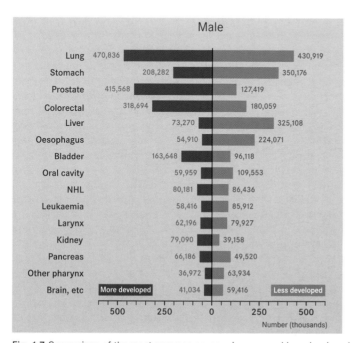
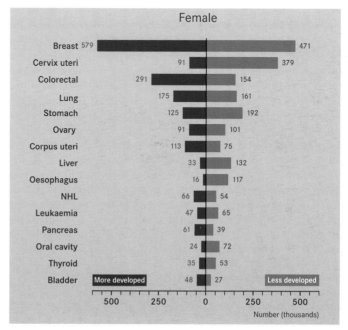

Fig. 1.7 Comparison of the most common cancers in more and less developed countries in 2000. NHL = Non-Hodgkin lymphoma.

Male

	More developed	Less developed
Lung	470,836	430,919
Stomach	208,282	350,176
Prostate	415,568	127,419
Colorectal	318,694	180,059
Liver	73,270	325,108
Oesophagus	54,910	224,071
Bladder	163,648	96,118
Oral cavity	59,959	109,553
NHL	80,181	86,436
Leukaemia	58,416	85,912
Larynx	62,196	79,927
Kidney	79,090	39,158
Pancreas	66,186	49,520
Other pharynx	36,972	63,934
Brain, etc	41,034	59,416

Number (thousands)

Female

	More developed	Less developed
Breast	579	471
Cervix uteri	91	379
Colorectal	291	154
Lung	175	161
Stomach	125	192
Ovary	91	101
Corpus uteri	113	75
Liver	33	132
Oesophagus	16	117
NHL	66	54
Leukaemia	47	65
Pancreas	61	39
Oral cavity	24	72
Thyroid	35	53
Bladder	48	27

Number (thousands)

Fig. 1.8 Incidence of cancer in twelve world regions.

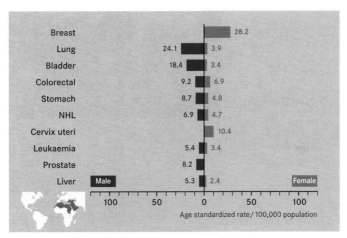

Incidence of cancer in North Africa and Western Asia.

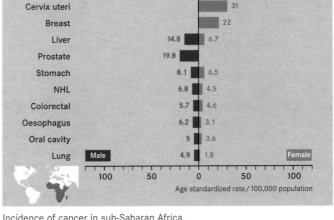

Incidence of cancer in sub-Saharan Africa.

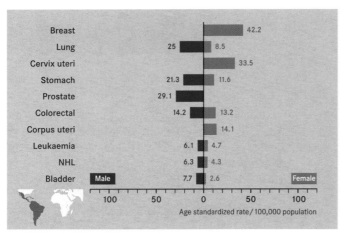

Incidence of cancer in South America and the Caribbean.

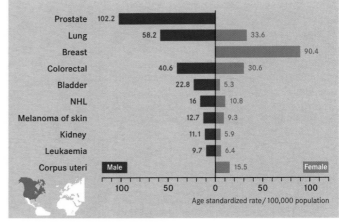

Incidence of cancer in North America.

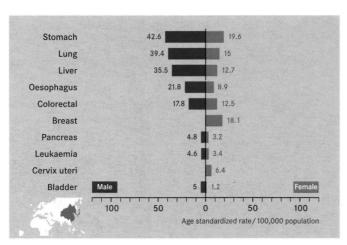

Incidence of cancer in Eastern Asia.

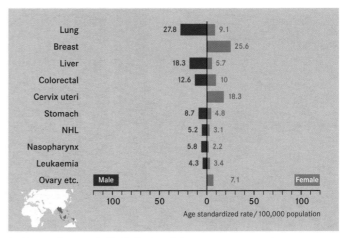

Incidence of cancer in South-Eastern Asia.

Fig. 1.8 Incidence of cancer in twelve world regions (continued).

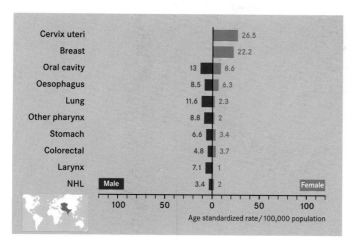

Incidence of cancer in South Central Asia.

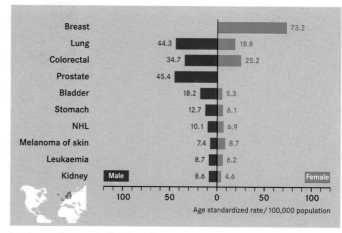

Incidence of cancer in Northern Europe.

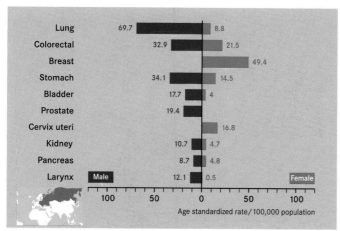

Incidence of cancer in Eastern Europe.

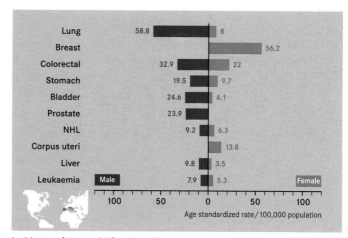

Incidence of cancer in Southern Europe.

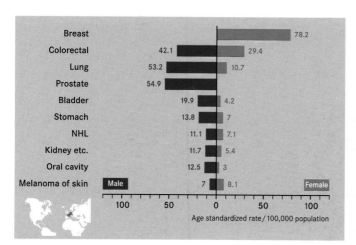

Incidence of cancer in Western Europe.

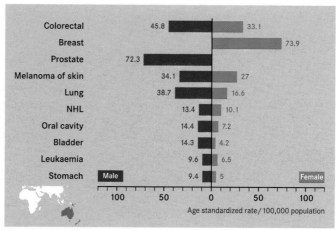

Incidence of cancer in Oceania.

TERMS USED IN CANCER EPIDEMIOLOGY

There are several statistics that may be used to measure the burden of cancer in a given community. The following discussion is presented specifically in relation to cancer, though in most instances the terms discussed have general application.

Cases are individual cancers. A person may have more than one cancer, giving rise to multiple cases in the same person, though this is relatively rare.

Incidence is the number of new cases which occur. It can be expressed as an absolute number of cases per year or as a rate per 100,000 persons per year. The latter provides an approximation of the average risk of developing a cancer, which is useful in making comparisons between populations (countries, ethnic groups, or different time periods within a country for example).

Mortality is the number of deaths occurring, and the mortality rate is the number of deaths per 100,000 persons per year. The number of deaths provides one measure of the outcome, or impact, of cancer. It represents the product of the incidence and the fatality of a given cancer. "Fatality", the inverse of survival, is the proportion of cancer patients who die. Mortality rates therefore measure the average risk to the population of dying from a specific cancer, while fatality (1 minus survival) represents the probability that an individual diagnosed with cancer will die from it.

Rate is a measure of the frequency of a phenomenon. Incidence, mortality and other data may be presented as rates, most often in relation to populations of 100,000.

Age-standardized rates (ASR) take into account differences in the age structure of the populations being compared. This is necessary because the risk of cancer is very powerfully determined by age; a population containing a high proportion of old people will generally have a higher incidence of cancer than one in which young people predominate. Standardization is a set of techniques used to remove the effects of differences in age when comparing two or more rates. Thus, standardization may be undertaken to allow comparison on the basis of populations having the same age structure for which a "world standard population" is commonly used.

Prevalence of cancer indicates the number of persons in whom the disease has been diagnosed and who are alive at a particular point in time. Thus prevalence may be characterized as the number of people living with cancer, although a precise meaning of this term is not agreed. Some authors understand "living with cancer" to refer to ever having been diagnosed, even if this was many years ago, and the disease no longer has any impact on the individual. The latter circumstances may be equated with cure. Probably what is sought from prevalence in most instances is the number of people being treated for cancer (or, at least, still needing some sort of medical supervision). Such data are not only difficult to obtain, but would certainly vary from one place to another, depending on medical practice. However, since cure is often but arbitrarily taken to equate with survival beyond five years, a useful compromise is to estimate prevalence as the number of people alive who have had a cancer diagnosed within the last five years.

Several other complex parameters are used to measure the impact of disease, and cancer specifically, particularly in relation to health economics. These parameters include *person-years of life lost* (how many years of normal life span are lost due to deaths from cancer). Economists often refine this measurement, by giving different values to life-years at different ages, so that a year saved at, for example, age 20, is more "valuable" than one at age 60. A further refinement is to calculate *quality-* or *disability-adjusted life-years lost (DALY)*, by giving a numerical score to the years lived with a reduced quality of life between diagnosis and death (where quality = 0) or cure (quality = 1). Such estimates require comprehensive data on incidence and survival as well as approximations about quality of life in different circumstances and cultures.

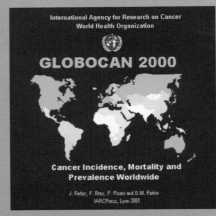

Fig. 1.9 The Globocan 2000 database is published as a CD and can be updated online.

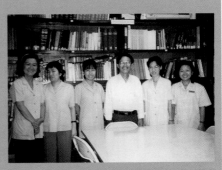

Fig. 1.10 A cancer registration team in Ho Chi Minh City, Viet Nam.

provides an opportunity for cancer prevention or early detection. This transition from documentation of disease to a basis for action may also be pursued in relation to treatment. Thus incidence, mortality and other data offer insight into prognosis and efficacy of treatment for particular cancer types.

The distribution of cancer changes with time, and specific assessments generally relate to a particular period. Irrespective of change in distribution, the burden of cancer remains. This burden involves the disruption, by suffering, of the lives of hundreds of millions of the world's population. As will be indicated throughout this volume, that burden may be progressively lessened by appropriate intervention.

REFERENCES

1. Ferlay J, Bray F, Parkin DM, Pisani P, eds (2001) *Globocan 2000: Cancer Incidence and Mortality Worldwide (IARC Cancer Bases No. 5)*, Lyon, IARCPress.

2. Parkin DM, Pisani P, Muñoz N, Ferlay J (1998) The global health burden of infection. In: Weiss RA, Beral,V, Newton, R eds, *Infections and Human Cancer (Vol. 33, Cancer Surveys)*, Cold Spring Harbor, Cold Spring Harbor Laboratory Press.

3. Parkin DM, Hakulinen T (1991) Analysis of survival. In: Jensen OM, Parkin DM, MacLennan R, Muir C, Skeet RG eds, *Cancer Registration, Principles and Methods (IARC Scientific Publications No. 95)*, Lyon, IARCPress, 159-176.

4. Parkin DM, Whelan SL, Ferlay J, Raymond L , Young J, eds (1997) *Cancer Incidence in Five Continents, Vol. VII (IARC Scientific Publications No. 143 and IARC Cancerbase No. 2)*, Lyon, IARCPress.

5. Sankaranarayanan R, Black RJ, Parkin DM, eds (1998) *Cancer Survival in Developing Countries (IARC Scientific Publications, No. 145)*, Lyon, IARCPress.

6. SEER (1997) *SEER Cancer Statistics Review 1973-1994 (NIH Publication No. 92-2789)*, Bethesda, MD, USA, US Dept. of Health and Human Services, NCI.

7. Berrino F, Sant M, Verdecchia A, Capocaccia R, Hakulinen T, Esteve J, eds (1995) *Survival of Cancer Patients in Europe: the Eurocare Study (IARC Scientific Publications, No. 132)*, Lyon, IARCPress.

8. United Nations (1998) *World Population Prospects: the 1998 Revision*, New York, United Nations.

9. Parkin DM, Bray F, Ferlay J, Pisani P (2001) Estimating the world cancer burden: Globocan 2000. *Int J Cancer*, 94: 153-156.

10. Pisani P, Parkin DM, Bray F, Ferlay J (1999) Estimates of the worldwide mortality from 25 cancers in 1990. *Int J Cancer*, 83: 18-29.

WEBSITES

IARC cancer epidemiology databases, including GLOBOCAN 2000 and the WHO Cancer Mortality Database: http://www-dep.iarc.fr/

ICD9 classification of disease: http://www.cdc.gov/nchs/about/otheract/abticd9.htm

2

The causes of cancer

Information on cancer causation has come from investigation of the patterns of cancer in human populations and the induction of tumours in experimental animals following treatment with cancer-causing agents. The most important human carcinogens include tobacco, asbestos, aflatoxins and ultraviolet light. Almost 20% of cancers are associated with chronic infections, the most significant ones being hepatitis viruses (HBV, HCV), papillomaviruses (HPV) and *Helicobacter pylori*. There is increasing recognition of the causative role of lifestyle factors, including diet, physical activity, and alcohol consumption. Genetic susceptibility may significantly alter the risk from environmental exposures.

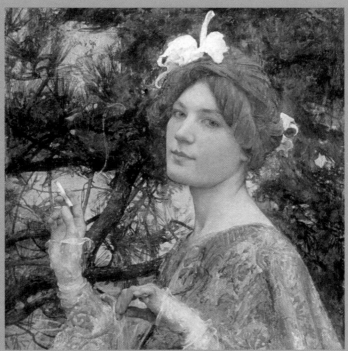

Detail from Edgard Maxence, Femme à l'orchidée, 1900 (RF 1989-41) Paris, musée d'Orsay.

TOBACCO

SUMMARY

> In addition to lung cancer, tobacco consumption causes tumours of the larynx, pancreas, kidney, bladder and, in conjunction with alcohol drinking, a high incidence of carcinomas of the oral cavity and the oesophagus. In most developed countries, tobacco accounts for as much as 30% of all malignant tumours.

> Lung cancer risk is determined by the amount of daily consumption of tobacco, duration of smoking and the depth of inhalation. For regular smokers, the relative risk for the development of lung cancer is more than 20 times higher than for non-smokers. Environmental tobacco smoke (passive smoking) is also carcinogenic but the risk is much smaller (relative risk 1.15-1.2).

> Tobacco smoke contains a great number of chemical carcinogens. The pattern of mutations in the *p53* tumour suppressor gene in smoking-associated lung tumours suggests that benzo(a)pyrene metabolites play a major role in the development of lung cancer.

> Cessation of smoking significantly reduces the risk of lung and other tobacco-associated cancers, even after many years of addiction. However, even ten or more years after stopping smoking, the risk is somewhat greater than that of never-smokers.

> Tobacco smoking is also the cause of various non-neoplastic ailments, including cardiovascular and obstructive lung diseases. The life expectancy of regular smokers is six to eight years less than that of people who have never smoked.

Use of tobacco has been identified by WHO as the major preventable cause of death of humankind. The topic is addressed here only in relation to cancer, although tobacco smoking causes a range of cardiovascular and respiratory diseases [1]. Tobacco smoking causes cancer of the lung and other organs and is the most intensively investigated environmental cause of cancer. Most information available involves the burden of smoking-related disease in more developed countries; far less is known in relation to less developed countries, though predictions can be made with confidence.

Preparation and use of tobacco

The main tobacco plant in the world is *Nicotiana tabacum*, although some varieties of *N. rustica* are also cultivated and used. Tobacco was imported from North America to Europe, Asia and Africa in the second half of the 16th century. By the mid-17th century, tobacco was being grown for commercial purposes not only in the American colonies, but also in Europe and East Asia. Industrial production of cigarettes started in the second half of the 19th century.

Tobacco needs to be cured before consumption. Two main curing processes are used. In flue-curing, the ripe leaves are cut and dried by artificial heat. Common names of flue-cured tobacco include "blond" and "Virginia". In air-curing, the entire plant is harvested and no artificial heat is used. Air-cured tobacco includes "Maryland" and "black". Cigars are also made of air-cured tobacco. Less important methods include sun-curing, fire-curing and various local adaptations. For "oriental" tobacco, sun- and air-curing are combined.

Cigarettes represent the most important tobacco product worldwide [2]. They are made from fine-cut tobacco wrapped in paper or maize leaf. The weight is between 0.5 and 1.2 g. Tobacco may be sprayed with sugar and other flavouring or aromatic agents. Other smoking tobacco products include cigars and cigarillos (which vary greatly in size, weight and flavour and have many local names, e.g. cheroots, chuttas, stumpen), tobacco for pipes and water pipes, bidis (flaked tobacco rolled in a piece of dried temburni leaf), as well as many other local products. Tobacco is also chewed, alone or with lime, betel nut or other compounds [3]. The habit is prevalent in the Indian region and South America, but also in North America and Northern Europe.

Tobacco snuff is taken in many countries, notably in Scandinavia, India and neighbouring countries, the Mediterranean and Southern Africa. The composition of chewing tobacco and snuff greatly varies geographically. In addition, other smokeless products are used in various parts of the world (e.g. "nass", a mixture of tobacco, lime, ash, and other ingredients, in Central Asia).

World production of tobacco is approximately seven million tonnes annually, China accounting for almost a third of this total [4]. Global trade in tobacco represents a major economic enterprise; although the USA and Europe lead the field, India and various nations of Africa are also major exporters (Table 2.1).

Exposure

The people most immediately exposed to the products of tobacco combustion are the

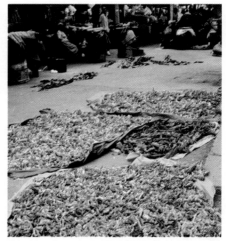

Fig. 2.1 Tobacco market in Zimbabwe. In the developing world, tobacco consumption is increasing rapidly.

users, that is, active smokers. The prevalence of smoking varies throughout the world and is subject to change (Fig. 2.8). The proportion of smokers is decreasing among men in industrialized countries. More than 70% of men born in Europe and North America during the first decades of the 20th century smoked during some time of their life, but this proportion has decreased in more recent times. There is an increasing proportion of ex-smokers in many countries, particularly within older age groups.

A different pattern is seen in women. In contrast to male smoking rates, smoking by women only became prevalent in the second half of the 20th century. While in some countries, such as the United Kingdom, the proportion of women who smoke has started to decrease in recent years, in most industrialized countries this proportion is still increasing [4].

In developing countries, less comprehensive data are available. It is clear, however, that a great increase in smoking has taken place during the last decade in many countries. The increase is particularly dramatic in China, where more than 60% of adult men are estimated to smoke, representing almost one-third of the total number of smokers worldwide. The prevalence of smoking among women in most developing countries is still low, although in many countries young women are taking up the habit. In India and its neighbouring countries, smokeless tobacco is widely used and "bidi" smoking is also common, this being the cheapest form of smoking available.

Non-smokers are exposed to environmental tobacco smoke, the extent of exposure being determined primarily by whether family members smoke and by workplace conditions. The amount of tobacco smoke inhaled as a consequence of atmospheric pollution is much less than that inhaled by an active smokers [5].

Location	Production (tonnes/annum)	Import (tonnes)	Export (tonnes)
USA	890,240	234,910	266,104
Europe	760,086	772,675	319,568
Russia	290,000	86,000	2,200
Africa	274,624	85,989	187,208
China	2,000,000	80,000	10,000
India	525,000	100	104,862
Global	6,660,000	1,512,638	1,484,144

Table 2.1 Tobacco production, imports and exports. In some regions, such as Africa and India, the export of tobacco is a major source of income.

Cancer risk

Tobacco smoking is the main known cause of human cancer-related death worldwide. Smoking most commonly causes lung cancer [6]. For a smoker, lung cancer risk is related to the parameters of tobacco smoking in accordance with the basic principles of chemical carcinogenesis: risk is determined by the dose of carcinogen, the duration of administration and the intensity of exposure. In respect of these determinants of lung cancer risk, women are at least as susceptible as men. An increase in risk of lung cancer (relative to a non-smoker) is consistently evident at the lowest level of daily consumption, and is at least linearly related to increasing

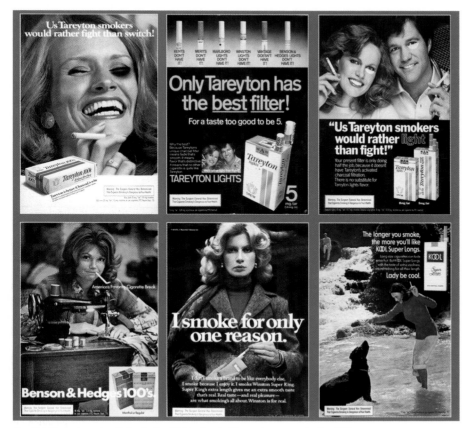

Fig. 2.2 Magazine advertising in the 1970s directed towards women in the USA.

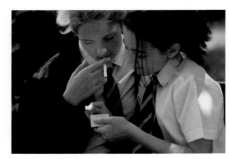

Fig. 2.3 Smoking by children is increasing world-wide.

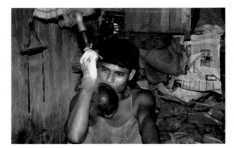

Fig. 2.4 A young man smoking a hookah (Bangladesh).

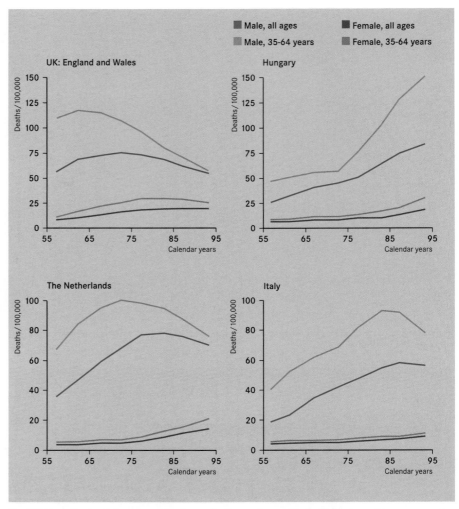

Fig. 2.5 Mortality due to lung cancer is decreasing in men in most industrialized countries, an exception being Hungary, which now has the highest rates of lung cancer mortality in the world.

consumption (Fig. 2.6). The risk is also proportional to the duration of smoking. Hence, the annual death rate from lung cancer among 55-64 year-olds who smoked 21-39 cigarettes daily is about three times higher for those who started smoking at age 15 than for those who started at age 25.

Intensity of exposure to tobacco smoke is determined by the smoking device used (cigarette, cigar, pipe, hookah, etc.) and, for any one method, may be determined by the "depth" of inhalation. Smoking of black tobacco cigarettes represents a greater risk for most tobacco-related cancers than smoking of blond cigarettes. Similarly, filtered and low-tar cigarettes entail a lower risk for most tobacco-related cancers than unfiltered and high-tar cigarettes. However, a "safe" cigarette does not exist; all smoking tobacco products entail a carcinogenic risk. Taken together, the epidemiological data summarized above establish "causation" because of the consistency of results, the strength of the relationship, its specificity, the temporal sequence between exposure and disease and the dose–response relationship.

Within many communities, smoking, and hence lung cancer, are sharply related to social class [7]. Between communities worldwide, incidence of lung cancer varies dramatically. High rates are observed in parts of North America, while developing countries have the lowest rates (Fig. 2.7). In the USA, Europe and Japan, 83-92% of lung cancer in men and 57-80% of lung cancer in women is tobacco-related. A maximal impact of lung cancer occurs when the population has attained a maximal prevalence of smoking that has continued throughout most of the life span of the smokers. As the prevalence of smoking increases, it is likely that an epidemic of

lung cancer will sweep the developing world in the coming decades [8].

In addition to lung cancer, smoking causes cancers of the larynx, oral cavity, pharynx, oesophagus, pancreas, kidney and bladder [2] (Table 2.3). Dose-response relationships between number of cigarettes smoked and risks for developing these cancers have been found consistently. Most data involve cigarette smoking but, for example, cigar and pipe smoking present a greater risk for cancer of the oral cavity than does cigarette smoking. For cancer of the bladder and kidney, risks vary with the duration and intensity of smoking, but are lower than those for lung cancer. In non-alcohol drink-

Substances	Tobacco smoke (per cigarette)	Smokeless tobacco (ng/g)
Volatile aldehydes		
Formaldehyde	20-105 µg	2,200-7,400
Acetaldehyde	18-1,400 µg	1,400-27,400
Crotonaldehyde	10-20 µg	200-2,400
N-Nitrosamines		
N-Nitrosodimethylamine	0.1-180 ng	0-220
N-Nitrosodiethylamine	0-36 ng	40-6,800
N-Nitropyrolidine	1.5-110 ng	0-337
Tobacco-specific nitrosamines		
N'-Nitrosonornicotine (NNN)	3-3,700 ng	400-154,000
4-(Methylnitrosamino)-1-(3-pyridyl)-1-butanone (NNK)	0-770 ng	0-13,600
4-(Methylnitrosamino)-1-(3-pyridyl)-1-butanol (NNAL)	+	+
N'-Nitrosoanabasine (NAB)	14-46 ng	0-560
Metals		
Nickel	0-600 ng	180-2,700
Cadmium	41-62 ng	700-790
Polonium 210	1-10 mBq	0.3-0.64 pci/g
Uranium 235 and 238	-	2.4-19.1 pci/g
Arsenic	40-120 ng	
Polycyclic aromatic hydrocarbons		
Benzo[a]pyrene	20-40 ng	>0.1-90
Benzo[a]anthracene	20-70 ng	-
Benzo[b]fluoranthene	4-22 ng	-
Chrysene	40-60 ng	-
Dibenzo[a,l]pyrene	1.7-3.2 ng	-
Dibenzo[a,h]anthracene	+	-

Table 2.2 Carcinogenic agents in tobacco smoke and smokeless tobacco. + = present, - = absent

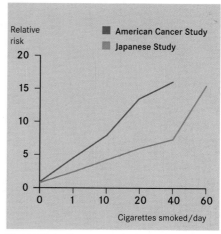

Fig. 2.6 Risk of lung cancer is determined by number of cigarettes smoked.

ing male smokers, risk of developing cancer of the oral cavity is about double that for non-drinking non-smokers. Elevations of ten-fold or more are evident for cancer of the larynx and five-fold or more for oesophageal cancer. The proportion of these cancers attributable to smoking varies with the tumour site and across communities, but is consistently high (80% or more) for laryngeal cancer specifically.

A common feature of lung and other smoking-induced cancers is the pattern of decreased risk which follows smoking cessation ("quitting") relative to continuing smoking [2]. The relative risk of cancer at most sites is markedly lower than that of current smokers after five years' cessation, although risks for bladder cancer and adenocarcinoma of the kidney appear to persist for longer before falling. Despite the clearly established benefit of cessation, the risk for ex-smokers does not decrease to that for "never smokers". Overall, decreased risk of lung and other cancers consequent upon quitting is further evidence (if any were needed) that smoking is causes the diseases in question (*Tobacco control*, p128).

Other cancer types may be a consequence of smoking [9]. These include cancer of the stomach, liver, nose and myeloid leukaemia. In contrast, some of the increased incidence of bowel and cervical cancer in smokers may be due to confounding. Exposure to environmental tobacco smoke causes lung cancer and possibly laryngeal cancer, although the burden of disease is much less than in active smokers; the relative risk has been estimated at about 1.15-1.2. Association of increased risk of breast cancer with exposure to environmental tobacco smoke is controversial [5].

Tobacco smoking has been estimated to cause approximately 25% of all cancers in men and 4% in women, and, in both genders, approximately 16% of cancer in more developed countries and 10% in less developed countries [11], although some estimates are as high as 30% [12]. The low attributable risk in women (and, to a lesser extent, in developing countries) is due to the low consumption of tobacco in past decades. A recent upward trend in smoking prevalence among women in many developing countries will result in a much greater number of attributable cancers in the future. Use of smokeless tobacco products has been associated with increased risk of head and neck cancer [10]. Since chewing of tobacco-containing products is particularly prevalent in Southern Asia, it represents a major carcinogenic hazard in that region.

Cancers positively associated with smoking	Sex	Standardized mortality per 100,000/year		Relative risk	Absolute excess risk per 100,000/year	Attributable proportion (%)*
		Life-long non-smoker	Current cigarette smoker			
Lung cancer	M	24	537	22.4	513	87
	F	18	213	11.9	195	77
Cancer of the upper respiratory sites	M	1	27	24.5	26	89
	F	2	10	5.6	8	58
Cancer of the bladder and other urinary organs	M	18	53	2.9	35	36
	F	8	21	2.6	13	32
Pancreatic cancer	M	18	38	2.1	20	25
	F	16	37	2.3	21	29
Oesophageal cancer	M	9	68	7.6	59	66
	F	4	41	10.3	37	74
Kidney cancer	M	8	23	3	15	37
	F	6	8	1.4	2	11

American Cancer Study. Men and women aged 35 yrs and more. *Attributable proportion is the proportion of all deaths from the specified disease which are attributable to cancer, assuming that 30% of the population are current smokers and that all the excess risk in smokers is due to smoking.

Table 2.3 Smoking increases the risk of many human cancers.

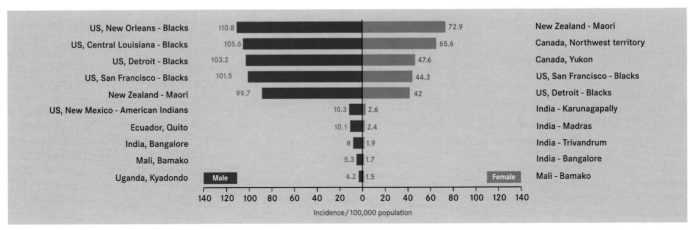

Fig. 2.7 The five highest and the five lowest recorded lung cancer incidence rates in males and females.

Interaction with other hazards

Alcohol consumption, exposure to asbestos and exposure to ionizing radiation interact with smoking in determining risk of some cancers [13]. For alcohol drinking and smoking, risks for cancer of the larynx, oesophagus and oral cavity increase multiplicatively in relation to the respective risks generated by either expo- sure in the absence of the other. For indi- viduals exposed to both asbestos and tobacco smoke (for example, insulation workers who smoke), risk of lung cancer is also increased multiplicatively, although smoking does not affect risk of mesothe- lioma (a tumour type specifically caused by asbestos). Quitting smoking can con- siderably lower the risk for lung cancer among people who were exposed to asbestos in the past.

Mechanisms of carcinogenesis

As tobacco is the most important human carcinogen, elucidation of mechanisms which result in cancer among humans exposed to tobacco smoke provides an important means for assessing some preventive options, and may be relevant to the prevention of other environmentally-induced cancer.

Mainstream smoke (the material inhaled by smokers) is an aerosol including approximately 4,000 specific chemicals and containing 10^{10} particles per ml. The particulate matter (tar) is made up of some 3,500 compounds, the most abundant being nicotine (0.1-2.0 mg per cigarette) and also including most of the polycyclic aromatic hydrocarbons occurring in the smoke [14]. Another class of carcinogens represented in tobacco smoke is N-nitroso compounds, particularly including the nitroso derivatives of nicotine and nornicotine [15]. Chemicals such as aromatic amines, benzene and heavy metals, independently established as carcinogenic for humans, are present in tobacco smoke (Table 2.2). Use of smokeless tobacco results in exposure to tobacco-related nitroso compounds, but not to polycyclic aromatic hydrocarbons, which are products of combustion.

Cancer causation by tobacco smoke is not attributable to any one chemical component, or any one class of chemicals present, but to an overall effect of the complex mixture of chemicals in smoke. Mechanistic inferences which can be made from epidemiological studies, together with relevant experimental data, indicate a scenario compatible with "multistage carcinogenesis" as understood at the cellular and molecular level (*Multistage carcinogenesis*, p84) [16].

Epidemiological studies indicate that for cancers of the lung, bladder and head and neck (data for other cancers are inadequate for such evaluation), the various carcinogens in tobacco smoke exert an effect on both early and late steps in the process of carcinogenesis. Evidence for early effects comes from the higher risk associated with early age at starting smoking and with increasing time since beginning smoking, while the continued elevated risk, albeit at decreasing levels over time, following quitting smoking is a strong argument for late effects.

Most chemical carcinogens in tobacco smoke require metabolic activation in order to exert a carcinogenic effect [17].

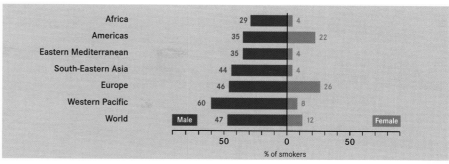

Fig. 2.8 Estimated prevalence of smoking among adults by region, in the early 1990s.

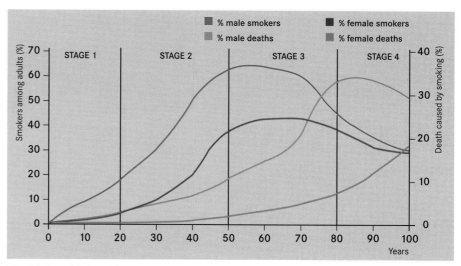

Fig. 2.9 A model describing stages of the tobacco epidemic based on data from developed countries. Note the time lag between increase in consumption and the manifestation of lung cancer

The requisite enzymes are present in lung and other "target" organs. Individual risk may be affected by the activity and levels of enzymes such as glutathione-S-transferase, cytochrome P450 and N-acetyl transferases. In the course of metabolism, reactive forms of polycyclic aromatic hydrocarbons, nitrosamines and aromatic amines are generated and become covalently bound to DNA in relevant tissues. Such DNA adducts, and the products of their repair, have been detected in tissues, bodily fluids and urine from smokers and from persons exposed to environmental tobacco smoke.

The molecular genetics of tobacco smoke-induced lung and other cancers are being progressively elucidated. An increasing number of genes are implicated as being relevant to a carcinogenic outcome [18]. The degree of current understanding is exemplified by studies of the pattern of mutation in the *p53* gene. When comparison is made of particular mutation frequencies in lung cancers from smokers and non-smokers, differences are evident. Using relevant experimental systems, mutations evident in smokers are attributable, at least in part, to the miscoding caused by the binding of some polycyclic aromatic hydrocarbons to DNA [19].

PHARMACOLOGICAL APPROACHES TO SMOKING ADDICTION

Quitting smoking is very difficult. Surveys show that 74% of smokers report a desire to quit and 70% of smokers have made previous attempts to quit smoking, yet success rates remain low (US Department of Health and Human Services, *Healthy People 2000 Review*, 1994). The difficulty that most smokers encounter reflects both a habit and a physiological addiction. In addition, cessation involves discontinuing a dependency that smokers acquired at a vulnerable period in their lives (*Tobacco control*, p128).

The low success rates associated with unaided attempts to quit suggest that pharmacological treatment be offered unless there is a medical contraindication. Treatments for smoking addiction include nicotine replacement therapies and non-nicotine therapy (Okuyemi KS et al., *Arch Family Med*, 9: 270-281, 2000; The Tobacco Use and Dependence Clinical Practice Guideline Panel, *JAMA*, 283: 3244-3254, 2000). Nicotine replacement therapies include nicotine polacrilex gum, transdermal nicotine patch, nicotine nasal spray, nicotine sublingual tablet, and nicotine inhaler but only about 25% of attempts involve the use of any nicotine replacement therapy.

The only approved non-nicotine therapy is the antidepressant bupropion hydrochloride. Other antidepressants such as nortriptyline and moclobemide have shown some promise but are not generally approved for use.

Combination of two nicotine replacement therapies (patch plus gum, spray, or inhaler) or a nicotine replacement therapy plus a non-nicotine drug (bupropion) may work better than single agents.

In summary, treatments help fewer than one in five smokers and are not being used by the majority of smokers trying to quit. Recent progress in the understanding of the neuropharmacological basis of nicotine addiction holds promise for the development of new treatments.

REFERENCES

1. Wald NJ, Hackshaw AK (1996) Cigarette smoking: an epidemiological overview. *Br Med Bull*, 52: 3-11.

2. IARC (1986) *Tobacco Smoking (IARC Monographs on the Evaluation of the Carcinogenic Risk of Chemicals to Humans, Vol. 38)*, Lyon, IARCPress.

3. IARC (1985) *Tobacco Habits Other Than Smoking; Betel-quid and Areca-nut Chewing; and Some Related Nitrosamines (IARC Monographs on the Evaluation of Carcinogenic Risks to Humans, Vol. 37)*, Lyon, IARCPress.

4. Corrao MA, Guindon GE, Sharma N, Shokoohi DF, eds (2000) *Tobacco Control Country Profiles*, Atlanta, Georgia, American Cancer Society.

5. Law MR, Hackshaw AK (1996) Environmental tobacco smoke. *Br Med Bull*, 52: 22-34.

6. Boyle P, Maisonneuve P (1995) Lung cancer and tobacco smoking. *Lung Cancer*, 12: 167-181.

7. Stellman SD, Resnicow K (1997) Tobacco smoking, cancer and social class. In: Kogevinas M, Pearce N, Susser M & Boffetta P, eds, *Social Inequalities and Cancer, (IARC Scientific Publications, No. 138)*, Lyon, IARCPress, 229-250.

8. Chen ZM, Xu Z, Collins R, Li WX, Peto R (1997) Early health effects of the emerging tobacco epidemic in China. A 16-year prospective study. *JAMA*, 278: 1500-1504.

9. Doll R (1996) Cancers weakly related to smoking. *Br Med Bull*, 52: 35-49.

10. Winn DM (1997) Epidemiology of cancer and other systemic effects associated with the use of smokeless tobacco. *Adv Dent Res*, 11: 313-321.

11. Parkin DM, Pisani P, Lopez AD, Masuyer E (1994) At least one in seven cases of cancer is caused by smoking. Global estimates for 1985. *Int J Cancer*, 59: 494-504.

12. Doll R, Peto R (1981) The causes of cancer: quantitative estimates of avoidable risk of cancer in the USA today. *J Natl Cancer Inst*, 66: 1191-1308.

13. Levi F (1999) Cancer prevention: epidemiology and perspectives. *Eur J Cancer*, 35: 1912-1924.

14. Rodgman A, Smith CJ, Perfetti TA (2000) The composition of cigarette smoke: a retrospective, with emphasis on polycyclic components. *Hum Exp Toxicol*, 19: 573-595.

15. Brunnemann KD, Prokopczyk B, Djordjevic MV, Hoffmann D (1996) Formation and analysis of tobacco-specific N-nitrosamines. *Crit Rev Toxicol*, 26: 121-137.

16. Shields PG (2000) Epidemiology of tobacco carcinogenesis. *Curr Oncol Rep*, 2: 257-262.

17. Hecht SS (1999) Tobacco smoke carcinogens and lung cancer. *J Natl Cancer Inst*, 91: 1194-1210.

18. Shields PG, Harris CC (2000) Cancer risk and low-penetrance susceptibility genes in gene-environment interactions. *J Clin Oncol*, 18: 2309-2315.

19. Hainaut P, Hollstein M (2000) p53 and human cancer: the first ten thousand mutations. *Adv Cancer Res*, 77: 81-137.

20. IARC (2003) *Tobacco Smoke and Involuntary Smoking (IARC Monographs on the Evaluation of Carcinogenic Risks to Humans, Vol. 83)*, Lyon, IARCPress. *In preparation*.

WEBSITES

Tobacco & Cancer, The American Cancer Society: http://www.cancer.org/docroot/PED/ped_10.asp?sitearea=PED

Tobaccopedia, an online tobacco encyclopaedia: http://tobaccopedia.org/

ALCOHOL DRINKING

SUMMARY

> Heavy alcohol drinking causes cancer of the oral cavity, pharynx, larynx, oesophagus, and liver, and may increase the risk of breast and colorectal cancer.

> Risk is linearly related to the mean daily consumption.

> Low levels of consumption appear to exert a protective effect against cardiovascular disease.

> In the oral cavity, pharynx, larynx and oesophagus, the risk is greatly increased by concurrent smoking.

Beverages containing alcohol (the common name for ethanol) as the product of the fermentation of carbohydrates have been produced in most human societies since ancient times. Despite great variety, most alcoholic beverages can be grouped as either beers (brewed by fermenting malted barley and typically containing 5% volume of alcohol), wines (made by fermenting grape juice or crushed grapes, containing 12% alcohol) or spirits (made by distilling fermented products of a variety of cereals, vegetables and fruits, containing 40% alcohol). Beverages that are less common and which are often limited to particular regions include cider, fortified wines and flavoured wines.

On a global scale, the consumption of alcoholic beverages by adults as calculated from official figures is equivalent to 4 L of alcohol per year (or 9 g/day), corresponding to approximately 3% of the average total intake of calories [1]. Unofficial consumption, however, is estimated to account for an additional amount corresponding to 20-100% of the official figures, depending on the country. Most "unofficial" alcohol is either sold illegally on the black market (usually to avoid taxation) or produced for private consumption. There is strong regional variability in consumption levels, with a minimum (<1 L/year) in Western and Southern Asia and Northern Africa and maximum (>12 L/year) in Central and Southern Europe. The distribution between each major type of beverage is also country-specific (Fig. 2.10). Official figures show a decrease in alcohol consumption in more developed countries and, over recent years, an increase in consumption in less developed countries.

Cancers caused

Through analytical epidemiological studies of cohort and case-control type conducted in many populations with different levels of consumption, the causal association of drinking alcohol has been definitely established in respect of oral, oesophageal, liver and other cancers [2]. In particular, studies of cancer risk in brewery workers and in alcoholic patients have provided important evidence on the carcinogenic role of alcohol. A causal association is also established in the case of breast cancer and is probable for colon and rectal cancer [2,3]. There have been suggestions of a possible carcinogenic effect of alcohol drinking on other organs, such as the lung, but the evidence is still inconclusive [4]. An association between alcohol intake and risk of head and neck cancer is indicated by the geographical pattern of these neoplasms; countries (and regions within countries) with heavy alcohol consumption are among those with the highest incidence of these neoplasms.

For all cancers caused by drinking alcohol, the risk of cancer is a linear function of the level of consumption, up to an intake of about 80 g/day (one litre of wine, a quarter of a litre of spirits), above which

Mean alcohol consumption	Relative risk (95% confidence)
No alcohol	1
> 0 to 30 g/day	1.2 (0.4 – 3.4)
> 30 to 60 g/day	3.2 (1.0 – 10.1)
> 60 g/day	9.2 (2.8 – 31.0)

*Adjusted for follow-up time, sex, education, body mass index (BMI), vegetable and fruit consumption, tobacco smoking and energy intake

Table 2.4 Consumption of alcohol increases the risk of cancer of the upper gastrointestinal tract.

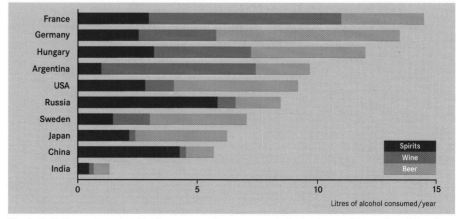

Fig. 2.10 Patterns of alcohol drinking, expressed as mean equivalent volumes of pure ethanol, in selected countries, 1996.

level the dose—response relationship is less clearly defined. The magnitude of increased risk associated with a particular rate of alcohol consumption varies for each tumour type. The risk of head and neck cancer is 5-10 times higher in heavy drinkers than in abstainers, the carcinogenic effect of alcohol appearing to be more potent in the oral cavity, pharynx and oesophagus and weaker in the larynx. The relative risk of breast cancer in women with a high consumption of alcohol is approximately two-fold.

Most available data concerning the carcinogenic role of alcohol in humans are derived from epidemiological studies based on interviews or similar approaches. Since alcohol drinking carries a strong social stigma in many populations, it is likely that individuals underestimate and under-report their intake of alcohol, particularly in the case of heavy consumption. Under-reporting of alcohol drinking, resulting in the classification of heavy drinkers as light- or non-drinkers, would result in underestimation of the actual carcinogenic effect of the habit. It is possible therefore that the role of alcohol in human cancer is greater than commonly perceived.

Alcohol drinking and tobacco smoking show a synergistic interaction in the etiology of cancers of the oral cavity, pharynx, larynx and oesophagus; the risk of cancer for heavy consumers of both products relative to that for subjects who neither smoke nor drink is higher than the product of the risks attributable respectively to heavy drinking and heavy smoking separately (Fig. 2.14) [5]. Very heavy drinkers (e.g. alcoholics), among whom alcohol can be the source of up to 30% of total calorie intake, tend to have a diet poor in fruit and vegetables, which may further enhance their risk of developing these cancers.

Relatively few studies have examined possible variations in risk attributable to different alcoholic beverages: evidence on

Region	% of deaths	Years of life lost	Disability-adjusted years life lost
Latin America	4.5	5.9	9.7
Sub-Saharan Africa	2.1	2.0	2.6
Other Asian countries	1.8	1.6	2.8
Former socialist countries	1.4	5.7	8.3
China	1.3	1.8	2.3
Industrialized countries	1.2	5.1	10.3
India	1.2	1.4	1.6
Middle East	0.1	0.2	0.4
Overall	1.5	2.1	3.5

Table 2.5 Percentage of the population dying from alcohol-associated diseases in different world regions, and the respective years of life lost .

Cancer	Men		Women	
	%	No. of cases	%	No. of cases
Oral cavity & pharynx	23	51,000	15	12,700
Oesophagus	24	51,800	14	14,500
Liver	10	30,100	6	7,300
Larynx	22	26,500	14	2,500
Breast	-	-	3	26,800
Total	4	159,400	2	63,800

Table 2.6 Percentage and number of cancer cases worldwide attributable to alcohol consumption, 1990.

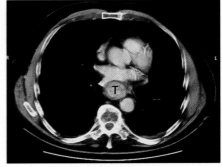

Fig. 2.11 Computed tomography (CT) scan of an oesophageal tumour (T). Heavy alcohol drinking is a major risk factor.

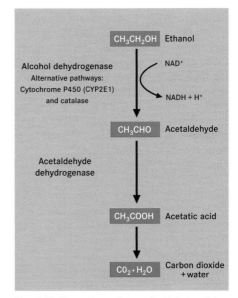

Fig. 2.12 The major pathway of alcohol metabolism in humans.

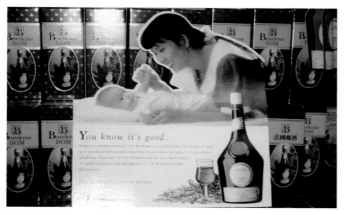

Fig. 2.13 Some advertising of alcohol (such as this poster from Malaysia) is directed specifically towards women. The liquor concerned is advertised as containing herbs traditionally taken by Chinese women after delivery of their baby. D. Jernigan

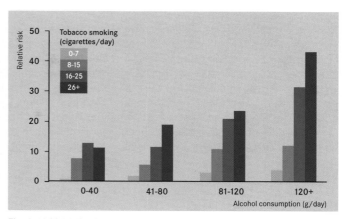

Fig. 2.14 Multiplicative increase in relative risk of laryngeal cancer as a consequence of both alcohol drinking and active smoking (colour coding approximates progressive doubling of risk as exposure increases). A.J. Tuyns et al. (1988) *Int J Cancer*, 41:483-91.

this issue is inconclusive at present. Similarly, there is no clear evidence as to whether the key factor in alcohol carcinogenesis is level of alcohol intake, or whether the pattern of drinking (e.g. regular intake of moderate quantities, typically at meals, versus intermittent intake of large quantities ("binge drinking") also plays a role.

Alcohol drinking is estimated to be involved in the etiology of 3% of all cancers (that is, 4% in men, 2% in women, Table 2.6). In women, approximately half of the neoplasms attributed to alcohol drinking are breast cancers. However, the actual burden of cancers attributable to alcohol consumption may be greater than these estimates, given that alcohol drinking may be a causative factor in cancers other than those presented, as well as the likely underestimation of the risk.

Mechanism of carcinogenesis and relevant model systems

The mechanism(s) of cancer causation by alcoholic beverages is not known. Ethanol has not been established as being carcinogenic to experimental animals. The compound does not appear to react with DNA in mammalian tissue. Among hypotheses proposed to explain the increased cancer risk are (i) a carcinogenic effect of chemicals other than ethanol present in alcoholic beverages (such as *N*-nitrosamines); (ii) a solvent action which facilitates absorption of other carcinogens (e.g. those in tobacco smoke); (iii) a carcinogenic role for acetaldehyde, the major metabolite of ethanol (Fig. 2.12). This last hypothesis is supported by evidence that acetaldehyde is carcinogenic in experimental animals, as well as by results of recent studies in populations exhibiting polymorphisms in genes encoding enzymes which are involved in the metabolism of alcohol. Genetic polymorphisms lead to variations in the level of activity of these enzymes between individuals (*Genetic susceptibility*, p71) such that varying quantities of acetaldehyde are found from the same intake of ethanol. Studies in Japan, where such polymorphisms are frequent, have shown an increased risk of cancer in subjects with a genetic profile that is associated with higher acetaldehyde levels following alcohol drinking [6]. Results from Western populations, however, are less clear-cut.

Apart from being associated with an increased risk of several types of cancer, overconsumption of alcohol causes alcoholism (alcohol addiction), alcohol psychosis, chronic pancreatitis, liver cirrhosis, hypertension, haemorrhagic stroke and low birth weight in babies born to alcoholic mothers. Furthermore, inebriation associated with alcohol drinking is responsible for a high proportion of all accidents and injuries (15-40%, according to the type of injury) and, in particular, traffic accidents. In global terms, immoderate consumption of alcohol is responsible for 1.5% of all deaths and 3.5% of disability-adjusted years of life lost (Table 2.5) [7]. In contrast, the regular consumption of a single alcoholic beverage per day has been clearly associated with a decreased risk of ischaemic heart disease [8]. This effect is likely to be due to an alcohol-induced increase in high-density

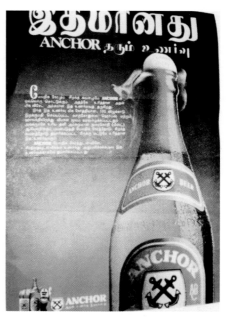

Fig. 2.15 An advertisement in the Tamil language targeted at Indian labourers in Malaysia.

lipoprotein-associated cholesterol, which exerts a protective effect against atherosclerosis. Protection is not evident for high levels of alcohol since the beneficial effect on cholesterol levels is probably offset by the alcohol-related increase in blood pressure, which increases the risk of ischaemic heart disease. Among British men in middle or old age, the consumption of an average of one or two units of alcohol per day is associated with significantly lower levels of risk of all causes of mortality, compared with consumption of no alcohol or with consumption of substantial amounts [8]. Cholelithiasis (gallstones) is another disease prevented by moderate alcohol consumption.

The global effect of alcohol on health in a given population depends therefore on the level of consumption. The health impact may be considered with reference to the increased risk of cancer, other diseases, and injuries, and also any decreased risk of ischaemic heart disease. Avoidance of excessive consumption of alcoholic beverages would prevent a range of cancers.

REFERENCES

1. World Health Organization (1999) *Global Status Report on Alcohol*, Geneva, WHO.

2. IARC (1988) *Alcohol Drinking (IARC Monographs on the Evaluation of Carcinogenic Risks to Humans, Vol. 44)*, Lyon, IARCPress.

3. Potter JD, ed. (1997) *Food, Nutrition and the Prevention of Cancer: a Global Perspective*, Washington, DC, American Institute for Cancer Research.

4. Bandera EV, Freudenheim JL, Vena JE (2001) Alcohol consumption and lung cancer: a review of the epidemiologic evidence. *Cancer Epidemiol Biomarkers Prev*, 10: 813-821.

5. Tuyns AJ, Esteve J, Raymond L, Berrino F, Benhamou E, Blanchet F, Boffetta P, Crosignani P, del Moral A, Lehmann W (1988) Cancer of the larynx/hypopharynx, tobacco and alcohol: IARC international case-control study in Turin and Varese (Italy), Zaragoza and Navarra (Spain), Geneva (Switzerland) and Calvados (France). *Int J Cancer*, 41: 483-491.

6. Matsuo K, Hamajima N, Shinoda M, Hatooka S, Inoue M, Takezaki T, Tajima K (2001) Gene-environment interaction between an aldehyde dehydrogenase-2 (ALDH2) polymorphism and alcohol consumption for the risk of esophageal cancer. *Carcinogenesis*, 22: 913-916.

7. Murray CJL, Lopez AD (1996) Quantifying the burden of disease and injury attributable to ten major risk factors. In: Murray CJL, Lopez AD eds, *The Global Burden of Disease*, Geneva, World Health Organization, 295-324.

8. Doll R, Peto R, Hall E, Wheatley K, Gray R (1994) Mortality in relation to consumption of alcohol: 13 years' observations on male British doctors. *BMJ*, 309: 911-918.

OCCUPATIONAL EXPOSURES

SUMMARY

> Many occupations and some specific chemicals encountered at work are associated with increased risk of cancer.

> Occupational cancer most often involves the lung; other sites affected include the skin, urinary tract, nasal cavity and pleura.

> Most occupational carcinogens have been eliminated from the workplace. However, in newly-industrialized countries, relevant exposures still pose a significant health risk.

> Some past exposures still carry a significant cancer burden; in most European countries, use of asbestos was banned in the 1990s, but the peak mesothelioma incidence will occur around 2020.

The first reports of associations between risk of cancer and employment in particular occupations appeared during the 18th century (scrotal cancer among chimney sweeps [1]) and 19th century (bladder cancer in workers exposed to dyes [2]). However, the majority of studies establishing a link between an increased risk of cancer and a particular working environment were published between 1950 and 1975 [3]. Relatively few occupational carcinogens have been identified in the last 25 years.

Identifying hazardous materials

The *IARC Monographs on the Evaluation of Carcinogenic Risks to Humans* evaluate data relevant to the carcinogenic hazard to humans as a consequence of exposure to particular chemical, physical and biological agents and mixtures [4]. Accordingly, evidence of carcinogenicity for most known or suspected occupational carcinogens has been evaluated in the *IARC Monographs* programme. At present, 25 chemicals, groups of chemi-

cals or mixtures for which exposures are mostly occupational, have been established as human carcinogens (Table 2.7). While some of these agents, such as asbestos, crystalline silica and heavy metals, are currently encountered in the workplaces of many countries, other agents have been phased out and are mainly of historical interest (e.g. mustard gas and 2-naphthylamine).

An additional 25 agents presenting a hazard on the basis of workplace exposure are classified as probably carcinogenic to humans. Most of these agents have been shown to be carcinogenic in experimental animals, and less than conclusive evidence of carcinogenicity in humans from epidemiological studies is available. They include chemicals and consequent exposures that are commonly in many countries, such as those associated with the use of formaldehyde and 1,3-butadiene (Table 2.8). In many instances, it is possible to associate

increased risk of cancer with a group of agents or a particular work environment rather than with a single compound. The hazard posed by polycyclic aromatic hydrocarbons is of particular interest. Although several individual polycyclic aromatic hydrocarbons are experimental carcinogens (three of them are listed in Table 2.8), human exposure always involves complex mixtures of these chemicals, often in variable proportions (e.g. soots, coal tars). Therefore, the determination of a hazard to humans must involve consideration of such mixtures and not the individual compounds. A large number of agents primarily encountered in an occupational context are classified as possibly carcinogenic to

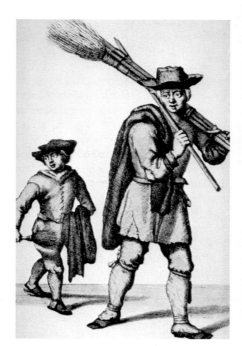

Fig. 2.16 The first cases of occupational cancer identified were scrotal cancers in chimney sweeps, in the late 18th century.

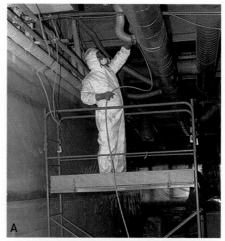

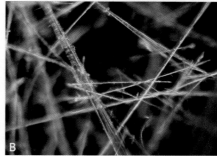

Fig. 2.17 Asbestos insulation is common in buildings and presents a hazard when disturbed during demolition. **(A)** Protective clothing must be worn to avoid contact with **(B)** asbestos fibres .

Agent	Cancer site/cancer	Main industry/use
4-Aminobiphenyl	Bladder	Rubber manufacture
Arsenic and arsenic compounds*	Lung, skin	Glass, metals, pesticides
Asbestos	Lung, pleura, peritoneum	Insulation, filter material, textiles
Benzene	Leukaemia	Solvent, fuel
Benzidine	Bladder	Dye/pigment manufacture
Beryllium and beryllium compounds	Lung	Aerospace industry/metals
Bis(chloromethyl) ether	Lung	Chemical intermediate/by-product
Cadmium and cadmium compounds	Lung	Dye/pigment manufacture
Chloromethyl methyl ether	Lung	Chemical intermediate/by-product
Chromium[VI] compounds	Nasal cavity, lung	Metal plating, dye/pigment manufacture
Coal-tar pitches	Skin, lung, bladder	Building material, electrodes
Coal-tars	Skin, lung	Fuel
Ethylene oxide	Leukaemia	Chemical intermediate, sterilising agent
Mineral oils, untreated and mildly-treated	Skin	Lubricants
Mustard gas (sulfur mustard)	Pharynx, lung	War gas
2-Naphthylamine	Bladder	Dye/pigment manufacture
Nickel compounds	Nasal cavity, lung	Metallurgy, alloys, catalyst
Shale-oils	Skin	Lubricants, fuels
Silica, crystalline	Lung	Stone cutting, mining, foundries
Soots	Skin, lung	Pigments
Strong-inorganic-acid mists containing sulfuric acid	Larynx, lung	Metal, batteries
Talc containing asbestiform fibres	Lung	Paper, paints
2,3,7,8-Tetrachlorodibenzo-*para*-dioxin (TCDD)	Several organs	Contaminant
Vinyl chloride	Liver	Plastics monomer
Wood dust	Nasal cavity	Wood industry

* This evaluation applies to the group of chemicals as a whole and not necessarily to all individual chemicals within the group.

Table 2.7 Chemicals classified as human carcinogens (IARC Group 1) for which exposures are mostly occupational.

humans, e.g. acetaldehyde, dichloromethane, inorganic lead compounds. For the majority of these chemicals, evidence of carcinogenicity comes from studies in experimental animals, and evidence of a carcinogenic outcome in humans is often lacking because human exposure occurs at the same time as exposure to many other agents, or for some other reason.

A number of industries and occupations have been subject to evaluation within the *Monographs* programme (Table 2.9). In some instances (e.g. wood dust in the wood industry), the agent(s) responsible for an increased risk of cancer is (are) well established, while in other cases (e.g. employment as a painter or in the rubber industry), an increased risk of cancer has been established, but no precise carcinogen has been identified. Furthermore, there are several agents known or suspected to cause cancer in humans to which humans are incidentally exposed in an occupational context (Table 2.10). Occupational exposure to

pharmaceutical drugs known or suspected to be carcinogenic can occur in pharmacies and during the administration of these drugs to patients by nursing staff (*Medicinal drugs*, p48). Hospital workers can be exposed to hepatitis B virus, food processors exposed to aflatoxins from contaminated foodstuff, outdoor workers exposed to ultraviolet radiation or diesel engine exhaust fumes and bar staff or waiters exposed to environmental tobacco smoke.

Current understanding of the relationship between occupational exposures and cancer is far from complete. For many chemicals known to cause cancer in experimental animals, no definitive evidence is available concerning route or extent of workplace exposure. Constructing and interpreting lists of

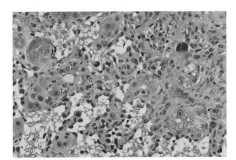

Fig. 2.18 Angiosarcoma of the liver caused by occupational exposure to vinyl chloride. The tumour is characterized by proliferation of vessel-like structures, lined by malignant, highly atypical endothelial cells.

Agent	Cancer site/cancer	Main industry/use
Acrylonitrile	Lung, prostate, lymphoma	Plastics, rubber, textiles, monomer
Benz[a]anthracene	Lung, skin	Combustion fumes
Benzidine-based dyes	Bladder	Paper, leather, textile dyes
Benzo[a]pyrene	Lung, skin	Combustion fumes
1,3-Butadiene	Leukaemia, lymphoma	Plastics, rubber, monomer
Captafol	-	Pesticide
Chlorinated toluenes (trichlorobenzene, benzal chloride, benzyl chloride, benzoyl chloride)	Lung	Chemical intermediates
para-Chloro-ortho-toluidine (and its strong acid salts)	Bladder	Dye/pigment manufacture, textiles
4-Chloro-ortho-toluidine	Bladder	Dye/pigment manufacture, insecticide
Creosotes	Skin	Wood preservation
Dibenz[a,h]anthracene	Lung, skin	Combustion fumes
Diethyl sulfate	-	Chemical intermediate
Dimethylcarbamoyl chloride	-	Chemical intermediate
Dimethyl sulfate	-	Chemical intermediate
Epichlorohydrin	-	Plastics/resins monomer
Ethylene dibromide	-	Chemical intermediate, fumigant, fuels
Formaldehyde	Nasopharynx	Plastics, textiles, laboratory agent
Glycidol	-	Chemical intermediate, sterilising agent
4,4'-Methylenebis(2-chloroaniline) (MOCA)	Bladder	Rubber manufacture
Methyl methanesulfonate	-	Laboratory research
ortho-Toluidine	Bladder	Dye/pigment manufacture
Polychlorinated biphenyls	Liver, bile ducts, leukaemia, lymphoma	Electrical components
Styrene oxide	-	Plastics, chemical intermediate
Tetrachloroethylene	Oesophagus, lymphoma	Solvent, dry cleaning
Trichloroethylene	Liver, lymphoma	Solvent, dry cleaning, metal
Tris(2,3-dibromopropyl) phosphate	-	Plastics, textiles, flame retardant
Vinyl bromide	-	Plastics, textiles, monomer

Table 2.8 Chemicals classified as probably carcinogenic to humans (IARC Group 2A) for which exposures are mostly occupational..

chemical or physical carcinogenic agents and associating these agents with specific occupations and industries is complicated by a number of factors:
- Information on industrial processes and consequent exposures is frequently poor, and does not allow a complete evaluation of the impact of specific exposures in different occupations or industries;
- Exposure to chemicals known to present a carcinogenic hazard, such as vinyl chloride monomer and benzene, may occur at markedly different levels in different occupational situations;
- Changes in work practice occur over time, either because identified carcinogenic agents are replaced by other agents or (more frequently) because new industrial processes or materials are introduced;
- Any list of occupations involving presumed exposure to an agent is likely to include only some of the situations in which a particular carcinogen may occur;
- Finally, the presence of a carcinogenic chemical in an occupational situation does not necessarily mean that workers are exposed to it. Conversely, the absence of identified carcinogens from a particular workplace does not exclude the possibility of a hazard and/or an as yet unidentified cause of cancer.

Particular chemicals and exposures
It is not possible to review here the carcinogenicity data for all recognized occupational carcinogens. Limited information on certain of these hazards is summarized below [4,5].

Aromatic amines
Many members of this class of compounds are established or implicated as causing occupational cancer. By the mid-1950s, studies of workers in the chemical industry revealed that benzidine and 2-naphthylamine caused bladder cancer. It was also recognized about this time that rubber workers were subject to this malignancy, attributable to aromatic amines and 4-aminobiphenyl in particular. Later studies on occupational exposure to aromatic amines have not definitively established single compounds as carcinogenic, in many cases because

Industry, occupation	Cancer site/cancer (suspected cancer sites in parentheses)
IARC Group 1	
Aluminium production	Lung, bladder
Auramine, manufacture of	Bladder
Boot and shoe manufacture and repair	Nasal cavity, leukaemia
Coal gasification	Skin, lung, bladder
Coke production	Skin, lung, kidney
Furniture and cabinet making	Nasal cavity
Haematite mining (underground) with exposure to radon	Lung
Iron and steel founding	Lung
Isopropanol manufacture (strong-acid process)	Nasal cavity
Magenta, manufacture of	Bladder
Painter (mainly in the construction industry)	Lung
Rubber industry (certain occupations)	Bladder, leukaemia
IARC Group 2A	
Art glass, glass containers and pressed ware (manufacture of)	(Lung, stomach)
Hairdresser or barber (occupational exposure as a)	(Bladder, lung)
Non-arsenical insecticides (occupational exposures in spraying and application of)	(Lung, myeloma)
Petroleum refining (occupational exposures in)	(Leukaemia, skin)
IARC Group 2B	
Carpentry and joinery	(Nasal cavity)
Dry cleaning (occupational exposures in)	(Bladder, oesophagus)
Textile manufacturing industry (work in)	(Nasal cavity, bladder)

Table 2.9 Industries and occupations classified as carcinogenic to humans (IARC Group 1), probably carcinogenic to humans (IARC Group 2A) or possibly carcinogenic to humans (IARC Group 2B).

workers were exposed to more than one such agent. Nonetheless, benzidine-based dyes and 4,4'-methylenebis (2-chloroaniline) (known as MOCA, a curing agent for plastics) are implicated. The manufacture of auramine has been shown to cause bladder cancer, but the causative agent is not known.

Benzene
Occupational exposure to benzene may occur in the chemical and petroleum industries; it is used as a solvent and intermediate. The compound is known to cause leukaemia, most relevant studies implicating non-lymphocytic leukaemia, and myelogenous leukaemia in particular [6].

Asbestos and other fibres
Cancer caused by inhalation of asbestos dust has been recognized since the 1950s. All forms of asbestos, including chrysotile and the amphibole, crocidolite, cause lung cancer and mesothelioma, an otherwise rare tumour derived from the lining of the peritoneum, pericardium or pleura. Apart from asbestos miners, those exposed include construction, demolition, shipbuilding, insulation and brake workers. Fibre size is a crucial factor determining the carcinogenicity of asbestos. Evidence suggests that insulation glass wool, rock wool and slag wool, which are used as replacements for asbestos in some applications, do not

cause increased risk of lung cancer or mesothelioma, although ceramic fibres and certain special-purpose glass wools are possible carcinogens [7].

Metals
Cancer of the lung can be caused by exposure to inorganic arsenic in mining and copper smelting. An increased incidence of lung cancer has also been recorded among workers in chromate-producing industries and among chromium platers and chromium alloy workers. Increased risk is predominantly associated with hexavalent chromium compounds. Nickel refining carries a carcinogenic risk in processes involving nickel (sub)sulfides, oxides and soluble nickel salts.

Coal tar, coal gas production and iron founding
Coal tar pitches and coal tar vapour are encountered in a variety of occupations including coke production, coal gasification and roofing. These mixtures produce cancers of the skin and at other sites including the urinary and respiratory systems. Work in iron and steel founding is also associated with an elevated risk of lung cancer; in addition to coal-related emissions, such work may involve exposure to silica, metal fumes and formaldehyde.

Wood work
Nasal adenocarcinomas are caused by exposures in the furniture- and cabinet-making industry, mainly among people exposed to wood dust.

Painting
Approximately 200,000 workers worldwide are employed in paint manufacture, and several million are believed to work as painters, including in specialist painting such as in vehicle production and repair. Painters are exposed to hydrocarbon and chlorinated solvents, dyes, polyesters, phenol-formaldehyde and polyurethane resins. A 40% excess risk of lung cancer has been consistently recorded, and cannot be explained by smoking alone.

Agent	Cancer site/cancer
IARC Group 1	
Aflatoxins	Liver
Chronic infection with hepatitis B virus	Liver
Chronic infection with hepatitis C virus	Liver
Erionite	Lung, pleura
Radon and its decay products	Lung
Solar radiation	Skin
Environmental tobacco smoke	Lung
IARC Group 2A	
Diesel engine exhaust	Lung, bladder
Ultraviolet radiation A	Skin
Ultraviolet radiation B	Skin
Ultraviolet radiation C	Skin

Table 2.10 Agents and mixtures which occur mainly in the general environment but to which exposure may also occur in an occupational context.

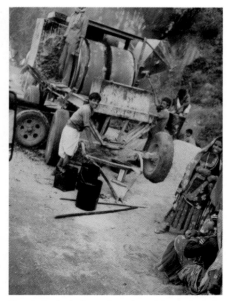

Fig. 2.19 Asphalt road-workers (shown here in India) are exposed to polycyclic aromatic hydrocarbons.

A worldwide problem

Evidence on occupational cancer has been obtained mainly in developed countries. To a large extent, the critical data concern the effects of high exposure levels as a consequence of industrial practice during the first half of the 20th century. Few studies have been conducted in developing countries, other than some in China. Since the period, twenty to thirty years ago, to which most studies pertain, there have been major changes in the geographical distribution of industrial production. These have involved extensive transfer of technology, sometimes obsolete, from highly-industrialized countries to developing countries in South America and in Asia. For example, the manufacture of asbestos-based products is relocating to countries such as Brazil, India, Pakistan and the Republic of Korea, where health and safety standards and requirements may not be so stringent (*Reduction of occupational and environmental exposures*, p135). Occupational exposures to carcinogenic environments are increasing in developing countries as a result of transfers of hazardous industries and the establishment of new local industries as part of a rapid global process of industrialization [8].

A particular problem in developing countries is that much industrial activity takes place in multiple small-scale operations. These small industries are often characterized by old machinery, unsafe buildings, employees with minimal training and education and employers with limited financial resources. Protective clothing, respirators, gloves and other safety equipment are seldom available or used. The small operations tend to be geographically scattered and inaccessible to inspections by health and safety enforcement agencies. Although precise data are lacking, the greatest impact of occupational carcinogens in developing countries is likely to be in the less organized sectors of the relevant industries. Examples include the use of asbestos in building construction, exposure to crystalline silica in mining and mining construction, and the occurrence of polycyclic aromatic hydrocarbons and heavy metals in small-scale metal workshops and in mechanical repair shops.

The most generally accepted estimates of the proportion of cancers attributable

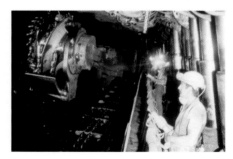

Fig. 2.20 In modern mines (such as those of Charbonnages de France), the prevention of occupational risk is a major concern, which is being addressed on both collective (reduction of dust, organization of transport) and individual (use of suitable protection equipment) levels.

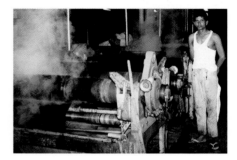

Fig. 2.21 Textile dyeing in Ahmedabad, India. Protection against occupational exposures is often suboptimal in developing countries.

to occupational exposures in developed countries are in the range of 4-5% [9,10]. Lung cancer is probably the most frequent of these cancers. However, the estimates do not apply uniformly to both sexes or to the different social classes. Among those actually exposed to occupational carcinogens (those doing manual work in mining, agriculture and industry, for example), the proportion of cancer attributable to such exposure is estimated to be about 20%.

REFERENCES

1. Pott P, ed. (1775) *Chirurgical Observations*, London, Hawes, Clarke and Collins.

2. Rhen L (1895) Blasengeschwülste bei Fuchsin-Arbeitern. *Arch Klin Chir*, 50: 588-600.

3. Monson R (1996) Occupation. In: Schottenfeld D, Fraumeni, JF eds, *Cancer Epidemiology and Prevention*, New York, Oxford University Press, 373-405.

4. IARC (1972-2001) *IARC Monographs on the Evaluation of Carcinogenic Risks to Humans, Vols 1-78*, Lyon, IARCPress.

5. Alderson M (1986) *Occupational Cancer*, Butterworths.

6. Hayes RB, Songnian Y, Dosemeci M, Linet M (2001) Benzene and lymphohematopoietic malignancies in humans. *Am J Ind Med*, 40: 117-126.

7. IARC (2002) *Man-made Vitreous Fibres, IARC Monographs on the Evaluation of Carcinogenic Risks to Humans Vol. 81*, Lyon, IARCPress.

8. Pearce N, Matos E, Vainio H, Boffetta P, Kogevinas M, eds (1994) *Occupational Cancer in Developing Countries (IARC Scientific Publications, No. 129)*, Lyon, IARCPress.

9. Harvard Center for Cancer Prevention (1996) Harvard report on cancer prevention. Causes of human cancer. Occupation. *Cancer Causes Control*, 7 Suppl 1: S19-S22.

10. Doll R, Peto R (1981) The causes of cancer: quantitative estimates of avoidable risks of cancer in the United States today. *J Natl Cancer Inst*, 66: 1191-1308.

WEBSITES

NCI Occupational Epidemiology Branch:
http://dceg.cancer.gov/ebp/oeb/

The American Conference of Governmental Industrial Hygienists:
http://www.acgih.org/home.htm

International Programme on Chemical Safety (IPCS):
http://www.who.int/pcs/index.htm

IARC Monographs programme:
http://monographs.iarc.fr

ENVIRONMENTAL POLLUTION

SUMMARY

> Pollution of air, water and soil is estimated to account for 1-4% of all cancers.

> A small proportion of lung cancer (<5%) is attributable to outdoor air pollution by industrial effluent, engine exhaust products and other toxins.

> Carcinogenic indoor air pollutants include tobacco smoke, and cooking fumes in particular regions, including parts of Asia.

> Chlorofluorocarbons cause destruction of the ozone layer and enhance the risk of skin cancer through increased ultraviolet radiation.

> Contamination of drinking water is not a general carcinogenic hazard, but high levels of arsenic and chlorination by-products in some communities carry a risk.

In a broad sense, "environmental factors" are implicated in the causation of the majority of human cancers [1]. In respect of many such environmental factors, such as active smoking, alcohol intake, sun exposure and dietary make-up, individuals exercise a degree of control over their level of exposure. However in the present context, "environmental pollution" refers to a specific subset of cancer-causing environmental factors; namely, contaminants of air, water and soil. One characteristic of environmental pollutants is that individuals lack control over their level of exposure. The carcinogenic pollutants for which most information is available include asbestos (referring here to non-occupational exposure), toxic agents in urban air, indoor air pollutants and chlorination by-products and other contaminants of drinking water. Relevant risk factors include place of residence: whether rural or urban, and the relationship to major industrial emission sources. Various determinations suggest that environmental pollution accounts for 1-4% of the total burden of cancer in developed countries [2,3].

Asbestos

Asbestos is one of the best characterized causes of human cancer in an occupational context (*Occupational exposures*, p33); the carcinogenic hazard associated with inhalation of asbestos dust has been recognized since the 1950s [1]. Non-occupational exposure to asbestos may occur domestically and as a consequence of localized pollution. Cohabitants of asbestos workers may be exposed to dust brought home on clothes. The installation, degradation, removal and repair of asbestos-containing products in the context of household maintenance represents another mode of domestic exposure. Further afield, whole neighbourhoods may be subject to outdoor pollution as a result of local asbestos mining or manufacture. The erosion of asbestos or asbestiform rocks may constitute a natural source of asbestos exposure in some parts of the world.

In common with occupational exposure, exposure to asbestos under domestic circumstances results in an increased risk of mesothelioma, a rare tumour derived from the cells lining the peritoneum, pericardium or pleura. Likewise, non-occupational exposure to asbestos may cause lung cancer, particularly among smokers [4]. A consequence of neighbourhood exposure, namely a very high incidence of mesothelioma, is evident among inhabitants of villages in Turkey where houses are built from erionite (a zeolite mineral).

Outdoor air pollution

Ambient air pollution has been implicated as a cause of various health problems, including cancer, and in particular as a cause of lung cancer. Air may be polluted by a complex mixture of different gaseous and particulate components. The concentrations of specific components vary greatly with locality and time. A critical exposure scenario is therefore hard to define, particularly as relevant biological mechanisms are largely unknown. It is, however, possible to attribute at least some carcinogenic risk to particular atmospheric pollutants, including benzo[a]pyrene, benzene, some metals, particulate matter (especially fine particles) in general, and possibly ozone.

Over recent decades, emission levels have been tending to decrease in developed countries, so that concentrations of traditional industrial air pollutants such as sulfur dioxide and particulate matter have fallen. However, vehicular exhaust remains a continuing or even increasing

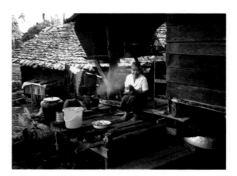

Fig. 2.22 Fuel used for heating and cooking, and high levels of cooking oil vapours are responsible for the high incidence of lung cancer among women in some parts of Asia.

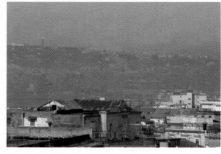

Fig. 2.23 Air pollution is common to many large cities throughout the world.

Air pollutant	WHO Air Quality Guideline, annual average	Number of cities with data	Population in those cities (millions)	% of population in those cities exposed above the AQG
Sulfur dioxide (SO_2)	50 µg/m³	100	61	14%
Black smoke	50 µg/m³	81	52	19%
Total suspended particles	60 µg/m³	75	25	52%

Table 2.11 The proportion of the population in Western European cities exposed to air pollutants at levels above the WHO Air Quality Guidelines (AQG), 1995.

problem. Engine combustion products include volatile organic compounds (benzene, toluene, xylenes and acetylene), oxides of nitrogen (NO_x) and fine particulates (carbon, adsorbed organic material and traces of metallic compounds). In developing countries, outdoor air pollution is likely to represent a greater public health problem than in more developed countries, because of poorly regulated use of coal, wood and biomass (e.g. animal dung, crop residues) for electricity production and heating, in addition to vehicle emissions in urban areas. Although the proportion of global energy derived from biomass fuels decreased from 50% in 1900 to about 13% in 2000, use of such fuels is now increasing in some impoverished regions [5].

Human exposure to air pollution is nevertheless hard to estimate. In a study based on air monitoring and population data for 100 Western European urban areas, the proportion of the population exposed ranged from 14% to 52%, depending on the indicator pollutant used (Table 2.11) [6].

Numerous studies have compared residence in urban areas, where air is considered to be more polluted, to residence in rural areas as a risk factor for lung cancer [7]. In general, lung cancer rates were higher in urban areas and, in some studies, were correlated with levels of specific pollutants such as benzo[a]pyrene, metals and particulate matter, or with mutagenicity of particulate extracts in bacterial assay systems. Other studies have attempted to address exposure to specific components of outdoor air, providing risk estimates in relation to quantitative or semi-quantitative exposure to pollutants. In general, these studies have provided evidence for an increased risk of lung cancer among residents in areas with higher levels of air pollution. Table 2.12 summarizes the results of three of the best designed studies (in particular these studies controlled for the possible concomitant effect of smoking): no matter which pollutant is considered, the results suggest a moderate increase in the risk of lung cancer.

Localized air pollution may be a hazard in relation to residence near to specific sources of pollution, such as petroleum refineries, metal manufacturing plants, iron foundries, incinerator plants and smelters. In general, an increased risk of lung cancer in the proximity of pollution sources has been demonstrated. In three Scottish towns, for example, increased lung cancer mortality occurred in the vicinity of foundries from the mid-1960s to the mid-1970s and later subsided in parallel with emission reductions [8]. Similar

Study	Population, follow-up	Number of subjects	Exposure range	Contrast / Controls	Relative risk of lung cancer (95% CI)
Dockery et al. 1993	6 Cities, USA, 1974-91	8,111	FP 11-30 µg/m³	Highest vs. lowest city	FP: 1.37 (1.11 - 1.68)
Pope et al. 1995	151 Areas, USA, 1982-89	552,138	FP 9-33 µg/m³ Sulfur dioxide: 3.6-23 µg/m³	Highest vs. lowest areas	FP: 1.03 (0.80 - 1.33) Sulfur dioxide: 1.36 (1.11 - 1.66)
Beeson et al. 1998	California, male non-smokers, 1977-82	2,278	FP 10-80 µg/m³ Sulfur dioxide: 0.6-11 ppb Ozone 4-40 ppb	Increment based on interquartile range (FP 24 µg/m³; Sulfur dioxide 3.7 ppb; Ozone 2.1 ppb)	FP: 5.21 (1.94 -13.99) Sulfur dioxide: 2.66 (1.62 - 4.39) Ozone: 2.23 (0.79 - 6.34)

Table 2.12 Studies indicating an increased risk of lung cancer associated with exposure to atmospheric pollutants. FP = fine particles.

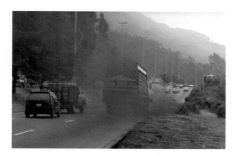

Fig. 2.24 Automobile emissions are a major source of atmospheric pollution.

results were obtained in studies focusing on industrial emission of arsenic from coal burning and non-ferrous metal smelting. The evidence for an increased risk of cancers other than lung cancer from outdoor air pollution is inconclusive at present.

Air pollution by chlorofluorocarbons (CFCs) is believed to be indirectly responsible for increases in skin cancers around the globe. These chemicals, including halons, carbon tetrachloride, and methyl chloroform, are emitted from home air conditioners, foam cushions, and many other products. Chlorofluorocarbons are carried by winds into the stratosphere, where the action of strong solar radiation releases chlorine and bromine atoms that react with, and thereby eliminate, molecules of ozone. Depletion of the ozone layer is believed to be responsible for global increases in UVB radiation (*Radiation*, p51) [9].

Indoor air pollution

Very high lung cancer rates occur in some regions of China and other Asian countries among non-smoking women who spend much of their time at home. Indoor air pollution occurs as a result of combustion sources used for heating and cooking, and may also be a consequence of cooking oil vapours. Three determinants of indoor air pollution ("smokiness") have been studied: (i) heating fuel (type of fuel, type of stove or central heating, ventilation, living area, subjective smokiness), (ii) cooking fuel (type of fuel, type of stove or open pit, ventilation of kitchen, location of cooking area in residence, frequency of cooking, smokiness) and (iii) fumes from frying oils (type of oil, frequency of frying, eye irrita-

tion when cooking). The evidence of carcinogenic hazard is particularly strong for cooking oil vapours from Chinese-style cooking and is supported by experimental data [10]. In circumstances of high exposure, more than 50% of cases of lung cancer among women can be attributed to indoor air pollution.

Tobacco smoke is an important source of indoor air pollution (*Tobacco*, p22). In adult non-smokers, chronic exposure to environmental tobacco smoke increases mortality from lung cancer by between 20% and 30% [11]. Among adults, exposure to environmental tobacco smoke has been linked to lung cancer and heart disease, whilst environmental exposure to tobacco smoke in children has been identified as a cause of respiratory disease, middle ear disease, asthma attacks and sudden infant death syndrome.

Water and soil pollution

Access to unpolluted water is one of the basic requirements of human health. The greatest concern relates to infectious disease. Water quality is influenced by seasons, geology of the soil, and discharges of agriculture and industry. Microbiological contamination of water is controlled by disinfection methods based on oxidants like chlorine, hypochlorite, chloramine, and ozone. In consequence, drinking water may contain a variety of potentially carcinogenic agents, including chlorination by-products and arsenic. It is desirable to reduce such contamination without reducing the rigour of disinfection procedures.

Chlorination by-products result from the interaction of chlorine with organic chemicals, the level of which determines the concentration of by-products. Among the many halogenated compounds that may be formed, trihalomethanes and chloroform are those most commonly found. Concentrations of trihalomethanes vary widely, mainly due to the occurrence of water contamination by organic chemicals [12]. Studies on bladder cancer have suggested an increased risk associated with consumption of chlorinated drinking water [13]. Doubts remain as to whether such associations are causal because of the way in which the studies measured expo-

sure [14]. Given the large number of people exposed to chlorination by-products, however, even a small increase in risk, if real, would result in a substantial number of cases attributable to this factor.

Arsenic causes cancer in the skin, lung and other organs [15]. The main source of environmental exposure to arsenic for the general population is through ingestion of contaminated water. High exposure to arsenic from drinking water is found in several areas of Alaska, Argentina, Bangladesh, Chile, India, Mexico, Mongolia, Taiwan and the USA. There is strong evidence of an increased risk of bladder, skin and lung cancers following consumption of water with high arsenic contamination [14]. The data on other cancers, such as those of the liver, colon and kidney, are less clear but suggestive of a systemic effect. The studies have been conducted in areas of high arsenic content (typically above 200 μg/L). The risk at lower arsenic concentrations (e.g. above 5 μg/L, a level to which 5% of the Finnish population is exposed, [16]) is not established, but an increased risk of blad-

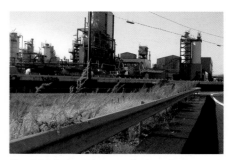

Fig. 2.25 Industrial atmospheric emissions may include carcinogens.

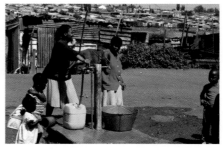

Fig. 2.26 Adequate supplies of clean water are essential for public health, including cancer prevention.

der cancer of the order of 50% is plausible. Several other groups of pollutants of drinking water have been investigated as possible sources of cancer risk in humans [14,17]. They include organic compounds derived from industrial, commercial and agricultural activities and in particular from waste sites, as well as nitrites, nitrates, radionuclides and asbestos. For most pollutants, the results are inconclusive. However, an increased risk of stomach cancer has been repeatedly reported in areas with high nitrate levels in drinking water, and an increased risk of leukaemia has been observed among residents in areas with elevated levels of radium in drinking water.

The atmosphere, and more particularly water and soil, may be polluted by a range of toxic organic compounds specifically including persistent pesticides, by-products of combustion, such as polychorinated dibenzo-*p*-dioxins (2,3,7,8-tetrachlorodibenzodioxin, TCDD, being of greatest concern) and dibenzofurans, and industrial products, such as polychlorinated biphenyls (PCBs) and polybrominated biphenyls (PBBs). These compounds are chemically stable, are often passed along the food chain and may accumulate in fatty tissue. In most case, they were recognized as a carcinogenic hazard to humans on the basis of increased cancer risk in small but relatively heavily exposed groups who were occupationally exposed, in some cases as a result of industrial breakdowns or malfunctions (*Occupational exposures*, p33). Therefore the hazard posed to the general population can only be determined on the basis of extrapolation using mathematical models.

REFERENCES

1. Tomatis L, Aitio A, Day NE, Heseltine E, Kaldor J, Miller AB, Parkin DM, Riboli E, eds (1990) *Cancer: Causes, Occurrence and Control (IARC Scientific Publications, No. 100)*, Lyon, IARCPress .

2. Doll R, Peto R (1981) The causes of cancer: quantitative estimates of avoidable risks of cancer in the United States today. *J Natl Cancer Inst*, 66: 1191-1308.

3. Harvard Center for Cancer Prevention (1996) Harvard report on cancer prevention. Causes of human cancer. Environmental pollution. *Cancer Causes Control*, 7 Suppl 1: S37-S38.

4. Health Effects Institute (1991) *Asbestos in Public and Commercial Buildings: A Literature Review and Synthesis of Current Knowledge*, Boston, MA, Health Effects Institute.

5. Bruce N, Perez-Padilla R, Albalak R (2000) Indoor air pollution in developing countries: a major environmental and public health challenge. *Bull World Health Organ*, 78: 1078-1092.

6. WHO European Centre for Environment and Health (1995) Air pollution. In: *Concern for Europe's Tomorrow: Health and the Environment in the WHO European Region*, Stuttgart, Wissenschaftliche Verlagsgesellschaft, 139-175.

7. Katsouyanni K, Pershagen G (1997) Ambient air pollution exposure and cancer. *Cancer Causes Control*, 8: 284-291.

8. Williams FL, Lloyd OL (1988) The epidemic of respiratory cancer in the town of Armadale: the use of long-term epidemiological surveillance to test a causal hypothesis. *Public Health*, 102: 531-538.

9. EPA (1999) *National Air Quality and Emissions Trends Report, 1999*. Office of Air Quality Planning & Standards. United States Environmental Protection Agency.

10. Zhong L, Goldberg MS, Parent ME, Hanley JA (1999) Risk of developing lung cancer in relation to exposure to fumes from Chinese-style cooking. *Scand J Work Environ Health*, 25: 309-316.

11. World Health Organization (2000) *Fact Sheet No. 187: Air Pollution*, WHO, Geneva.

12. IARC (1991) *Chlorinated Drinking-Water; Chlorination by-Products; Some Other Halogenated Compounds; Cobalt and Cobalt Compounds (IARC Monographs on the Evaluation of Carcinogenic Risks to Humans, Vol. 52)*, Lyon, IARCPress.

13. Morris RD, Audet AM, Angelillo IF, Chalmers TC, Mosteller F (1992) Chlorination, chlorination by-products, and cancer: a meta-analysis. *Am J Public Health*, 82: 955-963.

14. Cantor KP (1997) Drinking water and cancer. *Cancer Causes Control*, 8: 292-308.

15. IARC (1987) *Overall Evaluations of Carcinogenicity: An Updating of IARC Monographs Volumes 1 to 42 (IARC Monographs on the Evaluation of Carcinogenic Risks to Humans, Suppl. 7)*, Lyon, IARCPress.

16. Kurttio P, Pukkala E, Kahelin H, Auvinen A, Pekkanen J (1999) Arsenic concentrations in well water and risk of bladder and kidney cancer in Finland. *Environ Health Perspect*, 107: 705-710.

17. Cantor KP (1996) Arsenic in drinking water: how much is too much? *Epidemiology*, 7: 113-115.

WEBSITES

United States Environmental Protection Agency: http://www.epa.gov/

The Health Effects Institute (a partnership of the US Environmental Protection Agency and industry): http://www.healtheffects.org/index.html

United Nations Environment Programme: http://www.unep.org/

FOOD CONTAMINANTS

SUMMARY

> Food may be contaminated by natural or man-made toxins, including substances shown to be carcinogenic in experimental animals and, in some cases, in humans.

> Naturally-occurring carcinogens include mycotoxins, particularly aflatoxins, which contribute to causation of liver cancer in Africa and Asia.

> Food can be contaminated by residual pesticides. Small quantities of heterocyclic amines, which are mutagenic and carcinogenic in experimental animals, can be generated during food processing and cooking.

> Means to reduce and, in some cases, eliminate food contamination include storage hygiene, appropriately enforced by regulation.

> The burden of cancer attributable to food contamination is difficult to quantify, except in some defined instances (e.g. aflatoxin B$_1$).

Differences between diets eaten by diverse communities, in terms of amount and relative proportion of the major food groupings (vegetable content, fat content etc) exert a major influence on the distribution of cancers of the digestive tract and some other organs (*Diet and nutrition*, p62). By comparison, only a very minor part of the worldwide burden of cancer is attributable to contamination of foodstuffs by toxins recognized to be chemical carcinogens. Despite this global perspective, the issue warrants close attention because it may be a serious concern for particular communities and, irrespective of demonstrated cancer causation, food contamination can be rectified. Removal of carcinogenic contaminants requires that such contaminants are identified, and that ways are found to avoid their inclusion, or generation, in food. Such public health aims are amenable to regulation. Contamination of water is not included in the present discussion, but is considered elsewhere (*Environmental pollution*, p39).

Contamination of food may occur directly during its production, storage and preparation. For example, grains and cereals are subject to fungal growth and contamination by mycotoxins. Indirect contamination of food can occur when animals have been given contaminated feed or been otherwise treated with various products. The most contentious residues occurring in meat, milk and eggs are antibacterial drugs, hormonal growth promoters and certain pesticides, heavy metals and industrial chemicals. An additional category of contaminants comprises those generated in the course of food preparation.

Naturally occurring contaminants

Food may be contaminated by mycotoxins, the presence of one such agent being indicative of the possibility that others are also present. A single fungus can produce several mycotoxins and food or feed can be contaminated by several varieties of mycotoxin-producing fungi. Only a small number of mycotoxins have been categorized as carcinogenic hazards.

Aflatoxins

Aflatoxins are a family of related compounds (designated B$_1$, B$_2$, G$_1$, G$_2$ and M) which occur as food contaminants in hot, humid parts of the world, with particularly high levels in traditional diets based upon maize and groundnuts (peanuts) of sub-Saharan Africa, South-East Asia and South America. Aflatoxins are products of the *Aspergillus* fungi and particularly accumulate during storage of grains. In many countries, including Europe and North America, aflatoxin contamination is recognized as a hazard and aflatoxin levels in susceptible foods are subject to monitoring and associated regulatory control.

The detection of aflatoxin adducts on serum albumin is indicative of human exposure and, in regions where aflatoxins are a common food contaminant, such adducts are detectable in up to 95% of the population. In these regions, chronic hepatitis virus infection (essentially involving hepatitis B virus, HBV) occurs in up to 20% of the population. Together, aflatoxin exposure and HBV infection are the main risk factors accounting for the high incidence of hepatocellular carcinoma in some regions of Africa, Asia and South America [1].

Aflatoxin B$_1$ (the most common aflatoxin) causes liver cancer in experimental animals. In liver cells, aflatoxin B$_1$ is metabolized to form an epoxide which binds to the N7 position of specific guanines, leading to the formation of G to T transversions [2] (*Carcinogen activation and DNA repair*, p89). Mutations induced by aflatoxin B$_1$ are found in several genes involved in hepatocellular carcinogenesis. In particular, aflatoxin B$_1$ induces a typical

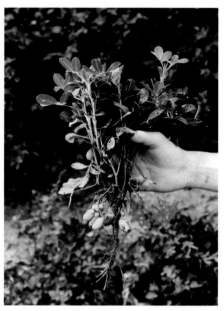

Fig. 2.27 Groundnuts (peanuts) are particularly susceptible to contamination with aflatoxins in some regions, such as West Africa.

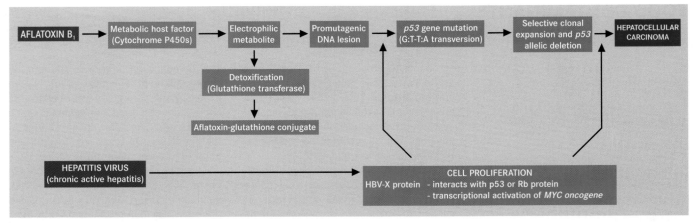

Fig. 2.28 Interaction between aflatoxin B_1 and HBV infection in the pathogenesis of human hepatocellular carcinoma.

mutation at codon 249 in the *p53* gene (AGG to AGT, arginine to serine) (Fig. 2.28). This mutation is rarely found in hepatocellular carcinomas in areas of low aflatoxin exposure, but occurs in up to 60% of hepatocellular carcinomas in regions of very high exposure to aflatoxins [3]. Naturally occurring aflatoxins are categorized by IARC as Group 1 carcinogens (causing cancer in humans).

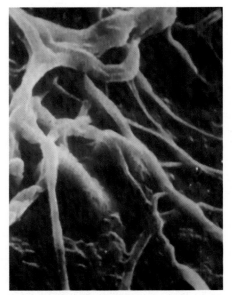

Fig. 2.29 The fungi *Aspergillus* and *Penicillium* produce ochratoxins in humid conditions on commodities used for the production of human or animal food.

Fusarium

Fusarium verticillioides (previously *F. monoliforme*), which is ubiquitous on maize, produces the toxins fumonisin B_1 and B_2 and fusarin C, under warm dry conditions. Incidence of oesophageal cancer incidence has been related to the occurrence of *F. verticillioides* or its toxins in maize. *Fusarium sporotrichioides* produces T-2 toxin, which may have played a significant role in large-scale human poisonings in Siberia in the last century and may be carcinogenic [4].

Ochratoxin

Ochratoxin A, also a fungal metabolite (Fig. 2.29), has been classed as a possible human carcinogen. This mycotoxin may contaminate grain and pork products and has been detected in human blood and milk. Several studies have suggested correlations between ochratoxin A and Balkan endemic nephropathy and between geographical distribution of Balkan endemic nephropathy and high incidence of urothelial urinary tract tumours. In mice, administration of ochratoxin A causes increased incidence of hepatocellular carcinomas and other tumour types [4,5].

Pyrrolizidine alkaloids

Pyrrolizidine alkaloids (including lasiocarpine and monocrotaline) are naturally occurring plant toxins which may be ingested by animals, and by humans eating some medicinal plants (e.g. comfrey) or honey, in some areas [6]. Several pyrrolizidine alkaloids have been found to cause DNA damage and show mutagenic properties *in vitro*. Chronic consumption of some pyrrolizidine alkaloids may cause liver tumours in rodents, but has not been associated with cancer in humans.

Bracken

Animals grazing on bracken (genus *Pteridium*) may show various signs of toxicity, including tumours in the upper gastrointestinal tract and bladder, which are attributable to the carcinogen ptaquiloside [7]. The corresponding glucoside may be present in bracken at a concentration of 13,000 ppm. Metabolism of this compound gives rise to alkylation adducts in DNA. Milk from cows fed on bracken fern causes cancer in experimental animals. Bracken may pose a carcinogenic hazard for humans in population identified as exposed in Japan, Costa Rica and the United Kingdom.

Contamination by industrial chemicals

Certain organochlorines, including DDT and other pesticides, are resistant to degradation, are very lipid-soluble and hence persist in the environment and are bioconcentrated up the human food chain. Related industrial chemicals such as polychlorinated biphenyls are subject to the same effect. DDT and a number of

MOLECULAR EPIDEMIOLOGY

In 1982, "molecular cancer epidemiology" was defined as "an approach in which advanced laboratory methods are used in combination with analytic epidemiology to identify at the biochemical or molecular level specific exogenous and/or host factors that play a role in human cancer causation" (Perera FP, Weinstein IB, *J Chron Dis* 35: 581-600, 1982). Four categories of biomarkers were described: internal dose, biologically effective dose, response, and susceptibility. The hope was that, by introducing biomarkers into epidemiology, researchers "should be able to predict human risks more precisely than hitherto possible". Since then, molecular cancer epidemiology has evolved rapidly, with special programmes in many schools of public health.

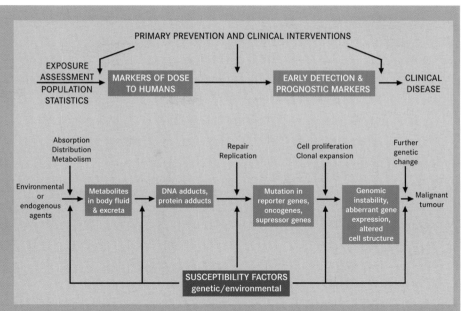

Potential molecular endpoints (specified in the lower section) that may serve as the basis for molecular epidemiological studies. These endpoints may be indicative of biological processes contributing to cancer development as shown in the upper section.

The stated goal of molecular cancer epidemiology is the prevention of cancer. Considerable molecular epidemiologic research has focused on environmental causes because many lines of evidence indicate that the factors that determine the great majority of cancers incidence are largely exogenous and hence preventable (Lichenstein P et al., *N Engl J Med* 343: 78-85, 2000). These include exposures related to lifestyle and occupation, and pollutants in air, water, and the food supply. This awareness has lent greater urgency to the search for more powerful tools in the form of early-warning systems to identify causal environmental agents and flag risks well before the malignant process is entrenched.

The potential contribution of molecular epidemiology includes: providing evidence that environmental agents pose carcinogenic risks, helping establish the causal roles of environmental factors in cancer, identifying environment-susceptibility interactions and populations at greatest risk and developing new intervention strategies. A recent review of the field (Perera F, *J Natl Cancer Inst*, 92: 602-612, 2000) critically evaluated the progress to date using as illustration research on tobacco smoke, polycyclic aromatic hydrocarbons, aflatoxin B_1, benzene and hepatitis B virus and their role in lung, breast, liver cancer and leukaemia. It concluded

that molecular epidemiology has identified a number of carcinogenic hazards, in some cases providing definitive etiologic data, furthering our understanding of individual genetic and acquired susceptibility to environmental carcinogens. However, molecular epidemiology has not yet led to broad policy changes to prevent or to reduce exposure to carcinogens. What is now needed is timely translation of existing data into risk assessment and public health policy as well as focused research to fill gaps in scientific knowledge.

other organochlorine pesticides cause liver cancer in rats. DDT in particular has been associated with increased risk of pancreatic cancer, breast cancer, lymphoma and leukaemia in humans. Some organochlorines exhibit sex steroid activity in relevant assay systems, and these pesticides are considered to have the potential to disrupt endocrine-regulated homeostasis. Attempts have been made to correlate levels of organochlorines and polychlorinated biphenyls in breast tissue with breast cancer risk in several communities, but without clear-cut results [8]. For the major pesticides, international regulations exist with regard to permissible amounts of residues in foods – the ADI, or acceptable daily intake, being the primary reference level for such exposures. ADI levels are determined by expert groups convened by WHO, and published as the *WHO Pesticide Residue Series*.

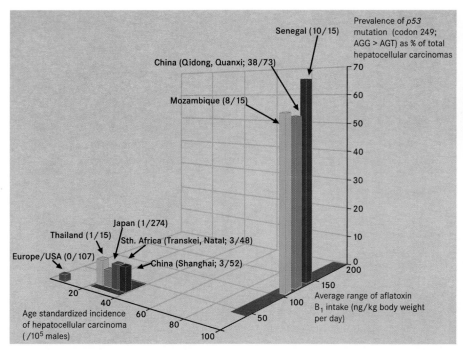

Fig. 2.30 Correlation between regional incidence of hepatocellular carcinoma, dietary exposure to aflatoxin B₁, and prevalence of G>T mutations at codon 249 of the *p53* tumour suppressor gene.

Labels on figure: Senegal (10/15); China (Qidong, Quanxi; 38/73); Mozambique (8/15); Japan (1/274); Thailand (1/15); Sth. Africa (Transkei, Natal; 3/48); Europe/USA (0/107); China (Shanghai; 3/52). Prevalence of *p53* mutation (codon 249; AGG > AGT) as % of total hepatocellular carcinomas. Average range of aflatoxin B₁ intake (ng/kg body weight per day). Age standardized incidence of hepatocellular carcinoma (/10⁵ males).

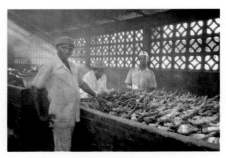

Fig. 2.31 Nitrosamines are present in smoked fish consumed in many parts of the world, including the Gambia.

Polychlorinated dibenzo-*para*-dioxins (which include 2,3,7,8-tetrachlorodibenzo-*para*-dioxin, TCDD) are ubiquitous pollutants in soil sediments and air (*Environmental pollution*, p39). Human exposure occurs through eating meat and related foods. The burden of cancer attributable to such exposure is unknown [9].

Chemicals generated during food preparation

Some chemicals formed during food preparation may present a carcinogenic hazard. The toxicity of these chemicals generally warrants the adoption of means to minimize their formation, particularly during industrialized food preparation. It has not been possible to attribute cancer causation in humans to hazards of this type specifically.

A possible pragmatic approach to the prioritization of chemical carcinogens occurring as food contaminants has been proposed. The highest priority category is chemical carcinogens that are believed to act by a genotoxic mechanism [10].

Heterocyclic amines

Certain heterocyclic amines are formed by pyrolysis of two amino acids, creatine and creatinine, during cooking of meat and fish at high temperature. Heterocyclic amines are carcinogenic in various organs of mice, rats and non-human primates, although their carcinogenic potential in humans has not yet been established [11]. Metabolism of heterocyclic amines can vary between individuals due to various genetic polymorphisms.

Polycyclic aromatic hydrocarbons

Polycyclic aromatic hydrocarbons can be generated in meat when it is fried, roasted or cooked over an open flame, and many members of this chemical class are carcinogenic. These compounds can also be formed during the curing and processing of raw foods prior to cooking. A number of polycyclic aromatic hydrocarbons, such as benzo[a]pyrene and benzanthracene, are present in smoke from the burning of fuels, tobacco and weeds.

N-Nitroso compounds

N-Nitroso compounds are a wide class of chemicals, many of which (particularly *N*-nitrosamines) are potent carcinogens in several species of experimental animals, and probably in humans [12]. Nitrosamines may be formed by chemical reactions in foods containing added nitrates and nitrites, such as salt-preserved fish and meat, and in foods processed by smoking or direct fire drying. The use of fertilizers may influence the level of nitrites in food, which may be a factor in determining generation of nitrosamines during food preparation and storage. Some industrial procedures, including brewing of beer, have been modified to reduce nitrosamine formation. Studies on volunteers consuming supplements of nitrate, or large portions of red meat, indicate that *N*-nitroso compounds can also be produced endogenously in the stomach and colon. Endogenous formation of nitrosamines is inhibited by several natural antioxidants, such as vitamins C and E, present in fruit and vegetables.

Metals

The hazard presented by dietary metals, whether regarded as essential nutrients or contaminants, is difficult to assess [13].

REFERENCES

1. Wild CP, Hall AJ (2000) Primary prevention of hepato-cellular carcinoma in developing countries. *Mutat Res*, 462: 381-393.

2. Smela ME, Currier SS, Bailey EA, Essigmann JM (2001) The chemistry and biology of aflatoxin B(1): from mutation-al spectrometry to carcinogenesis. *Carcinogenesis*, 22: 535-545.

3. Montesano R, Hainaut P, Wild CP (1997) Hepatocellular carcinoma: from gene to public health. *J Natl Cancer Inst*, 89: 1844-1851.

4. IARC (1993) *Some Naturally Occurring Substances: Food Items and Constituents, Heterocyclic Aromatic Amines and Mycotoxins (IARC Monographs on the Evaluation of Carcinogenic Risks to Humans, Vol. 56)*, Lyon, IARCPress .

5. Castegnaro M, Plestina R, Dirheimer G, Chernozemsky IN, Bartsch H, eds (1991) *Mycotoxins, Endemic Nephropathy and Urinary Tract Tumours (IARC Scientific Publications, No. 115)*, Lyon, IARCPress.

6. Prakash AS, Pereira TN, Reilly PE, Seawright AA (1999) Pyrrolizidine alkaloids in human diet. *Mutat Res*, 443: 53-67.

7. Shahin M, Smith BL, Prakash AS (1999) Bracken car-cinogens in the human diet. *Mutat Res*, 443: 69-79.

8. Department of Health (1999) Organochlorine insecti-cides and breast cancer. In: *1999 Annual Report of the Committees on Toxicity, Mutagenicity, Carcinogenicity of Chemicals in Food, Consumer Products and the Environment*, London, Department of Health (UK), 67-75.

9. van Leeuwen FX, Feeley M, Schrenk D, Larsen JC, Farland W, Younes M (2000) Dioxins: WHO's tolerable daily intake (TDI) revisited. *Chemosphere*, 40: 1095-1101.

10. McDonald AL, Fielder RJ, Diggle GE, Tennant DR, Fisher CE (1996) Carcinogens in food: priorities for regula-tory action. *Hum Exp Toxicol*, 15: 739-746.

11. Layton DW, Bogen KT, Knize MG, Hatch FT, Johnson VM, Felton JS (1995) Cancer risk of heterocyclic amines in cooked foods: an analysis and implications for research. *Carcinogenesis*, 16: 39-52.

12. O'Neill IK, Chen J, Bartsch H, Dipple A, Shuker DEG, Kadlubar FF, Segerbäck D, Bartsch H, eds (1991) *Relevance to Human Cancer of N-Nitroso Compounds, Tobacco Smoke and Mycotoxins (IARC Scientific Publications, No. 105)*, Lyon, IARCPress.

13. Rojas E, Herrera LA, Poirier LA, Ostrosky-Wegman P (1999) Are metals dietary carcinogens? *Mutat Res*, 443: 157-181.

WEBSITE

WHO Food Safety Programme:
http://www.who.int/fsf/index.htm

MEDICINAL DRUGS

SUMMARY

> Certain drugs used to treat malignant tumours, may rarely cause second primary tumours.

> Drugs with hormonal activity or which block hormonal effects may increase risk of some hormonally-responsive cancers, while reducing the risk of others.

> Drugs like diethylstilbestrol, which causes vaginal cancer following transplacental exposure, have been banned, while use of others, like phenacetin (which causes urothelial tumours), has been restricted.

Modern medicine has at its disposal hundreds of drugs, many of which are essential for the effective treatment of an enormous range of human diseases. A small fraction of such drugs has been found to have carcinogenicity to humans as a side-effect. This is most likely for some drugs that must be given at high doses or for prolonged periods. Where safer, non-carcinogenic alternatives exist, such drugs have been withdrawn from medical use. In certain cases, as in the treatment of otherwise fatal diseases such as disseminated cancer, the risk of using drugs that present a carcinogenic hazard is more than offset by an immediate benefit to the patient. Drugs that have been found to be carcinogenic to humans include some antineoplastic drugs and drug combinations [1], certain hormones and hormone antagonists [2,3], some immune suppressants and a small number of miscellaneous agents [1,4].

Anti-cancer drugs
Some antineoplastic agents and combined drug therapies have caused secondary cancers in patients (Table 2.13).

These agents have been evaluated by the *IARC Monographs on the Evaluation of Carcinogenic Risks to Humans* as carcinogenic to humans (IARC Group 1). Some of them are no longer used in medicine because more effective and less hazardous drugs have become available. Other agents have properties similar to the known carcinogens, and are likely to be carcinogenic to humans (IARC Group 2A) (Table 2.14). These agents all have in common the ability either to react chemically with DNA to produce genetic damage at the cellular level (e.g. procarbazine), or to interfere with DNA replication in ways that can produce genetic damage (e.g. etoposide) (*Medical oncology*, p281). The agents in Table 2.13 that have been studied in animal experiments all cause tumours. The potential of many effective anti-tumour drugs to cause secondary cancers in treated patients is well recognized. Medical oncologists have devoted much effort to optimizing the doses of these drugs, in order to maximize the anti-tumour effects while minimizing risk of secondary cancers.

Hormones
Hormones are potent regulators of bodily functions and hormonal imbalances can cause increased risk of certain cancers (*Reproductive factors and hormones*, p76). This can occur when natural or synthetic hormones are used for medical purposes, as in certain contraceptive preparations and in postmenopausal hormonal therapies. Certain drugs have been developed that counteract the effects of certain hormones in specific tissues. Some of these drugs have hormone-like effects in other tissues, however, and can increase risk of cancer at these sites. Tamoxifen, for example, is an antiestrogen that may be given to women with estrogen receptor-positive breast tumours to block estrogen from entering the breast tissues. It is an effective drug for prevention of contralateral breast cancer in breast cancer patients, but it also increases risk of cancer of the endometrium [5]. Diethylstilbestrol is a synthetic estrogen, originally prescribed to prevent miscarriage, which caused malformations of the reproductive organs and is associated with increased risk of vaginal adenocarcinoma in daughters exposed to the drug *in utero* (Fig. 2.32).

Other drugs and surgical implants
A small number of drugs that were used in medicine for many years for a variety of purposes other than antitumour, hormonal or immunosuppressive therapies have been found to present a risk of cancer in humans when used in very large quantities (e.g. phenacetin, contained in analgesic mixtures, Fig. 2.33) or for prolonged periods (e.g. Fowler's

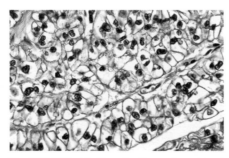

Fig. 2.32 Histopathology of a clear cell carcinoma of the vagina resulting from prenatal exposure to diethylstilbestrol.

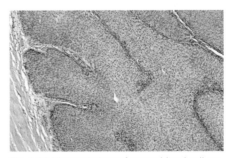

Fig. 2.33 Histopathology of a transitional cell carcinoma of the urinary tract caused by long-term abuse of phenacetin-based analgesics.

solution, containing a 1% solution of potassium arsenite in aqueous alcohol). The no-longer used radioactive X-ray contrast medium Thorotrast was associated with increased risk of angiosarcoma. Certain others have been found to be carcinogenic in experimental animals but have not been linked to cancers in humans despite extensive study. Some of these drugs have been withdrawn from clinical use (e.g. phenolphthalein), while others continue to be used because the benefit to individual patients is great and the risk of cancer is considered very slight (e.g. iron dextran, injectable; phenobarbital; phenytoin).

Some drugs that have been recently introduced into human medicine, including the antiretroviral drugs zidovudine (AZT) and zalcitabine (ddC), are carcinogenic in experimental animals and may possibly be carcinogenic to humans (IARC Group 2B), although there is as yet no direct evidence of increased cancer risk in treated patients [6].

Surgical implants of various kinds are widely used for both therapeutic and cosmetic purposes [7]. Foreign bodies of many kinds cause development of malignant tumours of connective tissue (sarcomas) when implanted in tissues or body cavities of experimental rodents and left in place for long periods. Foreign bodies include both metallic and non-metallic solid objects, and non-absorbable or very slowly absorbable liquid suspensions. Sarcomas develop in rodents immediately adjacent to the foreign body, in the soft connective tissues or in bone and/or cartilage. There have been more than 60 published case reports of sarcomas and other kinds of cancers that have developed in humans at the sites of surgical implants or other foreign bodies. However, there are no controlled studies that would allow a conclusion that these cancers were indeed caused by the pre-existing foreign body. Female breast implants have been extensively studied, and for silicone implants there is evidence suggesting lack of carcinogenicity for breast carcinoma in women who have received these implants.

Drug or drug combination	Cancer site/cancer
IARC Group 1	
Analgesic mixtures containing phenacetin	Kidney, bladder
Azathioprine	Lymphoma, skin, liver and bile ducts, soft connective tissues
N,N-bis(2-chloroethyl)-2-naphthylamine (Chlornaphazine)	Bladder
1,4-Butanediol dimethane-sulfonate (Myleran; Busulfan)	Leukaemia
Chlorambucil	Leukaemia
1-(2-Chloroethyl)-3-(4-methyl-cyclohexyl)-1-nitrosourea (Methyl-CCNU)	Leukaemia
Ciclosporin	Lymphoma, Kaposi sarcoma
Cyclophosphamide	Leukaemia, bladder
Diethylstilbestrol	Cervix, vagina
Etoposide in combination with cisplatin and bleomycin	Leukaemia
Fowler's solution (inorganic arsenic)	Skin
Melphalan	Leukaemia
8-Methoxypsoralen (Methoxsalen) plus ultraviolet radiation	Skin
MOPP and other combined [anticancer] chemotherapy including alkylating agents	Leukaemia
Estrogen therapy, postmenopausal	Breast, uterus
Estrogens, non-steroidal	Cervix/vagina
Estrogens, steroidal	Uterus, breast
Oral contraceptives, combined[a]	Liver
Oral contraceptives, sequential	Uterus
Tamoxifen[b]	Uterus
Thiotepa	Leukaemia
Treosulfan	Leukaemia

[a] There is also conclusive evidence that these agents have a protective effect against cancers of the ovary and endometrium.

[b] There is conclusive evidence that tamoxifen has a protective effect against second breast tumours in patients with breast cancer.

Table 2.13 Medicinal drugs that are classified as being carcinogenic to humans (IARC Group 1).

Drug or drug combination	Cancer
IARC Group 2A	
Androgenic (anabolic) steroids	Liver cancer
Bis(chloroethyl) nitrosourea (BCNU)	Leukaemia
Chloramphenicol	Leukaemia
1-(2-Chloroethyl)-3-cyclohexyl-1-nitrosourea (CCNU)	Leukaemia
Etoposide	Leukaemia
5-Methoxypsoralen	Skin cancer
Nitrogen mustard	Skin cancer
Procarbazine hydrochloride	Leukaemia
Teniposide	Leukaemia

Table 2.14 Medicinal drugs that are probably carcinogenic to humans (IARC Group 2A).

The recent past has not been marked by major discoveries in relation to cancer causation by drugs. This situation is attributable, at least in part, to the vigilance imposed by national authorities in relation to preclinical and clinical drug testing. Putative drugs exhibiting activity in relevant carcinogen-screening tests are unlikely to be carried forward to final development and marketing. Consequently, the prevention of cancer attributable to medical treatment is not identified as a major public health need.

REFERENCES

1. Selbey JV, Friedman GD, Herrinton LJ (1996) Pharmaceuticals other than hormones. In: Schottenfeld D, Fraumeni, JF eds, *Cancer Epidemiology and Prevention*, New York, Oxford University Press, 489-501.

2. Bernstein JF, Henderson BE (1996) Exogenous hormones. In: Schottenfeld D, Fraumeni, JF eds, *Cancer Epidemiology and Prevention*, New York, Oxford University Press, 462-488.

3. IARC (1998) *Hormonal Contraception and Post-Menopausal Hormonal Therapy (IARC Monographs on the Evaluation of Carcinogenic Risks to Humans, Vol. 72)*, Lyon, IARCPress.

4. IARC (1996) *Some Pharmaceutical Drugs (IARC Monographs on the Evaluation of Carcinogenic Risks to Humans, Vol. 66)*, Lyon, IARCPress.

5. White IN (2001) Anti-oestrogenic drugs and endometrial cancers. *Toxicol Lett*, 120: 21-29.

6. IARC (2000) *Some Antiviral and Antineoplastic Drugs and Other Pharmaceutical Agents (IARC Monographs on the Evaluation of Carcinogenic Risks to Humans, Vol. 76)*, Lyon, IARCPress.

7. IARC (1999) *Surgical Implants and Other Foreign Bodies (IARC Monographs on the Evaluation of Carcinogenic Risks to Humans, Vol. 74)*, Lyon, IARCPress.

WEBSITE

IARC Monographs programme, online search facility: http://monographs.iarc.fr

RADIATION

SUMMARY

> Exposure to ionizing radiation from natural as well as from industrial, medical and other sources, can cause a variety of neoplasms, including leukaemia, breast cancer and thyroid cancer.

> Sunlight is by far the most significant source of ultraviolet irradiation and causes several types of skin cancer, particularly in highly-exposed populations with fair skin, e.g. Australians of Caucasian origin.

> Extremely low frequency electromagnetic fields generated by electrical power transmission have been associated with an increased risk of childhood leukaemia, but the findings are not conclusive.

Natural and man-made sources generate radiant energy in the form of electromagnetic waves. Their interaction with biological systems is principally understood at the cellular level. Electromagnetic waves are characterized by their wavelength, frequency, or energy. Effects on biological systems are determined by the intensity of the radiation, the energy in each photon and the amount of energy absorbed by the exposed tissue.

The electromagnetic spectrum extends from waves at low frequency (low energy), referred to as "electric and magnetic fields", to those at very high frequencies, which are often called "electromagnetic radiation" (Fig. 2.38). The highest-energy electromagnetic radiation is X- and γ-radiation, which have sufficient photon energy to produce ionization (i.e. create positive and negative electrically-charged atoms or parts of molecules) and thereby break chemical bonds. Other forms of ionizing radiation are the sub-atomic particles (neutrons, electrons (β-particles) and α-particles) that make up cosmic rays and

are also emitted by radioactive atoms. Non-ionizing radiation is a general term for that part of the electromagnetic spectrum which has photon energies too weak to break chemical bonds, and includes ultraviolet radiation, visible light, infrared radiation, radiofrequency and microwave fields, extremely low frequency (ELF) fields, as well as static electric and magnetic fields.

Ionizing radiation

Exposure to ionizing radiation is unavoidable [1]. Humans are exposed both to X-rays and γ–rays from natural sources (including cosmic radiation and radioactivity present in rocks and soil) and, typically to a much lower extent, from man-made sources (Fig. 2.35). On average, for a member of the general public, the greatest contribution comes from medical X-rays and the use of radiopharmaceuticals, with lower doses from fallout from weapons testing, nuclear accidents (such as Chernobyl), and accidental and routine releases from nuclear installations. Medical exposures occur both in the diagnosis (e.g. radiography) of diseases and injuries and in the treatment (e.g. radiotherapy) of cancer and of some benign diseases. Occupational

exposure to ionizing radiation occurs in a number of jobs, including the nuclear industry and medicine. Airline pilots and crew are exposed to cosmic radiation.

Cancer causation
Ionizing radiation is one of the most intensely studied carcinogens [2-4].

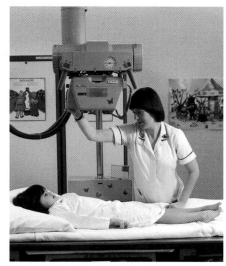

Fig. 2.34 Modern diagnostic radiology is no longer a significant source of exposure to ionizing radiation.

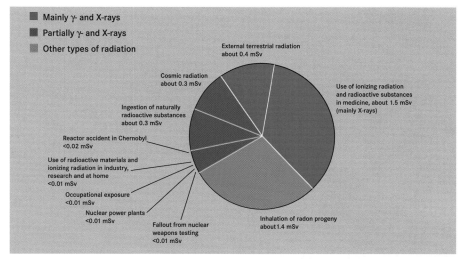

Fig. 2.35 Estimated annual dose of ionizing radiation received by a member of the general public.

Agent or substance	Cancer site/cancer
IARC Group 1: Carcinogenic to humans	
X-rays and gamma-radiation	Various – all sites
Solar radiation	Skin
Radon-222 and its decay products	Lung
Radium-224, -226, -228 and their decay products	Bone
Thorium-232 and its decay products	Liver, including haemangiosarcoma; leukaemia
Radioiodines (including iodine-131)	Thyroid
Plutonium-239 and its decay products (aerosols)	Lung, liver, bone
Phosphorus-32	Leukaemia
Neutrons	Various
Alpha (α) particle-emitting radionuclides	Various
Beta (β) particle-emitting radionuclides	Various
IARC Group 2A: Probably carcinogenic to humans	
Sunlamps and sun beds, use of	Skin
Ultraviolet radiation	Skin

Table 2.15 Various forms and sources of radiation that are carcinogenic to humans (IARC Group 1) or probably carcinogenic to humans (IARC Group 2A).

Frequency	Class	Type of device or service
30 - 300 kHz	LF (low)	LF broadcast and long-range radio
300 - 3,000 kHz	MF (medium)	AM radio, radio navigation, ship-to-shore
3 - 30 MHz	HF (high)	CB radio, amateurs, HF radio communications and broadcast
30 - 300 MHz	VHF (very high)	FM radio, VHF TV, emergency services
300 - 3,000 MHz	UHF (ultra high)	UHF TV, paging, mobile telephones, amateur radios
3 - 30 GHz	SHF (super high)	Microwaves, satellite communications, radar, point to point microwave communications
30 - 300 GHz	EHF (extremely high)	Radar, radioastronomy, short-link microwave communications

Table 2.16 Radiofrequency range: class and type of device or service.

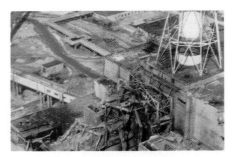

Fig. 2.36 The Chernobyl nuclear power plant following the accident in 1986.

Knowledge of associated health effects comes from epidemiological study of hundreds of thousands of exposed persons, including the survivors of the atomic bombings in Hiroshima and Nagasaki, patients irradiated for therapeutic purposes, populations with occupational exposures and people exposed as a result of accidents. These data are complemented by findings from large-scale animal experiments carried out to evaluate the effects of different types of radiation, taking account of variation in dose and exposure pattern, and with reference to cellular and molecular endpoints. Such experiments are designed to characterize the mechanisms of radiation damage, repair and carcinogenesis.

Survivors of the atomic bombings in Hiroshima and Nagasaki were exposed primarily to γ-rays. Amongst these people, dose-related increases in the risk of leukaemia, breast cancer, thyroid cancer and a number of other malignancies have been observed. Increased frequency of these same malignancies has also been observed among cancer patients treated with X-rays or γ-rays. The level of cancer risk after exposure to X-rays or γ-rays is modified by a number of factors in addition to radiation dose, and these include the age at which exposure occurs, the length of time over which radiation is received and the sex of the exposed person. Exposure to high-dose radiation increases the risk of leukaemia by over five-fold. Even higher relative risks have been reported for thyroid cancer following irradiation during childhood.

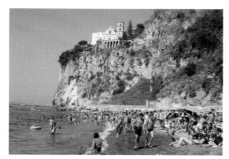
Fig. 2.37 Deliberate exposure to solar radiation in order to achieve a sun-tan.

Internalized radionuclides that emit α-particles and β-particles are carcinogenic to humans. For most people, exposure to ionizing radiation from inhaled and tissue-deposited radionuclides is mainly from naturally-occurring radon-222. Exposure to thorium-232, which occurs in soil, is less common. Cancers associated with exposure to particular nuclides, usually in an occupational context, include lung cancer, bone sarcomas, liver cancer, leukaemia and thyroid cancer.

The United Nations Scientific Committee on the Effects of Atomic Radiation [5] has estimated the lifetime risk of solid cancers and of leukaemia following an acute whole-body exposure to γ radiation, together with the corresponding estimated numbers of years of life lost per radiation-induced case (Table 2.17). The current recommendations of the International Commission for Radiological Protection are to limit exposures to the general public to 1 mSv per year, and doses to workers to 100 mSv over 5 years [6] (1 Sievert equals 1 joule per kilogram).

Ultraviolet radiation

The major source of human exposure to ultraviolet radiation is sunlight. Approximately 5% of the total solar radiation received at the surface of the earth is ultraviolet [7]. Intensity of solar terrestrial radiation varies according to geography, the time of day and other factors. The level of skin exposure to sunlight depends on many parameters including cultural and social behaviour, clothing, the position of the sun and the position of the body. Few measurements of personal exposure have been reported. Artificial sources of ultraviolet radiation are common and such devices are used to treat a number of diseases (e.g. psoriasis) as well as for cosmetic purposes.

Cancer causation

Solar radiation, and specifically the ultraviolet component of it, causes cutaneous malignant melanoma and non-melanocytic skin cancer (Fig. 2.39). Exposure of skin to ultraviolet radiation causes DNA damage (*Carcinogen activation and DNA repair*, p89) and also the conversion of *trans*-urocanic acid to *cis*-urocanic acid, which leads to cell injury and ultimately to cancer. Incidence of skin cancer is increasing rapidly among fair-skinned populations [7] (*Melanoma*, p253). In Canada, for example, occurrence of this disease has doubled over the past 25 years. IARC has estimated that at least 80% of all melanomas are caused by exposure to sunlight. Non-melanocytic skin cancer, which includes basal cell carcinoma and squamous cell carcinoma, is the most prevalent human malignancy: more people are living with this cancer than any other. In the USA and Australia, one of every two new cancers diagnosed is a non-melanocytic skin cancer. Use of sunlamps and sunbeds probably causes skin melanomas in humans.

Electromagnetic fields

Recent years have seen an unprecedented increase in the number and diversity of

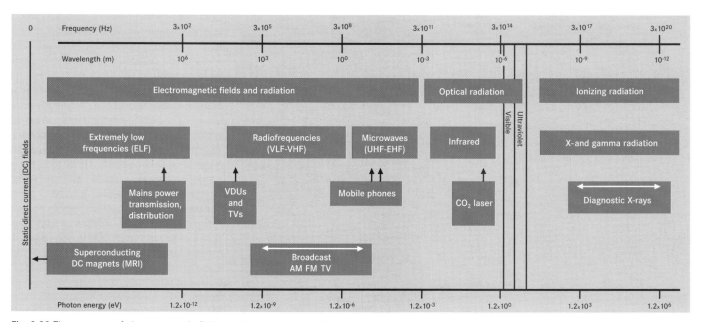
Fig. 2.38 The spectrum of electromagnetic fields and their use in daily life.

	Lifetime risk		Number of years of life lost per case	
	0.2 Sv	1 Sv	0.2 Sv	1 Sv
Solid cancers	2.4%	10.9%	11.2	11.6
Leukaemia	0.14%	1.1%	31	31

Table 2.17 Estimated risk of cancer following acute whole-body exposure to gamma radiation at two dose levels.

sources of electromagnetic fields [8], principally extremely low frequency and radiofrequency fields. Such sources include all equipment using electricity, television, radio, computers, mobile telephones, microwave ovens, anti-theft gates in large shops, radars and equipment used in industry, medicine and commerce. Static fields and extremely low frequency fields occur naturally, and also arise as a consequence of the generation and transmission of electrical power and through

the operation of a range of industrial devices and domestic appliances, the latter often at a greater field intensity. Exposure to extremely low frequency fields is mainly from human-made sources for the generation, transmission and use of electricity. Occupational exposure occurs, for example, in the electric and electronics industry, in welding and in use and repair of electrical motors. Environmental exposure to extremely low frequency fields occurs in residential settings due to prox-

imity to electricity transmission lines and use of electric appliances. Levels of exposure from many environmental sources are typically low [9].

Exposure to radiofrequency radiation can occur in a number of ways. The primary natural source of radiofrequency fields is the sun. Man-made sources, however, are the main source of exposure. Radiofrequency fields are generated as a consequence of commercial radio and television broadcasting and from telecommunications facilities (Table 2.16). Radiofrequency fields in the home are generated by microwave ovens and burglar alarms. Mobile telephones are now, however, the greatest source of radiofrequency exposure for the general public.

In respect of the work environment, employees working in close proximity to radiofrequency-emitting systems may receive high levels of exposure. This includes workers in the broadcasting, transport and communication industries, and in antenna repair, military personnel (e.g. radar operators) and police officers (utilizing traffic control radars). There are also industrial processes that use radiofrequency fields and these include dielectric heaters for wood lamination and sealing of plastics, industrial induction heaters and microwave ovens, medical diathermy equipment to treat pain and inflammation of body tissues, and electrosurgical devices for cutting and welding tissues.

Cancer causation

Several expert groups have recently reviewed the scientific evidence concerning the carcinogenicity of extremely low frequency fields e.g. [9,10]. A number of epidemiological studies on childhood leukaemia indicate a possible relationship between risk and exposure to extremely low frequency fields. Studies of adult cancers following occupational or environmental exposures to extremely low frequency fields are much less clear. There is little experimental evidence that these fields can cause mutations in cells. Mechanistic studies and animal experiments do not show any consistent positive

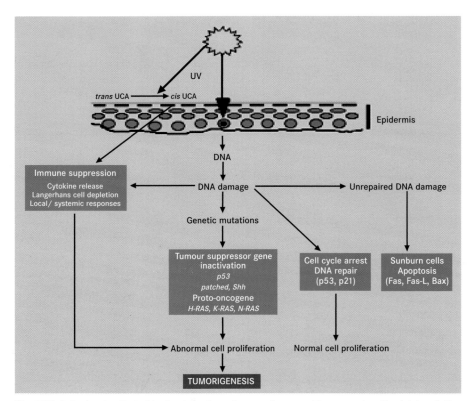

Fig. 2.39 Pathways implicated in the induction of non-melanoma skin cancer by ultraviolet radiation (UCA = urocanic acid).

results, although sporadic findings concerning biological effects (including increased cancers in animals) have been reported. IARC has classified extremely low frequency fields as possibly causing cancer in humans (Group 2B), based on childhood leukaemia findings [10].

The evidence for the carcinogenicity of radiofrequency fields is even less clear [11-14]. A few epidemiological studies in occupational settings have indicated a possible increase in the risk of leukaemia or brain tumours, while other studies indicated decreases. These studies suffer from a number of limitations. The experimental evidence is also limited, but suggests that radiofrequency fields cannot cause DNA mutations. The lack of reproducibility of findings limits the conclusions that can be drawn.

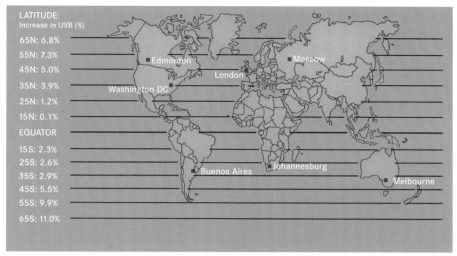

Fig. 2.40 Satellite-based analyses (1996) demonstrate increases in average annual levels of ultraviolet B (UVB) radiation reaching the Earth's surface over the past ten years. These changes are strongly dependent on latitude.

REFERENCES

1. IARC (2000) *Ionizing Radiation, Part 1: X- and Gamma Radiation and Neutrons (IARC Monographs on the Evaluation of Carcinogenic Risks to Humans, Vol. 75)*, Lyon, IARCPress .

2. United Nations Scientific Committee on the Effects of Atomic Radiation (2000) *Sources and Effects of Ionizing Radiation: 2000 Report*, Vienna, UNSCEAR.

3. US National Academy of Sciences (1998) *Health Effects of Radon and Other Internally Deposited Alpha-Emitters (US NAS, BEIR VI Report)*, Washington DC, US National Academy of Sciences.

4. US National Academy of Sciences (1990) *Health Effects on Populations of Exposure to Low Levels of Ionizing Radiation (US NAS BEIR V Report)*, Washington DC, US National Academy of Sciences.

5. United Nations Scientific Committee on the Effects of Atomic Radiation (1994) *Sources and Effects of Ionizing Radiation: 1994 Report*, Vienna, UNSCEAR.

6. International Commission on Radiological Protection (1991) *Recommendations of the International Commission on Radiological Protection (ICRP Report 60)*, Oxford, Pergamon Press.

7. IARC (1992) *UV and Solar Radiation (IARC Monographs on the Evaluation of Carcinogenic Risks to Humans, Vol. 55)*, Lyon, IARCPress .

8. Bernhardt JH, Matthes R, Repacholi M, eds (1997) *Non-Thermal Effects of RF Electromagnetic Fields (International Commission on Non-Ionizing Radiation Protection, WHO)*, Geneva, World Health Organization.

9. Bernhardt JH, Matthes R, Repacholi M, eds (1998) *Static and Extremely Low Frequency Electric and Magnetic Fields (International Commission on Non-Ionizing Radiation Protection, WHO)*, Geneva, World Health Organization.

10. US National Institute for Environmental Health Sciences (1999) *Report of the EMF-Rapid Programme*, NIEHS.

11. McKinlay A (1997) A possible health effect related to the use of radiotelephones. *Radiological Protection Bull*, 187: 9-16.

12. Repacholi MH (1998) Low-level exposure to radiofrequency electromagnetic fields: health effects and research needs. *Bioelectromagnetics*, 19: 1-19.

13. Royal Society of Canada (2000) *A Review of the Potential Health Risks of Radiofrequency Fields from Wireless Telecommunication Devices (RSC.EPR 1999-1)*, Ottawa, Royal Society of Canada.

14. Independent Expert Group on Mobile Phones (2000) *Mobile Phones and Health*, National Radiological Protection Board.

WEBSITES

ICNIRP (International Commission for Non-Ionizing Radiation Protection):
http://www.icnirp.de

National Council on Radiation Protection and Measurements (NCRP), USA:
http://www.ncrp.com

National Radiological Protection Board (NRPB), UK:
http://www.nrpb.org.uk

National Academy of Sciences USA, Committee on the Biological Effects of Ionizing Radiation (BEIR):
http://www.nas.edu

Radiation Effects Research Foundation (RERF), Hiroshima, Japan:
http://www.rerf.or.jp.

WHO International EMF Project:
http://www.who.int/peh-emf/

US National Institute for Environmental Health Sciences (NIEHS) report of EMF-rapid programme, 1998:
http://www.niehs.nih.gov/emfrapid/html/EMF_DIR_RPT/staff_18f.htm

US National Research Council report: Possible Health Effects of Exposure to Residential Electric and Magnetic Fields (1997):
http://books.nap.edu/books/0309054478/html

The Stewart report: Independent Expert Group on Mobile Phones: Report on Mobile Phones and Health, 2000, UK:
http://www.iegmp.org.uk/report/index.htm

The Royal Society of Canada report, 1999:
http://www.rsc.ca/english/RFreport.pdf

CHRONIC INFECTIONS

SUMMARY

> Infectious agents are one of the main causes of cancer, accounting for 18% of cases worldwide, the majority occurring in developing countries.

> The most frequently affected organ sites are liver (hepatitis B and C, liver flukes), cervix uteri (human papillomaviruses), lymphoid tissues (Epstein-Barr virus), stomach (*Helicobacter pylori*) and the urinary system (*Schistosoma haematobium*).

> The mechanism of carcinogenicity by infectious agents may be direct, e.g. mediated by oncogenic proteins produced by the agent (e.g. human papillomavirus) or indirect, through causating of chronic inflammation with tisssue necrosis and regeneration.

> Strategies for prevention include vaccination (hepatitis B virus), early detection (cervical cancer) and eradication of the infectious agent (*Helicobacter pylori*).

Infectious agents can cause cancer

That cancer can be caused by infectious agents has been known for more than 100 years. Early in the last century, Peyton Rous demonstrated that sarcomas in chickens were caused by an infectious agent, later identified as a virus [1]. However, the identification of infectious agents linked to human cancer has been slow, in part because of difficulties in detecting indicators of exposure. Progress has accelerated since the 1980s when advances in molecular biology made possible the detection of a very small quantity of infectious agent in biological specimens. A further difficulty is the fact that relevant infectious agents tend to persist silently for many years, before causing cancer in only a small proportion of chronically infected individuals.

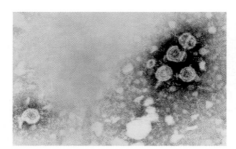

Fig. 2.41 Electron microscopy of hepatitis B virus particles.

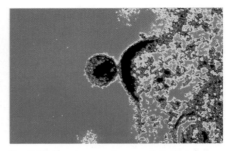

Fig. 2.42 The human immunodeficiency virus finds refuge in T-lymphocytes, as shown by the electron micrograph.

Today, experimental and epidemiological evidence indicates that a variety of infectious agents constitute one of the main causes of cancer worldwide [2]. Viruses are the principal ones, with at least eight different viruses associated with particular tumour types, with varying degrees of certainty. Other infectious agents involved in carcinogenesis are four parasites and one bacterium [3-7] (Table 2.18).

Hepatitis B and C viruses

Worldwide, about 2,000 million people have serological evidence of current or past hepatitis B virus (HBV) infection and about 350 million of them are chronic carriers of the virus. Infection can be transmitted from mother to child (vertical transmission), child to child (horizontal transmission), through sexual transmission and by contact with infected blood. Horizontal transmission is responsible for the majority of infections in the world, although the exact mechanisms of child to child transmission remain unknown. Close contact of young children is the primary risk factor and exposure to skin lesions, sharing food and utensils, tattooing and scarification procedures, and transmission by insects are some of the postulated mechanisms. The use of contaminated needles for medically-related injections may have played a role, probably via therapeutic injections rather than vaccination. Several case-control and cohort studies have clearly and consistently demonstrat-

ed that chronic carriers of HBV, identified by the presence of relevant antibodies in the sera, have around a 20 times higher risk of developing liver cancer than non-carriers [3]. It has been estimated that 60% of cases of primary liver cancer worldwide and 67% of cases in developing countries can be attributed to chronic persistent infection with HBV [2]. In many situations, exposure to aflatoxins is a related risk factor (*Food contaminants*, p43).

Hepatitis C virus (HCV) is the major cause of parenterally transmitted hepatitis worldwide. Strong associations with relative risks around 20 have been reported in several case-control studies. About 25% of cases of liver cancer in the world are attributable to HCV [3].

Human papillomavirus

Over 100 human papillomavirus (HPV) types have been identified and about 30 are known to infect the genital tract. Genital HPV types are subdivided into low-risk (e.g. 6 and 11) and high-risk or oncogenic types (e.g. 16, 18, 31 and 45) [5]. Dozens of molecular epidemiological studies [5, 8, 9] have consistently shown relative risks for invasive cervical cancer ranging from 20 to over 100. In fact, HPV DNA is found in virtually all invasive cervical cancers, indicating that HPV is a necessary cause [10] (*Cancers of the female reproductive tract*, p215). Moreover, about 80% of anal cancers and 30% of cancers of the vulva, vagina, penis

Infectious agent	IARC classification[1]	Cancer site/cancer	Number of cancer cases	% of cancer cases worldwide
H. pylori	1	Stomach	490,000	5.4
HPV	1, 2A	Cervix and other sites	550,000	6.1
HBV, HCV	1	Liver	390,000	4.3
EBV	1	Lymphomas and nasopharyngeal carcinoma	99,000	1.1
HHV-8	2A	Kaposi sarcoma	54,000	0.6
Schistosoma haematobium	1	Bladder	9,000	0.1
HTLV-1	1	Leukaemia	2,700	0.1
Liver flukes *Opisthorchis viverrini* *Clonorchis sinensis*	1 2A	Cholangiocarcinoma (biliary system)	800	
		Total infection-related cancers	1,600,000	17.7
		Total cancers in 1995	9,000,000	100

Table 2.18 The burden of cancer caused by infectious agents worldwide. [1]Group 1= carcinogenic to humans, Group 2A= probably carcinogenic to humans. [2]Applies only to cervical cancer.

and oro-pharynx can be attributed to HPV.

Epstein-Barr virus
Epstein-Barr virus (EBV) infection is ubiquitous. In developing countries, infection is acquired in childhood, while in developed countries infection is delayed until adolescence [7]. Individuals with high titres of antibodies to various early and late EBV antigens have a higher risk of developing Burkitt lymphoma and Hodgkin disease (*Lymphoma*, p237). Molecular evidence showing that EBV DNA and viral products are regularly detected (monoclonally) in cancer cells, but not in normal cells, provides a strong indication of a causal role for EBV in nasopharyngeal carcinoma and sinonasal angiocentric T-cell lymphoma. The association of EBV is associated with non-Hodgkin lymphoma mainly in patients with congenital or acquired immunodeficiency [7].

Human immunodeficiency virus
The prevalence of human immunodeficiency virus (HIV) infection is highest in sub-Saharan Africa (15-20%). High levels of infection are also seen among homosexual men, intravenous drug users and in subjects transfused with HIV-infected blood. An estimated 36 million people worldwide are currently living with HIV, and some 20 million people have died as a result of HIV-related disease [11]. HIV infection enhances the risk of Kaposi sarcoma by approximately 1,000-fold, of non-Hodgkin lymphoma by 100-fold, and of Hodgkin disease by 10-fold [6] (Box: *Tumours associated with HIV/AIDS*, p60). Increased risk of cancer of the anus, cervix and conjunctiva has also been observed. In all these cases, the role of HIV is probably as an immunosuppressive agent (*Immunosuppression*, p68) and hence indirect, the direct etiological agents being other cancer viruses (i.e. human herpesvirus 8 (HHV-8), EBV and HPV) [5-7].

Human T-cell lymphotropic virus
Human T-cell lymphotropic virus (HTLV-1) infection occurs in clusters in Japan, Africa, the Caribbean, Colombia and Melanesia [6]. As many as 20 million people worldwide may be infected with this virus. Spread of the virus is thought to occur from mother to child (mainly through breast-feeding beyond six months), via sexual transmission and as a result of transfusion of blood cell products, as well as through intravenous drug use. A strong geographical correlation suggests that HTLV-1 is the main etiological factor in adult T-cell leukaemia/lymphoma. This disease occurs almost exclusively in areas where HTLV-1 is endemic. In addition, laboratory evidence shows that the virus is clonally integrated into tumour cells. An association with tumours of the cervix, vagina and liver has been reported, but effects of confounding and bias cannot be excluded [6].

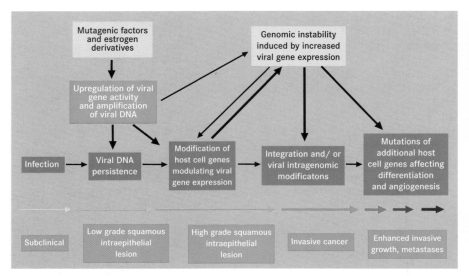

Fig. 2.43 Proposed pathogenetic mechanism by which human papillomavirus infection causes cervical cancer.

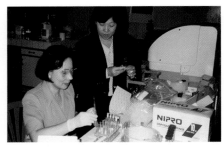

Fig. 2.44 Processing samples for HPV testing as part of a study of HPV prevalence in Thailand.

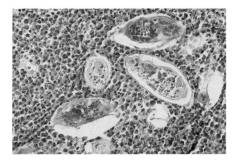

Fig. 2.45 The *Helicobacter pylori* bacterium structure as revealed by scanning electron microscopy.

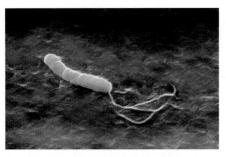

Fig. 2.46 Chronic infection of the bladder with *Schistosoma haematobium* causes an inflammatory reaction with dense eosinophilic infiltrates which may cause the development of a squamous cell carcinoma.

Human herpes virus 8

Human herpesvirus 8 (HHV-8) infection appears to be common in Africa and in some Mediterranean countries but rare elsewhere. HHV-8 DNA has been detected in over 90% of Kaposi sarcomas and rarely in control patients. Seropositivity rates are also higher in cases than controls, with relative risks over 10 in most studies. Accordingly, the evidence linking HHV-8 to Kaposi sarcoma is strong [9]. Certain lymphoproliferative diseases such as primary effusion lymphoma and Castleman disease have also been linked to HHV-8, but the evidence is very limited [7].

Helicobacter pylori

Infection with *Helicobacter pylori* is one of the most common bacterial infections worldwide. In developing countries, the prevalence of *H. pylori* among adults ranges from 80 to 90% whilst in developed areas it is around 50%. *H. pylori* is the main cause of gastritis and peptic ulcer; infection may be lifelong if not treated with antibiotics [12]. The relationship between gastric cancer and *H. pylori* has been difficult to determine due to the very high prevalence of *H. pylori* in most populations where the cancer is endemic and the very low bacterial load usually found in gastric cancer patients. It is clear that *H. pylori* plays a role in gastric cancer, but other cofactors (e.g. diet) are also contributory (*Stomach cancer*, p 194).

Parasites

Two liver flukes, *Opisthorchis viverrini* and *Clonorchis sinenesis*, have been associated with cholangiocarcinoma in parts of Asia (*Liver cancer*, p203). Infection by these flukes is acquired by eating raw or undercooked freshwater fish containing the infective stage of the fluke; the fluke matures and produces eggs in the small intrahepatic ducts [4]. The evidence for cancer causation by *O. viverrini*, a parasite mainly prevalent in Thailand, is stronger than for *C. sinensis*. The incidence of cholangiocarcinoma in areas where these liver flukes are non-endemic is very low.

Schistosomes are trematode worms. The cercarial stage infects humans by skin penetration. The worms mature and lay eggs in the bladder or intestine of the host, provoking symptoms of a disease known as bilharzia. *Schistosoma haematobium* infection is prevalent in Africa and the Middle East and has been identified as a cause of bladder cancer. *Schistosoma japonicum* infection is prevalent in Japan and China and has been associated with cancers of the liver, stomach and colorectum, but the evidence is weak and inconsistent [4].

Mechanisms of carcinogenicity

Two main pathogenic mechanisms have been invoked for infectious agents associated with cancer [13]. The first is a direct effect, when agents act directly on the cells which are ultimately transformed. HPV-induced cancer of the cervix is the best understood example of a "direct" effect in humans. The E5 oncoprotein expressed by high-risk HPV types may play a role in the early growth stimulation of infected cells, whilst oncoproteins E6 and E7 interfere with the functions of negative cellular regulators, including p53 and pRb (*Oncogenes and tumour suppressor genes*, p96). Integration of the viral genome, deregulation of oncogene expression and other cofactors may all contribute to malignant progression (Fig. 2.43).

A few other viruses are directly linked to human cancer, including EBV, HTLV-1 and HHV-8. EBV infects B lymphocytes and expression of viral protein is believed to induce what would otherwise be antigen-driven lymphocyte activation. The immortalization-associated viral proteins regulate the maintenance of the episomal viral DNA and the expression of viral genes, as well as driving cellular proliferation and blocking apoptosis. It is believed that a crucial role in the transformation and immortalization of infected cells is played by the EBNA-2 protein. Malarial infection may be a cofactor in the progression of Burkitt lymphoma. HTLV-1 is able to immortalize human T lymphocytes *in vitro*. Central to this property is the HTLV-1 Tax protein which, via interference with several classes of transcription factors, activates the expression of some cellular genes involved in the control of cellular proliferation. HHV-8 is the most recently-identified tumour-causing virus and its role in pathogenesis is still poorly understood [7, 13].

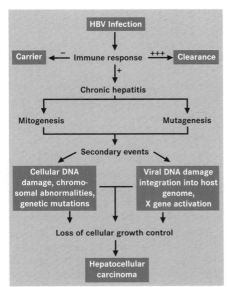

Fig. 2.49 Hepatitis B virus and the chronic injury hypothesis. A vigorous immune response to hepatitis B virus (+++) leads to viral clearance while an absent immune response (-) leads to the "healthy" carrier state and an intermediate response (+) produces chronic hepatitis which, via a multistep process, may eventually lead to hepatocellular carcinoma.

The second, or indirect, mechanism is the mode of action for some viruses (HBV, HCV, HIV), bacteria (*H. pylori*) and parasites. These agents provoke cancer by causing chronic inflammation and/or production of mutagenic compounds. The hepatitis viruses, for example, are unable to immortalize human cells *in vitro*, but infection may lead to cancer via induction of chronic liver injury and hepatitis (Fig. 2.49). Chronic hepatitis caused by an intermediate immune response to HBV infection is characterized by chronic liver cell necrosis which stimulates a sustained regenerative response. The inflammatory component includes activated macrophages which are a rich source of free radicals. The collaboration of these mitogenic and mutagenic stimuli has the potential to cause cellular and viral DNA damage, chromosomal abnormalities and genetic mutations that deregulate cellular growth control in a multistep process that eventually leads to hepatocellular carcinoma.

A prolonged process, lasting decades, precedes emergence of most gastric cancers. *H. pylori* is the most frequent cause of chronic gastritis. Gastritis and atrophy

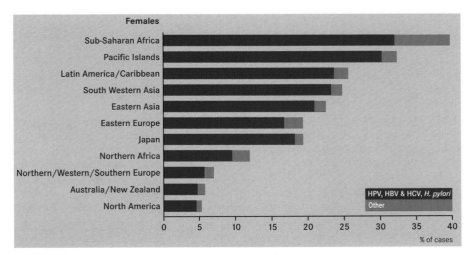

Fig. 2.47 The burden of cancer caused by infectious agents in women.

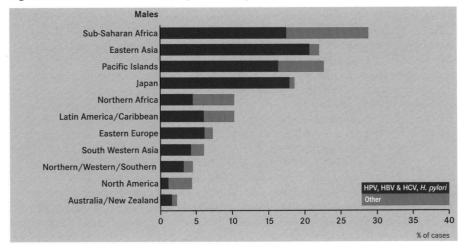

Fig. 2.48 The burden of cancer caused by infectious agents in men.

Approximately 30-40% of patients with HIV infection are likely to develop malignancies.

Kaposi sarcoma is the most common malignancy in patients with HIV infection. Since no current therapies have proven curative, both delivery of effective treatment and maintenance of adequate control of HIV and other infections remain the goals of current treatment. Several studies have shown benefits of highly active anti-retroviral treatment (HAART) on Kaposi sarcoma lesions. HAART might be a useful alternative both to immune response modifiers during less aggressive stages of this disease and to systemic cytotoxic drugs in the long term maintenance therapy of advanced Kaposi sarcoma (Tavio M et al., *Ann Oncol*, 9: 923, 1998; Tirelli U and Bernardi D, *Eur J Cancer*, 37: 1320-24, 2001). Liposomal anthracyclines are considered the standard treatment for patients with advanced stages of AIDS-related Kaposi sarcoma. Concomitant use of both HAART and haematological growth factors is needed, with the aim of reducing opportunistic infections and myelotoxicity.

Non-Hodgkin lymphoma in patients with HIV infection is about two hundred-fold more frequent than expected. One feature of AIDS-non-Hodgkin lymphoma is the widespread extent of the disease at initial presentation and the frequency of systemic B-symptoms (general symptoms such as night sweats, weight loss, temperature change). Whether intensive or conservative chemotherapy regimens are appropriate is still a matter of controversy. In fact, the poor bone marrow reserve and underlying HIV immunodeficiency make the management of systemic non-Hodgkin lymphoma very difficult. Intensive chemotherapy regimens may be given to low or intermediate risk category patients and conservative chemotherapy regimens to high or poor risk patients (Spina M et al., *Ann Oncol*, 10: 1271-1286, 1999). The prognosis of AIDS-non-Hodgkin lymphoma is very poor.

Hodgkin disease in patients with AIDS carries a relative risk much lower than that for non-Hodgkin lymphoma but the histological subtypes tend to be those with unfavourable prognosis and the response rate remains poorer than that of the general population. Outcome may be improved by an optimal combination of anti-neoplastic and HAART to improve control of the underlying HIV infection. The inclusion of growth factors may allow the use of higher doses of the drugs (Vaccher E et al., *Eur J Cancer*, 37: 1306-15, 2001)

Cervical intraepithelial neoplasia (CIN) has been increasingly diagnosed in HIV-infected women; *invasive cervical cancer* is currently an AIDS-defining condition. CIN in HIV-infected women is associated with high grade histology, more extensive and/or multifocal disease and disseminated lower genital tract HPV-related lesions (Mandelblatt JS et al., *AIDS*, 6: 173-178, 1992; Robinson W 3rd, *Semin Oncol*, 27: 463-470, 2000). Therapeutic recommendations are the same as for non-HIV-infected women, because most HIV-infected women will die from cervical cancer rather than other AIDS-related diseases.

Testicular cancer appears to be more frequent in HIV-seropositive homosexual men but the risk is not directly related to the

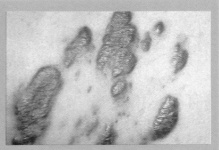

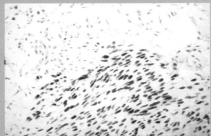

Fig. 2.51 Kaposi sarcoma of the skin in a patient with AIDS. The biopsy (below) reveals the presence of human herpes virus 8 (HHV-8) in tumour cell nuclei, demonstrated by immunohistochemistry (brown colour). Affected individuals are uniformly co-infected with HIV and HHV-8.

level of immune deficiency. Patients with HIV infection are offered the standard chemotherapy, since the majority can be cured of their tumour and have a good quality of life (Bernardi D et al., *J Clin Oncol*, 13, 2705-2711, 1995).

The spectrum of cancers in patients with HIV infection may further increase as these patients survive longer. Based on advances in current understanding of HIV viral dynamics and the availability of newer anti-retroviral therapies, continuation of HAART with prophylaxis against opportunistic infections in patients receiving chemotherapy may significantly improve treatment outcome.

---

alter gastric acid secretion, elevating gastric pH, changing the gastric flora and allowing anaerobic bacteria to colonize the stomach. These bacteria produce active reductase enzymes that transform food nitrate into nitrite, an active molecule capable of reacting with amines, amides and ureas to produce carcinogenic *N*-nitroso compounds. *H. pylori* acts as a gastric pathogen and thereby mediates a carcinogenic outcome involving soluble bacterial products and the inflammatory

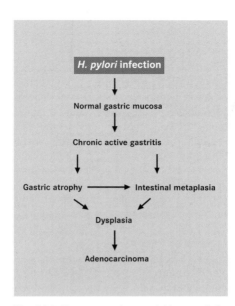

Fig. 2.50 The proposed natural history of the development of stomach cancer as a progressive process associated with atrophy and intestinal metaplasia with reduced acidity.

response generated by the infection (Fig. 2.50).

Infection by the liver fluke *O. viverrini* causes oedema, desquamation and acute inflammatory responses in the bile ducts in the early stages. Bile ducts of chronic carriers may exhibit metaplasia and adenomatous hyperplasia, which progress in some cases to cholangiocarcinoma [4]. Alternatively, such indirect agents may cause immunosuppression and the reactivation of latent oncogenic viruses. In fact, several virus-induced cancers occur almost exclusively under severe immunosuppression (*Immunosuppression*, p68) [6].

Global burden of cancer attributed to infectious agents

Recent estimates are that at least 1.6 million cases (18%) of the approximately 9 million new cases of cancer that occurred in the world in 1995 can be attributed to the infectious agents discussed (Table 2.18) [2]. The proportion of cancers attributed to infectious agents is higher in developing countries (23%) than in developed countries (9%). This proportion is greatest among women in Western, Eastern and Central Africa, where 40% of all cancers are associated with chronic infections, followed by South-American and Asian women in whom this proportion is around 25% (Fig. 2.47). A similar picture is seen among males but with lower attributable proportions (Fig. 2.48).

The realization that approximately one-quarter of all cancers occurring in the developing world can be attributed to infectious agents opens great hopes for prevention and treatment. This is particularly true for cancers of the cervix, stomach and liver (*Chapter 4*), which are very common in developing countries, where they represent 91% of the cancers associated with infectious agents.

REFERENCES

1. Rous P (1911) Transmission of malignant new growth by means of a cell-free filtrate. *J Am Med Assoc*, 56: 198.

2. Pisani P, Parkin DM, Muñoz N, Ferlay J (1997) Cancer and infection: estimates of the attributable fraction in 1990. *Cancer Epidemiol Biomarkers Prev*, 6: 387-400.

3. IARC (1994) *Hepatitis Viruses (IARC Monographs on the Evaluation of Carcinogenic Risks to Humans, Vol. 59)*, Lyon, IARCPress.

4. IARC (1994) *Schistosomes, Liver Flukes and Helicobacter Pylori (IARC Monographs on the Evaluation of Carcinogenic Risks to Humans, Vol. 61)*, Lyon, IARC

5. IARC (1995) *Human Papillomaviruses (IARC Monographs on the Evaluation of Carcinogenic Risks to Humans, Vol. 64)*, Lyon, IARCPress.

6. IARC (1996) *Human Immunodeficiency Viruses and Human T-Cell Lymphotropic Viruses (IARC Monographs on the Evaluation of Carcinogenic Risks to Humans, Vol. 67)*, Lyon, IARCPress .

7. IARC (1997) *Epstein-Barr Virus and Kaposi's Sarcoma Herpesvirus/Human Herpesvirus 8 (IARC Monographs on the Evaluation of Carcinogenic Risks to Humans, Vol. 70)*, Lyon, IARCPress.

8. Muñoz N, Bosch FX, de Sanjose S, Tafur L, Izarzugaza I, Gili M, Viladiu P, Navarro C, Martos C, Ascunce N (1992) The causal link between human papillomavirus and invasive cervical cancer: a population-based case-control study in Colombia and Spain. *Int J Cancer*, 52: 743-749.

9. Rolon PA, Smith JS, Muñoz N, Klug SJ, Herrero R, Bosch X, Llamosas F, Meijer CJ, Walboomers JM (2000) Human papillomavirus infection and invasive cervical cancer in Paraguay. *Int J Cancer*, 85: 486-491.

10. Walboomers JM, Jacobs MV, Manos MM, Bosch FX, Kummer JA, Shah KV, Snijders PJ, Peto J, Meijer CJ, Muñoz N (1999) Human papillomavirus is a necessary cause of invasive cervical cancer worldwide. *J Pathol*, 189: 12-19.

11. Piot P, Bartos M, Ghys PD, Walker N, Schwartlander B (2001) The global impact of HIV/AIDS. *Nature*, 410: 968-973.

12. Chey WD (1999) Helicobacter pylori. *Curr Treat Options Gastroenterol*, 2: 171-182.

13. zur Hausen H (1999) Viruses in human cancers. *Eur J Cancer*, 35: 1174-1181.

WEBSITES

National Center for Infectious Diseases (USA CDC): http://www.cdc.gov/ncidod/index.htm

WHO infectious disease information resources: http://www.who.int/health_topics/infectious_diseases/en

DIET AND NUTRITION

SUMMARY

> Up to 30% of human cancers are probably related to diet and nutrition.

> Excess salt intake causes arterial hypertension and an elevated risk of stomach cancer. Due to modern methods of food preservation, the incidence of stomach cancer is declining worldwide.

> A Western diet (highly caloric food rich in animal fat and protein), often combined with a sedentary lifestyle and hence energy imbalance, increases the risk of colon, breast, prostate, endometrial and other cancers.

> Physical activity, avoidance of obesity, and frequent daily intake of fresh fruit and vegetables reduce the risk of oral cavity, lung, cervix uteri and other cancers.

The incidence of most cancers varies worldwide and cancers of the breast, colorectum, prostate, endometrium, ovary and lung are generally much more frequent in the developed countries. These cancers are a major burden in countries of Europe, North America and in Australia. They are markedly less frequent in developing countries of Asia and Africa. In contrast, some cancers of the digestive system, including those of the stomach and liver, are more frequent in developing countries of Central and South America, Africa and Asia than they are in the developed world.

These observations, which were made more than 30 years ago with the publication of the first reliable data on cancer incidence from population-based cancer registries [1,2] are still substantially valid. They constitute one of the basic arguments for the hypothesis that environmental factors play an important role in cancer etiology. A principal environmental factor, now generally recognized as major

determinant of cancer incidence, is diet. Over the past 20 years, many epidemiological studies, particularly case-control studies and, more recently, large cohort studies, have investigated the role of habitual diet in relation to the risk of developing different types of cancer.

Vegetables and fruit

The most consistent finding on diet as a determinant of cancer risk is the association between consumption of vegetables and fruit and reduced risk of several cancers. Consumption of vegetables and fruit is associated with reduced risk of cancers of the pharynx, larynx, lung, oesophagus, stomach and cervix uteri, while only vegetables, but not fruit, seem to protect against cancers of the colon and rectum. During the last 30 years, over 250 epidemiological studies (case-control, cohort or ecological correlations) have been conducted around the world to investigate the relationship between fruit and vegetable consumption and cancer risk. About 80% of these

studies found a significant protective effect of overall consumption of vegetables and/or fruit, or at least of some types of vegetables and fruits [3]. Preliminary results from the large European Prospective Investigation into Cancer and Nutrition (EPIC) study confirm these results, suggesting, for example, that a daily consumption of 500 g of fruit and vegetables can decrease incidence of cancers of the digestive tract by as much as 25% [4].

Fruit and vegetables do not represent a major source of protein, fat, carbohydrates and therefore energy, but they can be major contributors of fibre, several vitamins, minerals and other biologically active compounds. Current hypotheses on mechanisms through which fruit and vegetables may protect against cancer invoke the interaction of micro-constituents with the processes of carcinogen metabolism, protection of DNA integrity and intercellular communication. Such mechanisms have been studied extensively in experimental systems.

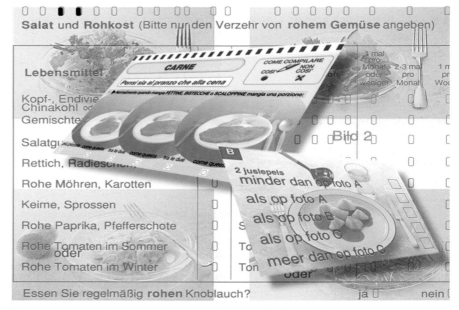

Fig. 2.52 Dietary questionnaires used to assess the quantity of different food types consumed by the participant in a nutritional study.

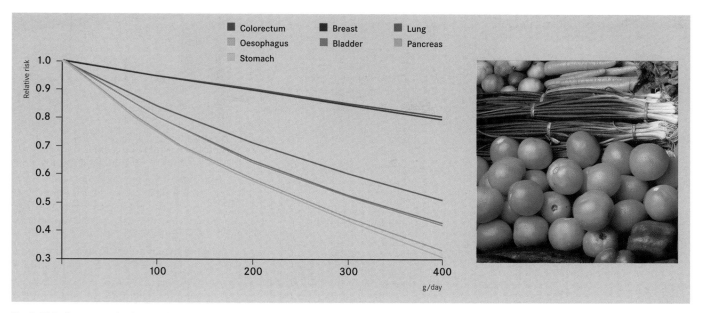

Fig. 2.53 Fruit consumption is associated with reduced risk of cancer (according to results of meta-analyses). Findings are essentially similar for vegetable consumption.

Legend: Colorectum, Oesophagus, Stomach, Breast, Bladder, Lung, Pancreas

Salt and salt-preserved foods

Consumption of salt added to food and salt-preserved foods has been investigated mainly in relation to cancers of the stomach, colorectum and nasopharynx. Several studies conducted in Europe, South America and Eastern Asia have reported increased relative risks of stomach cancer in relation to the consumption of salt and salt-preserved foods, particularly in populations with high stomach cancer incidence and high salt intake (Fig. 2.54). Salted, smoked, pickled and preserved food (rich in salt, nitrite and preformed N-nitroso compounds) are associated with increased risk of gastric cancer. Such high salt intake, together with *Helicobacter pylori* infection, may contribute to the development of atrophic gastritis, and hence gastric cancer. Domestic refrigeration and reduced salt consumption are likely to have contributed to the observed decreased stomach cancer incidence in developed countries during the 20th century [5].

Consumption of Chinese-style salted fish has been specifically associated with increased risk of nasopharyngeal cancer in South-East Asia [6], whereas European-style salted fish (e.g. anchovies and salmon) has not been found to be associated with any increase in cancer risk. Several biological mechanisms have been proposed to explain the association between Chinese-style salted fish and nasopharyngeal cancer, including partial fermentation and nitrosamine formation. The relationship of salt and salt-preserved foods with colorectal cancer seems to be of a different nature. Firstly, it has been observed particularly in Western populations and secondly, it mainly involves foods such as cooked and raw ham, various types of salami, European-style *charcuterie*, bacon and other salt-preserved pork (see next section).

Meat

Epidemiological studies on meat consumption and cancer risk support the existence of a specific association with colorectal cancer risk (Figs. 2.57, 2.58). This association, however, seems to have been found more consistently for consumption of red meat (beef, lamb and pork) and processed meat (ham, salami, bacon and other *charcuterie*) for which consumption of 80 g per day may increase colorectal cancer risk by 25 and 67%, respectively [7].

Several biological mechanisms have been investigated which could explain the possible effect of meat consumption on colorectal carcinogenesis. These include the influence of meat and/or fat consumption on the production and metabolism of bile salts and bile acids by gut flora [8]. Other hypotheses concern the potential carcinogenic effect of certain compounds that can be formed in meat during cooking, such as heterocyclic amines [9] and polycyclic aromatic hydrocarbons or as a consequence of preserved meat processing (nitrates and nitrites) or endo-intestinal metabolism (various N-nitroso compounds) (*Food contaminants*, p43).

Protein, carbohydrates and fat

The results of epidemiological studies on macro-nutrients (for example, proportion of total diet as protein) have so far been much less consistent in establishing an associated risk of cancer that those on foods. No clear risk patterns have emerged for consumption of protein. Some studies on oesophageal cancer in populations with high alcohol intake found

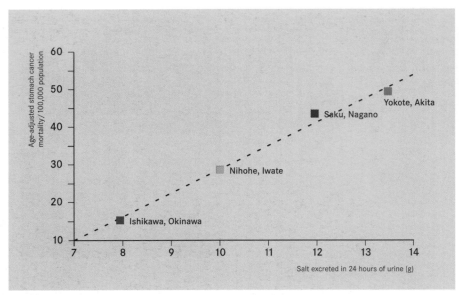

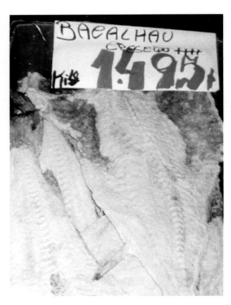

Fig. 2.54 The age-adjusted mortality rate for gastric cancer increases with increasing salt consumption, as measured by 24-hour urine sodium excretion, in selected regions of Japan.
S. Tsugane et al. (1991) *Cancer Causes Control*, 2:165-8.

Fig. 2.55 Consumption of salted fish (such as this salted cod) is associated with an increased risk of stomach cancer.

a protective effect of animal protein (and meat) while some studies on colorectal cancer found an increased risk for animal protein (and meat).

Results on carbohydrates are difficult to interpret because of inconsistencies in the way different food composition tables subdivide total carbohydrates into subfractions that have very different physiological and metabolic effects and which may affect carcinogenesis in opposite ways. The only pattern that seems to emerge so far is that consumption of simple sugars (mono- and disaccharides) may be associated with increased colorectal cancer risk, while consumption of complex polysaccharides, non-starch polysaccharides and/or fibre (partially overlapping categories based on different chemical and physiological definitions) is associated with lower cancer risk. Other less consistent findings suggest that a diet excessively rich in starchy foods (mainly beans, flour products or simple sugars) but also poor in fruit and vegetables, may be associated with increased gastric cancer risk.

The hypothesis that high fat intake is a major cancer risk factor of the Western-style diet has been at the centre of most epidemiological and laboratory experimental studies. The results are, however, far from clear and definitive. The positive association with breast cancer risk suggested by international correlation studies and supported by most case-control studies was not found in the majority of the prospective cohort studies conducted so far. Very few studies have investigated the effect of the balance between different types of fats, specifically as containing poly-unsaturated, mono-unsaturated and saturated fatty acids, on cancer risk in humans. The only moderately consistent result seems to be the positive association between consumption of fats of animal origin (except for fish) and risk of colorectal cancer. Additionally, olive oil in the context of the Mediterranean dietary tradition is associated with a reduced risk of cancer [10].

Food additives

Food additives are chemicals added to food for the purpose of preservation or to enhance flavour, texture or colour. Less than comprehensive toxicological data are available for most additives, although some have been tested for mutagenic or carcinogenic activity. In *in vitro* assay sys-

tems, some additives, such as dietary phenolics, have both mutagenic and anti-mutagenic effects [11]. In the past, some chemicals were employed as food additives before their carcinogenicity in animals was discovered, e.g. the colouring agent "butter yellow" (dimethylamino-azobenzene) and, in Japan, the preservative AF2 (2-(2-furyl)-3-(5-nitro-2-furyl) acrylamide). Saccharin and its salts have been used as sweeteners for nearly a century. Although some animal bioassays have revealed an increased incidence of urinary bladder cancer, there is inadequate evidence for carcinogenicity of saccharin in humans [12]. The proportion of

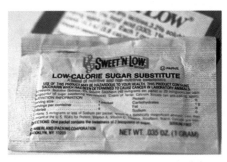

Fig. 2.56 Saccharin with a warning label recognizing a possible role in cancer causation.

dietary-related cancers considered attributable to food additives is very low [13].

Micronutrients

Research on vitamins and cancer in humans has focused mainly on carotenoids and vitamin A (retinol), vitamin E, vitamin C and some of the group of B vitamins (folic acid, B_6). The biological basis of the interest in these vitamins is their involvement in either of two metabolic mechanisms commonly called the antioxidant effect (carotenoids, vitamins C and E) and methyl donation (folic acid, B_6) (*Chemoprevention*, p151).

case-control studies based on dietary questionnaires and several small prospective cohort studies based on blood measurements have shown quite consistently that individuals with lower carotenoid levels have increased lung cancer risk. Less consistent and weaker protective effects of carotenoids have also been reported for cancers of the oesophagus, stomach, colorectum, breast and cervix. Low dietary intake of vitamin C has been found to be associated with increased risk of cancers of the stomach, mouth, pharynx, oesophagus and, less consistently, with cancers of the lung, pancreas and cervix. Although results on vitamin E and cancer are less strong and consistent than those on carotenoids and vitamin C, several

studies have suggested that low vitamin E intake is related to increased risk of cancers of the lung, cervix and colorectum.

Studies to investigate the effect of dietary supplementation with vitamins on cancer risk have had varying results (*Chemoprevention*, p151). Two large studies, ATBC and CARET [14], observed increases in lung cancer incidence of 18% and 28% respectively in the group receiving β-carotene (β-carotene plus vitamin A in CARET). In the ATBC study, the group receiving a vitamin E supplement had a 34% reduction in prostate cancer incidence, but deaths from cerebrovascular accidents doubled and there was no decrease in total mortality.

There is rising interest in the possible cancer-preventive effect of folic acid; some prospective studies have shown that high dietary intakes and higher blood levels may be associated with reduced risk of cancers and adenomatous polyps of the colorectum. Folates and vitamin B_6 are involved in the synthesis of methionine and choline as methyl donors. Folate deficiency leads to an accumulation of homocysteine. High homocysteine levels have recently been found to be strongly associated with death from myocardial infarction, total mortality and colon cancer risk [15].

Epidemiological studies conducted in populations with a high incidence of

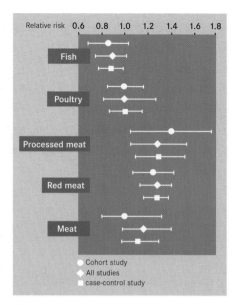

Fig. 2.57 Influence of the consumption of fish and different types of meat on the relative risk of developing colorectal cancer [7].

oesophageal cancer in China found that zinc deficiency was common in these populations. Some experimental studies also suggest that selenium deficiency may increase cancer risk [16]. Several epidemiological studies have examined the association between cancer risk and deficiencies of one of these minerals, with very variable results.

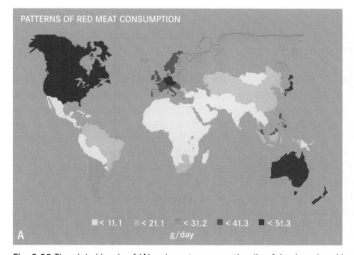

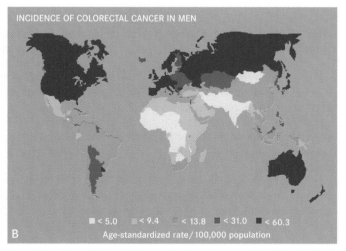

Fig. 2.58 The global levels of (A) red meat consumption (beef, lamb and pork) and its relationship to (B) the incidence of colorectal cancer. The biological basis of the correlation between these two variables is complex and not yet fully understood.

OVERWEIGHT, OBESITY AND PHYSICAL ACTIVITY

The body mass is most usefully measured as the body mass index (BMI), calculated by dividing the body weight in kilograms by the height in metres squared. The normal range is 18.5 to 25; overweight corresponds to BMI > 25 and obesity to a value greater than 30. In many developed countries, as much as half of the adult population may be overweight and more than 25% obese. Epidemiological studies have shown with varying degrees of consistency that excess body mass is associated with an increased cancer risk.

The strongest and most consistent association with body mass has so far been seen for endometrial cancer, the risk of which is increased two- to six-fold in obese compared to lean women, both before and after menopause. A possible biological explanation for this association is that adipose tissue is rich in aromatase, which converts androstenedione to estrone, thus increasing estrogenic stimulation of the endometrial mucosa. Several studies have investigated markers of fat distribution such as waist-to-hip ratio or subscapular-to-tight-skinfold ratio

in relation to endometrial cancer risk, with inconsistent results. Some studies found increased risk for markers of abdominal or android obesity (high waist-to-hip ratio or subscapular-to-tight-skinfold ratio) after adjustment for body mass index, while others did not.

The relationship between body mass index and breast cancer is even more complex. The majority of case-control and prospective studies found that high body mass index increased breast cancer risk in postmenopausal women, while it may slightly reduce risk in premenopausal women. A possible explanation for this apparent paradox is that overweight before menopause could be related to anovulatory cycles and fewer ovulatory cycles (as determined by pregnancy and lactation) are generally associated with lower breast cancer risk. After menopause, obesity may act as for endometrial cancer by enhancing the peripheral (as opposed to gonadal and adrenal) production of estrogens.

There is growing evidence that metabolic factors related to diet, nutritional status, anthropometry and physical activity have an influence on the development and clinical manifestation of various forms of can-

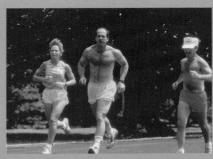

Fig. 2.59 Regular physical exercise appears to be correlated with decreased risk of cancer.

cer (*Weight Control and Physical Activity, IARC Handbooks of Cancer Prevention, Vol. 6*, 2001). Epidemiological studies suggest certain different dietary patterns may be specifically related to higher risk of particular types of cancer. The Western diet and lifestyle are generally associated with high incidence of cancers of the colorectum, breast, prostate and endometrium, but with low incidence of cancers of the stomach, oesophagus, liver and cervix uteri (see *Reproductive factors and hormones*, p76).

Caloric intake and other dietary-related factors

The results of animal experiments in which dietary restriction decreases the risk of cancer at some sites are not readily extrapolated to humans. While caloric intake can be employed as a single parameter of diet, caloric intake considered in isolation is an inadequate basis upon which to address a broad spectrum of studies concerning cancer risk. These studies indicate inter-relationships between caloric intake, body mass and physical activity. Thus it is argued that high energy intake *per se* is not a risk factor for cancer, but positive energy balance (energy balance being the difference

between caloric intake and caloric expenditure) leading to obesity is a cancer risk factor [17]. Data have accumulated suggesting that some metabolic factors related to nutritional status, such as obesity and physical activity, may also play a role by increasing the risk of certain cancers (Box: *Overweight, obesity and physical activity,* above).

Recently, several prospective studies have lent strong support to the hypothesis formulated decades ago regarding the prominent role of endogenous hormone levels in determining risk of cancer of the breast. It is also proposed that the insulin-resistance syndrome may underlie the relationship between obesity and hormone-

dependent cancers. Variations in the pattern of estrogens, androgens, insulin-like growth factor and their binding proteins are probably determined by both environmental and lifestyle factors, as well as by inherited genetic characteristics, as suggested by recent studies on polymorphisms of genes encoding for enzymes regulating steroid hormone metabolism and hormone receptors (*Reproductive factors and hormones*, p76)

Accordingly, the relationship between diet and cancer is proving to be more complex than was previously thought. Research based on a combination of laboratory investigations on human subjects and sound epidemiological projects of a prospective nature is likely to shed new light on the link between nutritionally related factors and cancer [18]. In the meantime, public health recommendations should focus on the benefits that can be expected from a diet rich in vegetables and fruit, the maintenance of a healthy weight and a physically active lifestyle.

REFERENCES

1. Doll R, Payne P, Waterhouse J, eds (1966) *Cancer Incidence in Five Continents - A Technical Report*, Berlin, Springer-Verlag.

2. Doll R, Muir C, Waterhouse J, eds (1970) *Cancer Incidence in Five Continents*, Berlin, Springer-Verlag.

3. WCRF/AICR (1997) *Food, Nutrition and the Prevention of Cancer: a Global Perspective*, World Cancer Research Fund/American Institute of Cancer Research.

4. Bueno-de-Mesquita HB, Ferrari P, Riboli E on behalf of EPIC (2002) Plant foods and the risk of colorectal cancer in Europe: preliminary findings. In Riboli E, Lambert R, Eds. *Nutrition and Lifestyle: Opportunities for Cancer Prevention (IARC Scientific Publication No. 156)*, Lyon, IARCPress.

5. Palli D (2000) Epidemiology of gastric cancer: an evaluation of available evidence. *J Gastroenterol*, 35 Suppl 12: 84-89.

6. IARC (1993) *Some Naturally Occurring Substances: Food Items and Constituents, Heterocyclic Aromatic Amines and Mycotoxins (IARC Monographs on the Evaluation of Carcinogenic Risks to Humans, Vol. 56)*, Lyon, IARCPress.

7. Norat T, Lukanova A, Ferrari P, Riboli E (2002) Meat consumption and colorectal cancer risk: dose response meta-analysis of epidemiological studies. *Int J Cancer*, 98: 241-256.

8. Reddy B, Engle A, Katsifis S, Simi B, Bartram HP, Perrino P, Mahan C (1989) Biochemical epidemiology of colon cancer: effect of types of dietary fiber on fecal mutagens, acid, and neutral sterols in healthy subjects. *Cancer Res*, 49: 4629-4635.

9. Layton DW, Bogen KT, Knize MG, Hatch FT, Johnson VM, Felton JS (1995) Cancer risk of heterocyclic amines in cooked foods: an analysis and implications for research. *Carcinogenesis*, 16: 39-52.

10. Trichopoulou A, Lagiou P, Kuper H, Trichopoulos D (2000) Cancer and Mediterranean dietary traditions. *Cancer Epidemiol Biomarkers Prev*, 9: 869-873.

11. Ferguson LR (1999) Natural and man-made mutagens and carcinogens in the human diet. *Mutat Res*, 443: 1-10.

12. IARC (1999) *Some Chemicals that Cause Tumours of the Kidney or Urinary Bladder in Rodents and Some Other Substances (IARC Monographs on the Evaluation of Carcinogenic Risks to Humans, Vol. 73)*, Lyon, IARCPress.

13. Doll R, Peto R (1981) The causes of cancer: quantitative estimates of avoidable risks of cancer in the United States today. *J Natl Cancer Inst*, 66: 1191-1308.

14. Goodman GE (2000) Prevention of lung cancer. *Crit Rev Oncol Hematol*, 33: 187-197.

15. Choi SW, Mason JB (2000) Folate and carcinogenesis: an integrated scheme. *J Nutr*, 130: 129-132.

16. Clark LC, Dalkin B, Krongrad A, Combs GF, Jr., Turnbull BW, Slate EH, Witherington R, Herlong JH, Janosko E, Carpenter D, Borosso C, Falk S, Rounder J (1998) Decreased incidence of prostate cancer with selenium supplementation: results of a double-blind cancer prevention trial. *Br J Urol*, 81: 730-734.

17. Willett WC (2001) Diet and cancer: one view at the start of the millennium. *Cancer Epidemiol Biomarkers Prev*, 10: 3-8.

18. Riboli E, Kaaks R (2000) Invited commentary: the challenge of multi-center cohort studies in the search for diet and cancer links. *Am J Epidemiol*, 151: 371-374.

WEBSITE

NCI Division of Cancer Prevention: Diet, food, nutrition: http://www.cancer.gov/prevention/lifestyle.html#diet

IMMUNOSUPPRESSION

SUMMARY

> Persistent suppression of the immune system results in an increased cancer risk.

> An increased incidence of malignant lymphomas, of which the majority contain the Epstein-Barr virus, is caused by immunosuppressive drugs used to prevent the rejection of organ transplants.

> Infectious agents that cause severe immune suppression, such as the human immunodeficiency virus (HIV), are associated with an increased incidence of several tumours, including non-Hodgkin lymphoma and Kaposi sarcoma.

Immunosuppression is a reduction in the capacity of the immune system to respond effectively to foreign antigens, and can be either transient or permanent.

Certain chemicals and drugs, ionizing radiation, and infection with particular viruses and parasites can cause immunosuppression. This phenomenon is observed in humans and in experimental animals. Immunosuppression after exposure to X-rays or other ionizing radiation is most pronounced when the entire body, rather than a limited area, is irradiated. Immunosuppression by chemicals or radiation is dose-dependent, the intensity and duration of the effect increasing with increasing dose or continuing exposure, and is generally reversible with cessation of exposure. In contrast, infection with certain pathogens, such as human immunodeficiency virus, is persistent and the immune deficiency that results is progressive, unless the infection is effectively treated.

Immunosuppression should be distinguished from various forms of immune deficiency resulting from certain genetic defects (e.g. ataxia telangiectasia, *ATM*; Wiskott-Aldrich Syndrome, *WASP*; X-linked severe combined immunodeficiency, *γc*). Persistent immunosuppression, especially when accompanied by continuing exposure to foreign antigens such as organ transplants, presents a risk for cancer, though not all tumour types arise with equal frequency. Ciclosporin and related compounds are widely used to facilitate organ transplantation by decreasing the risk of rejection. Risk is especially high for various forms of lymphoma and for certain other cancers that are associated with viral infections.

Immunosuppression mediated by drugs

Immunosuppression achieved by administration of drugs is used to treat autoimmune diseases (e.g. rheumatoid arthritis) and, usually involving the relevant drugs at much higher dosage, to maintain the functional and anatomic integrity of foreign tissues grafted to another individual. A graft from any individual except oneself or an identical twin will provoke an immune reaction against the grafted tissues, the intensity of which varies with the degree of antigenic difference between graft and host. In the absence of adequate immunosuppression, the host will destroy the graft. Whole organs (e.g. kidney, heart, liver, lung) can be transplanted with maintenance of function that may continue for a lifetime when appropriate levels of immunosuppression are maintained. The risk of cancer increases with increasing intensity and duration of immunosuppression [1].

Apart from deliberate suppression of the immune response in the context of organ transplantation, immunosuppression may arise as a side-effect of some drugs, and specifically many cytotoxic agents widely used in cancer chemotherapy. This action may contribute to the development of "second cancers", particularly in children. More generally, patients receiving cancer chemotherapy are vulnerable to infectious disease as a result of their immune system being compromised.

The suggested mechanisms of action of immunosuppressive agents [2] include:
- Interference with antigen-presentation mechanisms;
- Interference with T-cell function; inhibition of signal transduction or receptor actions (ciclosporin);

Drug or infectious agent	Cancer site/cancer
Azathioprine	Non-Hodgkin lymphoma, Kaposi sarcoma, squamous cell carcinoma of the skin, hepatobiliary cancers, mesenchymal tumours.
Cyclophosphamide	Bladder cancer
Ciclosporin	Non-Hodgkin lymphoma, Kaposi sarcoma
Human immunodeficiency virus-1 (HIV-1)	Non-Hodgkin (B-cell) lymphoma, Kaposi sarcoma (increased risk by coinfection with herpesvirus 8)
Epstein-Barr virus	Burkitt lymphoma (in conjunction with malaria infection), non-Hodgkin (B-cell) lymphoma in immunosuppressed patients, Hodgkin disease, smooth muscle tumours in immunosuppressed individuals
Human herpesvirus 8	Kaposi sarcoma
Human papillomaviruses	Cancers of cervix, vulva and anus

Table 2.19 Immunosuppressive agents associated with development of cancer.

- Interference with B-cell function;
- Interference with proliferation; clonal expansion (cyclophosphamide, methotrexate).

Organ transplant recipients receiving immunosuppressive drugs are at increased risk of non-Hodgkin lymphoma and some other cancers, especially non-melanoma skin cancer and Kaposi sarcoma (Table 2.19). Some such tumour types exemplify the manner in which immunosuppression has been otherwise linked to malignancy. Thus, a factor in the development of skin cancer is the ability of ultraviolet B radiation to suppress the immune response. Such immunomodulation may be by multiple mechanisms but generally manifests in an antigen-presenting cell defect and an altered cytokine environment in the draining lymph nodes [3]. Consistent with a role of immunosuppression in the etiology of these tumours, immunosuppression profoundly influences the prevalence of skin disorders in transplant patients: skin tumours occur with high incidence in such patients and constitute a major part of transplantation-related morbidity and mortality. On the other hand, evidence of immune system abnormalities is lacking in most patients with mature B-cell neoplasms. Nonetheless, immunosuppressed patients have a markedly increased incidence of such non-Hodgkin lymphoma [4].

More than 95% of all human beings are infected with the oncogenic herpesvirus, Epstein-Barr virus (EBV), which rarely causes clinically apparent disease except in immunocompromised individuals, including organ transplant recipients. Epstein-Barr virus-associated lymphoproliferative diseases in immunocompromised patients include a spectrum of mainly B-cell diseases that range from polyclonal lymphoproliferative diseases, which resolve when immunosuppression is halted, to highly malignant lymphomas [5]. EBV transforms lymphoid cells and the neoplastic cells can survive and proliferate to produce lymphomas very rapidly in an immunocompromised individual [6]. Because of the synergistic effects of EBV and immunosuppressive drugs in the cau-

sation of these lymphomas, both EBV and some of the drugs listed in Table 2.19 are classified in Group 1 (carcinogenic to humans) by the *IARC Monographs on the Evaluation of Carcinogenic Risks to Humans*. Cancers of the anogenital region are caused by infections with human papillomaviruses, and the incidence of such cancers is greatly increased in organ transplant recipients.

Autoimmune conditions for which immunosuppressive therapy is indicated include rheumatoid arthritis and lupus erythematosis and others. Milder therapy and, often, less potently immunosuppressive drugs (e.g. steroids such as prednisone) are generally used than for organ transplant recipients. Generally there are elevated risks for the same cancers as occur in excess in organ transplant recipients, but these risks are much lower in patients without an organ transplant. Prednisone and related immunosuppressive steroid drugs have not been shown to be carcinogenic.

Immunosuppression that will allow transplanted normal tissues to survive in a foreign host can also allow occult tumours within the transplanted tissues to survive and grow in the transplant recipient. Such transplanted cancers regress when immunosuppressive therapy is withdrawn [7].

Immunosuppression by carcinogens

As implied by the number of malignancies which emerge once the immune system is compromised, growth of tumours generally may be perceived as requiring a degree of failure by the immune response. Generally, chemical carcinogens are not characterized as immunotoxic. However, particular substances may exert some degree of immunosuppressive activity that may thus affect tumour growth in a manner comparable to that exerted by ultraviolet light in the etiology of skin cancer [2]. Thus TCDD (2,3,7,8-tetrachlorodibenzo-*para*-dioxin) is immunotoxic in primates, suggesting that humans exposed to this pollutant may be similarly affected, although no direct evidence was found to support this in a study of exposed residents living in a contaminated area in Seveso, Italy.

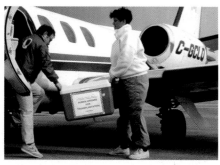

Fig. 2.60 Transport of an organ for transplantation. Immunosuppressed transplant patients exhibit an increased incidence of tumours, particularly lymphomas.

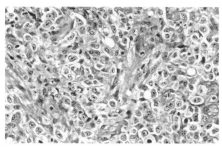

Fig. 2.61 An Epstein-Barr virus-positive, diffuse large B-cell lymphoma of soft tissue, arising in a patient with rheumatoid arthritis treated with methotrexate.

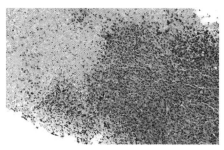

Fig. 2.62 A liver biopsy showing partial replacement of hepatocytes by diffuse large B-cell lymphoma of the immunoblastic variant, a lymphoproliferative disease which arose after organ transplant.

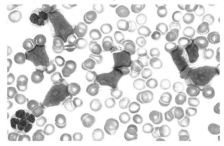

Fig. 2.63 Bone marrow smear of an acute myeloid leukaemia arising in a cancer patient treated with alkylating agents. Note the increased numbers of basophils.

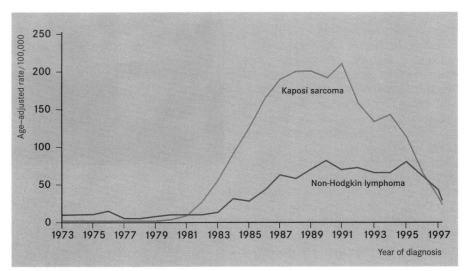

Fig. 2.64 Cancer following immunosuppression as a result of infection. The annual incidence of Kaposi sarcoma and non-Hodgkin lymphoma in San Francisco, USA, 1973-1998. Incidence increased dramatically between 1982 and 1990 as a result of the AIDS/HIV epidemic. Recent declines are partly attributable to the introduction of HAART therapy, although long-term risks remain unclear (Box: *Tumours associated with AIDS/HIV*, p60). C. Clarke (2001) *AIDS*, 15: 1913-1914

Immunosuppression caused by infectious agents

Immunosuppression as a consequence of infection is especially severe in individuals infected with human immunodeficiency virus (HIV), the cause of acquired immune deficiency syndrome (AIDS). Certain cancers are characteristic of AIDS and in fact are AIDS-defining conditions in HIV-infected individuals [8]. These include non-Hodgkin lymphoma, especially of the brain, associated with EBV co-infection, and Kaposi sarcoma, which is associated with co-infection with another oncogenic herpesvirus, human herpesvirus 8 (Box: *Tumours associated with HIV/AIDS*, p60). The incidence of such tumours is increasing, partly as a result of the AIDS epidemic (Fig. 2.64). Both EBV and HIV-1, the principal cause of AIDS, are classified as Group 1 - carcinogenic to humans - in the *IARC Monographs*.

REFERENCES

1. Kinlen LJ (1996) Immunologic factors, including AIDS. In: Schottenfeld D, Fraumeni, JF eds, *Cancer Epidemiology and Prevention*, New York, Oxford University Press, 532-545.

2. Neubert R, Neubert D (1999) Immune system. In: Marquardt H, Schafer SG, McClellan RO, Welsch F eds, *Toxicology*, San Diego, Academic Press, 371-436.

3. Hart PH, Grimbaldeston MA, Finlay-Jones JJ (2001) Sunlight, immunosuppression and skin cancer: role of histamine and mast cells. *Clin Exp Pharmacol Physiol*, 28: 1-8.

4. Penn I (2000) Cancers in renal transplant recipients. *Adv Ren Replace Ther*, 7: 147-156.

5. Mosier DE (1999) Epstein-Barr virus and lymphoproliferative disease. *Curr Opin Hematol*, 6: 25-29.

6. IARC (1997) *Epstein-Barr Virus and Kaposi's Sarcoma Herpesvirus / Human Herpesvirus 8 (IARC Monographs on the Evaluation of Carcinogenic Risks to Humans, Vol. 70)*, Lyon, IARCPress.

7. Wilson RE, Hager EB, Hampers CL, Corson JM, Merrill JP, Murray JE (1968) Immunologic rejection of human cancer transplanted with a renal allograft. *N Engl J Med*, 278: 479-483.

8. IARC (1996) *Human Immunodeficiency Viruses and Human T-Cell Lymphotropic Viruses (IARC Monographs on the Evaluation of Carcinogenic Risks to Humans, Vol. 67)*, Lyon, IARCPress.

WEBSITES

International Association of Physicians in AIDS Care: http://www.iapac.org/

The Transplantation Society: http://www.transplantation-soc.org/

The United Network for Organ Sharing: http://www.unos.org/

GENETIC SUSCEPTIBILITY

SUMMARY

> Inherited cancer syndromes, usually involving germline mutations in tumour suppressor or DNA repair genes, may account for up to 4% of all cancers.

> Inherited mutations of the *BRCA1* gene account for a small proportion of all breast cancers, but affected family members have a greater than 70% lifetime risk of developing breast or ovarian cancer.

> Identification of a germline mutation allows for preventive measures, clinical management and counselling.

> Environmental factors may modify the cancer risk of individuals affected by inherited cancer syndromes.

> Altered cancer susceptibility may be mediated by genetic variations in genes which, while not causing cancer, affect metabolism of carcinogens such as tobacco smoke.

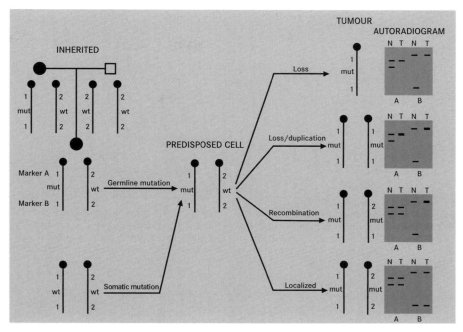

Fig. 2.65 Knudson's hypothesis, explaining the development of an inherited cancer caused by the inactivation of a suppressor gene. Tumours of the eye (retinoblastoma) in individuals who have inherited a mutation in one allele of the retinoblastoma gene on chromosome 13 ("mut" rather than the normal wild-type "wt"), almost always occur in both eyes, due to inherited susceptibility. When this tumour type occurs spontaneously in a single retinal cell ("sporadic") by a somatic mutation, only one eye is affected. The mechanisms by which the tumour arises can be determined by analysing the genotypes produced from normal ("N") and tumour ("T") tissues.

The genetic basis of cancer may be understood at two levels. Firstly, malignant cells differ from normal cells as a consequence of the altered structure and/or expression of oncogenes and tumour suppressor genes, which are found in all cancers. In this case, "the genetic basis of cancer" refers to acquired genetic differences (somatic) between normal and malignant cells due to mutation in the one individual. Secondly, the same phrase, "the genetic basis of cancer" may be used to refer to an increased risk of cancer that may be inherited from generation to generation. This section is concerned with the latter phenomenon. In many instances, the genes concerned have been identified, and have also sometimes been found to play a role in sporadic cancers as well.

Interplay between genes and environmental factors

The influence of lifestyle factors (especially smoking), occupational exposures, dietary habits and environmental exposures (such as air pollution, sun exposure or low levels of radiation) on the development of cancer is clear; such factors account for a specific fraction of cancers. Another large fraction of cancers is caused by viral and other infectious agents, this being particularly relevant to the developing world. Carcinogenic agents, as diverse as chemicals, radiation and viruses, act primarily by damaging DNA in individual cells. Such damage has broad ramifications when it involves disruption of genes which control cell proliferation, repair of further DNA damage, and ability of cells to infiltrate (invade) surrounding tissue

(*Chapter 3*). Because each of these changes is relatively rare, the chance that the necessary combination of such events occurs to allow a normal cell to progress into a fully malignant tumour is small. However, the risk to an individual over his or her lifetime can be as large as 10% for cancers of the breast or prostate (that is, in some instances, 10% of the population will suffer from one of these cancer types in their lifetime). Genetic alterations accumulate gradually either through random events and/or by the action of specific environmental carcinogens, and thus most cancers in the population occur in middle-aged and elderly individuals. Some individual cancers can be attributed to particular environmental factors. In the absence of apparent causative factors, a cancer is described as "sporadic" or "spontaneous".

Syndrome	Gene	Location	Cancer site/cancer
Familial retinoblastoma	RB1	13q14	Retinoblastoma, osteosarcoma
Multiple endocrine neoplasia II	RET	10q11	Medullary thyroid carcinoma, phaeochromocytoma
Multiple endocrine neoplasia I	MEN1	11q13	Adrenal, pancreatic islet cells
Neurofibromatosis type I	NF1	17q11	Neurofibromas, optic gliomas, phaeochromocytoma
Neurofibromatosis type II	NF2	22q2	Bilateral acoustic neuromas, meningiomas, cerebral astrocytomas
Bloom syndrome	BLM	15q26	Leukaemia, lymphoma
Familial adenomatous polyposis	APC	5q21	Colorectal, thyroid
Von Hippel-Lindau	VHL	3p25	Renal cell carcinoma, phaeochromocytoma
Familial Wilms tumour	WT1	11q	Wilms tumour (kidney)
Xeroderma pigmentosum	XP(A-D)	9q, 3p, 19q, 15p	Basal cell carcinoma, squamous cell carcinoma, melanoma (skin)
Fanconi anaemia	FAC	16q, 9q, 3p	Acute leukaemia
Li-Fraumeni syndrome	p53	17p13,	Breast and adrenocortical carcinomas, bone and soft tissue sarcomas, brain tumours, leukaemia
Cowden syndrome	PTEN	10q22	Breast, thyroid
Gorlin syndrome	PTCH	9q31	Basal cell carcinoma
X-linked proliferative disorder	XLP	Xq25	Lymphoma
Peutz-Jeghers syndrome	LKB1	19p	Breast, colon
Ataxia telangiectasia	ATM	11q22	Leukaemia, lymphoma

Table 2.20 Inherited cancer syndromes caused by a single genetic defect. The lifetime risk of cancer is high. There are usually recognizable phenotypic features that make the syndromes easy to identify clinically.

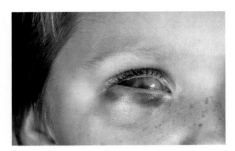

Fig. 2.66 Child with retinoblastoma, a malignant tumour of the eye, which arises from retinal germ cells. In the familial form it is caused by an autosomal dominant mutation of the retinoblastoma gene.

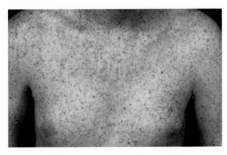

Fig. 2.67 Patient with xeroderma pigmentosum, a rare inherited (autosomal recessive) disease, exhibiting spots of hyperpigmentation in sun-exposed portions of the skin, which are prone to develop into multiple skin cancers. The disease is caused by mutations in genes involved in DNA repair.

Although most cancers arise through somatically acquired mutations (which are found uniformly only in relevant tumour cells), about 5% of all cancers can be attributed to inherited gene alterations which are common to every cell in an affected individual. Such a genetic change may be present in, and hence inherited from, one parent or may have occurred in a germ cell (egg or sperm cell) before fertilization, and may, in turn, be passed on to the next generation. These alterations, in every cell, constitute a partial commitment to cancer which may be completed either by random processes or as a result of environmental insults. This theory of why tumour development preferentially occurs in individuals with a genetic predisposition was first proposed by Alfred Knudson in 1971 in the context of a childhood eye tumour, familial retinoblastoma [1] (Figs. 2.65, 2.66). In general, inherited forms of cancer occur at an earlier age than sporadic or environmentally-caused tumours. Thus although only a relatively small fraction of all cancers are attributable to inherited mutations in cancer susceptibility genes, such "germline" alterations account for a significant fraction of cancers occurring at young ages. It is also likely that individual differences in the ability to detoxify or metabolize carcinogens (Carcinogen activation and DNA repair, p89) or regulate levels of hormones (Reproductive factors and hormones, p76) are under some degree of genetic control. Both of these forms of variation would modify the effects of environmental exposures and the consequent cancer risk.

Cancer genes

The fact that cancer can "run in families" has been recognized for over a century. Among the earliest recorded evidence for inherited susceptibility is a description by a Parisian physician, Paul Broca, of a family with many cases of early onset breast cancer, liver cancer or other tumours [2]. Such families have proven to be key resources in establishing the inheritance of disease from generation to generation. By analysing DNA extracted from a blood or tumour sample from members of these families, the inheritance of cancer susceptibility within a family can be tracked to determine whether the disease is transmitted from parent to child together with a "genetic marker", that is, a gene sequence which may not have any clinical significance but which is highly variable between individuals. If this is the case, and if this is also true for a sufficient number of other families, the approximate location of the gene causing the disease can be determined. From there, it is a matter of using more molecular-based strategies to home in on and identify the specific gene involved and localize the predisposing gene to a small region within the overall human genome. This allows the identification of the specific genes involved and of the alterations in those genes predisposing an individual to cancer [3].

Specific genes involved in susceptibility to many forms of cancer, both rare tumours such as retinoblastoma, and more common cancers such as breast and colon, have been identified and are designated as "tumour suppressor genes" or "oncogenes" (*Oncogenes and tumour suppressor genes*, p96). For other forms of inherited cancer, only the chromosomal location of a putative susceptibility gene is known; the specific gene involved has not yet been identified. Many of the early successes involved identifying the genetic defects, and subsequently the genes responsible for specific cancer-associated syndromes such as neurofibromatosis, familial adenomatous polyposis and Li-Fraumeni syndrome. Neurofibromatosis types are respectively associated with *NF1* and *NF2* genes: neurofibromatosis type 1 suffer from particular skin pigmentation and risk

Gene	Location	Associated tumours
BRCA1	17q	Breast, ovary, colon, prostate
BRCA2	13q	Breast, ovary, pancreas, prostate
p16 INK4A	9p	Melanoma, pancreas
CDK4	6q	Melanoma, other tumours (rarely)
hMLH1	3p	Colorectal, endometrial, ovarian cancer
hMSH2	2p	Colorectal, endometrial, ovarian cancer
hMSH6	2p	Colorectal, endometrial, ovarian cancer
PMS1	2q	Colorectal cancer, other tumours (rarely)
PMS2	7p	Colorectal cancer, other tumours (rarely)
HPC2	17p	Prostate (rarely)

Table 2.21 High-risk susceptibility genes and their chromosomal location. Inherited mutations in these genes are associated with some common cancers.

of phaeochromocytoma, neurofibroma, gliomas and other tumours, while type 2 patients develop schwannomas and some other brain tumours [4]. Individuals afflicted with adenomatous polyposis, which is attributable to alterations in the *APC* gene, suffer from multiple premalignant lesions in the colon [5] (*Multistage carcinogenesis*, p84). In some, but not all such instances, the genes in question are also involved in sporadic cancers. Although the functions of these genes are not completely characterized, many appear to be involved either in key cellular processes such as control of the cell cycle, programmed cell death, or in repair and/or detection of DNA damage. In the rarer inherited cancer syndromes for which lifetime risks are very high, usually there are recognizable phenotypic features which make the syndrome easy to identify clinically, and a single genetic defect accounts for the majority of occurrences (Table 2.20). Other genes are associated with more common cancers, where there is a predominant type of cancer without other distinguishing clinical characteristics (Table 2.21). For some such genes, the actual genetic defect is not known but convincing evidence for a chromosomal localization has been reported. It should be noted that such distinction between the rarer inherited cancer syndromes and more common cancers is sometimes arbitrary.

Prevalence, risks and impact of inherited cancer

The lifetime risks of cancer due to mutations in cancer predisposition genes can be very high; a woman who carries a mutated *BRCA1* gene has a lifetime risk of approximately 70% of developing either breast or ovarian cancer, compared with women lacking such mutations [6]. For some of the rare syndromes, risks of cancer can be even higher. Nonetheless, mutations in cancer predisposition genes are relatively unusual, ranging from 1/100,000 for very rare diseases such as Cowden syndrome, to 1/10,000 for germline *p53* gene mutations involved in Li-Fraumeni syndrome to 1/1,000 for genes like *BRCA1* and *MLH1* (involved in DNA mismatch repair). However, in some populations which have arisen from a relatively small number of founders, expanded rapidly and remained genetically isolated, these genes can achieve higher frequencies and therefore account for a larger fraction of cancers. For example, in the Jewish population, two specific mutations (one in *BRCA1*, one in *BRCA2*) are present. One in a hundred Jewish individuals carry one of these two mutations and they may account for as much as 40% of all ovarian cancer cases and 20% of all breast cancer cases diagnosed under age 40 in this population. Identification of genetically susceptible individuals, confirmation of a gene defect and provision of appropriate clinical care has led to development of specialist familial cancer clinics within comprehensive cancer care centres. Families now regularly seen in such clinics include those with inherited cancer due to the relatively common *BRCA1* gene alterations (Figs. 2.68, 2.69) and those which have the syndrome of multiple endocrine neoplasia type II (MEN2) [7]. As genetic testing for mutations in cancer susceptibility genes becomes more widespread, especially with regard to common, later-onset types of cancer, there are an increasing number of ethical, legal, and social issues to consider [8] (Box: *Ethics in cancer*, p322). Much of the discussion centres on issues regarding genetic discrimination, that is, the denial of health or life insurance or a job, based on a person's genetically-determined risk of developing a serious disease.

Even for cancers where direct gene testing is available, there are some difficulties in interpreting the results. While in many cases the sequence variants are clearly deleterious, since they can lead, for exam-

ple, to truncated or absent protein products, other variants which simply change one amino acid in a complex protein cannot be clearly associated with increased risk. When no defect in a particular cancer gene is found in a member of a high-risk family in which the inherited defect has not been identified, the risk of cancer may still be high due to an undiscovered mutation in the same or another gene. In contrast, if the gene defect responsible for the cancer in an affected family has been identified, any member of that family who is found not to carry this defect will simply face the overall population risk of the cancer, which, for example, may be very low for retinoblastoma but as high as 1 in 11 for breast cancer [9]. Even when an individual is identified to carry a known deleterious mutation with a high lifetime cancer risk, intervention strategies may be limited. The psychological and social consequences of genetic testing for later-onset diseases, including breast and colon cancer are under investigation. Family members found to carry a predisposing mutation may suffer from increased

anxiety and depression from this knowledge, and parents may experience guilt in having transmitted the mutation to their children. Even individuals who are found not to carry the mutation otherwise present in their families sometimes suffer from adverse psychological effects arising from having been spared the misfortune.

Gene-environment interactions

Some recent information indicates that some environmental factors may pose a particular hazard to individuals who have inherited a very high risk of cancer. For example, risk of breast cancer in women who have *BRCA1* mutations is influenced by certain environmental factors, indicating that such tumours are subject to hormonal influence, as are sporadic breast cancers [10,11].

The role of genes known to confer high cancer risks cannot explain all the familial risk for the relevant cancers and it is likely that there are other loci which are involved but which individually do not give rise to detectable familial clustering. These loci will be difficult, if not impossible to detect using traditional

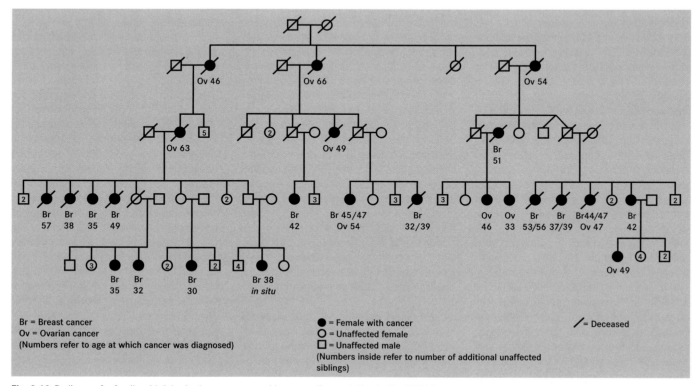

Br = Breast cancer
Ov = Ovarian cancer
(Numbers refer to age at which cancer was diagnosed)

● = Female with cancer
○ = Unaffected female
□ = Unaffected male
(Numbers inside refer to number of additional unaffected siblings)

╱ = Deceased

Fig. 2.68 Pedigree of a family with inherited cancers caused by a germline mutation in the *BRCA1* gene.

linkage studies in high-risk families. More likely, these loci, which may be associated with a two or three-fold increased risk of cancer (or even less), are more amenable to examination using either population-based or family-based case-control studies. One alternative approach is to focus on the fact that for any given environmental exposure, individual differences in susceptibility may have a genetic basis. Knowledge of the specific genetic polymorphism conferring this susceptibility should provide more power for the detection and characterization of the environmental risk factors through stratification of the sample according to the underlying genetic make-up. Likewise, there may be environmental factors that are associated with cancer (e.g. smoking and bladder cancer) in all individuals, but with a much stronger effect in individuals who have a reduced capacity to metabolize the relevant carcinogens (e.g. *N*-acetyltransferase-2, *NAT2* slow acetylators [7] or glutathione *S*-transferase, *GSTM1*-null individuals [12]). Two cytochrome P450 enzymes, CYP2D6 and CYP2A6, are associated with nicotine

metabolism [13,14]. Persons with a genetic deficiency in these enzymes smoke fewer cigarettes and can quit smoking more easily compared to individuals with normal activity of these enzymes. Drugs that inhibit the activity of these enzymes reduce a smoker's urge for cigarettes [15].

Genes relevant in this regard may be associated with a particular cancer or may be associated with basic cellular or physiological processes and include:
- genes coding for enzymes involved in the metabolism and detoxification of carcinogens including the cytochrome P450[16] and glutathione *S*-transferase (GST) [17] families;
- genes involved in the repair of DNA damage;
- genes related to cell growth and differentiation or steroid hormone pathways;
- known high-risk genes, such as *p16* [INK4A], *BRCA1* or *hMLHI*.

It is hoped that a more unified approach to cancer epidemiology and genetics will identify those combinations of genetic susceptibility and environmental exposures that lead to significant increases in risk at the individual

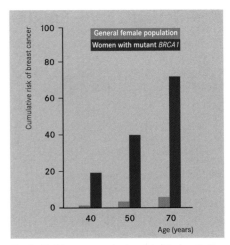

Fig. 2.69 Women carrying an inherited mutation in the *BRCA1* gene have a greatly increased risk of developing breast cancer.

and population level. This in turn could lead to reduction of the cancer burden by lifestyle modification and avoidance of specific exposures in genetically susceptible individuals.

REFERENCES

1. Knudson AG, Jr. (1971) Mutation and cancer: statistical study of retinoblastoma. *Proc Natl Acad Sci USA*, 68: 820-823.

2. Steel M, Thompson A, Clayton J (1991), Genetic aspects of breast cancer. *Br Med Bull*, 47: 504-518.

3. Russo A, Zanna I, Tubiolo C, Migliavacca M, Bazan V, Latteri MA, Tomasino RM, Gebbia N (2000) Hereditary common cancers: molecular and clinical genetics. *Anticancer Res*, 20: 4841-4851.

4. Gutmann DH (2001) The neurofibromatoses: when less is more. *Hum Mol Genet*, 10: 747-755.

5. Fearnhead NS, Britton MP, Bodmer WF (2001) The ABC of APC. *Hum Mol Genet*, 10: 721-733.

6. Eeles RA (1999) Screening for hereditary cancer and genetic testing, epitomized by breast cancer. *Eur J Cancer*, 35: 1954-1962.

7. Learoyd DL, Delbridge LW, Robinson BG (2000) Multiple endocrine neoplasia. *Aust N Z J Med*, 30: 675-682.

8. Evans JP, Skrzynia C, Burke W (2001) The complexities of predictive genetic testing. *BMJ*, 322: 1052-1056.

9. Nathanson KN, Wooster R, Weber BL (2001) Breast cancer genetics: what we know and what we need. *Nat Med*, 7: 552-556.

10. Rebbeck TR, Wang Y, Kantoff PW, Krithivas K, Neuhausen SL, Godwin AK, Daly MB, Narod SA, Brunet JS, Vesprini D, Garber JE, Lynch HT, Weber BL, Brown M (2001) Modification of BRCA1- and BRCA2-associated breast cancer risk by AIB1 genotype and reproductive history. *Cancer Res*, 61: 5420-5424.

11. King MC, Wieand S, Hale K, Lee M, Walsh T, Owens K, Tait J, Ford L, Dunn BK, Costantino J, Wickerham L, Wolmark N, Fisher B (2001) Tamoxifen and breast cancer incidence among women with inherited mutations in BRCA1 and BRCA2: National Surgical Adjuvant Breast and Bowel Project (NSABP-P1) Breast Cancer Prevention Trial. *JAMA*, 286: 2251-2256.

12. Brockton N, Little J, Sharp L, Cotton SC (2000) N-acetyltransferase polymorphisms and colorectal cancer: a HuGE review. *Am J Epidemiol*, 151: 846-861.

13. Nakajima M, Yamagishi S, Yamamoto H, Yamamoto T, Kuroiwa Y, Yokoi T (2000) Deficient cotinine formation from nicotine is attributed to the whole deletion of the CYP2A6 gene in humans. *Clin Pharmacol Ther*, 67: 57-69.

14. Bartsch H, Nair U, Risch A, Rojas M, Wikman H, Alexandrov K (2000) Genetic polymorphism of CYP genes, alone or in combination, as a risk modifier of tobacco-related cancers. *Cancer Epidemiol Biomarkers Prev*, 9: 3-28.

15. Sellers EM, Kaplan HL, Tyndale RF (2000) Inhibition of cytochrome P450 2A6 increases nicotine's oral bioavailability and decreases smoking. *Clin Pharmacol Ther*, 68: 35-43.

16. Ingelman-Sundberg M (2001) Genetic susceptibility to adverse effects of drugs and environmental toxicants. The role of the CYP family of enzymes. *Mutat Res*, 482: 11-19.

17. Strange RC, Spiteri MA, Ramachandran S, Fryer AA (2001) Glutathione-S-transferase family of enzymes. *Mutat Res*, 482: 21-26.

WEBSITES

UICC Familial Cancer and Prevention Project:
http://www.uicc.org/programmes/epid/familial.shtml

GeneClinics, a clinical information resource:
http://www.geneclinics.org/

REPRODUCTIVE FACTORS AND HORMONES

SUMMARY

> Female sex steroid hormone metabolism, reproductive factors and menopausal status affect the development of endometrial, ovarian and breast cancer.

> Use of combined oral contraceptives accounts for a slight increase in risk of breast cancer, but is protective against ovarian and endometrial cancers.

> Hormone replacement therapy isassociated with increases in risk of breast and endometrial cancers, but may relieve other health problems associated with menopause.

> Energy imbalance due to a Western lifestyle causes increased serum levels of insulin-like growth factor I (IGF-I) which is predictive of an elevated risk for prostate cancer.

There is overwhelming evidence that sex steroids (androgens, estrogens, progestogens) can have an important role in the development of human tumours, especially of the female reproductive organs (endometrium, ovary) and breast.

Cancers of the breast, endometrium and ovary

For breast cancer, incidence rates rise more steeply with age before menopause than after, when ovarian synthesis of estrogens and progesterone ceases and ovarian androgen production gradually diminishes. Furthermore, breast cancer risk is increased in women who have early menarche, or who have late menopause, whereas an early age at first full-term pregnancy and high parity are associated with reduced risk of the three forms of cancer [1]. The rise in incidence rates of endometrial cancer also appears to flatten off at older age, but this change is related

less markedly to the menopausal transition than is the case with breast cancer. Ovarian cancer risk does not show strong relationships with menstrual history, but is clearly and inversely related to parity [2]. Obesity (related to various alterations in plasma levels of total and bioavailable sex steroids) is a strong risk factor for endometrial cancer, as well as for breast cancer in postmenopausal women. Circulating levels of sex steroids are regulated by a range of factors, including insulin and insulin-like growth factors (IGFs), which thus provide a possible link between many observations regarding excessive energy intake and increased risk of cancer (Box: *IGF-1 and cancer*, p79). Together, these observations suggest that alterations in endogenous sex steroid metabolism, and notably the ovarian synthesis of sex steroids, can be an important determinant of risk for each of the three forms of cancer in women.

Breast cancer risk is increased in postmenopausal women with a hyperandrogenic (excess of androgens) plasma hormone profile, characterized by increased plasma levels of testosterone and Δ-4 androstenedione, reduced levels of sex hormone-binding globulin and increased levels of total estradiol, and bioavailable estradiol not bound to sex hormone-binding globulin [e.g. 3-5]. Similarly, postmenopausal women are at increased risk from endometrial cancer. The situation for breast cancer in premenopausal women is less clear [6,7].

Oral contraceptives

Oral contraceptives, in the form of estrogen-progestogen combinations, were introduced in the early 1960s, and rapidly found very widespread use in most developed countries. Over 200 million women are estimated to have used oral contraceptives since their introduction and about 60 million women are currently using them [8].

Preparations of oral contraceptives have undergone substantial changes over time,

including reductions in the potency and dosage of the estrogens, addition of different progestogens (progesterone analogues), and introduction (in 1983) of biphasic and triphasic pills that vary in the amounts of estrogen and progestogen throughout the month. A progestogen-only pill ("minipill") was first marketed in the USA in 1973, but has never been used widely. Sequential pills, with two weeks of estrogen alone followed by a combination of estrogen and progestogen for five days, were removed from the consumer market in the 1970s after concern about a possible association with endometrial cancer.

There is a small increase in the risk of breast cancer in current and recent users of combined oral contraceptives containing both estrogen and progestogen [8]. This association, however, is unrelated to duration of use or type and dose of preparation and, 10 years after cessation of use, is no longer present (Fig. 2.71). The association of breast cancer with oral contraceptive use may be a result of detection bias, due to increased attention to the occurrence of breast tumours in women regularly visiting a physician for contraceptive prescriptions.

Risk of endometrial cancer is approximately halved in women using combination-type oral contraceptives, the reduction in risk being stronger the longer the contraceptives are used [8]. The reduction in risk persists for at least ten years

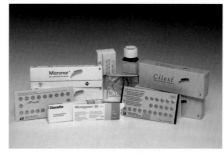

Fig. 2.70 Varieties of oral contraceptives. Use of the contraceptive pill reduces the risk of cancers of the ovary and endometrium, but is associated with a slightly increased risk of breast cancer.

after cessation of use. Interestingly, however, use of sequential oral contraceptives, containing progestogens only in the first five days of a cycle, is associated with an increased risk of endometrial cancer. For ovarian cancer, risk is reduced in women using combined oral contraceptives, the reduction being about 50% for women who have used the preparations for at least five years (Table 2.22). Again, this reduction in risk persists for at least 10-15 years after cessation of use. It has also been suggested that long-term use of oral contraceptives (more than five years) could be a cofactor that increases risk of cervical carcinoma in women who are infected with human papillomavirus [9].

Postmenopausal hormone replacement therapy
Clinical use of estrogen to treat the symptoms of menopause (estrogen replacement therapy or hormone replacement therapy) began in the 1930s, and became widespread in the 1960s. Nowadays, up to 35% of menopausal women in the USA and many European countries have used replacement therapy at least for some period. The doses of oral estrogen prescribed decreased over the period 1975-83 and the use of injectable estrogens for estrogen replacement therapy has also diminished. On the other hand, the use of transdermally administered estrogens has increased progressively to about 15% of all estrogen replacement therapy prescriptions in some countries. In the 1960s, some clinicians, especially in Europe, started prescribing combined estrogen-progestogen therapy, primarily for better control of uterine bleeding. The tendency to prescribe combined estrogen-progestogen hormonal replacement therapy was strengthened when first epidemiological studies showed an increase in endometrial cancer risk in women using estrogens alone.

A small increase in breast cancer risk is correlated with longer duration of estrogen replacement therapy use (five years or more) in current and recent users [8]. The increase seems to cease several years after use has stopped. There appears to be no material difference in breast cancer risk between long-term users of all hor-

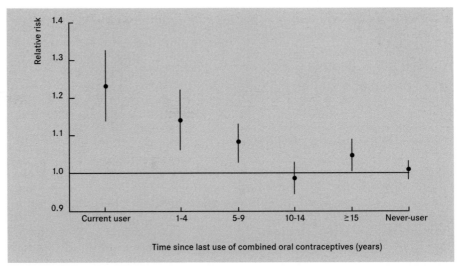

Fig. 2.71 Estimated risk of breast cancer by time since last use of combined oral contraceptives, relative to never-users. Data adjusted by age at diagnosis, parity, age at first birth and age at which risk of conception ceased. Vertical bars indicate 95% confidence interval.

mone replacement therapy and users of estrogens alone. Nevertheless, one large cohort study and a large case-control study have provided strong evidence for a greater increase in breast cancer risk in women using hormone replacement therapy than in women using estrogens alone [10,11].

For endometrial cancer, there is an increase in risk among women using estrogen replacement therapy, the risk increasing further with longer duration of use [8]. In contrast, women using hormone replacement therapy have only a mild increase in risk compared to women who have never used any postmenopausal hormone replacement and this increase is much smaller than that of women who used estrogens alone. There seems to be no relationship between risk of ovarian cancer and postmenopausal estrogen use, while data on ovarian cancer risk in relation to hormone replacement therapy use are too scarce to evaluate.

Prostate cancer
Normal growth and functioning of prostatic tissue is under the control of testosterone through conversion to dihydroxytestosterone [12]. Dihydroxytestosterone is bound to the androgen receptor, which

translocates the hormone to the nucleus. There have been conflicting findings as to whether patients with prostate cancer have higher levels of serum testosterone than disease-free controls. Diminution of testosterone production, either through estrogen administration, orchidectomy or treatment with luteinizing hormone-releasing hormone agonists, is used to manage disseminated prostate cancer.

Mechanisms of tumorigenesis
Breast cancer
The role of endogenous hormones in breast cancer development suggests the "estrogen excess" hypothesis, which stipulates that risk depends directly on breast tissue exposure to estrogens. Estrogens increase breast cell proliferation and inhibit apoptosis *in vitro*, and in experimental animals cause increased rates of tumour development when estrogens are administered. Furthermore, this theory is consistent with epidemiological studies [4,15] showing an increase in breast cancer risk in postmenopausal women who have low circulating sex hormone-binding globulin and elevated total and bioavailable estradiol.

The "estrogen-plus-progestogen" hypothesis [15,16] postulates that, compared

PHYTO-ESTROGENS AND CANCER PEVENTION

Plant foods contain phyto-estrogens, lignans and isoflavones, which are structurally similar to the mammalian estrogen, estradiol-17β. The significance of the structural similarity of the lignans and isoflavones to mammalian estrogens and possible cancer preventive effects were first promulgated in the early 1980s (Setchell KDR et al., *Am J Clin Nutr*, 40, 569, 1984; Adlercreutz H, *Gastroenterology*, 86, 761-6, 1984). The isoflavones are diphenols and include daidzein, equol and genistein, all of which have been shown to bind to α- and especially β-estrogen receptors (Kuiper GG et al., *Endocrinology*, 138, 863-870, 1997). In common with many other weak estrogens, the isoflavones have been shown to be anti-estrogens, competing for estradiol at the receptor complex, yet failing to stimulate a full estrogenic response after binding to the nucleus. In animal models, inclusion of soy in the feed, a rich source, reduces mammary tumorigenicity. The lignans enterolactone and enterodiol are derived from microbial fermentation of secoisolariciresinol and matairesinol in foods, and excreted in urine. These have

also been shown to be weakly estrogenic and anti-estrogenic, and supplements have been shown to reduce tumorigenesis in a rodent model of breast cancer. However, proliferative effects of phytoestrogens on the human breast have also been suggested (reviewed in Bingham SA et al., *Br J Nutr*, 79, 393-406, 1998).

The cancers most closely linked to plant estrogens are the hormone-related carcinomas of breast and prostate, which appear to be less common in soy-consuming populations. However, in the most recent and largest prospective study of 34,759 women in Hiroshima and Nagasaki, there was no association between breast cancer risk and soya foods (Key TJ et al., *Br J Cancer*, 81, 1248-1256, 1999). Some recent epidemiological studies include biomarkers of intake, e.g. urine excretion of plant estrogens. One recent case-control study showed that tumour patients excreted significantly less equol and enterolactone in 72 hour urine collections than matched controls, but genistein was not measured (Ingram D et al., *Lancet*, 350, 990-992, 1997). A second study showed that overnight urine total isoflavonoid excretion, especially of glycetein, was significantly lower in cancer cases compared

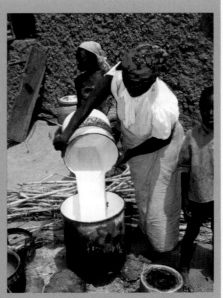

Fig. 2.72 A Nigerian woman boiling milk from strained soya beans to make soy curd. This is becoming a substitute for a cheese traditionally made from more expensive cows' milk.

with controls (Zheng W et al., *Cancer Epidemiol Biomarkers Prev*, 8 35-40, 1999). Messina MJ et al. (*Nutr Cancer* 21, 113-131, 1994) reviewed the evidence relating to the impact of soy on cancers at sites other than the breast.

---

to an exposure to estrogens alone (as in postmenopausal women not using any exogenous hormones), risk of breast cancer is increased further in women who have elevated plasma and tissue levels of estrogens in combination with progestogens. This theory is supported by observations that postmenopausal women using estrogen-plus-progestogen preparations for hormone replacement therapy have a greater increase in breast cancer risk than women using estrogens alone [10,11]. In premenopausal women, the estrogen-plus-progestogen theory may explain why obesity is associated with a mild reduction in breast cancer risk [16], because obesity may cause chronic anovulation and decreases in luteal-phase progesterone levels.

Endometrial cancer
Most observations relating endometrial cancer risk to endogenous and exogenous sex steroids, as well as to other risk factors (obesity, ovarian hyperandrogenism syndromes; see below) are explicable by the "unopposed estrogen" hypothesis [13,14]. This stipulates that risk is increased among women who have high plasma levels of bioavailable estrogens and low plasma progesterone, so that the effect of estrogens is insufficiently counterbalanced by that of progesterone. The hypothesis is supported by observations that proliferation of endometrial cells, a necessary condition for cells to accumulate genetic mutations and to expand clonally with selective growth advantage, occurs at greater rates during the follicu-

lar phase of the menstrual cycle (when the ovary produces estrogens but very little progesterone), than during the luteal phase (when the ovaries produce both estrogens and progesterone). Furthermore, there are frequent case reports of ovarian hyperandrogenism (polycystic ovary syndrome) in women developing endometrial cancer before the age of 40 and other studies showing an increased risk of endometrial cancer in polycystic ovary syndrome patients [13]. Polycystic ovary syndrome is a relatively frequent endocrine disorder, with an estimated prevalence of 4-8%, and in premenopausal women is associated with frequent anovulatory menstrual cycles and hence with impaired luteal-phase progesterone synthesis. Finally, the theory explains why

IGF-1 AND CANCER

Insulin-like growth factors (IGFs) are a family of peptide hormones which have been found to reflect excess energy intake associated with the Western lifestyle and an increased risk of several hormonally-responsive tumours.

IGFs have direct effects on tumour development. IGF-1 has been found to be involved in the stimulation of cell proliferation and differentiation and suppression of apoptosis in organs such as the breast, prostate gland, colon and lung (Yu H et al., *J Natl Cancer Inst*, 92: 1472-1489, 2000). IGFs are overexpressed in certain cancers, and cancer cells with a strong tendency to metastasize have higher expression of IGFs. Many molecules known to be involved in cancer interact with IGFs, for example, the tumour suppressor p53, and the products of the *WT1* and *PTEN* genes, and also tumour viruses, e.g. HBV. Estrogens increase the cell-proliferative effects of IGF-1, induce IGF-1 expression and promote production of the IGF-1 receptor in breast cancer cells. Conversely, IGF-1 can strongly stimulate expression of the estrogen receptor in estrogen-receptor positive breast cancer cell lines (Yee D et al., *J Mammary Gland Biol Neoplasia*, 5: 107-15, 2000).

Blood and tissue concentrations of insulin, IGF-1 and IGF-binding proteins are intimately linked to energy balance and nutritional status (Kaaks R et al., *Proc Nutr Soc*, 60: 91-106, 2001). The primary factor influencing production of IGFs is growth hormone, whilst insulin appears to regulate levels according to nutritional conditions. Circulating IGFs in the blood are mainly bound to IGF-binding proteins (IGFBPs), in particular IGFBP-3, and are subject to elaborate systems of regulation. The bioactivity of IGF-1 is increased by insulin, which both promotes its synthesis and decreases production of certain IGF-binding proteins. Prolonged fasting or insulin-dependent diabetes mellitus (low plasma insulin levels) decrease the synthesis of IGF-1, whereas obesity and non-insulin dependent diabetes mellitus (high insulin levels) are characterized by reduced levels of IGFBPs-1 and -2, and increased levels of IGF-1. Brief periods of physical exercise in adults appear to increase levels of IGF-1 and IGFBP-1, although activities such as marathon running can decrease levels of IGF-1 for several days. IGF-1 and insulin are also directly involved in the regulation of circulating levels of sex steroids. This is achieved by the inhibition of synthesis of sex hormone-binding globulin, as well as stimulation of the production of sex steroids, especially androgens.

The role of IGFs may thus help to explain associations between energy imbalance and cancer risk discovered in epidemiological studies. Some cancers, including those of the endometrium and colon, have been linked to a history of type 2 diabetes, characterized by insulin resistance and chronic hyperinsulinaemia (excessive blood levels of insulin). Increased risk of several cancers, including those of the breast, prostate, endometrium and colon, is associated with excessive energy intake relative to expenditure (as a result of low physical activity or a diet rich in fats and carbohydrates.

Studies to date suggest a link between raised levels of IGF-1 and increased risk of breast, colon, prostate and lung cancers and childhood leukaemia, and a decreased risk associated with high levels of another IGF binding protein, IGFBP-3 (Yu H et al., *J Natl Cancer Inst*, 92: 1472-1489, 2000).

Further research is necessary to determine the influences of lifestyle factors on IGF levels and how these interact with genetic susceptibility. Such information could be used in the development and targeting of intervention programmes to prevent and control cancer.

---

endometrial cancer risk is increased in women taking high-estrogen/low-progestogen oral contraceptives or estrogen replacement medication without progestogens, whereas combination-type oral contraceptives containing estrogens plus progestogens protect against endometrial cancer, and hormonal replacement therapy with estrogens plus progestogens causes only a weak increase risk.

Ovarian cancer
Ovarian cancer may develop in two stages. In the first stage, ovarian surface epithelium is entrapped into the stroma in the form of inclusion cysts, that are believed to form as a result of repeated damage and remodelling of the ovarian epithelial surface induced by regular ovulations [16]. In the second stage, the inclusion cysts gradually transform to tumour cells, under the influence of hormonal factors. One hormonal factor strongly implicated is excessive stimulation by luteinizing hormone [2] which may act either directly, through the activation of luteinizing hormone-responsive genes, or indirectly, through over-stimulation of ovarian production of androgens. There is at least one study showing an increased ovarian cancer risk in women with poly-cystic ovary syndrome, who generally have increased pituitary luteinizing hormone secretion. Oral contraceptive use, pregnancies and lactation all cause a suppression of pituitary luteinizing hormone secretion, and are also related to reduced ovarian androgen production, especially in women with a tendency to become hyperandrogenic.

Prostate cancer
Risk of prostate cancer may be increased in men with high intra-prostatic concentrations of dihydrotestosterone. Dihydrotestosterone is formed from testosterone in the prostate and binds and activates the

Indicator	Number of oral contraceptive users among		Relative risk (95% confidence interval)
	Ovarian cancer cases	Controls	
Age (years)			
< 45	48	221	0.6 (0.3-1.0)
45-54	30	92	0.5 (0.3-1.0)
55-64	2	11	0.6 (0.4-0.9)
Parity			
0	21	67	0.6 (0.4-0.8)
1	15	75	0.6 (0.4-0.9)
≥ 2	44	182	0.3 (0.1-1.4)

Table 2.22 Estimated relative risk of ovarian cancer for women who have used oral contraceptives at any period in their lives, given for different ages and number of births. S. Franceschi et al. (1991) *Int J Cancer*, 49: 61-65.

androgen receptor with a four times higher affinity than testosterone [18]. One determinant of intra-prostatic dihydrotestosterone formation may be variation in the activity of intraprostatic (type II) 5-α-reductase (SRD5A2), that catalyses the testosterone-dihydrotestosterone conversion. Another possible determinant, which could provide a physiological link between prostate cancer risk and nutritional lifestyle factors, is an increase in circulating levels of bioavailable testosterone unbound to sex hormone binding globulin, that can freely diffuse into the prostatic cells.

The androgen hypothesis originated from observations that surgical or medical castration can often dramatically improve the clinical course of advanced metastatic prostate cancer patients. Furthermore, Japanese and Chinese migrants to the USA have lower incidence rates of prostate cancer than men of African or European ancestry, and at the same time have been found to have lower 5-α-reductase activity; there are positive associations of prostate cancer risk with specific genetic polymorphisms in the SRD5A2 gene. Finally, polymorphisms in the androgen receptor gene causing increased receptor transactivation have also been found associated with an increase in prostate cancer risk [12,19].

On the basis of the above observations, one can predict an increase in prostate cancer risk in men with elevated blood levels of bioavailable testosterone, as well as with levels of androstanediol-glucuronide, a major breakdown product of dihydrotestosterone and a possible marker of intraprostatic androgen activity. These predictions, however, have received only very limited support from epidemiological studies [20]. There is little evidence as yet for any association between circulating estrogen levels and prostate cancer risk.

REFERENCES

1. Kelsey JL, Gammon MD, John EM (1993) Reproductive factors and breast cancer. *Epidemiol Rev*, 15: 36-47.

2. Weiss NS, Cook LS, Farrow DC, Rosenblatt KA (1996) Ovarian cancer. In: Schottenfeld D, Fraumeni JF, eds, *Cancer Epidemiology and Prevention*, New York, Oxford University Press, 1040-1057.

3. Secreto G, Zumoff B (1994) Abnormal production of androgens in women with breast cancer. *Anticancer Res*, 14: 2113-2117.

4. Thomas HV, Reeves GK, Key TJ (1997) Endogenous estrogen and postmenopausal breast cancer: a quantitative review. *Cancer Causes Control*, 8: 922-928.

5. Thomas HV, Key TJ, Allen DS, Moore JW, Dowsett M, Fentiman IS, Wang DY (1997) A prospective study of endogenous serum hormone concentrations and breast cancer risk in postmenopausal women on the island of Guernsey. *Br J Cancer*, 76: 401-405.

6. Helzlsouer KJ, Alberg AJ, Bush TL, Longcope C, Gordon GB, Comstock GW (1994) A prospective study of endogenous hormones and breast cancer. *Cancer Detect Prev*, 18: 79-85.

7. Rosenberg CR, Pasternack BS, Shore RE, Koenig KL, Toniolo PG (1994) Premenopausal estradiol levels and the risk of breast cancer: a new method of controlling for day of the menstrual cycle. *Am J Epidemiol*, 140: 518-525.

8. IARC (1998) *Hormonal Contraception and Post-Menopausal Hormonal Therapy (IARC Monographs on the Evaluation of Carcinogenic Risks to Humans, Vol. 72)*, Lyon, IARCPress.

9. Moreno V, Bosch FX, Muñoz N, Meijer CJLM, Shah KV, Walboomers JMM, Herrero R, Franceschi S (2002) Effect of oral contraceptives on risk of cervical cancer in women with human papillomavirus infection: the IARC multi-centric case-control study. *Lancet*, 359: 1085-1092.

10. Ross RK, Paganini-Hill A, Wan PC, Pike MC (2000) Effect of hormone replacement therapy on breast cancer risk: estrogen versus estrogen plus progestin. *J Natl Cancer Inst*, 92: 328-332.

11. Schairer C, Lubin J, Troisi R, Sturgeon S, Brinton L, Hoover R (2000) Menopausal estrogen and estrogen-progestin replacement therapy and breast cancer risk. *JAMA*, 283: 485-491.

12. Bosland MC (2000) The role of steroid hormones in prostate carcinogenesis. *J Natl Cancer Inst Monogr*, 39-66.

13. Grady D, Ernster VL (1996) Endometrial cancer. In: Schottenfeld D, Fraumeni JF,eds, *Cancer Epidemiology and Prevention*, New York, Oxford University Press, 1058-1089.

14. Key TJ, Pike MC (1988) The dose-effect relationship between "unopposed" oestrogens and endometrial mitotic rate: its central role in explaining and predicting endometrial cancer risk. *Br J Cancer*, 57: 205-212.

15. Bernstein L, Ross RK (1993) Endogenous hormones and breast cancer risk. *Epidemiol Rev*, 15: 48-65.

16. Cramer DW, Welch WR (1983) Determinants of ovarian cancer risk. II. Inferences regarding pathogenesis. *J Natl Cancer Inst*, 71: 717-721.

17. Fathalla MF (1971) Incessant ovulation — a factor in ovarian neoplasia? *Lancet*, 2: 163.

18. Bosland MC (1996) Hormonal factors in carcinogenesis of the prostate and testis in humans and in animal models. *Prog Clin Biol Res*, 394: 309-352.

19. Ross RK, Pike MC, Coetzee GA, Reichardt JK, Yu MC, Feigelson H, Stanczyk FZ, Kolonel LN, Henderson BE (1998) Androgen metabolism and prostate cancer: establishing a model of genetic susceptibility. *Cancer Res*, 58: 4497-4504.

20. Eaton NE, Reeves GK, Appleby PN, Key TJ (1999) Endogenous sex hormones and prostate cancer: a quantitative review of prospective studies. *Br J Cancer*, 80: 930-934.

WEBSITE

The Endocrine Society:
http://www.endo-society.org/about/index.cfm

3

Mechanisms of tumour development

The phenotypic changes which a cell undergoes in the process of malignant transformation is a reflection of the sequential acquisition of genetic alterations. This multi-step process is not an abrupt transition from normal to malignant growth, but may take place over 20 years or more. The mutation of critical genes, including suppressor genes, oncogenes and genes involved in DNA repair, leads to genetic instability and progressive loss of differentiation. Tumours enlarge because cancer cells lack the ability to balance cell division by cell death (apoptosis) and by forming their own vascular system (angiogenesis). The transformed cells lose their ability to interact with each other and exhibit uncontrolled growth, invade neighbouring tissues and eventually spread through the blood stream or the lymphatic system to distant organs.

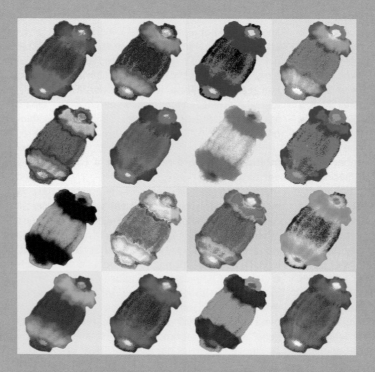

MULTISTAGE CARCINOGENESIS

SUMMARY

> Tumours consist of cells whose growth and morphological characteristics are markedly different from those of normal cells. Criteria for malignancy include increased cell proliferation, loss of differentiation, infiltrative growth and metastasis to other organs.

> Malignant transformation is a multistage process, typically a progression from benign lesions (e.g. adenoma) to malignant tumours (e.g. carcinoma). This evolution of malignant cells is caused by the sequential accumulation of alterations in genes responsible for the control of cellular proliferation, cell death and the maintenance of genetic integrity.

> The development of cancer may be initiated by environmental agents (chemical carcinogens, radiation, viruses) and inherited genetic factors (germline mutations).

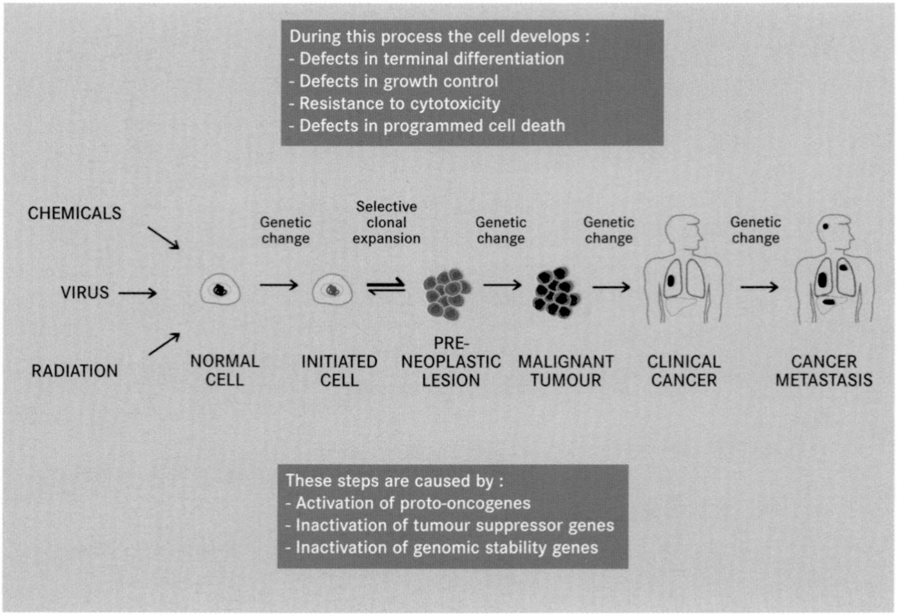

Fig. 3.1 Carcinogenesis is a multistage process involving multiple genetic and epigenetic events in proto-oncogenes, tumour suppressor genes and anti-metastasis genes.

Cancer arises from a single cell

Malignant tumours (or "cancers") are described as monoclonal, meaning that each tumour arises from a single cell. The development of a malignant tumour from a normal cell usually occurs over a considerable fraction of our lifetime. Such a long period is reflected, for example, by the difference between the age at which people start smoking and the age at which diagnosis of lung cancer most often occurs. The long "latent period" in lung cancer and almost all other malignancies is not explicable on the basis of a single-step transition from a normal cell to malignant one. Rather, the tumour is the outcome of an evolutionary process involving successive generations of cells, which are progressively further advanced towards cancerous growth [1].

Human histopathological observations support this scenario, and a range of pre-malignant lesions have been identified [2]. Likewise, in experimental animals, specific cell populations may be identified as marking a commitment towards malignancy, and these may be exploited as an early indicator in the context of carcinogen testing [3]. Thus, wholly on morphological grounds, cancer may be perceived as the outcome of a complex biological process.

Multiple steps are required for a cancer to arise

Animal "models" of cancer development, most commonly involving treatment of rodents with carcinogenic chemicals or other cancer-inducing agents, have provided clear evidence that specific stages in malignant transformation can occur discretely [4]. Chemicals which cause cancer in animals without the need for other treatment are sometimes called "complete carcinogens" (although "carcinogens" would be appropriate). Most such carcinogens cause damage to DNA of cells or tissues exposed to them. DNA-damaging activity may be identified on the basis of defined protocols (sometimes called "short-term tests", to emphasize their difference from chronic lifetime bioassay in rodents). Chemicals which exhibit mutagenic activity in short-term tests, which typically involve sensitive bacterial strains and cell-free extracts to catalyse metabolism of the test compound, are characterized as "genotoxic" [5]. Genotoxic agents may be complete carcinogens, but can also act as "initiating agents". After a single treatment with an initiating agent, tumour growth may be facilitated by chemicals (or treatments) which stimulate cell proliferation, sometimes by inducing mild toxic damage in exposed tissue. These agents are termed "promoters" (Table 3.1). As well as these genotoxic chemicals, a range of non-genotoxic agents can cause cancer in humans and/or experimental animals [6].

The stages in tumorigenesis have been designated "initiation", which encompasses damage to, and then division of exposed cells such that their growth potential is changed irreversibly, and "progression", denoting multiple rounds of cell replication mediating the gradual transition of an initiated cell towards autonomous, cancerous, growth. Ultimate spread of malignant cells resulting in multiple tumour sites has been termed "metastasis". The unequivocal identification by the mid-1970s of these various phases was one indication that carcinogenesis is a multistage process. Arguably, the greatest achievement of cancer research during the last decades of the 20th century has been the elucidation of multistage carcinogenesis at the molecular genetic level.

The molecular basis of tumour pathology

In a seminal publication, Vogelstein and colleagues [7] provided evidence that the different stages in the cellular evolution of colon cancer in humans, histologically identified as hyperplasia, early-stage adenoma, late-stage adenoma etc., could be identified with specific successive genetic changes (Fig. 3.2). The genetic changes included oncogene activation by mutation at specific sites and loss of chromosomal regions (necessarily involving multiple genes) which were subsequently shown to be the location of tumour suppressor genes. Since that initial description, knowledge of the molecular genetic basis for human colon cancer has been massively extended (*Colorectal cancer*, p198). For most tumours, the genetic changes are not inherited from our parents but arise in a previously normal cell. The progeny of this cell after cell division carry the same genetic change but the surrounding cells remain normal. Because these genetic changes affect only the cancer cells, they are not passed on to the children of cancer patients. However, in a minority of cases some critical changes are inherited, giving a familial predisposition to colon or other cancers.

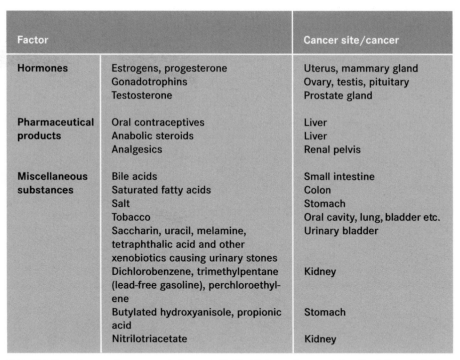

Factor		Cancer site/cancer
Hormones	Estrogens, progesterone	Uterus, mammary gland
	Gonadotrophins	Ovary, testis, pituitary
	Testosterone	Prostate gland
Pharmaceutical products	Oral contraceptives	Liver
	Anabolic steroids	Liver
	Analgesics	Renal pelvis
Miscellaneous substances	Bile acids	Small intestine
	Saturated fatty acids	Colon
	Salt	Stomach
	Tobacco	Oral cavity, lung, bladder etc.
	Saccharin, uracil, melamine, tetraphthalic acid and other xenobiotics causing urinary stones	Urinary bladder
	Dichlorobenzene, trimethylpentane (lead-free gasoline), perchloroethylene	Kidney
	Butylated hydroxyanisole, propionic acid	Stomach
	Nitrilotriacetate	Kidney

Table 3.1 Promoting agents: non-genotoxic agents that facilitate carcinogenesis by stimulating cell division. Tobacco smoke also contains genotoxic carcinogens.

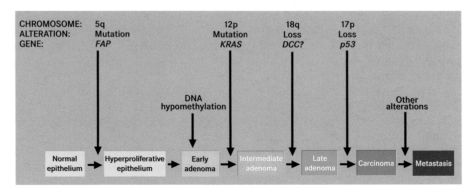

Fig. 3.2 The original Vogelstein model for the genetic and histological evolution of colon cancer. (*Colorectal cancer*, p198).

Commonality and heterogeneity

The molecular biological basis of multistage carcinogenesis initially described for colon cancer appears to have application to all tumour types, although there is marked variation in the extent to which genes relevant to particular tumours have been identified [8]. Some genes, and the corresponding change associated with tumorigenesis (mutation, overexpression, deletion and/or amplification) are common to a number of tumour types. However, each tumour type is associated with a distinctive set of gene alterations. The genes in question are discussed under the subheading *Pathology and genetics* for each of the tumour types included in Chapter 5. Such enumeration of relevant genes necessitates a degree of simplification. There is clear heterogeneity between individual tumours of the same type. In

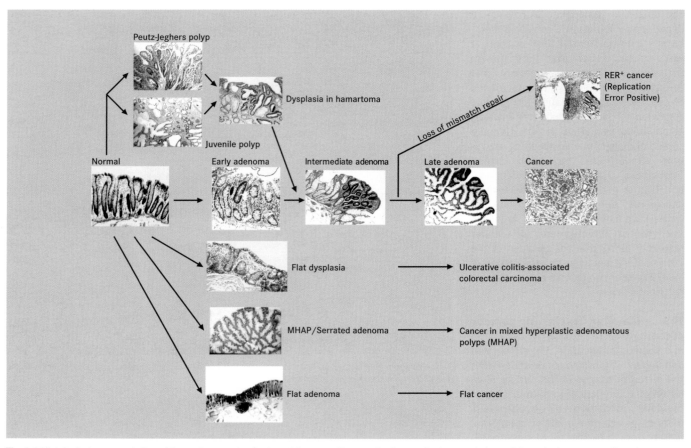

Fig. 3.3 Histological representation of the pathogenesis of colorectal cancer. Phenotypic changes in the morphology of the colonic mucosa reflect the sequential acquisition of genetic alterations.

other words, not every tumour will necessarily exhibit all the genetic changes established for the tumour type in question. Moreover, there is often marked heterogeneity within an individual tumour: adjacent cells differ. Mapping and identification of genes involved in malignant transformation has been a major component of the study of the molecular mechanisms of carcinogenesis.

Multiple genetic changes required

The emergence of a malignant cell population is understood to be the cumulative effect of multiple (perhaps five, ten or more) genetic changes, such changes being accumulated in the course of the evolution of the cell from normal to malignant. The genes designated as oncogenes and tumour suppressor genes (*Oncogenes*

and tumour suppressor genes, p96) have been identified in terms of their biological function [9]. Such genes are among those that facilitate transmission of growth control signals from the cell membrane to the nucleus (that is, signal transduction), that mediate cell division, differentiation or cell death and, perhaps most critical of all, that maintain the integrity of genetic information by DNA repair and similar processes (*Carcinogen activation and DNA repair*, p89). Since mutations are normally infrequent events, it seems unlikely that in the course of a human lifetime a cell would acquire all the mutations necessary for cancer to develop, unless at some point the developing cell lost its ability to protect itself against mutation and gained what is called a "mutator" phenotype [10]. Thus, alterations in gene structure and expression which bring about carcinogen-

esis are being progressively identified [11]. As noted earlier, members of some cancer-susceptible families inherit mutations in particular genes that contribute to cancer development, and hence to their individual risk of disease. However, with most cancers, the genetic change critical to carcinogenesis results from damage to DNA by chemicals, radiation and viruses (Fig. 3.1). This damage is not entirely and perhaps not predominantly produced by exogenous agents but by natural processes, such as the production of reactive oxygen species or the spontaneous deamination of the 5-methylcytosine naturally present in DNA [13]. Furthermore, as shown as the second step in Fig. 3.2, biological change that is heritable may result from non-genetic processes including the modulation of gene expression by hypermethylation [12].

PRECURSOR LESIONS IN CHEMOPREVENTION TRIALS

Trials of agents for chemopreventive activity which are based on assessment of malignant disease are almost unmanageable because of the long period of time (perhaps decades) potentially involved. Attention has therefore been focused on lesions, either cellular or molecular, demonstrated to be valid indicators of the subsequent development of malignancy. A trial may then evaluate the effect of the putative chemopreventive agent on such precursor lesions.

The best-validated precursor lesions are benign tumours, such as colorectal adenomas. It is established that adenoma number, size, and severity of dysplasia are predictive factors for colorectal cancer incidence. It has been estimated that 2-5% of all colorectal adenomas progress to adenocarcinomas if not removed or treated. The risk is greater for large and severely dysplastic polyps. Cancer risk is decreased by polyp removal, and a strong correlation exists between the relative prevalence of adenomas and cancers across populations (Winawer SJ et al., *N Engl J Med*, 328: 901-906, 1993). Several epidemiological studies have shown that regular use of aspirin or related drugs is associated with a reduced adenoma incidence (*IARC Handbooks of Cancer Prevention. Vol. 1*, Lyon, 1997). This provides further confirmation that adenomas are precursor lesions for colon cancer, since aspirin is known to reduce the incidence of malignant colon cancer.

Potential precursor lesions of carcinogenesis include both phenotypic and genotypic markers (Miller AB et al. *Biomarkers in Cancer Chemoprevention, IARC Scientific Publications 154*, Lyon, 2001). Thus oral leukoplakia is a recognized precursor for cancer of the oral cavity. Histological modulation of a precancer (often called intraepithelial neoplasia) has been used as a precursor lesion in prevention trials (Kelloff GJ et al., *Cancer Epidemiol Biomarkers Prev, 9*: 127-137, 2000). Additionally, genetic lesions such as progressive genomic instability as measured by loss of heterozygosity or amplification at specific microsatellite loci, have been considered (Califano J et al. *Cancer Res*, 56: 2488-2492, 1996). Other potential precursor endpoints include proliferation and differentiation markers, specific gene and general chromosomal damage, cell growth regulatory molecules, and biochemical activities (e.g. enzyme inhibition). Serum proteins are of special interest because of their availability. Thus prostate-specific antigen (PSA) is being used as a "surrogate" marker for prostate cancer. It is expected that the number and variety of biomarkers for precursor lesions will continue to expand In parallel with the advances in understanding of the genetic and cellular basis of carcinogenesis.

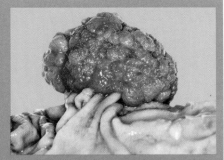

Fig. 3.6 Tubular adenoma of the colon is a precursor lesion for colorectal cancer.

Ageing
Apart from multistage development, certain other processes are fundamental to malignant disease. Principal amongst these is ageing, which can be considered both in relation to the whole individual, and

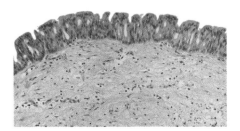

Fig. 3.4 Severe intraepithelial neoplasia (dysplasia) in the epithelium of an intrahepatic large bile duct, a condition caused by hepatolithiasis.

also at the cellular level. In humans, as well as in other mammals, the incidence of cancer rises dramatically with age. An exponential increase occurs from mid-life [14]. Passage of time is also critical to cell biology. Normal cells do not divide indefinitely due to senescence (Box: *Telomeres and Telomerase*, p108). Senescent cells cannot be stimulated to divide further, become resistant to apoptotic cell death and acquire differentiated functions. Senescence may be an anti-cancer mechanism that limits accumulation of mutations. However, when maintained in culture, cells treated with carcinogenic chemicals or infected with oncogenic viruses may avoid senescence and proliferate indefinitely. Such cell populations are described as being "transformed" and when further maintained in culture, once-normal cells acquire the same characteristics as cells cultured from malignant tumours. These and various other alterations in growth characteristics are recognized as the experimental counterpart of multistage carcinogenesis through which tumours develop in intact animals or humans. The genetic basis for senescence, and its relationship to malignancy, is a subject of intense investigation [15].

Preventing cancer
The significance of multistage carcinogenesis extends beyond facilitating understanding of how a transition from normal to malignant cell growth occurs. The fundamental cellular studies outlined earlier provide a basis for preventing can-

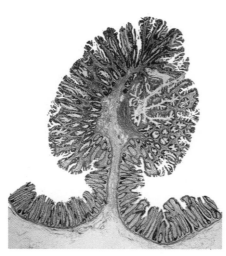

Fig. 3.5 Pedunculated hyperplastic polyp of the colon.

cer (see chapter 4). The fact that particular patterns of cell morphology and growth precede emergence of an unequivocally malignant cell population is the basis of secondary prevention of cancer.

Examples include detection of polyps in the large bowel (Fig. 3.5) and of morphological change which is the basis of the Papanicolaou smear test for early detection of cervical cancer. Moreover, dietary or pharmaceutical interventions calculated to prevent or reverse such lesions are the basis of chemoprevention [16]. Most importantly, knowledge of the genetic basis underlying tumour growth should provide new criteria for individual determination of diagnosis and prognosis. The mechanisms now known to operate in the proliferation of cancer cells provide a basis for the development of new, more efficient therapies without the side-effects that currently often afflict cancer patients [17].

REFERENCES

1. Foulds L, ed. (1969) *Neoplastic Development,* Vol. 1, London, Academic Press.

2. Correa P (1996) Morphology and natural history of cancer precursors. In: Schottenfeld D, Fraumeni JF, eds, *Cancer Epidemiology and Prevention,* New York, Oxford University Press, 45-64.

3. Ito N, Imaida K, Asamoto M, Shirai T (2000) Early detection of carcinogenic substances and modifiers in rats. *Mutat Res,* 462 : 209-217.

4. Weinstein IB (1982) Carcinogenesis as a multistage process—experimental evidence. In: Bartsch H, Armstong B, eds, *Host Factors in Human Carcinogenesis (IARC Scientific Publications No. 39)* Lyon, IARCPress, 9-25.

5. Vainio H, Magee PN, McGregor DB, McMichael AJ, eds (1992) *Mechanisms of Carcinogenesis in Risk Identification (IARC Scientific Publications No. 116),* Lyon, IARCPress.

6. Yamasaki H, Ashby J, Bignami M, Jongen W, Linnainmaa K, Newbold RF, Nguyen-Ba G, Parodi S, Rivedal E, Schiffmann D, Simons JW, Vasseur P (1996) Nongenotoxic carcinogens: development of detection methods based on mechanisms: a European project. *Mutat Res,* 353: 47-63.

7. Vogelstein B, Fearon ER, Hamilton SR, Kern SE, Preisinger AC, Leppert M, Nakamura Y, White R, Smits AM, Bos JL (1988) Genetic alterations during colorectal-tumor development. *N Engl J Med,* 319: 525-532.

8. Balmain A, Harris CC (2000) Carcinogenesis in mouse and human cells: parallels and paradoxes. *Carcinogenesis,* 21: 371-377.

9. Evan GI, Vousden KH (2001) Proliferation, cell cycle and apoptosis in cancer. *Nature,* 411: 342-348.

10. Loeb LA (2001) A mutator phenotype in cancer. *Cancer Res,* 61: 3230-3239.

11. Hahn WC, Counter CM, Lundberg AS, Beijersbergen RL, Brooks MW, Weinberg RA (1999) Creation of human tumour cells with defined genetic elements. *Nature,* 400: 464-468.

12. Esteller M, Corn PG, Baylin SB, Herman JG (2001) A gene hypermethylation profile of human cancer. *Cancer Res,* 61: 3225-3229.

13. Marnett LJ, Plastaras JP (2001) Endogenous DNA damage and mutation. *Trends Genet,* 17: 214-221.

14. Armitage P, Doll R (1954) The age distribution of cancer and a multistage theory of carcinogenesis. *Br J Cancer,* 8: 1-12.

15. Wynford-Thomas D (1999) Cellular senescence and cancer. *J Pathol,* 187: 100-111.

16. Bartsch H (2000) Studies on biomarkers in cancer etiology and prevention: a summary and challenge of 20 years of interdisciplinary research. *Mutat Res,* 462: 255-279.

17. Kallioniemi OP, Wagner U, Kononen J, Sauter G (2001) Tissue microarray technology for high-throughput molecular profiling of cancer. *Hum Mol Genet,* 10: 657-662.

CARCINOGEN ACTIVATION AND DNA REPAIR

SUMMARY

>Many chemical carcinogens require spontaneous or enzymatic activation to produce reactive intermediates which bind to DNA. The resulting carcinogen-DNA adducts may be eliminated from DNA by various enzyme-mediated repair processes.

>In cells and tissues with deficient DNA repair, replication of carcinogen-damaged DNA may result in the mutation of genes that regulate cell growth and differentiation in target cell populations. Such genetic alterations typically lead to progressive genetic instability resulting in uncontrolled growth, loss of differentiation, invasion and metastasis.

Experimental studies in rodents and in cultured cells have led to the classification of chemical carcinogens into two broad classes: genotoxic and non-genotoxic. Genotoxic carcinogens alter the structure of DNA, mostly by covalent binding to nucleophilic sites. These lesions, that is, the chemical entity of carcinogen bound to DNA, are called DNA "adducts". The replication of DNA containing unrepaired adducts may result either in the generation of sequence changes (mutations) in the newly synthesized daughter strands of DNA or in DNA rearrangements evident as chromosome aberrations.

This critical, irreversible genetic event can thus result in fixation of the original structural change in DNA as permanent, transmissible, genetic damage, or in the loss of genetic information through alterations in chromosomes. Such heritable change has the potential to perturb growth control in the affected cell, and is sometimes referred to as the "initiation" step of the tumorigenic process (Fig. 3.7).

Carcinogen activation

The first indication that certain cancers were associated with exposure to chemicals arose from observations by clinicians in the 18th and 19th centuries. The field of experimental chemical carcinogenesis started in 1915 with the experiments of Yamagiwa and Ichikawa, who showed that application of tar to the ears of rabbits induced skin tumours. In the 1940s, experiments on mouse skin demonstrated the stepwise evolution of cancer and allowed the characterization of two classes of agents, initiators and promoters [1]. Most chemical carcinogens are subject to metabolism that results in their elimination, but in the course of which reactive intermediates are generated. Such metabolic activation results in the modification of cellular macromolecules (nucleic acids and proteins) [2]. Accordingly, mutagenicity tests using bacteria and mammalian cells in culture were developed and are extensively used to identify potential carcinogens. Not all chemicals known to cause cancer, however, can be demonstrated to bind to DNA and hence be classified as "genotoxic".

Activation of chemical carcinogens in mammalian tissue mostly occurs through oxidation by microsomal mono-oxygenases (cytochromes P450, phase I enzymes). Cytochromes P450 are located in the endoplasmic reticulum (internal membranes of the cell) and constitute a superfamily of proteins; about 50 are now known in humans. The oxidation products are substrates for other families of enzymes (transferases, phase II enzymes) which link the carcinogen residues to a glutathione, acetyl, glucuronide or sulfate group; the resulting conjugates are hydrophilic and thus can be easily excreted. Carcinogenic electrophilic metabolites arise as by-products of these metabolic reactions. The metabolic pathways are well characterized for the major classes of chemical carcinogens (Fig. 3.8), including polycyclic aromatic hydro-carbons, aromatic amines, N-nitrosamines, aflatoxins and vinyl halides, which yield electrophilic species through phase I activation [3]. Other metabolic pathways are known. For example, dihaloalkanes are activated to carcinogenic metabolites by glutathione transferases.

Understanding of carcinogen-DNA interactions (Fig. 3.9) has resulted largely from the development of sensitive and specific methods for determining DNA adducts [4]. The most frequently used methods include immunoassays using adduct-specific anti-sera or antibodies, 32P-postlabelling, fluorescence spectroscopy, electrochemical detection and mass spectrometry. Measurement of carcinogen-DNA adducts in rodents has revealed correlations between the concentration of the carcinogen in the environment, DNA adduct levels in tissues where tumours may arise and cancer incidence. It is therefore accepted that DNA adducts may be used as indicators

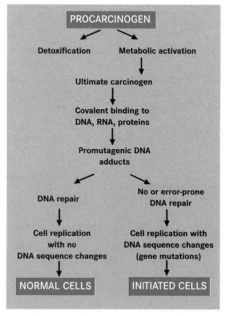

Fig. 3.7 Critical stages in the process of initiation by genotoxic chemicals.

of the effective biological exposure, and hence of carcinogenic risk in humans [5]. However, analysis of DNA adducts in human cells and tissues remains difficult, due to the very low levels of adducts present in DNA (typically, one adduct per 10^7-10^8 parent nucleotides).

Activities of the enzymes involved in carcinogen metabolism vary greatly between individuals due to induction and inhibition processes or to gene polymorphisms that can affect activity. These variations can affect the formation of carcinogen-DNA adducts, together with other genetic determinants that regulate DNA repair or cell cycle control, for example, and thus affect the outcome of exposure to DNA-damaging agents and influence cancer risk in different individuals [6]. Many studies have sought to correlate genetic polymorphisms, adduct levels and cancer risk in human populations (*Genetic susceptibility*, p71). These studies have hitherto provided some correlations for risk prediction at the population level. However, due to the great number of enzymes and polymorphisms involved, large-scale studies and high throughput assays (based on DNA microchips, for example) will be required to fully elucidate the complex nature of such gene-environment interactions.

Mutational spectra

Adducts of DNA and proteins can be used as early markers of exposure to carcinogens as indicated. However, because adducts only persist for a short time (typically, for a few hours or days for DNA

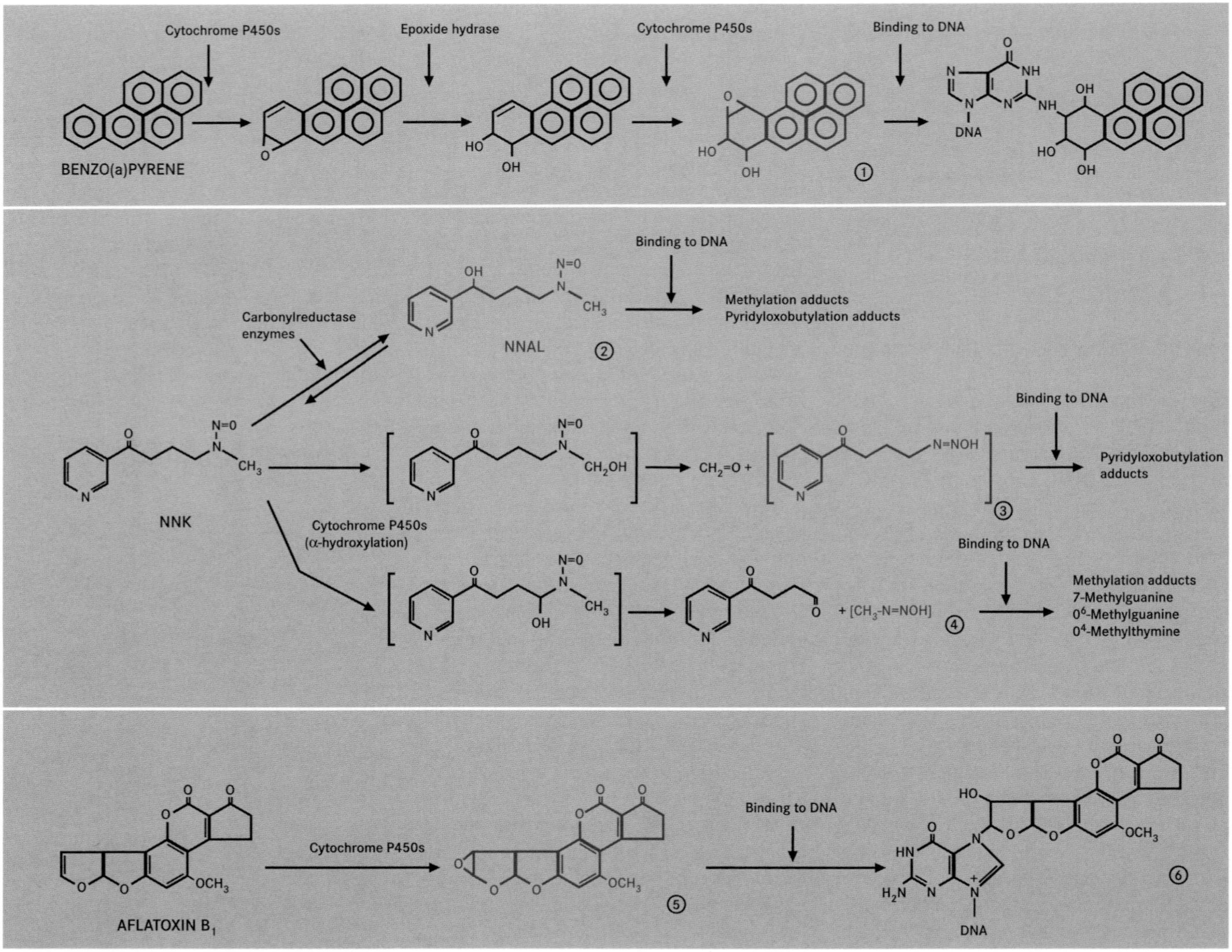

Fig. 3.8 Carcinogen activation by mammalian enzymes: reactions catalysed during metabolism of benzo[a]pyrene and NNK (4-(methylnitrosamino)-1-(3-pyridyl)-1-butanone), both contained in tobacco, and of aflatoxin B_1, produce reactive intermediates (ultimate carcinogens, in box), which bind to DNA. Other reaction pathways leading to the formation of glucuronides and other esters, which are excreted, are not shown. **1.** Benzo[a]pyrene-7, 8-diol-9, 10-epoxide; **2.** 4-(methylnitrosamino)-1-(3-pyridyl)-1-butanol; **3.** Diazohydroxide; **4.** Diazohydroxide; **5.** Aflatoxin B_1-8,9-oxide; **6.** 2,3-Dihydro-2-(N^7- guanyl)-3-hydroxyaflatoxin B_1.

adducts, a few weeks or months for albumin or haemoglobin adducts), their usefulness as exposure markers is limited. Mutations in specific genes can be used as longer-term "biomarkers" of early biological effects or of disease [7]. Indeed, gene mutation patterns are probably the only biological marker that can be characteristic of a past exposure to a carcinogenic agent or mixture. Study of such mutations will increasingly assist in the identification of etiologic agents, in risk prediction and in cancer prevention studies. Mutation spectra can be analysed either in normal tissues (including blood cells) or in tumour tissues. Analysis of mutations in normal tissues remains difficult, because the mutant cell or DNA must be identified against a background of a very large excess of non-mutant cells or DNA, and a selection or an enrichment step is required. In contrast, mutations in tumour cells often favour growth and are amplified due to clonal expansion of the tumour cell population.

A few genes are suitable markers ("reporters") of mutation induction in experimental animals and in humans. Thus the hypoxanthine-guanine phospho-ribosyl-transferase gene *HPRT*, when inactivated by mutation, renders cells resistant to growth inhibition by 6-thioguanine; such mutant cells can therefore be isolated by culture in the presence of this agent. Studies in humans have associated increases in the frequency of *HPRT* mutations (measured in circulating lymphocytes) with exposure to environmental genotoxic agents. However, in contrast to observations made in rodents, in which mutation profiles often reflect the relatively extreme DNA damage that induced them, characteristic *HPRT* mutation spectra (i.e. the types and positions of the base changes within the DNA sequence of the *HPRT* gene) are more difficult to observe in humans.

The identification of oncogenes and tumour suppressor genes (*Oncogenes and tumour suppressor genes*, p96) has led to the characterization of gene mutations which are more directly associated with carcinogenesis. The *RAS* family of oncogenes was among the first that was recognized as being mutated in a wide variety of human cancers. *p53* is the most commonly altered tumour suppressor gene in human cancer, being mutated in over 50% of almost all tumour types. A large database of *p53* mutations has been generated. Mutational spectra have been identified that provide evidence for the direct action of environmental carcinogens in the development of certain cancers (i.e. in these cases, cancer can be linked causally to past exposure to a defined carcinogenic agent). These mutations, which could in principle be used to identify exposure to particular agents, have been termed "signature" mutations. They result from the formation of specific DNA adducts. For example, *p53* mutations characteristic of the known or suspected etiological agent occur in lung cancer (attributable to benzo[a]pyrene in tobacco smoke) and hepatocellular carcinomas (due to aflatoxin B$_1$ in contaminated food) (Box: *Geographic variation in mutation patterns*, p102). In general, however, it is often not practical to obtain DNA from healthy tissue to analyse for potentially tumorigenic mutations, as invasive methods of sampling are required. Fortunately, the protein products of the mutated genes and, even the mutated DNA itself, can be detected and measured in body fluids or secretions, such as blood plasma, that have been in contact with the malignant tissue.

Presumed signature mutations have also been identified in "normal" tissues (non-pathological but probably containing initiated cells) from exposed individuals. For example, the *p53* mutation associated with exposure to aflatoxin B$_1$ has been found in liver tissue and in plasma DNA from healthy subjects (without cancer) who have consumed food contaminated with aflatoxins. Therefore, mutations in cancer genes could be used, in certain cases, as early indicators of risk before disease diagnosis.

DNA repair

The 3×10^9 nucleotides of the DNA within each human cell are constantly exposed to an array of damaging agents of both environmental origin, exemplified by sunlight and tobacco smoke, and of endogenous origin, including water and oxygen [8] (Table 3.2). This scenario necessitates constant surveillance so that damaged

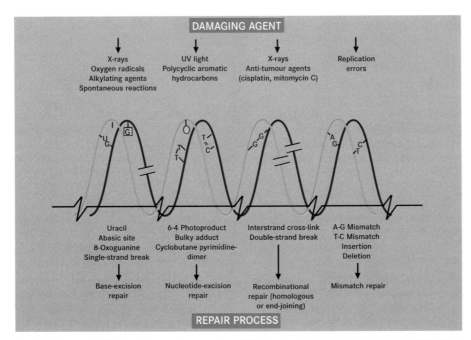

Fig. 3.9 Common DNA damaging agents, examples of DNA lesions induced by these agents and the most important DNA repair mechanism responsible for the removal of these lesions.

nucleotides may be removed and replaced before their presence in a DNA strand at the time of replication leads to the generation of mutations [9]. Restoration of normal DNA structure is achieved in human cells by one of several DNA repair enzymes that cut out the damaged or inappropriate bases and replace them with the normal nucleotide sequence. This type of cellular response is referred to as "excision repair" and there are two major repair pathways which function in this manner: "base excision repair" which works mainly on modifications caused by endogenous agents and "nucleotide excision repair" which removes lesions caused by environmental mutagens. UV light is probably the most common exogenous mutagen to which human cells are exposed and the importance of the nucleotide excision repair pathway in protecting against UV-induced carcinogenesis is clearly demonstrated in the inherited disorder xeroderma pigmentosum. Individuals who have this disease lack one of the enzymes involved in nucleotide excision repair and have a 1,000 times greater risk of developing skin cancer following exposure to sunlight than normal individuals. The genes in question have been named *XPA*, *XPB*, etc. [10].

One of the great achievements of the last two decades has been the isolation and characterization of the genes, and their protein products, involved in base excision repair and nucleotide excision repair. It has become apparent that certain proteins so identified are not exclusively involved in DNA repair but play an integral part in other cellular processes such as DNA replication and recombination.

Excision repair

The first step in both base excision repair and nucleotide excision repair is the recognition of a modification in DNA by enzymes that detect either specific forms of damage or a distortion in the DNA helix. Recognition of damage is followed by an excision step in which DNA containing the modified nucleotide is removed. Gap-filling DNA synthesis and ligation of the free ends complete the repair process.

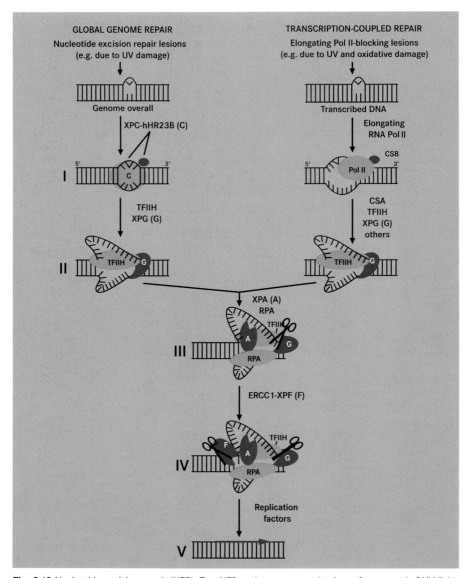

Fig. 3.10 Nucleotide excision repair (NER). Two NER pathways are predominant for removal of UV light- and carcinogen-damaged DNA. In global genome NER, the lesion is recognized by the proteins XPC and hHR23B while in transcription-coupled NER of protein-coding genes, the lesion is recognized when it stalls RNA polymerase II. Following recognition, both pathways are similar. The XPB and XPD helicases of the multi-subunit transcription factor TFIIH unwind DNA around the lesion (II). Single-stranded binding protein RPA stabilizes the intermediate structure (III). XPG and ERCC1-XPF cleave the borders of the damaged strand, generating a 24-32 base oligonucleotide containing the lesion (IV). The DNA replication machinery then fills in the gap (V).

Nucleotide excision repair may occur in the non-transcribed (non-protein-coding) regions of DNA (Fig. 3.10, steps I to V). A distortion in DNA is recognized, probably by the XPC-hHR23B protein (I). An open bubble structure is then formed around the lesion in a reaction that uses the ATP-dependent helicase activities of XPB and XPD (two of the subunits of TFIIH) and also involves XPA and RPA (II-III). The XPG and ERCC1-XPF nucleases excise and release a 24- to 32-residue oligonu-

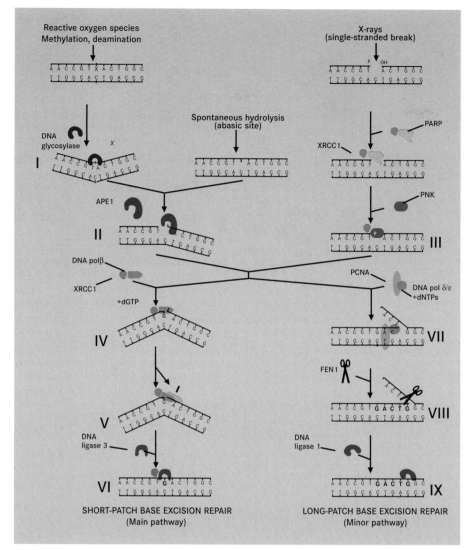

Fig. 3.11 Stages of base excision repair. Many glycosylases, each of which deals with a relatively narrow spectrum of lesions, are involved. The glycosylase compresses the DNA backbone to flip the suspect base out of the DNA helix. Inside the glycosylase, the damaged base is cleaved, producing an "abasic" site (I). APE1 endonuclease cleaves the DNA strand at the abasic site (II). In the repair of single-stranded breaks, poly(ADP-ribose)polymerase (PARP) and polynucleotide kinase (PNK) may be involved. In the "short-patch" pathway, DNA polymerase β fills the single nucleotide gap and the remaining nick is sealed by DNA ligase 3. The "long-patch" pathway requires the proliferating cell nuclear antigen (PCNA) and polymerases β, ε and δ fill the gap of 2–10 nucleotides. Flap endonuclease (FEN-1) is required to remove the flap of DNA containing the damage and the strand is sealed by DNA ligase 3.

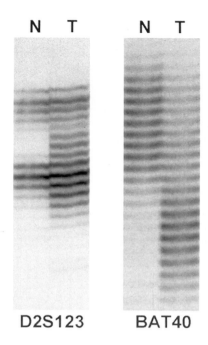

Fig. 3.12 In the human genome there are numerous places where short sequences of DNA are repeated many times. These are called microsatellites. In DNA from a patient with hereditary nonpolyposis colorectal cancer, there are changes in the number of repeats in the microsatellites. Note the difference in the microsatellite pattern between normal (N) and tumour tissue (T) from the same patient. This microsatellite instability is caused by errors in post-replicative DNA mismatch repair.

cleotide (IV) and the gap is filled in by PCNA-dependent polymerases (POL) epsilon and delta and sealed by a DNA ligase, presumed to be LIG1 (V). Nucleotide excision repair in regions which are transcribed (and hence code for proteins) requires the action of TFIIH [11].

DNA base excision repair (Fig. 3.11, steps I to VI or steps III to IX) involves the removal of a single base by cleavage of the sugar-base bond by a damage-specific DNA glycosylase (e.g. hNth1 or uracil DNA glycosylase) and incision by an apurinic/apyrimidinic nuclease (human

AP1) [12]. Gap-filling may proceed by replacement of a single base or by resynthesis of several bases in the damaged strand (depending on the pathway employed).

More complex and unusual forms of damage to DNA, such as double strand breaks, clustered sites of base damage and noncoding lesions that block the normal replication machinery are dealt with by alternative mechanisms. Inherited human diseases in which the patient shows extreme sensitivity to ionizing radiation and altered processing of strand breaks, such as ataxia telangiectasia and Nijmegen breakage syndrome, constitute useful models to study the repair enzymes involved in these processes. Indeed, if elucidation of base excision repair and nucleotide excision repair was the great achievement of the late 1990s, then understanding strand

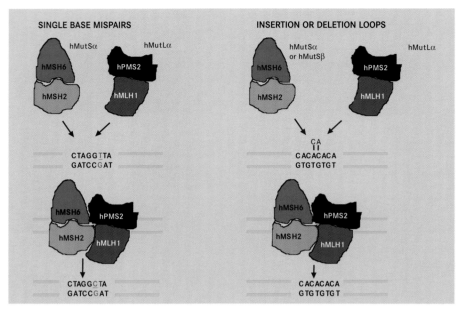

SINGLE BASE MISPAIRS

hMutSα   hMutLα

hMSH6   hPMS2

hMSH2   hMLH1

CTAGG**T**TA
GATCCGAT

hMSH6   hPMS2

hMSH2   hMLH1

CTAGG**C**TA
GATCCGAT

INSERTION OR DELETION LOOPS

hMutSα
or hMutSβ   hMutLα

hMSH6   hPMS2

hMSH2   hMLH1

C A
CACACACA
GTGTGTGT

hMSH6   hPMS2

hMSH2   hMLH1

CACACACA
GTG TGTG T

Fig. 3.13 Mismatch repair pathways: after DNA synthesis, base pairing mistakes that have escaped the editing function of DNA polymerase are recognized by mismatch repair proteins.

Other repair pathways

Human cells, in common with other eukaryotic and prokaryotic cells, can also perform one very specific form of damage reversal, the conversion of the methylated adduct, O^6-methylguanine, in DNA back to the normal base (Fig. 3.14). O^6-Methylguanine is a miscoding lesion: both RNA and DNA polymerases "read" it incorrectly when they transcribe or replicate a DNA template containing it. As this modified base can pair with both the base cytosine (its correct partner) and the base thymine (an incorrect partner), its presence in DNA can give rise to transition mutations by mispairing of relevant bases. A specific protein, O^6-alkylguanine-DNA-alkyltransferase, catalyses transfer of the methyl group from the guanine base to a cysteine amino acid residue located at the active site of the protein [13]. This error-free process restores the DNA to its original state but results in the inactivation of the repair protein. Consequently, repair can be saturated when cells are exposed to high doses of alkylating agents and synthesis of the transferase protein is required before repair can continue.

Mismatched bases in DNA arising from errors in DNA replication, for instance guanine paired with thymine rather than cytosine, are repaired by several pathways involving either specific glycosylases,

break repair will probably be the great achievement of the next decade. This will have important consequences. Certain cancers are often treated with radiotherapy (*Radiotherapy*, p277) and a small percentage of patients show considerable sensitivity to their treatment, with the result that treatment schedules are reduced to try to avoid adverse reactions. A better understanding of the possible causes of this radiosensitivity, including characterization of the enzymes involved in the repair of DNA damage produced by ionizing radiation, may lead to better tailoring of radiotherapy doses to individual patients.

Agent	Mutation hotspot	Type of mutation (> = changes to)	Tumours associated
Benzo[a]pyrene (tobacco smoke)	Codons 157, 158, 248, 273	G>T transversions	Lung, larynx
4-Aminobiphenyl (aromatic dyes, tobacco smoke)	Codons 280, 285	G>C transversions G>A transitions	Bladder
Aflatoxin B_1	Codon 249	AGG>AGT (arginine > serine)	Hepatocellular carcinoma
Ultraviolet (UV)	Codons 177-179, 278	C>T transitions CC>TT transitions	Skin cancer (not melanoma)
Vinyl chloride	Several codons	A>T transversions	Angiosarcoma of the liver
Endogenous mechanism (enhanced by nitric oxide)	Codons 175, 248, 273, 282	C>T transitions at CpG dinucleotides	Colon, stomach Brain cancers

Table 3.2 Spectra of *p53* mutations caused by environmental carcinogens or endogenous mechanisms.

which remove the mismatched bases, or long-patch mismatch repair involving homologues of the bacterial genes *MUTS* and *MUTL* (Fig. 3.13). Insertion or deletion loops at microsatellite sequences can be recognized by hMutSα (a heterodimer of hMSH2 and hMSH6) or hMutSβ (a heterodimer of hMSH2 and hMSH3). Subsequent recruitment of hMutLα (a heterodimer of hMLH1 and hPMS2) to the altered DNA targets the area for repair, which requires excision, resynthesis, and ligation. Single nucleotide mispairing events require hMutSα function for recognition. One important requirement of such repair processes is that they are able to distinguish the correct base from the incorrect one in the mispair. Since both bases are normal constituents of DNA, this cannot be achieved by an enzyme that

scans the DNA for a lesion or structure that is not a normal constituent of the DNA. Defects in at least four of the genes whose products are involved in mismatch repair, namely hMSH2, hMLH1, hPMS1 and hPMS2, have been associated with hereditary nonpolyposis colorectal cancer. This is one of the most common genetic diseases and affects as many as 1 in 200 individuals and may account for 4-13% of all colorectal cancers (*Colorectal cancer*, p198). Affected individuals also develop tumours of the endometrium, ovary and other organs. The DNA of hereditary non-polyposis colorectal cancer tumours is characterized by instabilities in simple mono-, di- and trinucleotide repeats which are common in the human genome (Fig. 3.12). This instability is also seen in certain sporadic colorectal tumour cells and arises

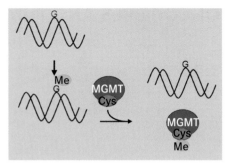

Fig. 3.14 The repair of O^6-methylguanine by O^6-alkylguanine-DNA-alkyltransferase.

directly from alterations in the proteins involved in mismatch repair [14]. Generally speaking, genomic instability is considered an indicator of, and fundamental to the nature of, malignant cell growth.

REFERENCES

1. Miller EC, Miller JA (1979) Milestones in chemical carcinogenesis. *Semin Oncol*, 6: 445-460.

2. Miller JA, Miller EC (1977) Ultimate chemical carcinogens as reactive mutagenic electrophiles. In: Hiatt HH, Watson, JD, Winsten, JA eds, *Origins of Human Cancer* (Book B), Cold Spring Harbor, Cold Spring Harbor Laboratory, 605-627.

3. Guengerich FP (2000) Metabolism of chemical carcinogens. *Carcinogenesis*, 21: 345-351.

4. Hemminki K, Dipple A, Shuker DEG, Kadlubar FF, Segerbäck D, Bartsch H, eds (1994) *DNA Adducts. Identification and Biological Significance* (IARC Scientific Publications No. 125), Lyon, IARCPress.

5. Toniolo P, Boffetta P, Shuker DEG, Rothman N, Hulka B, Pearce N, eds (1997) *Application of Biomarkers in Cancer Epidemiology* (IARC Scientific Publications No. 142), Lyon, IARCPress.

6. Vineis P, Malats N, Lang M, d'Errico A, Caporaso N, Cuzick J, Boffetta P, eds (1999) *Metabolic Polymorphisms and Susceptibility to Cancer* (IARC Scientific Publications No. 148), Lyon, IARCPress.

7. McGregor DB, Rice JM, Venitt S, eds (1999) *The Use of Short- and Medium-Term Tests for Carcinogens and Data on Genetic Effects in Carcinogenic Hazard Evaluation* (IARC Scientific Publications No. 146), Lyon, IARCPress.

8. Friedberg EC, Walker GC, Siede W, eds (1995) *DNA Repair and Mutagenesis*, Washington DC, ASM Press.

9. Lindahl T (2000) Suppression of spontaneous mutagenesis in human cells by DNA base excision-repair. *Mutat Res*, 462: 129-135.

10. de Boer J, Hoeijmakers JH (2000) Nucleotide excision repair and human syndromes. *Carcinogenesis*, 21: 453-460.

11. Benhamou S, Sarasin A (2000) Variability in nucleotide excision repair and cancer risk: a review. *Mutat Res*, 462: 149-158.

12. Cadet J, Bourdat AG, D'Ham C, Duarte V, Gasparutto D, Romieu A, Ravanat JL (2000) Oxidative base damage to DNA: specificity of base excision repair enzymes. *Mutat Res*, 462: 121-128.

13. Pegg AE (2000) Repair of O^6-alkylguanine by alkyltransferases. *Mutat Res*, 462: 83-100.

14. Pedroni M, Sala E, Scarselli A, Borghi F , Menigatti M, Benatti P, Percesepe A, Rossi G, Foroni M, Losi L, Di Gregorio C, De Pol A, Nascimbeni R, Di Betta E, Salerni B, de Leon MP, Roncucci L (2001) Microsatellite instability and mismatch-repair protein expression in hereditary and sporadic colorectal carcinogenesis. *Cancer Res*, 61: 896-899.

WEBSITES

A comprehensive listing of human DNA repair genes:
http://www.sciencemag.org/cgi/content/abstract/291/5507/1284

DNA Repair Interest Group (NCI):
http://www.nih.gov:80/sigs/dna-rep/

ONCOGENES AND TUMOUR SUPPRESSOR GENES

SUMMARY

> Human cells become malignant through the activation of oncogenes and inactivation of tumour suppressor genes. The pattern of genes involved varies markedly at different organ sites.

> Oncogenes stimulate cell proliferation and may be overexpressed by gene amplification (e.g. *MYC*). In addition, oncogenes may be activated by mutations (e.g. the *RAS* gene family).

> Tumour suppressor genes are typically inactivated by gene mutations in one allele (gene copy), followed by loss of the intact allele during cell replication (two-hit mechanism). This leads to loss of expression and abolition of the suppressor function, which is particularly important in cell cycle control.

> Mutational inactivation of suppressor genes in germ cells is the underlying cause of most inherited tumour syndromes. The same type of mutation may arise through mutations occurring during an individual's lifetime.

Definitions

The multi-step nature of carcinogenesis has long been recognized (*Multistage carcinogenesis*, p84). Over the past 20 years, experimental studies in animals and molecular pathological studies have converged to establish the notion that each step in malignant transformation is determined by a limited number of alterations in a small subset of the several thousands of cellular genes [1]. The terms "oncogene" and "tumour suppressor gene" are commonly used to identify the sets of genes involved in such sequences of events [2]. Both groups of genes are extremely diverse in terms of nature and function. An oncogene is a gene whose function is activated in cancer. This can be achieved by a number of simple molecular mechanisms, including point mutations that constitutively activate an enzyme, deletions that remove negative regulatory regions from proteins, or increased expression resulting from promoter deregulation or from multiplication of the number of copies of the gene (a phenomenon called "amplification" [3]). Activation of an oncogene is a dominant mechanism, since alteration of a single allele is sufficient to confer a gain of function for cancer onset or progression. The non-activated counterpart of an oncogene is sometimes called a "proto-oncogene". A proto-oncogene is in fact a "normal" gene in all respects, often with important functions in the control of the signalling of cell proliferation, differentiation, motility or survival.

A tumour suppressor gene is a gene whose alteration during carcinogenesis results in the loss of a functional property essential for the maintenance of normal cell proliferation. Loss of function of a tumour suppressor gene is typically a recessive mechanism. Indeed, in many instances both copies of the gene need to be inactivated in order to switch off the corresponding function. Inactivation of tumour suppressor genes proceeds by loss of alleles (most often through the loss of entire chromosomal sections encompassing several dozen genes), small deletions or insertions that scramble the reading frame of the gene, transcriptional silencing by alteration of the promoter region, or point mutations that change the nature of residues that are crucial for the activity of the corresponding protein. Recently, it has emerged that tumour suppressor genes can be conveniently subclassified into two major groups. The genes of the first group are nicknamed "gatekeepers". Their products control the gates on the pathways of cell proliferation. Typically, gatekeeper genes are negative regulators of the cell cycle, acting as "brakes" to control cell division. The genes of the second group are called "caretakers", as their primary function is not to control the speed or timing of cell division but rather its accuracy. Caretaker genes are usually involved in DNA repair and in the control of genomic stability. Their inactivation does not enhance cell proliferation *per se* but primes the cell for rapid acquisition of further genetic changes [4]. The combined activation of oncogenes and inactivation of tumour suppressor genes drive the progression of cancer. The most evident biological consequences of these alterations are autonomous cell proliferation, increased ability to acquire genetic alterations due to deregulated DNA repair, ability to grow in adverse conditions due to decreased apoptosis, (*Apoptosis*, p113) capacity to invade tissues locally and to form distant metastases, and ability to activate the formation of new blood vessels (a process called angiogenesis). Together, these five biological phenomena may be caricatured as pieces of the "cancer jigsaw" [5] (Fig. 3.15). None alone is sufficient in itself, but cancer arises when they interact together into a chain of coordinated events that profoundly modifies the normal cellular pattern of growth and development.

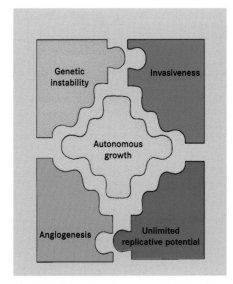

Fig. 3.15 The cancer jigsaw: multiple functions must be altered for tumorigenesis to occur.

Common human oncogenes

Many common proto-oncogenes encode components of the molecular cascades that regulate the cellular response to mitogenic signals [6]. They include growth factors (e.g. *TGFA*), growth factor receptors (e.g. the receptors for epidermal growth factor, *EGF* and its close homologue, *ERBB2*), receptor-coupled signal transduction molecules (in particular, several small guanosine triphosphate (GTP)-binding proteins located on the inner face of the cell membrane, such as the various members of the *RAS* family), kinases (*SRC*, *ABL*, *RAF1*), regulatory subunits of cell cycle kinases (*CCND1* and *CCNA*), phosphatases (*CDC25B*), anti-apoptotic molecules (*BCL2*) and transcription factors (*MYC*, *MYB*, *FOS*, *JUN*). The cumbersome nomenclature of these genes (Box: *Naming genes and proteins*, p101) owes much to the way they were discovered and identified. The *SRC* gene, for example, was the first oncogene identified, in 1976, as a modified version of a cellular gene incorporated in the genome of a highly transformant chicken retrovirus, the Rous sarcoma virus. The *MYC* gene was also originally identified in the genome of an avian retrovirus inducing promyelocytic leukaemia. The *RAS* genes were first identified as activated genes capable of inducing the formation of rat sarcomas, and various members of the family were found in different murine retroviruses, such as the Harvey sarcoma virus (*HRAS*) and the Kirsten sarcoma virus (*KRAS*).

The most commonly activated oncogenes in human cancers are *ERBB2* (in breast and ovarian cancers), members of the *RAS* family (in particular *KRAS* in lung, colorectal and pancreatic cancers, and *MYC* (in a large variety of tumours such as cancers of the breast and oesophagus and in some forms of acute and chronic leukaemia). These three examples give an excellent illustration of the diversity of the mechanisms of oncogene activation and of their consequences for cell growth and division.

ERBB2

In the case of *ERBB2*, oncogenic activation is almost always the result of amplification of the normal gene [7] (Fig. 3.16). This

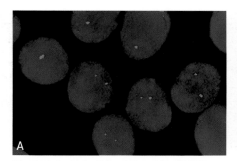
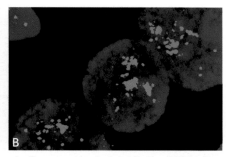

Fig. 3.16 Analysis of the status of the *ERBB2* oncogene by fluorescent in situ hybridization (FISH) with a rhodamine-labelled *ERBB2* probe (pink). In breast tumour cells without amplification of the gene, each nucleus possesses two copies of *ERBB2* (A). In tumour cells with high-level amplification of the gene, numerous signals are evident in each nucleus (B).

gene is located within a region of the genome which is amplified in about 27% of advanced breast cancers, leading to a spectacular increase in the density of the molecule at the cell surface. *ERBB2* encodes a transmembrane protein with the structure of a cell-surface receptor, the intracellular portion of which carries a tyrosine kinase activity. Overexpression of *ERBB2* leads to constitutive activation of the growth-promoting tyrosine phosphorylation signal. The elucidation of this mechanism has led to the development of neutralizing antibodies and specific chemical inhibitors of tyrosine kinase activity as therapeutic approaches to the blocking of *ERBB2* action.

RAS

The *RAS* genes are located one step downstream of *ERBB2* in growth signalling cascades. The protein products of the *RAS* genes are small proteins anchored at the cytoplasmic side of the plasma membrane by a lipidic moiety. They indirectly interact with activated tyrosine kinases and act as "amplifiers" to increase the strength of the signal generated by the activation of cell-surface receptors [8]. In their active form, ras proteins bind guanosine triphosphate (GTP) and catalyse its hydrolysis into guanosine diphosphate (GDP) returning to their inactive form. Oncogenic forms of activated *RAS* genes often carry missense mutations at a limited number of codons within the GTP-binding site of the enzyme, making it unable to hydrolyse GTP and thus trapping it in the active form. Activation of *RAS* genes thus induces the cell to behave as if the upstream, Ras-coupled receptors were being constantly stimulated.

MYC

The *MYC* oncogene may be seen as a prototype of the family of molecules which lies at the receiving end of the signal transduction cascades. *MYC* encodes a transcription factor which is rapidly activated after growth stimulation and which is required for the cell to enter into cycle [9].

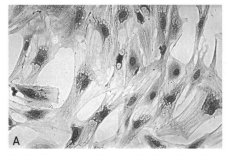
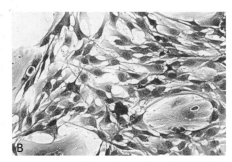

Fig. 3.17 In cell cultures, activation of a single oncogene may result in a changed morphology from "normal" (A) to "transformed" (B) and this often corresponds to a change in growth properties. Malignant transformation appears to require the co-operation of at least three genes.

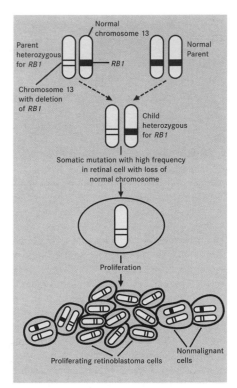

Fig. 3.18 The retinoblastoma gene is a paradigm for tumour suppressor genes: if a child inherits a mutation or deletion of one copy ("allele") of the retinoblastoma gene, the remaining normal copy tends to be lost at a high frequency in cells of the retina, resulting in loss of function and in the formation of tumours. The diagram shows loss of the whole normal chromosome but the normal allele can also be lost by mutation, deletion, gene conversion or mitotic recombination.

Myc transactivates a number of other cellular genes and has a wide spectrum of molecular effects (a phenomenon that may explain why Myc is activated in many different types of cancer cells). Activation of Myc often proceeds through amplification of the region containing the gene on chromosome 8, but Myc is also commonly activated by chromosomal translocation in some forms of B-cell leukaemia (*Leukaemia*, p242).

BCL2

The *BCL2* gene (activated in B cell lymphomas) exemplifies another kind of oncogene. Initially identified as a gene located within a chromosomal breakpoint in some forms of leukaemia, *BCL2* was found to encode a protein capable of extending the life span of a cell by preventing the onset of programmed cell death, or apoptosis [10] (*Apoptosis*, p113). Biochemical studies have revealed that *BCL2* encodes a regulator of the permeability of the mitochondrial membrane. Mitochondrial damage and cytoplasmic leakage of mitochondrial components is one of the important signals that lead a cell to apoptosis. By helping to keep the mitochondrial permeability pores closed, Bcl-2 protein prevents this leakage and thus allows the survival of cells that would otherwise have been eliminated by a physiological process.

Tumour suppressor genes: history of a concept

Whereas the study of retroviruses and gene transfection experiments were the keys to the discovery of oncogenes, tumour suppressor genes were identified through the study of large DNA viruses and the analysis of familial tumour syndromes.

Retinoblastoma

In 1971, Knudsen proposed the now popular "two hits" hypothesis to explain the inheritance of retinoblastoma, a rare childhood tumour type [11,12] (*Genetic susceptibility*, p71). He postulated that, in a familial setting, individuals may inherit only one normal copy of the gene (localized by linkage studies to chromosome 13q14), the other being either lost, partially deleted or otherwise inactivated. Consequently, these individuals would just need one additional mutagenic step to switch off the remaining copy of the gene, thus totally losing the corresponding function (Fig. 3.18). The very same type of cancer may also occur in a sporadic manner, but in this case it would require two consecutive "hits" (mutagenic events) to inactivate the two copies of the gene in the same cell. This theory paved the way for the modern concept of recessive tumour suppressor genes. In 1988, the gene responsible for familial retinoblastoma was identified [13]. The *RB1* gene encodes a protein that binds and inactivates transcription factors that are essential for the progression of the cell cycle, thus fulfilling the functions of a molecular "brake" on cell division.

Large DNA viruses

In parallel with events previously outlined, it became evident that many DNA viruses associated with cancer encode complex viral proteins that are capable of sequestering and inactivating cellular proteins [14]. This is the case of a tumorigenic simian virus, SV40, of several adenoma and polyoma viruses and of oncogenic forms of human papillomaviruses. In the case of SV40, the virus encodes a large protein (called LT for Large Tumour antigen) which binds two cellular proteins, the

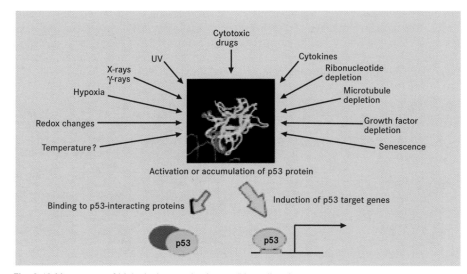

Fig. 3.19 Many types of biological stress lead to a p53-mediated response.

product of the *RB1* gene (pRb) and an ubiquitous protein that was conservatively called p53. In the case of oncogenic human papillomaviruses, the viruses encode two distinct proteins, E7 (which neutralizes pRb) and E6 (which neutralizes p53). Thus it was suggested that pRb and p53 might have similar, complementary functions, operating jointly in the control of cell division.

The "missing link" in this conceptual edifice was the discovery of alterations in the gene encoding p53. This was achieved in 1989, when it emerged that the *p53* gene was often mutated and/or deleted in many forms of cancers [15]. In 1991, inherited loss of *p53* was found to be associated with a rare familial syndrome of multiple cancers, the Li-Fraumeni syndrome, in which afflicted family members suffer vastly increased incidence of many tumour types [16]. Today, about 215 families worldwide affected by this syndrome have been described and the *p53* mutations they exhibit are compiled in a database maintained at IARC.

Tumour suppressor genes and familial cancer syndromes

Most familial cancer syndromes are inherited as a recessive trait, and correspond to the constitutive inactivation of an important tumour suppressor gene, as described above in the case of familial retinoblastoma. Over the past 15 years, many loci containing tumour suppressor genes have been identified by linkage studies in cancer-prone families.

Colorectal cancer

In colorectal cancers, two different familial cancer syndromes have been found to be associated with the constitutive alteration of two distinct sets of tumour suppressor genes (*Colorectal cancer*, p198). Patients with familial adenomatous polyposis, a disease that predisposes to the early occurrence of colon cancer, often carry alterations in one copy of the adenomatous polyposis coli (*APC*) gene [17]. This gene plays a central role in a signalling cascade that couples cell-surface receptors, calcium-dependent adhesion

molecules and transcription factors that regulate cell proliferation. Loss of APC function sets these transcription factors free, an event that favours not only the formation of polyps but also their transformation into adenomas and carcinomas.

Breast cancer

Two genes have been identified as involved in familial breast cancer risk, *BRCA1* and *BRCA2* [18]. These genes encode large proteins with complex functions in many aspects of cell regulation, such as cell cycle control and DNA repair. However, how their inactivation contributes to the onset or development of breast cancer is still largely unknown.

Others

In the case of hereditary Wilms tumours, a rare type of kidney cancer, the gene identified encodes a protein essential for the correct differentiation of the nephron. This very specific role may explain why the hereditary loss of this gene does not seem to be associated with cancers at any other site.

This short overview gives only a few examples of the diversity of tumour suppressor genes, and there is little doubt that many still remain to be identified. Given the breadth of the concept of "tumour suppressors", many genes encoding components of stress response pathways have the potential to behave in this fashion (as their alteration may prevent cells from mounting an adequate response to genotoxic, potentially

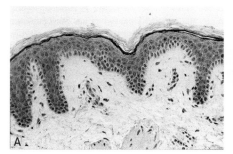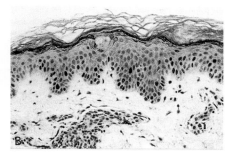

Fig. 3.20 Accumulation of p53 in human epidermis after exposure to sunlight. Unexposed skin shows no immunostaining against p53 protein (A). Exposed skin (B) shows a dense dark nuclear coloration of epidermal cells due to positive immunostaining for p53 protein.

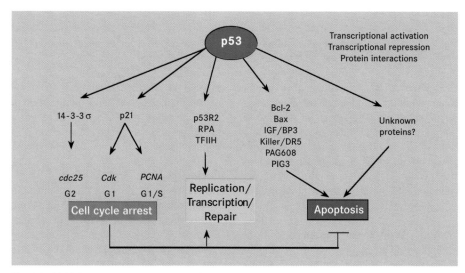

Fig. 3.21 Multiple response pathways are triggered by the accumulation of p53 in the cell nucleus.

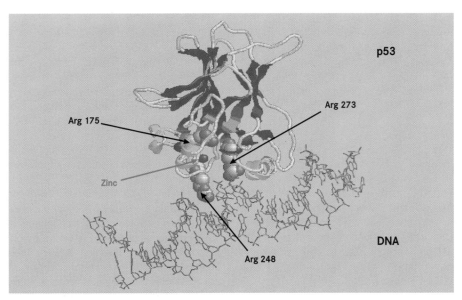

Fig. 3.22 Molecular modelling of part of the p53 protein (DNA-binding domain), showing its interaction with DNA. The amino acids labelled (arginine 175, 248, 273) are important for maintaining biological activity and are among the "hotspots" for mutations in cancer. The zinc atom is required for stabilizing the complex three-dimensional structure of the p53 oligomer.

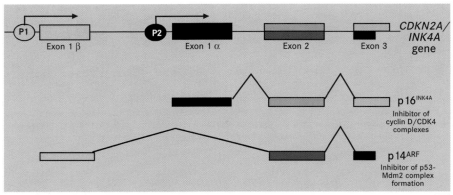

Fig. 3.23 Generally, a single segment of DNA codes for a single protein. However, the p16 and p14^{ARF} proteins are both encoded by a single region of DNA. P = promoter.

oncogenic forms of stress). The genes responsible for complex inherited diseases such as ataxia telangiectasia or xeroderma pigmentosum (*Carcinogen activation and DNA repair*, p89) belong to this category [19]. Alteration of such genes results in many defects, including hypersensitivity to radiation and therefore to the development of cancers such as skin tumours.

Tumour suppressor genes and sporadic cancers

Many of the tumour suppressor genes associated with familial cancer syndromes are also mutated at variable rates in many forms of sporadic cancer. However, two of them, *p53* and *CDKN2A*, are very commonly altered in almost every kind of human cancer.

p53, the guardian of the genome

The *p53* gene encodes a phosphoprotein of molecular weight 53,000 daltons, which accumulates in the nucleus in response to various forms of stress, in particular, DNA damage (Fig. 3.20). In this context, p53 acts as a transcriptional regulator, increasing or decreasing the expression of several dozen genes involved in cell cycle control, in the induction of apoptosis, in DNA repair and in differentiation control. Together these genes exert complex, anti-proliferative effects (Fig. 3.21). Essentially, when cells are subjected to tolerable levels of DNA-damaging agents, activation of p53 will result in cell cycle arrest, temporarily removing the cells from the proliferative pool or mediating differentiation. However, when faced with highly damaging levels of genotoxic stress, p53 will induce apoptosis, a programmed form of suicide that eliminates cells with potentially oncogenic alterations. This complex role in the protection of the cell from DNA damage has resulted in p53 being described as the "guardian of the genome" [20]. Loss of this function by mutation, as often occurs during carcinogenesis, will allow cells with damaged DNA to remain in the proliferative population, a situation that is essential for the expansion of a clone of cancer cells.

The *p53* gene differs from most other tumour suppressors in its mode of inactivation in human cancers. Whereas most tumour suppressors are altered by loss of alleles or inactivating deletions or insertions, *p53* is commonly the target of point mutations within the portion of the gene that encodes the DNA-binding domain of the protein (Fig. 3.22). These mutations prevent the correct folding of this protein domain, and therefore disrupt the interactions of p53 with its specific DNA targets. However, the mutant proteins are often extremely stable and therefore accumulate to high levels within the nucleus of cancer cells. This accumulated protein can often be detected by immunohistochemistry in primary tumours as well as in distant metastases. Although not all mutations induce accumulation of the protein, p53 accumulation provides a convenient tool for pathologists to assess the possibility of a p53 dysfunction in cancer specimens [21].

Mutation is not the only way to alter p53 protein in cancer. In cervical cancers, *p53* gene mutations are infrequent, but the protein is inactivated by binding of the viral protein E6 which is produced by human papillomavirus. This protein creates a molecular bridge between p53 and the protein degradation machinery, resulting in the rapid degradation and effective elimination of p53 protein. This interaction plays an important role in cervical cancer (*Cancers of the female reproductive tract,* p215). In normal cells, the degradation of p53 is regulated by the Mdm2 protein. Mdm2 ("murine double minute gene 2") was originally identified in the mouse as the product of a gene amplified in aberrant chromosome fragments called "double minute chromosomes". Amplification of *MDM2* is common in osteosarcomas and is sometimes detected in other cancers, such as carcinomas or brain tumours. *MDM2* thus behaves as an oncogene, since its activation by amplification causes the inactivation of a tumour suppressor gene [22].

The *p53* gene (and its product) is one of the most studied genes in human cancer. In the 20 years since its discovery in 1979, more than 15,000 publications have addressed its structure, function and alteration in cancers. There have been many attempts to exploit this knowledge in the development of new therapies based on the control of p53 activity in cancer cells. Experimental gene therapy has shown that it may be possible to restore p53 function in cells that have lost the gene. More recently, drugs designed to specifically target and restore the function of mutant *p53* have shown promising results in experimental systems. As knowledge of the *p53* pathway improves, it is anticipated that this central molecular event in human cancer will provide a basis for developing new forms of therapy.

CDKN2A: one locus, two genes
CDKN2, or "cyclin dependent kinase inhibitor 2", is known under several names, including *INK4A* (inhibitor of kinase 4A) and *MTS1* (multiple tumour suppressor 1). The *CDKN2A* locus is located at the extremity of the short arm of chromosome 9, the letter "A" serving to distinguish it from the *CDKN2B* gene, which is located just 20 kilobases away.

This gene is unique in that it contains two distinct reading frames, with two different promoters, the same DNA being used to synthesize two proteins that do not have a single amino acid sequence in common [23] (Fig. 3.23). The first reading frame to be discovered encodes p16, an inhibitor of cyclin-dependent kinases 4 and 6, which associates with cyclin D1 in G1 phase of the cell cycle (*The cell cycle,* p104). The p16 protein is thus an archetypal cell cycle "brake", its loss leading to increased cell proliferation and, more specifically, to escape from replicative senescence and extended cellular life span. The other reading frame, named p14ARF for "alternative reading frame" (often called by the same name as its mouse homologue, p19ARF), is synthesized from a different portion of the *CDKN2A* locus but shares one exon (exon 2) with p16. However, although the DNA sequence encoding the two products is identical, p16 and p14ARF use different reading frames of exon 2, such that their amino acid sequences are completely different. p14ARF is a protein that controls Mdm2, which in turn regulates p53 protein stability. Activation of p14ARF blocks Mdm2 and therefore results in p53 protein accumulation and activation. Thus the *CDKN2A* locus behaves as two unrelated but interlocked genes. The first gene, encoding p16, directly controls cell cycle progression and senescence. The second, encoding p14ARF, controls p53 and all its downstream anti-proliferative functions.

The *CDKN2A* locus is often altered by loss of alleles (which removes both p16 and p14ARF), by mutation (most frequently in exon 2, common to both gene products), and by hypermethylation. Increased methylation of specific regions of the DNA within the promoters and some of the coding regions prevents adequate transcription and decreases the levels of protein synthesized. Loss of expression due to hypermethylation may be the most frequent way of altering the *CDKN2A* locus in many forms of cancers, particularly carcinomas.

NAMING GENES AND PROTEINS

Conventionally, a gene (that is, a specific segment of DNA) is identified by a single name, in upper case and italicized (e.g. the oncogene *RAS*) that is indicative of the character or function of the protein encoded, which is designated by the same name, in lower case (ras in the case of the present example). Proteins are also named by reference to their molecular weight, with the corresponding gene in superscript (e.g. p21WAF1). The names of genes are often based on acronyms, and are generally the prerogative of the successful investigator. Identification of a novel gene is often followed by discovery of structurally related or "homologous" genes (and corresponding proteins) and these may be given names closely related to the first member of the "family" identified. Such an approach to nomenclature may be inadequate, for example, in those instances in which a single DNA segment encodes multiple proteins through alternative splicing of messenger RNA. Multiple names for the same gene or protein may arise because of independent discovery (and hence, naming) by different investigators. Thus, the cyclin-dependent kinase inhibitor *WAF1* is also known as *CDKN1A, CAP20, MDA-6, PIC-1* and *SDI-1*. In scientific writing, all such names are given in the first instance, after which a single name is used consistently in any one document. The latest estimates from the Human Genome Project suggest that there may be about 30,000 human genes.

Conventions for the naming of genes and proteins are subject to international agreement and are continuously subject to review (HUGO Gene Nomenclature Committee, http://www.gene.ucl.ac.uk/nomenclature/).

GEOGRAPHIC VARIATION IN MUTATION PATTERNS

Mutations in cancer genes are the direct consequence of attack on DNA by exogenous or endogenous agents or of errors in DNA repair systems. By analysing the type and the sequence context of such mutations, it is possible to form hypotheses regarding the nature of the mutagenic mechanism involved. The most interesting genes in this respect are those altered by missense point mutations, such as members of the *RAS* family, *CDKN2A/INK4A*, and, in particular, the *p53* gene.

The *p53* gene is the most frequently mutated gene in human cancer, with over 16,000 mutations reported and compiled in a database maintained at IARC (http://www.iarc.fr/p53). The diversity of these mutations allows the identification of patterns which vary depending on the tumour type, the geographic origin and the risk factors involved. These are often specific for particular agents that have caused these mutations. Thus *p53* gene mutations in cancers may be seen as "fingerprints" left by carcinogens in the human genome, which may help to identify the particular carcinogen involved.

A typical example of such a "fingerprint" is the mutation at codon 249 observed in liver cancers of patients from sub-Saharan Africa and Eastern Asia. In these regions, liver cancer is a consequence of chronic infection by hepatitis viruses and of dietary poisoning with aflatoxins, a

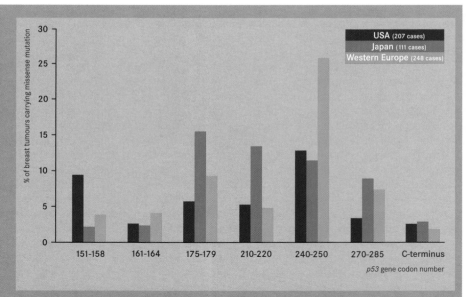

Fig. 3.24 Geographic variations in the prevalence of *p53* gene mutations in breast cancers.

class of mycotoxins which contaminates traditional diets (groundnuts) (*Food contaminants*, p43). Experiments in animals and in cell culture have shown that aflatoxins can directly induce the mutation at codon 249. This particular mutation is not found in liver cancers in areas of the world, such as the USA, where exposure to aflatoxins is low.

Specific mutations have also been observed in lung cancers from smokers (due to tobacco carcinogens). In skin cancers, the mutations bear typical chemical signatures of the damage inflicted to DNA by exposure to solar ultraviolet radiation. In other instances, exemplified by patterns of mutation in breast cancer, marked differ-

ences have been observed between geographical areas, which may provide information on the nature of risk factors involved.

In many other cancers, mutation patterns also vary from one region of the world to another. This variability may give clues about the genetic heterogeneity of populations, as well as about the diversity of agents involved in causing cancers. For example, in oesophageal cancers, mutation types widely differ between high-incidence and low-incidence regions, suggesting that specific mutagens are at work in causing the excess incidence seen in some parts of the world, such as Northern Iran and Central China.

Lesions in the p16INK4A–cyclin D, CDK4-pRb and p14ARF-Mdm2-p53 pathways occur so frequently in cancer, regardless of patient age or tumour type, that they appear to be fundamental to malignancy [24].

Prospects for the molecular analysis of cancer
More than 200 genes that are altered at variable proportions in different human

cancer types have been characterized. Most of these have a powerful impact on tumour growth. However, it is very likely that many critical genes with less penetrant phenotypes remain to be identified. In particular, the genes involved in stress reponses, in the control of oxygen metabolism and in the detoxification of xenobiotics are all candidates for a role as cofactors in the

cancer process. Moreover, many biological alterations leading to cancer may not be detectable at the DNA level. Cancer-causing changes may result from modification of RNA levels or processing, and of protein structure and function through a variety of epigenetic phenomena. The systematic profiling of gene expression in cancer cells will probably reveal a whole new set of potential cancer genes altered through less conspicuous mechanisms. Apart from expression studies, the whole territory of protein structure, dynamics and interactions is still largely unexplored. An understanding of such processes will provide a basis for the development of new means for treatment and diagnosis.

REFERENCES

1. Fearon ER, Vogelstein B (1990) A genetic model for colorectal tumorigenesis. *Cell*, 61: 759-767.

2. Weinberg RA (1995) The molecular basis of oncogenes and tumor suppressor genes. *Ann N Y Acad Sci*, 758: 331-338.

3. Savelyeva L, Schwab M (2001) Amplification of oncogenes revisited: from expression profiling to clinical application. *Cancer Lett*, 167: 115-123.

4. Kinzler KW, Vogelstein B (1997) Cancer-susceptibility genes. Gatekeepers and caretakers. *Nature*, 386: 761, 763.

5. Hanahan D, Weinberg RA (2000) The hallmarks of cancer. *Cell*, 100: 57-70.

6. Hunter T (1991) Cooperation between oncogenes. *Cell*, 64: 249-270.

7. Hung MC, Lau YK (1999) Basic science of HER-2/neu: a review. *Semin Oncol*, 26: 51-59.

8. Wiesmuller L, Wittinghofer F (1994) Signal transduction pathways involving Ras. Mini review. *Cell Signal*, 6: 247-267.

9. Henriksson M, Luscher B (1996) Proteins of the Myc network: essential regulators of cell growth and differentiation. *Adv Cancer Res*, 68: 109-182.

10. Antonsson B, Martinou JC (2000) The Bcl-2 protein family. *Exp Cell Res*, 256: 50-57.

11. Knudson AG (1996) Hereditary cancer: two hits revisited. *J Cancer Res Clin Oncol*, 122: 135-140.

12. Knudson AG, Jr. (1971) Mutation and cancer: statistical study of retinoblastoma. *Proc Natl Acad Sci U S A*, 68: 820-823.

13. Bartek J, Bartkova J, Lukas J (1997) The retinoblastoma protein pathway in cell cycle control and cancer. *Exp Cell Res*, 237: 1-6.

14. Lukas J, Muller H, Bartkova J, Spitkovsky D, Kjerulff AA, Jansen-Durr P, Strauss M, Bartek J (1994) DNA tumor virus oncoproteins and retinoblastoma gene mutations share the ability to relieve the cell's requirement for cyclin D1 function in G1. *J Cell Biol*, 125: 625-638.

15. Baker SJ, Fearon ER, Nigro JM, Hamilton SR, Preisinger AC, Jessup JM, vanTuinen P, Ledbetter DH, Barker DF, Nakamura Y (1989) Chromosome 17 deletions and p53 gene mutations in colorectal carcinomas. *Science*, 244: 217-221.

16. Birch JM (1994) Li-Fraumeni syndrome. *Eur J Cancer*, 30A: 1935-1941.

17. Bresalier RS (1997) The gatekeeper has many keys: dissecting the function of the APC gene. *Gastroenterology*, 113: 2009-2010.

18. Zheng L, Li S, Boyer TG, Lee WH (2000) Lessons learned from BRCA1 and BRCA2. *Oncogene*, 19: 6159-6175.

19. Shiloh Y, Rotman G (1996) Ataxia-telangiectasia and the ATM gene: linking neurodegeneration, immunodeficiency, and cancer to cell cycle checkpoints. *J Clin Immunol*, 16: 254-260.

20. Lane DP (1992) Cancer. p53, guardian of the genome. *Nature*, 358: 15-16.

21. Hainaut P, Hollstein M (2000) p53 and human cancer: the first ten thousand mutations. *Adv Cancer Res*, 77: 81-137.

22. Momand J, Jung D, Wilczynski S, Niland J (1998) The MDM2 gene amplification database. *Nucleic Acids Res*, 26: 3453-3459.

23. Chin L, Pomerantz J, DePinho RA (1998) The INK4a/ARF tumor suppressor: one gene—two products—two pathways. *Trends Biochem Sci*, 23: 291-296.

24. Sherr CJ (2000) The Pezcoller lecture: cancer cell cycles revisited. *Cancer Res*, 60: 3689-3695.

WEBSITES

American Tissue Type Collection:
http://www.atcc.org/

Centers for Disease Control and Prevention, Atlanta:
http://www.cdc.gov/

Cancer Genome Anatomy Project:
http://www.ncbi.nlm.nih.gov/ncicgap/

European Bioinformatics Institute:
http://www.ebi.ac.uk/

HotMolecBase (Weizmann Institute, Israel):
http://bioinformatics.weizmann.ac.il/hotmolecbase/

IARC p53 database:
http://www.iarc.fr/p53/homepage.htm

Kyoto encyclopedia of genes and genomes:
http://www.genome.ad.jp/kegg/kegg.html

OMIM (Online Mendelian Inheritance in Man):
http://www3.ncbi.nlm.nih.gov/omim/

Protein Data Bank (a protein structure database):
http://www.rcsb.org/pdb/

THE CELL CYCLE

SUMMARY

> The control of cell division is critical to normal tissue structure and function. It is regulated by a complex interplay of many genes that control the cell cycle, with DNA replication (S phase) and mitosis as major checkpoints.

> The cell cycle is tightly regulated to minimize transmission of genetic damage to subsequent cell generations.

> Progression through the cell cycle is primarily controlled by cyclins, associated kinases and their inhibitors. Retinoblastoma (*RB*) and *p53* are major suppressor genes involved in the G1/S checkpoint control.

> Cancer may be perceived as the consequence of loss of cell cycle control and progressive genetic instability.

Classically, the "cell cycle" refers to the set of ordered molecular and cellular processes during which genetic material is replicated and segregates between two newly generated daughter cells via the process of mitosis. The cell cycle can be divided into two phases of major morphological and biochemical change: M phase ("mitosis"), during which division is evident morphologically and S phase ("synthesis"), during which DNA is replicated. These two phases are separated by so-called G ("gap") phases. G1 precedes S phase and G2 precedes M phase.

During progression through this division cycle, the cell has to resolve a number of critical challenges. These include ensuring that sufficient ribonucleotides are available to complete DNA synthesis, proof-reading, editing and correcting the newly-synthesized DNA; that genetic material is not replicated more than once; that the spatial organization of the mitotic spindle apparatus is operational; that the packing and the condensation of chromosomes is optimal; and that there is equal distribu-tion of cellular materials between the daughter cells. Moreover, immediately before or after the cell cycle, various factors interact to determine whether the cell divides again or whether the cell becomes committed to a programme of differentiation or of cell death. Therefore, the term "cell cycle" is often used in a broad sense to refer to, as well as the basic, self-replicating cellular process, a number of connected processes which determine pre- and post-mitotic commitments. These may include the commitment to stop dividing in order to enter a quiescent state, to undergo senescence or differentiation, or to leave the quiescent state to re-enter mitosis.

Molecular architecture of the cell cycle

The molecular ordering of the cell cycle is a complex biological process dependent upon the sequential activation and inactivation of molecular effectors at specific points of the cycle. Most current knowledge of these processes stems from experiments carried out in the oocyte of the frog, *Xenopus laevis,* or in yeast, either *Saccharomyces cerevisiae* (budding yeast) or *Schizosaccharomyces pombe* (fission yeast). The *Xenopus* oocyte is, by many criteria, one of the easiest cells to manipulate in the laboratory. Its large size (over a millimetre in diameter) means that cell cycle progression can be monitored visually in single cells. Microinjections can be performed for the purpose of interfering with specific functions of the biochemical machinery of the cell cycle. The *Xenopus* oocyte has proven to be an invaluable tool in the study of the biochemistry of the cell cycle, allowing, among other findings, the elucidation of the composition and regulation of maturation promoting factor (MPF), a complex enzyme comprising a kinase (p34cdc2) and a regulatory subunit (cyclin B), which drives progression from G2 to M phase [1]. In contrast, the exceptional genetic plasticity of yeast has allowed the identification of scores of mutants with defects in cell cycle progression; in mam-malian cells, these mutations would have been lethal and it would therefore have been impossible to characterize them. These mutants were called "cdc", for cell division cycle mutants, and many of them have been accorded wider recognition through the application of their names to the mammalian homologues corresponding to the yeast genes.

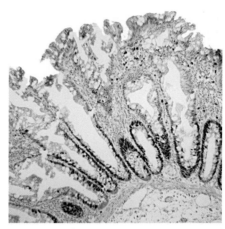

Fig. 3.25 Proliferating cells in the basal parts of the colonic crypts, visualized by immunohisto-chemistry (stained brown).

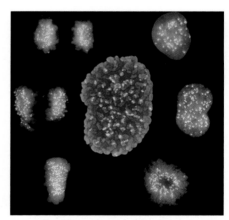

Fig. 3.26 A human osteosarcoma cell nucleus during mitosis. Cell division proceeds clockwise from upper right through interphase, prophase (centre), prometaphase, metaphase, anaphase and telophase. During the cycle, the chromo-somes are replicated, segregated and distributed equally between the two daughter cells.

One of the earliest genes to be identified in this way was *cdc2*. Isolated in *S. pombe*, *cdc2* was determined to be able to correct a G2 cell cycle arrest defect. The product of this gene, a serine-threonine kinase of molecular weight 32-34,000 daltons, was subsequently shown to be the yeast homologue of the kinase contained in the *Xenopus* MPF. This enzyme became the paradigm of a class of enzymes now called cyclin-dependent kinases, or CDKs. In their active form, CDKs form heterodimers with cyclins, a class of molecules synthesized in a time-dependent manner during the cell cycle. The progression of the cell cycle depends upon the sequential activation and inactivation of cyclin/CDK complexes [2], a process which requires the synthesis of cyclins, the formation of a complex between a specific cyclin and a CDK and post-translational modification of the CDK to convert the enzyme to an active form (Fig. 3.27).

Progression through the cell cycle as mediated by cyclins is, in turn, determined by factors categorized as having either regulatory (upstream) or effector (downstream) roles. Upstream of cyclin/CDKs are regulatory factors called cyclin-dependent kinase inhibitors (CDKIs), that regulate the assembly and the activity of cyclin/CDK complexes. Downstream of cyclin/CDKs are effector molecules, essentially transcription factors, which control the synthesis of proteins that mediate the molecular and cellular changes occurring during each phase.

CDKIs are small proteins that form complexes with both CDKs and cyclins [3]. Their role is primarily to inhibit the activities of cyclin/CDK complexes and to negatively regulate cell cycle progression. They constitute the receiving end of many of the molecular cascades signalling growth promotion or suppression of growth. Thus CDKIs may be considered as the interface between the cell cycle machinery and the network of molecular pathways which signal proliferation, death or stress responses. However, by virtue of their complexing properties, some CDKIs also play a positive role in cell cycle progression by facilitating the assembly of cyclin/CDK complexes. For example, p21, the product of the *CDKN1A* gene (also known as WAF1/CIP1), promotes the assembly of cyclin D/cdk2 complexes in G1 at a stoichiometric 1:1 ratio, but inhibits the activities of these complexes when expressed at higher levels. There are three main families of CDKIs, each with distinct structural and functional properties: the WAF1/CIP1 family (p21), the KIP family (p27, p57) and the INK4 family (p16, p15, p18) (Fig. 3.27).

Downstream effectors of cyclin/CDKs include proteins mediating three main functional categories: (1) those involved in the control of the enzymes responsible for DNA replication, proof-reading and repair, (2) those involved in chromosome and chromatin remodelling and in the control of genomic integrity and (3) those involved in the mechanics of cell division (including the formation of the centrosome and the mitotic spindle, and in the resorption of the nuclear membrane). These processes require the coordinated synthesis of hundreds of cellular proteins. Transcription factors of the E2F family play a critical role in the control of gene transcription during cell cycle progression (Fig. 3.28). In G1, factors of the E2F family are bound to their DNA targets but are maintained in a transcriptionally inactive state by the binding of proteins of the retinoblastoma (pRb) protein family. At the G1/S transition, the sequential phosphorylation of pRb by several cyclin/CDKs dissociates pRb from the complexes, allowing E2Fs to interact with transcription co-activators and to initiate mRNA synthesis [4].

Gene (chromosome)	Product	Type of alteration	Role in cell cycle	Involvement in cancer
p53 (17p13)	p53	Mutations, deletions	Control of p21, 14-3-3σ, etc.	Altered in over 50% of all cancers
CDKN2A (9p22)	p16 and p19ARF	Mutations, deletions, hypermethylation	Inhibition of CDK4 and 6	Altered in 30-60% of all cancers
RB1 (13q14)	pRb	Deletions	Inhibition of E2Fs	Lost in retinoblastomas, altered in 5-10% of other cancers.
CCND1	Cyclin D1	Amplification	Progression into G1	10-40% of many carcinomas
CDC25A, CDC25B	cdc25	Overexpression	Progression in G1, G2	10-50% of many carcinomas
KIP1	p27	Down-regulation	Progression in G1/S	Breast, colon and prostate cancers

Table 3.3 Cell cycle regulatory genes commonly altered in human cancers.

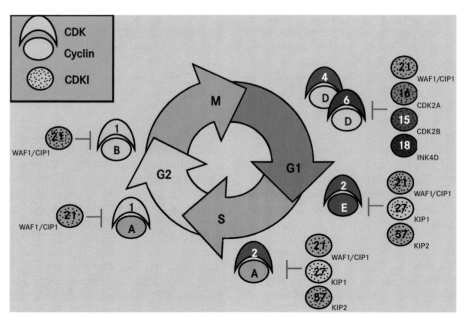

Fig. 3.27 The progression of the cell cycle depends upon the sequential activation and inactivation of cyclin/CDK complexes. This process requires the synthesis of cyclins, the formation of a complex between a specific cyclin and a CDK, and modification of the CDK to convert this enzyme to an active form. The enzyme's activity may be disrupted by a specific inhibitor, a CDKI.

Through this mechanism, E2Fs exert a dual function both as transcriptional repressors in G1, when bound to pRb, and as transcriptional activators in G1/S and in S phase, after dissociation of pRb from the complex. Recent observations suggest that transcriptional repression by E2Fs is essential to prevent the premature activation of cell cycle effectors, which would scramble the temporal sequence of molecular events and preclude cell cycle progression.

Cell cycle checkpoints

The notion of "cell cycle checkpoints" is also derived from early studies in *Xenopus* oocytes and in yeast mutants. In *S. cerevisiae*, commitment to the mitotic cycle requires the crossing of a "restriction point" called the *start* transition. Failure to cross this transition results in cells being blocked in the G1 phase of the cycle. Another control point has been clearly identified after S phase, at the transition between G2 and M phases. Cells unable to cross this checkpoint may remain blocked in a pre-mitotic, tetraploid state. Physiologically, this checkpoint is active in

germ cells during the second division of meiosis: cells that have undergone the first, asymmetric division of the meiotic cycle arrest in G2 until completing the second division, which is triggered by fertilization. This concept of "cell cycle checkpoints" was later extended to all mammalian cells [5]. It is now common to envisage the mammalian cell cycle as a succession of checkpoints that have to be negotiated in order for division to be achieved. There is no clear agreement on how many such checkpoints exist in the mammalian cell cycle, or on their exact position.

Control of cdk1 at G2/M transition

The regulation of the complex between cdk1 (also called p34cdc2) and cyclin B exemplifies how different factors co-operate to control the activation of cyclin/CDK complexes at a cell cycle checkpoint. This activation process requires co-operation between three levels of regulation: association between the two partners of the complex, post-translational modifications of the kinase and of the cyclin, and escape from the negative regulation exerted by the CDKIs.

In early G2, cdk1 is in an inactive form. Its activation requires first association with cyclin B, followed by post-translational modification of the kinase itself. This modification includes phosphorylation of a conserved threonine residue (Thr161) by a kinase complex called CAK (CDK-activating kinase), as well as dephosphorylation of two residues localized within the active site of the enzyme, a threonine (Thr14) and a tyrosine (Tyr15). The removal of these phosphate groups is carried out by the dual-specificity phosphatases of the cdc25 group, comprising three isoforms in humans (A, B and C). Activation of these phosphatases is therefore crucial for the activation of cyclin B/cdk1 complexes. The phosphatase is directly controlled by a number of regulators, including plk1 (polo-like kinase), an activating kinase, pp2A, (protein phosphatase 2A), an inhibitory phosphatase and 14-3-3s, a signal transduction molecule which complexes with cdc25, sequesters it in the cytoplasm and thus prevents it from dephosphorylating its nuclear targets. Of course, the action of cdc25 phosphatases is counteracted by kinases that restore the phosphorylation of Thr14 and Tyr15, named wee1 and mik1 [6].

Following the activation process outlined above, the cyclin B/cdk1 complex is potentially able to catalyse transfer of phosphates to substrate proteins. However, in order to achieve this, it has to escape the control exerted by CDKIs, such as p21. The function of this CDKI is itself controlled by several activators, including BRCA1, the product of a breast cancer susceptibility gene (*Oncogenes and tumour suppressor genes,* p96). The p21 protein is removed from the complex by a still poorly understood phosphorylation process, which also drives rapid degradation of the protein by the proteasome. This leaves the cyclin B/cdk1 complex ready to function, after a final step of autophosphorylation, in which cdk1 phosphorylates cyclin B. The complex is now fully active and ready to phosphorylate many different substrates, such as nuclear lamins, during entry into mitosis.

Regulation of the cell cycle and control of genetic stability

During the cell cycle, a number of potential problems may result in damage to the genome. These problems may arise at three distinct stages: (1) during DNA replication, especially if the cell is under conditions of stress that favour the formation of DNA damage (irradiation, exposure to carcinogens etc.), (2) following the termination of DNA replication, when the cell effectively "switches off" its DNA synthesis machinery and (3) during M phase, when the cell has to negotiate the delicate task of segregating chromatids equally. A tight coupling between these processes and cell cycle regulation is therefore crucial to allow the cell to pause during the cell cycle in order to afford the time necessary for the successful completion of all the operations of DNA and chromosome maintenance. Failure to do this may result in both genetic and genomic instabilities, which are hallmarks of cancer. Genetic instability is characterized by an increased rate of gene mutation, deletion or recombination (essentially due to defects in DNA repair). Genomic instability results in chromosome translocations, loss or duplication of large chromosome fragments and aberrant chromosome numbers (aneuploidy).

Tens of molecules have been identified as components of the signalling cascades which couple detection of DNA damage and regulation of the cell cycle. One of these is the product of the tumour suppressor gene *p53* (*Oncogenes and tumour suppressor genes*, p96). *p53* is specifically activated after various forms of direct DNA damage (such as single or double strand breaks in DNA) and regulates the transcription of several inhibitors of cell cycle progression, particularly at the G1/S and G2/M transitions [7]. Other important molecules in this coupling process include the checkpoint kinases chk1 and chk2. Chk1 is activated after replication blockage during S-phase. In turn, chk1 activates wee1 and mik1, two kinases that counteract the action of cdc25 and keep cdk1 in an inactive form. Thus, through activation of chk1, the cell triggers an emergency mechanism that ensures that cells with incompletely replicated DNA cannot enter mitosis.

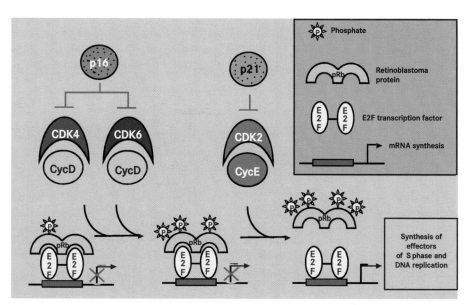

Fig. 3.28 Progression from G1 to S phase is regulated by phosphorylation of the retinoblastoma protein (pRb), in the absence of which DNA replication cannot proceed.

The cell cycle and cancer

Genes involved in cell cycle control are important among those subject to the genetic alterations that give rise to cancer [8]. However, the proliferation of cancer cells requires that the cells retain functional cell cycle processes. The cell cycle alterations seen in cancer are mainly confined to two major sets of regulators: those involved in the negative control of cell cycle progression (inactivation of which leads to accelerated and unchecked cell proliferation) and those involved in coupling the maintenance of genome integrity to the cell cycle (inactivation of which results in cells having gene alterations that progressively accumulate during carcinogenesis) (Table 3.3) [9]. Most of the genes corresponding to these two categories fall within the group of tumour suppressors, and many of them are also direct participants in DNA repair processes.

The gene which encodes p16 (*CDKN2A/ INK4A*) has been established as a tumour suppressor gene [10], and mutations and deletions at this site are commonly found in primary human tumours, especially melanoma (although the contribution of another protein encoded by the same locus on chromosome 9p, p14[ARF], to sup-

pressor activity remains to be determined). Unlike the *CDKN2A/INK4A* gene, the *CDKN1A* gene (encoding p21) is rarely disrupted in cancer. As p21 plays many roles in the negative regulation of almost all phases of the cell cycle, loss of this function might be expected to result in uncontrolled cell division. This is apparently not the case, as mice lacking the *CDKN1A* gene do not show an increased frequency of cancer. This observation illustrates one of the most important characteristics of cell cycle regulatory mechanisms: there is a large degree of redundancy and overlap in the function of any particular effector. Therefore, cancer-causing deregulation of the cell cycle requires a combination of many alterations in genes encoding proteins that, either alone or in concert, are critical for the control of cell division.

Apart from inactivation of negative regulators, a few cell cycle genes may be activated as oncogenes, in that their alteration results in enhanced activity leading to accelerated cell proliferation. The best example of such a cell cycle oncogene is *CCND1*, the gene encoding cyclin D1, a G1-specific cyclin [11]. This gene is located on chromosome 11p13, within a large region that is amplified in up to 20% of several carcinomas (e.g. breast, head and neck, oesophageal and lung cancers). There is also limited evidence for transcriptional activation of cyclin A (an S-phase cyclin) and for activating mutations of CDK4 (one of the partners of cyclin D1) in some cancers. Indeed, the high complexity of cell cycle effectors provides an extremely diverse range of possibilities for cancer-associated alterations. In this respect, cancer can be seen as, fundamentally, a disease of the cell cycle.

TELOMERES AND TELOMERASE

The ends of eukaryotic chromosomes are referred to as telomeres. These contain many copies of a repetitive DNA sequence, which in vertebrates is the hexanucleotide TTAGGG. The telomeres of normal human somatic cells shorten by 50 to 150 base pairs every time cell division occurs. This appears to act as a cell division counting mechanism: when a cell's telomeres have shortened below a critical length, the cell exits permanently from the cell cycle. Normal cells thus have a limited proliferative capacity, and this acts as a major barrier against carcinogenesis. Cells that have accumulated some carcinogenic changes are unable to form clinically significant cancers unless this proliferation barrier is breached. More than 85% of all cancers achieve this by expressing an enzyme, telomerase, that synthesizes new telomeric DNA to replace the sequences lost during cell division (Shay JW, Bacchetti S, *Eur J Cancer*, 33A: 787-791, 1997).

Telomerase assays have not yet entered routine clinical practice, but there is considerable interest in their possible use for cancer diagnosis and prognosis. For example, telomerase assays of urine sediments may be useful for diagnosis of urinary tract cancer (Kinoshita H et al., *J Natl Cancer Inst*, 89: 724-730, 1997), and telomerase activity levels may be a predictor of outcome in neuroblastoma (Hiyama E et al., *Nature Medicine*, 1: 249-255, 1995).

The catalytic subunit of human telomerase, hTERT, was cloned in 1997 (Lingner J, Cech TR, *Curr Opin Genet Dev* 8: 226-232, 1998). It has subsequently been shown that genetic manipulations of hTERT which result in inhibition of telomerase activity in tumour cells limit their proliferation and often result in cell death. This raises the possibility that telomerase inhibitors may be a very useful form of therapy for many or most types of cancer. However, in tumours with long telomeres, it may take many cell divisions before telomerase inhibitors exert an anti-tumour effect. When such drugs are developed they will therefore need to be carefully integrated with other anticancer treatments.

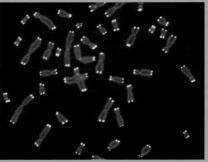

Fig. 3.29 Telomeres contain repetitive DNA sequences that cap the ends of chromosomes. Quantitative fluorescence *in situ* hybridization analysis of human metaphase chromosome spreads is shown, using oligonucleotide probes specific for telomere (white) and centromere (red) DNA sequences, and the DNA dye DAPI (blue). From the laboratory of Drs J.W. Shay and W.E. Wright.

A potential challenge facing telomerase research is the finding that some cancers maintain their telomeres by a mechanism that does not involve telomerase, referred to as alternative lengthening of telomeres, ALT (Bryan TM et al., *Nature Medicine*, 3: 1271-1274, 1997; Reddel RR, *J Clin Invest*, 108: 665-667, 2001).

REFERENCES

1. Hunt T (1989) Maturation promoting factor, cyclin and the control of M-phase. *Curr Opin Cell Biol*, 1: 268-274.

2. Pines J (1995) Cyclins and cyclin-dependent kinases: a biochemical view. *Biochem J*, 308 (Pt 3): 697-711.

3. Sherr CJ, Roberts JM (1999) CDK inhibitors: positive and negative regulators of G1-phase progression. *Genes Dev*, 13: 1501-1512.

4. Weinberg RA (1995) The retinoblastoma protein and cell cycle control. *Cell*, 81: 323-330.

5. Hartwell LH, Weinert TA (1989) Checkpoints: controls that ensure the order of cell cycle events. *Science*, 246: 629-634.

6. Zeng Y, Forbes KC, Wu Z, Moreno S, Piwnica-Worms H, Enoch T (1998) Replication checkpoint requires phosphorylation of the phosphatase Cdc25 by Cds1 or Chk1. *Nature*, 395: 507-510.

7. Hainaut P, Hollstein M (2000) p53 and human cancer: the first ten thousand mutations. *Adv Cancer Res*, 77: 81-137.

8. Hartwell LH, Kastan MB (1994) Cell cycle control and cancer. *Science*, 266: 1821-1828.

9. Kinzler KW, Vogelstein B (1997) Cancer-susceptibility genes. Gatekeepers and caretakers. *Nature*, 386: 761, 763.

10. Strohmaier H, Spruck CH, Kaiser P, Won KA, Sangfelt O, Reed SI (2001) Human F-box protein hCdc4 targets cyclin E for proteolysis and is mutated in a breast cancer cell line. *Nature*, 413: 316-322.

11. Schuuring E (1995) The involvement of the chromosome 11q13 region in human malignancies: cyclin D1 and EMS1 are two new candidate oncogenes—a review. *Gene*, 159: 83-96.

WEBSITES

Animation of the phases of the cell cycle and of mitosis: http://www.cellsalive.com/

Nature Reviews, "Focus on cell division": http://www.nature.com/ncb/celldivision/

The Forsburg laboratory home pages, a guide to the cell cycle and DNA replication in *S. pombe*: http://pingu.salk.edu/~forsburg/lab.html

CELL-CELL COMMUNICATION

SUMMARY

> Cells communicate by means of secreted molecules which affect neighbouring cells carrying appropriate receptors, and also by direct cell contact, including specifically includes gap junctions.

> Cell contact-mediated communication through gap junctions is controlled by connexin genes and is often disrupted in cancer. This may contribute to uncontrolled and autonomous growth.

> Interventions restoring gap junction communication may provide a basis for therapy.

In complex organisms, neighbouring cells behave and function in harmony for the benefit of the whole organism through the operation of cell-cell communication. During evolution, various types of intercellular communication have developed, which in mammals take two forms: (1) humoral communication and (2) cell contact-mediated communication (Fig. 3.30). Humoral communication is typically mediated by molecules, such as growth factors and hormones, excreted from certain cells and received by receptors of other cells. Intercellular communication based on direct cell-cell contact is mediated by various junctions, including adherence junctions, desmosomes and gap junctions. During multistage carcinogenesis, genes critically involved in cell growth are altered [1]. Most such genes are known to be directly or indirectly involved in the control of cell replication (*The cell cycle*, p104) or in the death of individual cells [2] (*Apoptosis*, p113). Genes involved in intercellular communication control cellular growth at another level. These genes function to maintain cell growth in harmony with that of the surrounding tissue. Since most cancer cells do not proliferate in har-

mony with normal neighbouring cells, it is not surprising that the function of genes involved in intercellular communication mechanisms is disrupted in many tumours. Thus, several oncogenes (*Oncogenes and tumour suppressor genes*, p96) encode products involved in humoral intercellular communication: c-erb, c-erbB2 and c-SIS [3]. It has also become clear that cell contact-mediated intercellular communication plays a crucial role in cell growth control [4] and genes involved are often classified as tumour suppressor genes [5]. Cell adhesion molecules are also involved in cell-cell recognition. There are several lines of evidence which suggest that aberrant functions of cell adhesion may be involved in tumour invasion and metastasis [6].

Gap junctional intercellular communication and cancer

Gap junctional intercellular communication is the only means by which cells exchange signals directly from the interior of one cell to the interior of surrounding cells [7]. Since the extent to which tumour cells deviate from cells which exhibit tissue homeostasis is fundamen-

tal to the nature of malignancy, it has long been postulated that gap junctional intercellular communication is disturbed in cancer. The first confirmatory evidence was the observation that of a reduced level of gap junctional intercellular communication in one tumour type [8]. This phenomenon has now been observed in almost all tumours [4]. Cell lines established from tumours, as well as cells transformed *in vitro*, usually exhibit impaired function in respect of gap junctional intercellular communication. Gap junctional intercellular communication between transformed cells and neighbouring normal counterparts is selectively defective in murine embryonic BALB/c3T3 cells (Fig. 3.31). A lack of heterologous gap junctional intercellular communication between transformed and normal cells has been observed using rat liver epithelial cell lines and rat liver tumour *in vivo*. It appears that reduced gap junctional intercellular communication is common to many tumour cells. Further studies with multistage models of rat liver and mouse skin carcinogenesis have revealed that there is, in general, a progressive decrease in the level of gap

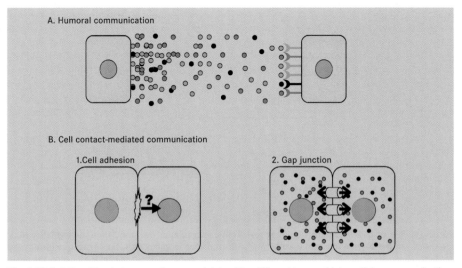

Fig. 3.30 Relationships between cells are maintained by different types of intercellular communication, which may (**B**) or may not (**A**) require cell contact.

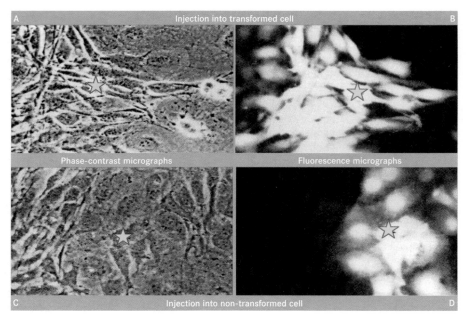

Fig. 3.31 Selective gap junctional communication: cells transformed by a chemical carcinogen (spindle-shaped and criss-crossed) communicate among themselves, but not with their surrounding non-transformed counterparts. When a gap junction-diffusible fluorescent dye is microinjected into a single cell (marked with star) of a transformed focus there is communication between transformed cells but not with the surrounding non-transformed cells (A, B). Injection of the dye into a non-transformed cell which is located near a transformed focus results in communication between non-transformed cells, but not with transformed cells (C, D).

junctional intercellular communication during carcinogenesis and tumour progression.

Another line of evidence, that implies a causal role for blockage of intercellular communication in carcinogenesis, is that agents or genes involved in carcinogenesis have been shown to modulate gap junctional intercellular communication. The mouse skin tumour-promoting agent 12-O-tetradecanoylphorbol 13-acetate (TPA) inhibits gap junctional intercellular communication. Many other tumour-promoting agents inhibit gap junctional intercellular communication [9]. In addition to such chemicals, other tumour-promoting stimuli, such as partial hepatectomy and skin wounding, have been demonstrated to inhibit gap junctional intercellular communication. Activation of various oncogenes, including those which encode src, SV-40 T antigen, c-erbB2/neu, raf, fps and ras, also results in inhibition of gap junctional intercellular communication. Conversely, some chemopreventive agents enhance gap junctional intercellular communication [10].

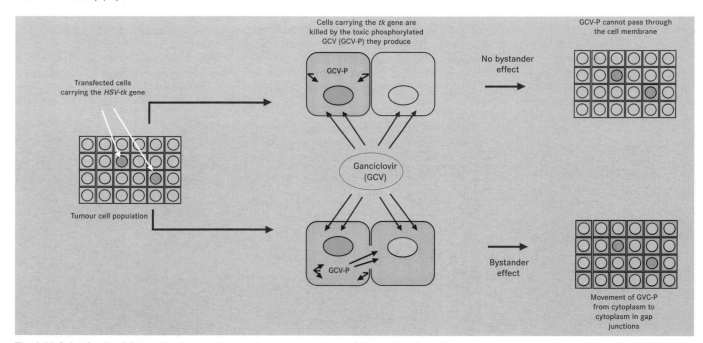

Fig. 3.32 Role of cell-cell interaction in gene therapy. In a tumour cell population, only a few cells can be reached by vectors carrying the HSV-tk gene. Expression of the tk gene (orange) makes these cells sensitive to ganciclovir: they produce phosphorylated ganciclovir, which is toxic. As phosphorylated ganciclovir cannot pass through the cell membrane, theoretically only cells expressing the tk gene will die as a result of ganciclovir treatment. Transmembrane diffusion of phosphorylated ganciclovir from cytoplasm to cytoplasm can induce a bystander effect sufficient to eradicate a tumour cell population, even if only a few cells express the tk gene [13].

Connexin genes and tumour suppression

The first indication that normal cells may suppress the growth of malignant cells with which they are in contact came from the work of Stoker and colleagues [11]. More recent evidence for such a direct role of gap junctional intercellular communication in tumour suppression has come from experiments in which connexin genes were transfected into gap junctional intercellular communication-deficient malignant cell lines. In many cases, connexin gene expression reduced or eliminated tumorigenicity of recipient cells [10].

Although tumour suppressor genes, most notably p53, are mutated in a high proportion of tumours, few mutations of connexin genes have yet been found in rodent tumours and none has been reported for any human cancer. Although this suggests that connexin gene mutations are rare in carcinogenesis, only a few studies (all from one laboratory) on a limited number of connexin genes (Cx32, Cx37[α4] and Cx43) have been conducted. Several polymorphisms in connexin genes in humans and rats have been described, although there was no apparent correlation between such polymorphisms and the cancer sites examined [10].

Enhancement of cancer therapy by cell-cell communication

A decade ago it was demonstrated that gap junctional intercellular communication could be exploited to distribute therapeutic agents among cancer cells and thereby enhance cancer therapy [12]. One principle of gene therapy is the mediation of selective cytotoxicity by the introduction, into malignant cells, of a gene that activates an otherwise innocuous drug. In practice, only a fraction of the total number of tumour cells sought to be eliminated, are successfully transfected with the gene in question. However, at least in the case of brain tumour therapy based upon the thymidine kinase gene from herpes simplex virus (HSV-tk), not only are the cells transfected with the gene affected by treatment with the drug ganciclovir, but neighbouring cells are also killed in the presence of ganciclovir. Several studies have provided strong evidence that this phenomenon, termed "the bystander effect" (Fig. 3.32), is due to connexin-mediated gap junctional intercellular communication; that is, ganciclovir phosphorylated by HSV-tk can diffuse through gap junctions and even those cells without HSV-tk gene can be killed. The role of connexin genes in this effect has been confirmed [13].

Signal transduction from intercellular network

The main physiological function of gap junctional intercellular communication is probably to maintain homeostasis by keeping the level of signals mediated by agents of low molecular weight at equilibrium among cells linked by gap junctions. This implies that intercellular communication may control cell growth indirectly. As already noted, such an activity is distinct from that mediated by genes which are directly involved in cell growth and death. One particularly important pathway linking intercellular interaction to signal transduction involves the cell adhesion molecule β-catenin. If the level of β-catenin in the cytoplasm and nucleus rises, it activates transcription factors of the TCF(T-cell factor)/LEF family and increases activity of genes including C-MYC, cyclin D1 and connexin-43. Normally the levels of β-catenin in the cytoplasm and nucleus are kept very low because a complex of proteins including the APC gene product (adenomatous polyposis coli, Colorectal cancer, p198), axin and glycogen synthesis kinase 3β bind the free β-catenin and put a phosphate group onto it which marks it for destruction [14].

In normal cells the level of free β-catenin is regulated by the Wnt ("wingless homologue") signal from outside the cell, which

Gene	Cancer site/cancer	Changes observed
Integrin	Skin, liver, lung, osteosarcoma	Reduced expression
E-cadherin	Stomach, colon, breast, prostate	Mutations: reduced expression
α-catenin	Stomach, colon, breast, prostate, oesophagus, kidney, bladder, etc	Reduced expression
β-catenin	Melanoma, colon	Mutations: reduced expression
γ-catenin	Breast, colon	Loss of expression, translocation into nuclei
Connexins	Liver, skin etc	Reduced expression, aberrant localization

Table 3.4 Examples of cell-cell interaction genes involved in carcinogenesis [10].

increases the level by transiently reducing the activity of the kinase. However, mutations in either the *APC* gene or in the part of the β-catenin (*CTNNB1*) gene which codes for the part of the molecule which accepts the phosphate allow the levels of β-catenin to rise; when this happens the TCF/LEF-controlled genes are permanently activated. The fact that mutations of the *CTNNB1*, *AXIN1*, *AXIN2* and *APC* genes occur in many cancers, including those of the colon, breast and endometrium, shows the importance of this pathway and emphasizes the connection between cell-cell contact and signal transduction.

REFERENCES

1. Fearon ER, Vogelstein B (1990) A genetic model for colorectal tumorigenesis. *Cell*, 61: 759-767.

2. Kinzler KW, Vogelstein B (1997) Cancer-susceptibility genes. Gatekeepers and caretakers. *Nature*, 386: 761, 763.

3. Heldin CH (1996) Protein tyrosine kinase receptors. *Cancer Surv*, 27: 7-24.

4. Krutovskikh V, Yamasaki H (1997) The role of gap junctional intercellular communication (GJIC) disorders in experimental and human carcinogenesis. *Histol Histopathol*, 12: 761-768.

5. Hirohashi S (1998) Inactivation of the E-cadherin-mediated cell adhesion system in human cancers. *Am J Pathol*, 153: 333-339.

6. Birchmeier EJ, Behrens J (1994) Cadherin expression in carcinoma: Role in the formation of cell junctions and prevention of invasiveness. *Biochim Biophys Acta*, 1198: 11-26.

7. Bruzzone R, White TW, Paul DL (1996) Connections with connexins: the molecular basis of direct intercellular signaling. *Eur J Biochem*, 238: 1-27.

8. Loewenstein WR, Kanno Y (1966) Intercellular communication and the control of tissue growth: lack of communication between cancer cells. *Nature*, 209: 1248-1249.

9. Trosko JE, Chang CC, Madhukar BV, Klaunig JE (1990) Chemical, oncogene and growth factor inhibition gap junctional intercellular communication: an integrative hypothesis of carcinogenesis. *Pathobiology*, 58: 265-278.

10. Yamasaki H, Omori Y, Zaidan-Dagli ML, Mironov N, Mesnil M, Krutovskikh V (1999) Genetic and epigenetic changes of intercellular communication genes during multistage carcinogenesis. *Cancer Detect Prev*, 23: 273-279.

11. Stoker MG (1967) Transfer of growth inhibition between normal and virus-transformed cells: autoradiographic studies using marked cells. *J Cell Sci*, 2: 293-304.

12. Yamasaki H, Katoh F (1988) Novel method for selective killing of transformed rodent cells through intercellular communication, with possible therapeutic applications. *Cancer Res*, 48: 3203-3207.

13. Mesnil M, Yamasaki H (2000) Bystander effect in herpes simplex virus-thymidine kinase/ganciclovir cancer gene therapy: role of gap-junctional intercellular communication. *Cancer Res*, 60: 3989-3999.

14. Behrens J, Jerchow BA, Wurtele M, Grimm J, Asbrand C, Wirtz R, Kuhl M, Wedlich D, Birchmeier W (1998) Functional interaction of an axin homolog, conductin, with beta-catenin, APC, and GSK3beta. *Science*, 280: 596-599.

APOPTOSIS

SUMMARY

> The term apoptosis refers to a type of cell death that occurs both physiologically and in response to external stimuli, including X-rays and anticancer drugs.

> Apoptotic cell death is characterized by distinctive morphological changes different from those occurring during necrosis, which follows ischaemic injury or toxic damage.

> Apoptosis is regulated by several distinct signalling pathways. Dysregulation of apoptosis may result in disordered cell growth and thereby contribute to carcinogenesis.

> Selective induction of apoptosis in tumour cells is among current strategies for the development of novel cancer therapies.

Apoptosis is a mode of cell death that facilitates such fundamental processes as development (for example, by removal of unwanted tissue during embryogenesis) and the immune response (for example, by elimination of self-reactive T cells). This type of cell death is distinguished from necrosis both morphologically (Fig. 3.33) and functionally. Specifically, apoptosis involves single cells rather than areas of tissue and does not provoke inflammation. Tissue homeostasis is dependent on controlled elimination of unwanted cells, often in the context of a continuum in which specialization and maturation is ultimately succeeded by cell death in what may be regarded as the final phase of differentiation. Apart from elimination in a physiological context, cells that have been lethally exposed to cytotoxic drugs or radiation may be subject to apoptosis.

The process of apoptosis can be described by reference to distinct phases, termed "regulation", "effector" and "engulfing" respectively [1]. The regulatory phase includes all the signalling pathways that culminate in commitment to cell death. Some of these pathways regulate only cell death, but many of them have overlapping roles in the control of cell proliferation, differentiation, responses to stress and homeostasis. Critical to apoptosis signalling are the "initiator" caspases (including caspase-8, caspase-9 and caspase-10) whose role is to activate the more abundant "effector" caspases (including caspase-3 and caspase-7) which, in turn, brings about the morphological change indicative of apoptosis. Finally, the engulfing process involves the recognition of cellular "remains" and their elimination by the engulfing activity of surrounding cells.

Identification of genes mediating apoptosis in human cells has been critically dependent on definition of the *ced* genes in the nematode *Caenorhabditis elegans*, members of this gene family being variously homologous to human *BCL2* (which suppresses apoptosis), *APAF-1* (which mediates caspase activation) and the caspases themselves (proteases which mediate cell death). The centrality of apoptosis to cancer biology is indicated by excess tumorigenesis in *BCL2*-transgenic and *p53*-deficient mice. An appreciation of apoptosis provides a basis for the further development of novel and conventional cancer therapy

The role of cell death in tumour growth

Apoptosis, or lack of it, may be critical to tumorigenesis [2]. *BCL2*, a gene mediating resistance to apoptotic stimuli, was discovered at the t(14:18) chromosomal

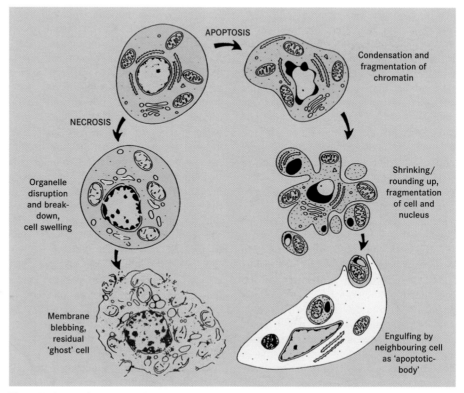

Fig. 3.33 Apoptosis and necrosis are distinguished by characteristic morphological changes.

translocation in low grade B cell non-Hodgkin lymphoma. It thus became apparent that neoplastic cell expansion could be attributable to decreased cell death rather than rapid proliferation. Defects in apoptosis allow neoplastic cells to survive beyond senescence, thereby providing protection from hypoxia and oxidative stress as the tumour mass expands. Growth of tumours, specifically in response to chemical carcinogens, has been correlated with altered rates of apoptosis in affected tissues as cell populations with altered proliferative activity emerge. Paradoxically, growth of some cancers, specifically including breast, has been positively correlated with increasing apoptosis [3].

Interrelationships between mitogenic and apoptotic pathways

A dynamic relationship between regulation of growth/mitosis and apoptosis may be demonstrated using a variety of relevant signalling pathways. Many differing promoters of cell proliferation have been found to possess pro-apoptotic activity [4]. Thus, ectopic expression of the *C-MYC* oncogene (normally associated with proliferative activity) causes apoptosis in cultured cells subjected to serum deprivation (which otherwise prevents proliferation). Oncogenes that stimulate mitogenesis can also activate apoptosis. These include oncogenic *RAS*, *MYC* and *E2F*. Mutations in *E2F* that prevent its interaction with the retinoblastoma protein (pRb) accelerate S phase entry and apoptosis. A function of pRb is to suppress apoptosis: pRb-deficient cells seem to be more susceptible to p53-induced apoptosis.

Agents such as radiation or cytotoxic drugs cause cell cycle arrest and/or cell death [5]. The DNA damage caused by radiation or drugs is detected by various means (Fig. 3.34). DNA-dependent protein kinase and the ataxia-telangiectasia mutated gene (*ATM*) (as well as the related ATR protein) bind to damaged DNA and initiate phosphorylation cascades to transmit damage signals. DNA-dependent protein kinase is believed to play a key role in the response to double-stranded DNA breaks. ATM plays an important part in the response to DNA

damage caused by ionizing radiation, controlling the initial phosphorylation of proteins such as p53, Mdm2, BRCA1, Chk2 and Nbs1. Other sensors of DNA damage include mammalian homologues of the PCNA-like yeast proteins Rad1, Rad9 and Hus1, as well as the yeast homologue of replication factor C, Rad17. Specific molecules detect nucleotide mismatch or inappropriate methylation. Following exposure of mammalian cells to DNA-damaging agents, p53 is activated and among many "targets" consequently upregulated are the cyclin-dependent kinase inhibitor p21 (which causes G1 arrest) and Bax (which induces apoptosis). Thus, the tumour suppressor gene *p53* mediates two responses to DNA damage by radiation or cytotoxic drugs: cell cycle arrest at the G1 phase of the cell cycle and apoptosis (*Oncogenes and tumour suppressor genes*, p96). The serine/threonine kinase Chk2 is also able to positively interact with p53 and BRCA1. Chk2 and the functionally related Chk1 kinase appear to have a role in the inhibition of entry into mitosis via inhibition of the phosphatase Cdc25 (*The cell cycle*, p104).

The regulatory phase

Two major apoptotic signalling pathways have been identified in mammalian cells (Fig. 3.37). The "extrinsic" pathway

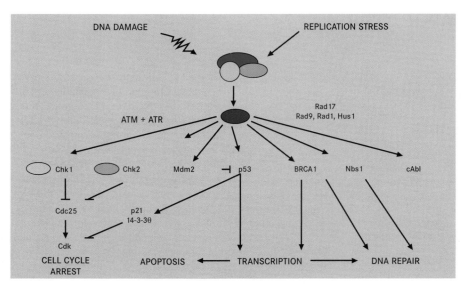

Fig. 3.34 Response to DNA damage is mediated by several signalling pathways and may include apoptosis.

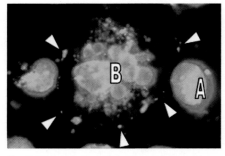

Fig. 3.35 Apoptotic cell death requires gap junctional intercellular communication. Expression and subcellular location of connexin 43 in healthy (A) and in apoptotic (B) rat bladder carcinoma cells. Arrows indicate location of connexin 43 in areas of intercellular contact between apoptotic (B) and non-apoptotic (A) cells. Counterstaining of DNA with propidium iodide reveals fragmentation of the nucleus typical of apoptosis (B).

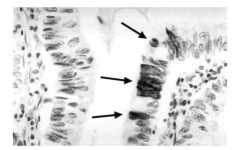

Fig. 3.36 Apoptotic cells in an adenoma, visualized by immunohistochemistry (red). Apoptosis is restricted to single cells, unlike necrosis, which typically involves groups of cells. Apoptosis does not produce an inflammatory response.

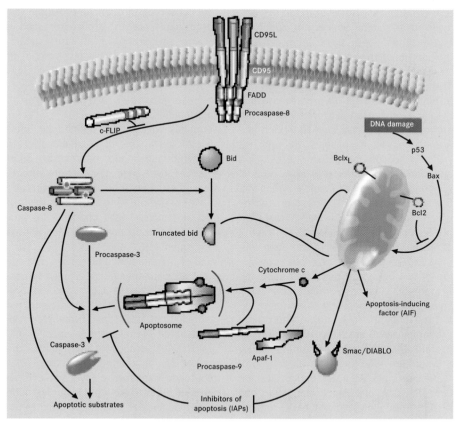

Fig. 3.37 Apoptosis occurs when specific proteases (caspases) digest critical proteins in the cell. The caspases are normally present as inactive procaspases. Two pathways lead to their activation. The death receptor pathway (at the top and left side of the figure) is triggered when ligands bind to death receptors such as CD95/Fas. The mitochondrial pathway is triggered by internal insults such as DNA damage as well as by extracellular signals. In both pathways, procaspases are brought together. They then cleave each other to release active caspase. The binding of ligand (FasL or CD95L) to CD95 brings procaspase 8 molecules together; release of mitochondrial components bring procaspases 9 together. The active caspase 8 and 9 then activate other procaspases such as procaspase 3.

depends upon the conformational change in certain cell surface receptors following the binding of respective ligands. The "intrinsic" pathway involves mitochondrial function and is initiated by growth factor deprivation, corticosteroids or DNA damage induced by radiation or cytotoxic drugs.

Cell surface receptors
Apoptosis may be induced by signalling molecules, usually polypeptides such as growth factors or related molecules, which bind to "death" receptors on the cell surface [6]. Such cell death was initially investigated in relation to the immune response, but has much wider ramifications. The best-characterized receptors belong to the tumour necrosis factor (*TNF*) receptor gene superfamily [7]. In addition to a ligand-binding domain, death receptors contain homologous cytoplasmic sequence termed the "death domain". Members of the family include Fas/APO-1/CD95 and TNF-1 receptor (which binds TNFα). Activation of the Fas (or CD95) receptor by its specific ligand (FasL or CD95L) results in a conformational change such that the "death domain" interacts with the adaptor molecule FADD which then binds procaspase-8. In some cell types, drug-induced apoptosis is associated with Fas activation. Ultraviolet irradiation directly

activates the Fas receptor in the absence of ligand. TRAIL (TNF-related apoptosis-inducing ligand, Apo-2L) has 28% amino acid identity to FasL. TRAIL induces cell death only in tumorigenic or transformed cells and not in normal cells [8].

The regulation of apoptosis by BCL2 family genes
While the members of the "death receptor" family and their ligands have structural elements in common, agents and stimuli initiating the mitochondrial pathway to apoptosis are diverse. Common to these stimuli, however, is a change in mitochondrial function, often mediated by members of the *BCL2* family [9]. In humans, at least 16 homologues of *BCL2* have been identified. Several family members (including Bcl-2, Bcl-x_L, Bcl-W) suppress apoptosis, while others induce apoptosis and may be subdivided on the basis of their ability to dimerize with Bcl-2 protein (Bad, Bik, Bid) or not (Bax, Bak). Phosphorylation of Bad protein by a specific (Akt/PKB) and other kinases prevents dimerization with Bcl-2 and promotes cell survival. At least two distinct mechanisms of action are recognized: the binding of Bcl-2 (or other members of the family) with either pro- or anti-apoptotic members of the Bcl-2 family or the formation of pores in mitochondrial membranes. Bcl-x_L is a potent death suppressor that is upregulated in some tumour types. Bax is a death promoter that is inactivated in certain types of colon cancer, stomach cancer and in haematopoietic malignancies. By dint of relevant binding sites, Bax is under the direct transcriptional control of p53.

Involvement of mitochondria
Apoptosis induced by cytotoxic drugs is accompanied by critical changes in mitochondria. Such apoptotic stimuli induce translocation of Bax from cytosol to mitochondria, which induces release of cytochrome c. Loss of transmembrane potential follows cytochrome c release and is dependent on caspase activation (see below), whereas cytochrome c release is not. Bcl-2 and Bcl-x_L reside chiefly in the outer mitochondrial mem-

brane. Bcl-2, Bcl-x$_L$ and Bax can form ion channels when they are added to synthetic membranes, and this may be related to their impact on mitochondrial biology [10]. In the cytosol after release from mitochondria, cytochrome c activates the caspases through formation of a complex (the "apoptosome") with Apaf-1 (apoptotic-protease activating factor-1), procaspase-9 and ATP. It appears that Bcl-2/Bcl-x$_L$ may suppress apoptosis by either preventing release of cytochrome c or interfering with caspase activation by cytochrome c and Apaf-1. Sustained production of nitric oxide (NO) may cause the release of mitochondrial cytochrome c into the cytoplasm and thus contribute to the activa-

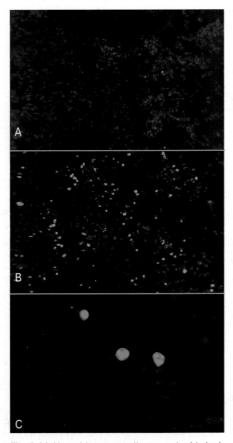

Fig. 3.38 Neuroblastoma cells treated with ionizing radiation undergo apoptosis. The TUNEL assay was used to visualize apoptotic cells (green), before (**A**) and 24 hours after (**B**) treatment with X-rays (5 Gray). Close-up shows that the nuclei of the apoptotic cells are fragmented (**C**).

tion of caspases. However, nitric oxide is involved in several aspects of apoptosis and may act both as a promoter and inhibitor depending on conditions [11].

The effector and engulfing phases
In mammals at least 13 proteases which mediate the breakdown of cell structure during apoptosis have been identified and are designated caspases-1 through -13 [12]. All possess an active site cysteine and cleave substrates after aspartic acid residues. They exist as inactive zymogens, but are activated by different processes which most often involve cleavage of their pro-forms (designated procaspase-8, etc.) at particular sites, thereby generating subunits which form active proteases consisting of two large and two small subunits. Proteolytic cascades may occur with some caspases operating as upstream initiators (which have large N-terminal prodomains and are activated by protein-protein interaction) and others being downstream effectors (activated by protease cleavage). As noted earlier, at least two pathways of caspase activation can be discerned: one involving FADD or similar protein-protein complexes and the other mediated by release of cytochrome c. In the former, affinity labelling suggests that caspase-8 activates caspases-3 and -7 and that caspase-3 in turn may activate caspase-6. On the other hand, release of cytochrome c into the cytoplasm results in the activation of caspase-9 which in turn activates caspase-3.
Though the intrinsic pathway to caspase-3 activation may be distinguished from the extrinsic pathway (i.e. that activated by Fas, etc.), some interaction is demonstrable. Thus, caspase-9 is able to activate caspase-8. Nonetheless, the pathways are separate to the extent that caspase-8 null animals are resistant to Fas- or TNF-induced apoptosis while still susceptible to chemotherapeutic drugs; cells deficient in caspase-9 are sensitive to killing by Fas/TNF but show resistance to drugs and dexamethasone. Finally, death of some cells may occur independently of caspase-3. Caspases-3, -7 and −9 are inactivated by proteins of the inhibitor of apoptosis family (IAPs) which are suppres-

sors conserved throughout evolution. The IAP protein "survivin" is overexpressed in a large proportion of human cancers. Little is known about the involvement of caspase mutations in cancer.

Caspase substrates and late stages of apoptosis
Apoptosis was initially defined by reference to specific morphological change. In fact, both mitosis and apoptosis are characterized by a loss of substrate attachment, condensation of chromatin and phosphorylation and disassembly of nuclear lamins. These changes are now attributable to caspase activation and its consequences.
Most of the more than 60 known caspase substrates are specifically cleaved by caspase-3 and caspase-3 can process procaspases-2, -6, -7 and -9 [13]. Despite the multiplicity of substrates, protease activity mediated by caspases is specific and seems likely to account for much of the morphological change associated with apoptosis. Caspases cleave key components of the cytoskeleton, including actin as well as nuclear lamins and other structural proteins. Classes of enzymes cleaved by caspases cover proteins involved in DNA metabolism and repair exemplified by poly(ADP-ribose) polymerase and DNA-dependent protein kinase. Other classes of substrates include various kinases, proteins in signal transduction pathways and proteins involved in cell cycle control, exemplified by pRb. Cleavage of some substrates is cell-type specific. Caspase activity accounts for internucleosomal cleavage of DNA, one of the first characterized biochemical indicators of apoptosis. ICAD/DFF-45 is a binding partner and inhibitor of the CAD (caspase-activated DNAase) endonuclease, and cleavage of ICAD by caspase-3 relieves the inhibition and promotes the endonuclease activity of CAD.

Therapeutic implications
In theory, knowledge of critical signalling or effector pathways which bring about apoptosis provides a basis for therapeutic intervention, including the development of novel drugs to activate particular path-

ways. Several options are under investigation [14]. More immediately, attempts are being made to exploit knowledge of apoptotic processes to increase the efficacy or specificity of currently available therapy. Simple answers have not emerged. Thus, for example, relatively increased expression of Bcl-2 (which, under many experimental conditions, inhibits apoptosis) is not necessarily indicative of poor prognosis and the reverse appears true for some tumour types. In experimental systems, cells acquiring apoptosis defects (e.g. *p53* mutations) can more readily survive hypoxic stress and the effects of cytotoxic drugs [15]. However, clinical studies have not consistently established that mutation of *p53* is associated with poor response to chemotherapy [16].

The function of Bcl-2 family members may be subject to interference by small molecules [17]. In preclinical animal models, suppression of Bcl-2 by an antisense oligonucleotide has been shown to retard tumour growth and the approach is currently subject to clinical trial. Likewise, antisense oligonucleotides directed at "survivin" are being evaluated. The possibility of using recombinant TRAIL to induce apoptosis in malignant cells is under investigation. TRAIL is implicated as the basis of *all-trans*-retinoic treatment of promyelocytic leukaemia [18]. Also note-

DRUGS TARGETING SIGNAL TRANSDUCTION PATHWAYS

In complex multicellular organisms, cell proliferation, differentiation and survival are regulated by a number of extracellular hormones, growth factors and cytokines. These molecules are ligands for cellular receptors and communicate with the nucleus of the cell through a network of intracellular signalling pathways. In cancer cells, key components of these signal transduction pathways may be subverted by proto-oncogenes through over-expression or mutation, leading to unregulated cell signalling and cellular proliferation. Because a number of these components may be preferentially over-expressed or mutated in human cancers, the cell signalling cascade provides a variety of targets for anticancer therapy (Adjei AA, *Current Pharmaceutical Design*, 6: 471-488, 2000).

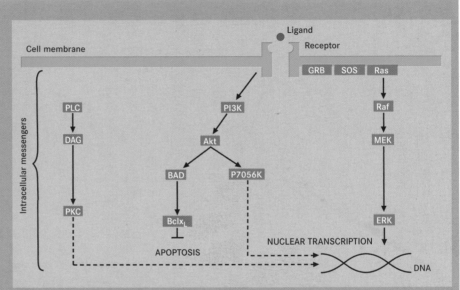

Fig. 3.39 Signaling pathways targeted by anticancer agents. PI3K = phosphoinositide-3-kinase; PLC = phospholipase C; PKC = protein kinase C; MEK = mitogen-activated protein kinase kinase; ERK = extracellular signal-regulated kinase; Akt = protein kinase B (PKB); BAD = Bcl-XL/Bcl-2-associated death protein; VEGF = vascular endothelial growth factor; HER = human epidermal growth factor receptor family; PDGF = platelet derived growth factor; FGF = fibroblast growth factor; SOS = son of sevenless guanine nucleotide exchange protein; GRB = growth factor receptor-bound protein.

Different approaches have been used to attack these targets and include classical cytotoxic agents as well as small molecule drug inhibitors. In addition, antisense oligonucleotides, vaccines, antibodies, ribozymes and gene therapy approaches have been utilized.

The diagram illustrates cell signalling pathways that are targeted by anticancer agents currently undergoing clinical testing. The drug Gleevec is already in clinical use (*Leukaemia*, p242). It is hoped that in future, a combination of agents targeting parallel pathways, as well as combinations with classical cytotoxic agents will improve the outcome of cancer patients.

Classes of agents and their potential targets include:
> *Inhibitors of ligands*, such as recombinant human antibody to VEGF (rHu mAbVEGF)
> *Receptors*, anti-receptor antibodies and tyrosine kinase receptor inhibitors
> *RAS* farnesyltransferase inhibitors
> *RAF inhibitors*
> *MEK inhibitors*
> *Rapamycin analogues*
> *Protein kinase C (PKC) inhibitors*
> *Inhibitors of protein degradation*
> *Inhibitors of protein trafficking*

worthy is the development of caspase inhibitors for the treatment of certain degenerative (non-cancerous) diseases characterized by excess apoptosis.

Drugs shown to induce apoptosis specifically include chemopreventive agents (*Chemoprevention*, p151), exemplified by 4-hydroxyphenylretinamide. Butyrate, a short-chain fatty acid produced by bacterial fermentation of dietary fibre, inhibits cell growth *in vitro* and promotes differentiation; it also induces apoptosis. Both roles may contribute to its prevention of colorectal cancer. Moreover, cyclo-oxygenase enzyme (COX-2) expression may modulate intestinal apoptosis via changes in Bcl-2 expression. Aspirin and similar drugs which inhibit COX-2 may promote apoptosis and prevent tumour formation.

REFERENCES

1. Strasser A, O'Connor L, Dixit VM (2000) Apoptosis signaling. *Annu Rev Biochem*, 69: 217-245.

2. Kaufmann SH, Gores GJ (2000) Apoptosis in cancer: cause and cure. *Bioessays*, 22: 1007-1017.

3. Parton M, Dowsett M, Smith I (2001) Studies of apoptosis in breast cancer. *BMJ*, 322: 1528-1532.

4. Choisy-Rossi C, Yonish-Rouach E (1998) Apoptosis and the cell cycle: the p53 connection. *Cell Death Differ*, 5: 129-131.

5. Rich T, Allen RL, Wyllie AH (2000) Defying death after DNA damage. *Nature*, 407: 777-783.

6. Peter ME, Krammer PH (1998) Mechanisms of CD95 (APO-1/Fas)-mediated apoptosis. *Curr Opin Immunol*, 10: 545-551.

7. Yeh WC, Hakem R, Woo M, Mak TW (1999) Gene targeting in the analysis of mammalian apoptosis and TNF receptor superfamily signaling. *Immunol Rev*, 169: 283-302.

8. Griffith TS, Lynch DH (1998) TRAIL: a molecule with multiple receptors and control mechanisms. *Curr Opin Immunol*, 10: 559-563.

9. Gross A, McDonnell JM, Korsmeyer SJ (1999) BCL-2 family members and the mitochondria in apoptosis. *Genes Dev*, 13: 1899-1911.

10. Matsuyama S, Llopis J, Deveraux QL, Tsien RY, Reed JC (2000) Changes in intramitochondrial and cytosolic pH: early events that modulate caspase activation during apoptosis. *Nat Cell Biol*, 2: 318-325.

11. Chung HT, Pae HO, Choi BM, Billiar TR, Kim YM (2001) Nitric oxide as a bioregulator of apoptosis. *Biochem Biophys Res Commun*, 282: 1075-1079.

12. Kumar S (1999) Regulation of caspase activation in apoptosis: implications in pathogenesis and treatment of disease. *Clin Exp Pharmacol Physiol*, 26: 295-303.

13. Porter AG, Janicke RU (1999) Emerging roles of caspase-3 in apoptosis. *Cell Death Differ*, 6: 99-104.

14. Nicholson DW (2000) From bench to clinic with apoptosis-based therapeutic agents. *Nature*, 407: 810-816.

15. Zhou BB, Elledge SJ (2000) The DNA damage response: putting checkpoints in perspective. *Nature*, 408: 433-439.

16. Brown JM, Wouters BG (1999) Apoptosis, p53, and tumor cell sensitivity to anticancer agents. *Cancer Res*, 59: 1391-1399.

17. Zheng TS (2001) Death by design: the big debut of small molecules. *Nat Cell Biol*, 3: E43-E46.

18. Altucci L, Rossin A, Raffelsberger W, Reitmair A, Chomienne C, Gronemeyer H (2001) Retinoic acid-induced apoptosis in leukemia cells is mediated by paracrine action of tumor-selective death ligand TRAIL. *Nat Med*, 7: 680-686.

WEBSITE

The European Cell Death Organization: http://www.ecdo.dote.hu/

INVASION AND METASTASIS

SUMMARY

> The ability of tumour cells to invade and colonize distant sites is a major feature distinguishing benign growths from malignant cancer.

> Most human tumours lead to death through widespread metastasis rather than the adverse local effects of the primary neoplasm.

> Often, metastatic spread first involves regional lymph nodes, followed by haematogenous spread throughout the body. Metastases may become clinically manifest several years after surgical resection of the primary tumour.

> Current methods are inadequate for the routine detection of micrometastases and the search for effective, selective therapies directed toward metastatic growth remains a major challenge.

Metastasis (from the Greek meaning "change in location") refers to growth of secondary tumours at sites distant from a primary neoplasm. Metastasis thus distinguishes benign from malignant lesions and is the ultimate step in the multistage process of tumour progression. Metastatic growth is the major cause of treatment failure and the death of cancer patients. Although secondary tumours may arise by shedding of cells within body cavities, the term metastasis is generally reserved for the dissemination of tumour cells via the blood or lymphatics. Spread in the cerebrospinal fluid and transcoelomic passage may also occur. Most (60-70%) cancer patients have overt or occult metastases at diagnosis, and the prognosis of the majority of these patients is poor (Box: *TNM Classification of Malignant Tumours*, p124).

There is a critical need to identify reliable indicators of metastatic potential, since clinical detection of metastatic spread is synonymous with poor prognosis. Current methods of detecting new tumours, including computed tomography (CT) scans or magnetic resonance imaging (MRI), ultrasound, or measurement of circulating markers such as carcinoembryonic antigen (CEA), prostate-specific antigen (PSA) or cancer antigen 125 (CA125) are not sufficiently sensitive to detect micrometastases. A greater understanding of the molecular mechanisms of metastasis is required. It is clear that metastatic growth may reflect both gain and loss of function, and indeed the search for "metastasis suppressor" genes has been more fruitful than identification of genes which specifically and reliably potentiate metastasis [1].

The genetics of metastasis

With the publication of the human genome sequence, and various major initiatives such as the Cancer Genome Project in the UK and the Cancer Genome Anatomy Project in the USA, the search for genes selectively upregulated, mutat-

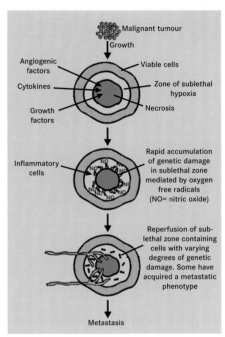

Fig. 3.40 The hypoxia hypothesis suggests that the progression of malignant tumours to a metastatic phenotype is mediated by deficiency of oxygen and resulting tumour necrosis.

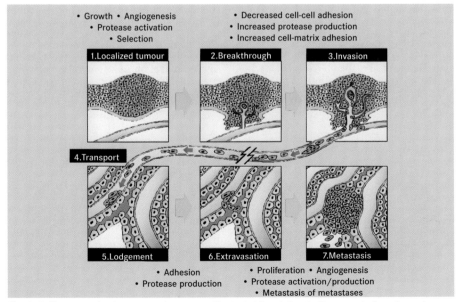

Fig. 3.41 The stages in the metastatic process, illustrated in relation to the spread of a primary tumour from a surface epithelium to the liver.

Gene	Cancer type(s)	Mechanism
nm23 Family (H1-6) of nucleoside diphosphate kinases	Breast (liver, ovary, melanoma)	Cell migration? Signalling via G proteins, microtubule assembly
PTEN/MMAC1	Prostate, glioma, breast	Migration, focal adhesions
KAI1/CD82/C33	Prostate, stomach, colon, breast, pancreas, lung	Cell-cell adhesion, motility
CAD1/E-cadherin	Many adenocarcinomas	Cell-cell adhesion, epithelial organization
MKK4/SEK1	Prostate	Cellular response to stress?
KiSS-1	Melanoma, breast cancer	Signal transduction? Regulation of MMP-9?
BRMS1	Breast	Cell communication, motility
DPC4	Colon, pancreas	?

Table 3.5 Putative metastasis suppressor genes.

ed or lost in metastatic cancers (Table 3.5) has gained momentum. It is now possible, using laser capture microdissection and serial analysis of gene expression (SAGE), to isolate invasive cancer cells and compare their gene or protein expression with non-invasive or normal cells from the same patient [2]. Prior to this, transfection of chromosomes or DNA from metastatic to non-metastatic cells (or vice versa), subtractive hybridization/differential display PCR, cDNA array and other strategies resulted in identification of some genes specifically linked to

metastasis, although many others so identified are also associated with tumour growth or developmental processes.

The events which lead to cancer metastasis include changes in cell-cell and cell-matrix adhesion, alterations in cell shape, deformability and motility, invasion of surrounding normal tissues, gaining access to lymphatic or vascular channels, dissemination via blood or lymph, survival of host defence mechanisms, extravasation and colonization of secondary sites (Fig. 3.41). There are now many features of cancer cells recognized to potentiate

metastasis, and a great deal is known about the cellular and molecular events that underlie the process. However the ability to predict which patient has occult micrometastases, and the discovery of effective, selective therapies for metastatic disease, remain major challenges in oncology.

The biology of metastasis

Growth of tumours beyond a few millimetres in diameter cannot progress without neovascularization, and there is a growing appreciation of how this phenomenon is linked to metastasis [3]. Many genetic changes associated with malignant progression (mutation of HRAS, over-expression of ERBB2 oncogenes, loss of p53) induce an angiogenic phenotype (developing blood vessels) via induction of cytokines, such as vascular endothelial growth factor (VEGF-A). VEGF-A is also upregulated by hypoxia in tumours, partly by host cells such as macrophages. The presence of hypoxic areas is a characteristic of solid tumours and has been related to poor response to conventional therapies (Fig. 3.40). In addition, activation of epithelial growth factor receptor (EGFR) and other oncogenic signalling pathways can also upregulate VEGF-C, a known lymphangiogenic cytokine [4]. The receptors for these cytokines (Flk-1 and Flk-4) are expressed on tumour vasculature, and both (in addition to acting as potent mitogens for endothelial cells) also enhance vessel permeability. Thus activation of these signalling pathways may potentiate both vascular and lymphatic invasion and tumour spread. Basic fibroblast growth factor (bFGF) is often upregulated in cancers, particularly at the invasive edge where tumour cells interact with host cells [5].

Epithelial cells are normally bounded by basement membranes which separate them from the underlying stroma and mesenchymal compartments. Breaching this barrier is the first step in the transition from carcinoma in situ to invasive and potentially metastatic carcinoma. Basement membrane is composed of a variety of structural proteins including collagen IV (the major component),

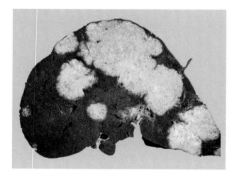

Fig. 3.42 Multiple metastatic growths of an intestinal carcinoma in the liver.

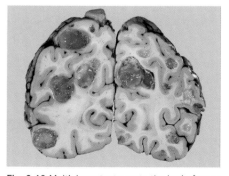

Fig. 3.43 Multiple metastases to the brain from a lung carcinoma.

laminin, entactin and also heparan sulfate proteoglycans. Interactions of tumour cells with the basement membrane have been considered to comprise three steps, which can readily be demonstrated *in vitro*: adhesion, matrix dissolution/proteolysis and migration [6].

Epithelial cells are normally polarized and firmly attached to each other via desmosomes, tight junctions and intercellular adhesion molecules such as E-cadherin, and also bound to the basement membrane via other adhesion molecules including integrins. Changes in cell-cell and cell-matrix adhesive interactions are common in invasive cancer (*Cell-cell communication*, p109). Indeed, E-cadherin may be designated a tumour suppressor gene, since its loss or functional inactivation is one of the most common characteristics of metastatic cancer, and its reintroduction into cells can reverse the malignant phenotype. The adenomatous polyposis coli gene (*APC*), which is mutated in many inherited and sporadic colon cancers, normally regulates the expression of β-catenin, a protein which interacts with E-cadherin. Mutations in *APC* (or β-catenin) increase cellular levels of the latter and facilitate interactions with transcription factors such as T-cell factor/lymphoid enhancer factor (TCF/LEF) which drive the expression of genes involved in inhibiting apoptosis and stimulating cell proliferation. Other genes commonly lost in cancers (e.g. *DCC*, Deleted in Colon Carcinoma) also encode adhesion molecules.

Integrins

Integrins are heterodimeric proteins that mediate adhesion between cells and the extracellular matrix or other cellular elements. Ligand specificity is determined by the subunit composition; many integrins bind multiple substrates and others are more selective. Far from being an inert "glue", they are capable of transmitting important signals regulating cell survival, differentiation and migration [7]. Many differences in integrin expression between benign and malignant cells have been documented, but the patterns are complex. In addition, their expression and binding

affinity can be profoundly influenced by the local microenvironment and soluble factors, enabling the tumour cell to respond to different conditions encountered throughout the metastatic cascade.

Other molecules involved in adhesion

Other adhesion molecules implicated in cancer progression include selectins such as sialyl Le[x] and members of the immunoglobulin superfamily, including intercellular adhesion molecules (ICAM-1, ICAM-2, VECAM and PECAM). The latter are upregulated on activated endothelial cells, and can interact with integrins on leukocytes and circulating tumour cells, assisting their arrest and extravasation. CD44 is another adhesion molecule utilized during lymphocyte "homing", and a change from the standard "epithelial" pattern to expression of splice variants associated with haematopoietic cells has been proposed to assist carcinoma cells in haematogenous dissemination. Thrombospondin may mediate adhesion between circulating tumour cells, platelets and endothelial cells, promoting embolization (vessel obstruction) and arrest. Tumour cells then gain access to the subendothelial basement membrane when endothelial cells retract in response to these emboli, and can adhere to exposed proteins. Synthetic peptides containing sequences of amino acids which compete with binding to laminin or fibronectin can inhibit colonization of the lung by intra-

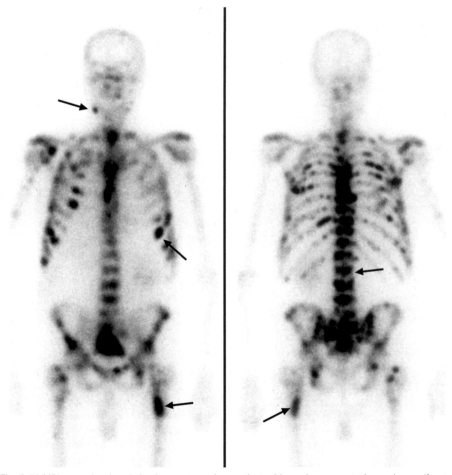

Fig. 3.44 MRI scan showing skeletal metastases in a patient with a primary prostatic carcinoma (front and back views). Some of the larger metastases are marked by arrows. Note the numerous metastases in the ribs and in the spine.

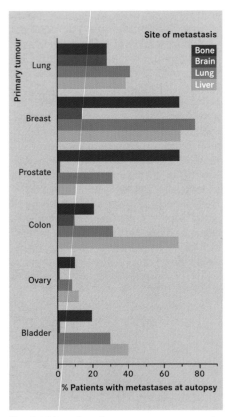

Fig. 3.45 Location of metastases at autopsy for some common cancers, indicating that the site of metastasis is not random.

Primary tumour	Site of metastasis
Bronchial cancer	Adrenal (often bilateral)
Breast ductal carcinoma	Liver
Breast lobular carcinoma	Diffuse peritoneal seeding
Breast	Bone, ovary
Lung	Brain
Ocular melanoma	Liver
Prostate	Bone
Melanoma	Brain

Table 3.6 Some sites of metastasis which are not explicable by circulatory anatomy.

venously injected cells in experimental models.

RHO

The *RHO* gene family of small GTP-hydrolysing proteins contains several members known to be involved in cell migration via regulation of actomyosin-based cytoskeletal filament contraction and the turnover of sites of adhesion. Overexpression of RhoC alone in melanoma cells is sufficent to induce a highly metastatic phenotype [8].

Enzyme functions in invasion and metastasis

Invasive tumour cells show increased expression of many enzymes due to upregulation of genes, enhanced activation of pro-enzymes or reduced expression of inhibitors such as tissue inhibitors of metalloproteinases (TIMPs). In addition, tumour cells may also induce expression of enzymes by neighbouring host cells and "hijack" these to potentiate invasion.

Matrix metalloproteinases

One important group is the matrix metalloproteinases (MMP). Different cancers may show different patterns of expression; for instance squamous carcinomas frequently have high levels of gelatinase B (MMP-9), stromelysins 1-3 (MMP-3, MMP-10 and MMP-11, normally stromal enzymes, but also expressed by these carcinomas) and matrilysin (MMP-7). Adenocarcinomas such as breast may have increased levels of gelatinase A (MMP-2) and colon carcinomas commonly overexpress MMP-7. In addition, MT1-MMP, which activates MMP-2, is often upregulated in tumour and/or neighbouring host tissues. The major substrate of the gelatinases is collagen IV, a major component of the basement membrane, whereas the stromelysins prefer laminin, fibronectin and proteoglycans, and can also activate procollagenase (MMP-1), which in turn degrades the fibrillar collagens of the interstitial tissues. Urokinase plasminogen activator (uPA) is also frequently upregulated in cancer. It controls the synthesis of plasmin, which degrades

laminin and also activates gelatinases. Thus, upregulation of these enzymes in cancers leads to proteolytic cascades and potential for invasion of the basement membrane and stroma.

Metalloproteinases also contribute to tumour growth and metastasis by other means [9]. During angiogenesis, "invasion" of capillary sprouts requires local proteolysis (mediated in part by upregulated MMP-2 and MMP-9 together with uPA) and in addition MMP-9 has been implicated in the "angiogenic switch" by releasing VEGF from sequestration in the extracellular matrix [10]. Furthermore, these proteases can contribute to the sustained growth of tumours by the ectodomain cleavage of membrane-bound pro-forms of growth factors, and the release of peptides which are mitogenic and chemotactic for tumour cells.

Heparanase

Apart from the structural proteins cleaved by metalloproteinases in the basement membrane and extracellular matrix, the other major components are glycosaminoglycans, predominantly heparan sulfate proteoglycan (HSPG). Heparanase is an important enzyme which degrades the heparan sulfate side-chains of HSPGs and, like the proteases described above, not only assists in the breakdown of extracellular matrix and basement membrane, but is also involved in the regulation of growth factor and cytokine activity. Basic fibroblast growth factor (bFGF, another potent mitogen and chemotactic factor for endothelial cells) and other heparin-binding growth factors are sequestered by heparan sulfate, providing a localized depot available for release by heparanase. Similarly, uPA and tissue plasminogen activator (tPA) can be released from heparan sulfate by heparanase, further potentiating proteolytic and mitogenic cascades.

Tissue-specific growth factors

Finally, it is possible that release of tissue-specific growth factors may play a role in organ selectivity of metastasis. For example, colorectal carcinoma cells over-expressing EGFR have a predilection for

Target	Example of agent	Comments
Adhesion/attachment	RGD-toxin constructs and RGD-targeted gene therapy	Have not reached clinical trials
	Anti-avfl3 monoclonal antibody (Vitaxin, Medi522)	Cytostasis in patients; anti-tumour and anti-angiogenic in animal models
Proteolysis	Matrix metalloproteinase inhibitors	Cytostatic in patients; rare occurence of tumour partial regressions; stromal fibrosis; activity seen in multiple animal models and in combination with chemotherapy; new agents with varied MMP specificity under development
Motility	No selective agents	
Signal pathways	Squalamine (NHE-3 inhibitor)	Selective for endothelial cells
	PDGFR, KDR and EGFR small molecule inhibitors	Active *in vitro* in animal models; preclinical activity in combinations; phase I trials completed for several agents, some tumour stabilization or regression
	Anti-EGFR monoclonal antibody (C225)	Neutralizing antibody; active *in vitro* in animal models; phase I trials ongoing
	Anti-VEGF antibody	Blocking antibody; active *in vitro* in animal models; preclinical activity alone and in combination; phase I-III trials ongoing
	CAI (non-voltage-gated Ca^{++} uptake inhibitor)	Active *in vitro* in animal models; preclinical activity in combinations; phase I trials of single agents and combinations, some tumour stabilization or regression
Extracellular matrix	Pirfenidone	Suppresses stromal/inflammatory cell Remodelling by stromal expression of TGF-β Phase I trials for pulmonary fibrosis

Table 3.7 Therapeutic agents directed towards stroma-tumour interactions.

growth in the liver where there are high concentrations of its ligands. All of these require proteolytic cleavage for activation. Other enzymes which have been implicated in metastasis include the cysteine proteinases, notably cathepsins B and D. For most of the enzymes described, there are active research programmes seeking selective inhibitors (some of which have reached phase II and III clinical trials) to prevent or treat metastatic disease.

Motility, coupled with proteolysis, is the basis of tumour cell invasion, and is also important during intravasation and extravasation of blood and lymphatic vessels. Many motility factors have been described which may be tumour- or host-derived. Many growth factors, such as transforming growth factor alpha, epidermal growth factor and platelet-derived growth factor, can induce chemotactic responses in tumour cells expressing the cognate receptors. Scatter factor (also known as hepatocyte growth factor, HGF) is a potent host-derived motility factor, and tumour cells themselves secrete a variety of autocrine motility factors including autotaxin and neuroleukin/phosphohexose isomerase.

Organ preference of metastases
The organ distribution of metastases depends on the type and location of the primary tumour, with 50-60% of the secondary sites being dictated by the anatomical route followed by the dissemi-nating cells. Most metastases occur in the first capillary bed or lymph node encountered. The number of involved nodes is a key prognostic factor for many cancers, and this has led to efforts to identify "sentinel" lymph nodes in order to improve predictions of cancer spread. Lymphatic channels present less of a challenge to tumour cell entry than capillaries since they have scanty basement membrane. Once in the lymphatics, tumour cells are carried to the subcapsular sinus of draining nodes, where they may arrest and grow, succumb to host defences, or leave the node via the efferent lymphatics. The propensity for a tumour cell to generate a lymphatic metastasis may depend upon its ability to

TNM CLASSIFICATION OF MALIGNANT TUMOURS

The TNM system for the classification of malignant tumours (http://tnm.uicc.org/) is a form of clinical shorthand used to describe the anatomic extent (staging) of a cancer in terms of:

T - the primary tumour
N - regional lymph nodes
M - distant metastases

These components are given a number that reflects the absence or presence and extent of the disease. For example, a tumour of the colon that is classified as T2N1M0 would have extended into the colon's muscular wall, spread to 1 to 3 regional lymph nodes but without evidence of distant metastasis. Evaluation by the TNM system can therefore help in the planning of treatment by the oncologist and in monitoring the efficacy of this treatment, as well as giving some indication of prognosis. Moreover, the use of a standardized system facilitates the dissemination of information in the clinical community.

The TNM system was developed by Pierre Denoix (President of the UICC, 1973-1978) between 1943 and 1952 (Sobin LH, TNM − principles, history and relation to other prognostic factors. *Cancer*, 91:1589-92, 2001). In 1968, a series of brochures published by UICC describing the classification of cancers at 23 body sites were combined to produce the *Livre de Poche*, which has been subject to regular re-edition, enlargement and revision over subsequent years. In order to prevent unwanted variations in the classification by its users, in 1982 it was agreed that a single international TNM classification should be formulated. This is achieved via meetings of experts that update existing classifications, as well as develop new ones. The present TNM edition (Eds. Sobin LH and Wittekind Ch, *TNM Classification of Malignant Tumours, 6th Edition*, Wiley, 2002) contains guidelines for classification and staging that correspond exactly with those of the 6th edition of the *AJCC Cancer Staging Manual* (2002). TNM, now the most widely used system to classify tumour spread, is published in 12 languages and is accompanied by an illustrated *TNM Atlas* (Eds. Hermanek P et al., 4th Edition, Springer-Verlag, 1997), *a TNM Mobile Edition* (Wiley, 2002) and a TNM supplement (Eds. Wittekind Ch et al., *TNM Supplement 2001. A Commentary on Uniform Use, 2nd Edition*, Wiley 2001) with rules and explanations.

The challenge for the future is the incorporation into TNM of information from new diagnostic and imaging technologies (such as endoscopic ultrasound, magnetic resonance imaging, sentinel node biopsy, immunohistochemistry and polymerase chain reaction). There is an expanding array of known and potential prognostic factors (Eds. Gospodarowicz M et al., *Prognostic Factors in Cancer*, Wiley, 2001) with which TNM could be integrated to form a comprehensive prognostic system. Such integration could potentially be exploited to enhance the prediction of prognosis, and individualize cancer patient treatment.

T = primary tumour	
TX	Primary tumour cannot be assessed
T0	No evidence of primary tumour
Tis	Carcinoma *in situ*
T1	Tumour invades submucosa
T2	Tumour invades muscularis propria
T3	Tumour invades through muscularis propria into subserosa or into non-peritonealized pericolic or perirectal tissues
T4	Tumour directly invades other organs or structures and/or perforates visceral peritoneum
N = regional lymph nodes	
NX	Regional lymph nodes cannot be assessed
N0	No regional lymph node metastasis
N1	Metastasis in 1 to 3 regional lymph nodes
N2	Metastasis in 4 or more regional lymph nodes
M = distant metastasis	
MX	Distant metastasis cannot be assessed
M0	No distant metastasis
M1	Distant metastasis

Table 3.8 TNM classification of cancer of the colon and rectum.

adhere to reticular fibres in the subcapsular sinus. These fibres contain laminin, fibronectin and collagen IV, and different integrins expressed by different tumour cells may be responsible for adhesion to these structures and to the lymphatic endothelial cells [11].

Sarcomas tend to metastasize to lungs because the venous drainage returns there; colon carcinoma cells enter the portal circulation which delivers cells to the liver, and so on (Fig. 3.45). However, a non-random element in metastatic patterns has long been recognized (Table 3.6). Stephen Paget developed the "seed and soil" hypothesis in 1889, based on his observations from autopsies of over 700 women with breast cancer. He proposed that specific cancer cells (the seed) had an affinity for certain organs (the soil).

In experimental systems there are many examples showing that primary tumours are heterogeneous, and that cloned cells can vary in their ability to metastasize to different sites. Some of the patterns relate to the ability of malignant cells to adhere to the endothelial cells in target organs, and to respond to local growth factors once they have extravasated. It used to be thought that escape from the primary tumour and survival in the circulation were the major rate-limiting steps for successful metastasis. However, while there is a good deal of attrition at these stages, both in experimental models and in man, many tumour cells reach distant sites but may remain dormant, either due to lack of appropriate growth factors, or their failure to induce neoangiogenesis. Indeed, using sensitive assays such as immunocytochemistry and polymerase chain reaction (PCR), individual tumour cells (or specific genetic markers) can be found in blood, nodes, bone marrow, body fluids etc, but the significance of "positive" results, and whether they can be used to predict subsequent overt metastases is not yet established.

REFERENCES

1. Yoshida BA, Sokoloff MM, Welch DR, Rinker-Schaeffer CW (2000) Metastasis-suppressor genes: a review and perspective on an emerging field. *J Natl Cancer Inst*, 92: 1717-1730.

2. Simone NL, Paweletz CP, Charboneau L, Petricoin EF, Liotta LA (2000) Laser capture microdissection: Beyond functional genomics to proteomics. *Mol Diagn*, 5: 301-307.

3. Fidler IJ (2000) Angiogenesis and cancer metastasis. *Cancer J Sci Am*, 6 Suppl 2: S134-S141.

4. Eccles SA (2000) Cell biology of lymphatic metastasis. The potential role of c-erbB oncogene signalling. *Recent Results Cancer Res*, 157: 41-54.

5. Fidler IJ (1999) Critical determinants of cancer metastasis: rationale for therapy. *Cancer Chemother Pharmacol*, 43 Suppl: S3-10.

6. Stracke ML, Liotta LA (1992) Multi-step cascade of tumor cell metastasis. *In Vivo*, 6: 309-316.

7. Berman AE, Kozlova NI (2000) Integrins: structure and functions. *Membr Cell Biol*, 13: 207-244.

8. Ridley A (2000) Molecular switches in metastasis. *Nature*, 406: 466-467.

9. McCawley LJ, Matrisian LM (2000) Matrix metalloproteinases: multifunctional contributors to tumor progression. *Mol Med Today*, 6: 149-156.

10. Bergers G, Brekken R, McMahon G, Vu TH, Itoh T, Tamaki K, Tanzawa K, Thorpe P, Itohara S, Werb Z, Hanahan D (2000) Matrix metalloproteinase-9 triggers the angiogenic switch during carcinogenesis. *Nat Cell Biol*, 2: 737-744.

11. Brodt P (1991) Adhesion mechanisms in lymphatic metastasis. *Cancer Metastasis Rev*, 10: 23-32.

WEBSITE

The Metastasis Research Society (UK):
http://www.metastasis.icr.ac.uk

4

Prevention and screening

The majority of cancers are preventable. The goal of primary prevention is to avoid the development of cancer by reducing or eliminating exposure to cancer-causing factors. These include environmental carcinogens as well as lifestyle factors such as nutrition and physical activity. Secondary prevention aims at early detection at a stage when curative treatment is still possible. This is achieved by frequent medical check-ups of individuals or by population-based screening programmes to which all those belonging to a certain age group are invited. Chemoprevention seeks to reduce the risk of cancer development through the use of pharmaceuticals.

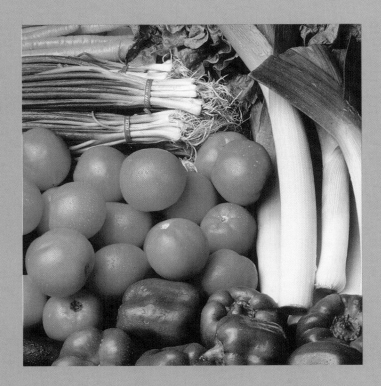

TOBACCO CONTROL

SUMMARY

> Tobacco-induced death and disease are preventable: halving current smoking rates would avoid 20-30 million deaths before 2025 and 150 million by 2050.

> Smoking cessation is very effective in reducing the risk of lunb cancer even in later life.

> The greatest saving of life would result if rates of smoking uptake by children and adolescents were decreased.

> Comprehensive tobacco control, including implementation of regulatory measures and encouraging personal commitment, requires coordinated involvement of government and community organizations, health care professionals and planners.

> The hazard posed by environmental tobacco smoke is significant. This justifies the demand for a tobacco-free environment, particularly at work and in public places.

Tobacco usage was estimated to account for an annual death toll of more than three million in 1990 (Table 4.1). The latest estimates from WHO put the annual number of deaths today at more than four million. If current smoking patterns continue, the total is predicted to increase to more than eight million in 2020 (Table 4.2). Thus current cigarette smoking will cause about 450 million deaths worldwide in the next 50 years. Accordingly, smoking is recognized as the most preventable cause of death of humankind. Apart from lung and several other cancers, respiratory heart disease, chronic obstructive lung disease, stroke, pneumonia, aortic aneurysm and ischaemic heart disease are caused by smoking and are, to that extent, preventable, as are a range of non-fatal diseases (Table 4.3) [1-3].

Attributable risk and years of life potentially saved

Apart from knowing the diseases caused by tobacco, increasingly definitive estimates may now be made of the number of lives lost and the extent to which those lives were shortened. For a time, knowledge of attributable risk and years of life lost was restricted to quite specific populations: the British doctors constituting the cohort established by Doll and Hill in 1951 and monitored thereafter [2] and the cohort of volunteers from the American Cancer Society [4]. Extrapolation from these relatively limited databases to, in some instances, the population of the whole world was inappropriate because, despite validity of the respective studies, the populations involved were predominantly male white upper class Western populations. Although this selection of the population may not invalidate establishing the list of diseases linked to use of tobacco, extrapolation is more uncertain in relation to quantitation of risk. The key quantities that need to be measured include the relative risk (measuring how much more frequent the disease is in tobacco smokers than in non-smokers) and the attributable risk in the total population (measuring the proportion of people suffering from the disease in the population whose disease may be attributed to smoking). Granted the limitations already noted, follow-up of the British doctors for 40 years [2] indicates that one smoker out of three died from a smoking-related illness, losing on average 7.5 years of life (Fig. 4.1). It should be noted that the outlook for smokers worsens the longer the follow-up lasts. Thus, based on the first 20 years of the study, the estimate was five years of life lost, but the period became 7.5 years when the result for the last 20 years were added. Most probably the final estimate will be close to ten years, with perhaps the death of one in two smokers being attributable to the habit. The impact of smoking on survival is dose-dependent; smokers of 25 or more cigarettes per day have a survival of

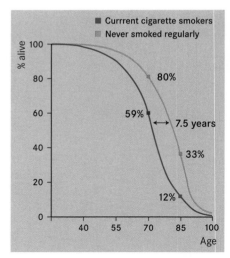

Fig. 4.1 Smoking significantly reduces overall survival. British Doctors Study. Estimates based on age-specific death rates for the entire 40-year period.[2]

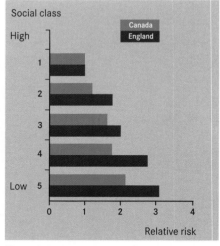

Fig. 4.2 Lung cancer mortality among men in Canada and England, late 1980s, by social class.

only about 50% at around the age of 70 years, whereas 80% of non-smokers are still alive.

World estimates for mortality caused by all diseases linked to tobacco have been produced [5] (Table 4.1). For the present, the most affected regions of the world remain

Europe and North America, but the burden is already high in China and recent studies suggest that there the disease and death toll will be heavy (Fig. 4.5). While in the United Kingdom and the USA, tobacco is responsible for about a third of all deaths at ages 35 to 69 years [6], for China the current estimate for men is about 12% to 20% but is predicted to increase to 33% by 2030 [7,8] with, for the time being, about equal proportions of lung cancers, other cancers and other diseases.

The numbers of lives lost to tobacco-induced disease and the extent to which lives are shortened may be regarded as indicative, at least in theory, of what could be saved by cessation of smoking. The effectiveness of preventive activity may often be assessed in terms of the number of lives able to be saved and these data taken into account when determining the allocation of resources. Clearly, total and immediate cessation of smoking is unachievable and can be set aside as a realistic goal. Even reducing current smoking rates by 50% would avoid 20-30 million premature deaths in the first quarter of the current century and about 150 million in the second quarter. The affected numbers of individuals in virtually all communities are so great that any incremental decrease in smoking rates will affect large numbers of individuals and have direct repercussions, for example, on health budgets .Accordingly, the efforts directed toward smoking cessation should not be balanced solely against an assessment of the numbers of lives saved, but must involve consideration of total community health care resources and the avenues through which such finite resources are most usefully expended.

Nature of intervention

Beyond being a primary concern for individual users, smoking or tobacco use has ramifications for the whole community. Therefore all sectors of society have to be mobilized against it. As a means of influencing an individual's decision to smoke, or to continue to smoke, responsibility has traditionally been accorded to doctors and public health specialists. However, a critical influence may be exercised by teachers and all professionals in schools. In terms of action at a community level, a critical role may fall to legislators, who are responsible for design of legislation controlling tobacco use, and politicians, who enact relevant legislation.

Tobacco usage has massive economic ramifications for governments who derive benefits from taxes on tobacco trade, but these may be considered to be offset by the costs of diagnosing and treating diseases linked to tobacco, as well as other less direct costs. The broad economic impact of tobacco use involves traders dealing on world or national scales. The economic ramifications of tobacco control may involve agronomy insofar as alternative crops must be considered. Finally, the wider community may be influenced by the manner in which relevant issues are presented through the media [9].

Legislation is a crucial aspect of tobacco control and WHO has proposed a framework convention on this topic [10]. Key

Region	Deaths due to tobacco use (1,000s)	% of total deaths (all causes)	Years of life lost due to tobacco use (1,000s)	% of total years of life lost (all causes)
Established market economies	1,063	14.9	11,607	11.7
Former socialist economies of Europe	515	13.6	7,803	12.5
India	129	1.4	1,719	0.6
China	820	9.2	8,078	3.9
Other Asian countries and islands	223	4.0	2,638	1.5
Sub-Saharan Africa	78	0.9	1,217	0.4
Latin America and the Caribbean	99	3.3	1,340	1.4
Middle East	111	2.4	1,779	1.2
World	3,038	6.0	36,182	2.6
Developed regions	1,578	14.5	19,410	12.1
Developing regions	1,460	3.7	16,772	1.4

Table 4.1 The estimated burden of mortality attributable to tobacco use in 1990. Numbers of deaths and years of life lost due to tobacco use are shown. These figures are also expressed as a percentage of the total numbers of deaths and years of life lost from all causes.

Region	Deaths due to tobacco use (1,000s)	% of total deaths (all causes)	Years of life lost due to tobacco use (1,000s)	% of total years of life lost (all causes)
Established market economies	1,286	14.9	11,607	21.2
Former socialist economies of Europe	1,101	22.7	10,072	26.3
India	1,523	13.3	18,183	12.0
China	2,229	16.0	23,418	18.0
Other Asian countries and islands	681	8.8	7,475	7.7
Sub-Saharan Africa	298	2.9	3,945	1.7
Latin America and the Caribbean	447	9.4	4,888	8.8
Middle East	817	12.3	9,477	9.2
World	8,383	12.3	88,129	10.3
Developed regions	2,387	17.7	20,742	23.4
Developing regions	5,996	10.9	67,386	8.7

Table 4.2 The estimated burden of mortality attributable to tobacco use in 2020. Numbers of deaths and years of life lost due to tobacco use are shown. These figures are also expressed as a percentage of the total numbers of deaths and years of life lost from all causes.

areas include pricing, smuggling, tax-free products, advertising and sponsorship, the Internet, test methods, package design and labelling, agriculture and information sharing. These topics partly overlap with those necessary for any national tobacco control legislation, particularly actions to limit supply, including those calculated to modify the product and limit its availability or by modifying people's attitudes [11]. In respect of affecting supply, and apart from banning the product, options include modifying the composition of tobacco and in particular setting limits for selected constituents (tar content), changing the presentation (information provided, health warning, generic packaging), controlling advertising and sales promotion, and increasing the price paid by consumers through taxation. So far as demand is concerned, steps may be taken to restrict smoking in public places and at the workplace, to prevent youth from smoking and to make health education compulsory. Elements of legislation of special importance for young people

include restriction of advertising, banning of smoking in schools and other places where children and adolescents congregate and, finally, educating children. Approaches to control of tobacco-related cancer can be divided between those directed towards health protection and those acting through health promotion.

Health protection
Health protection approaches have been effective in reducing tobacco consumption in many countries. A 1% increase in the price of tobacco products is followed by a 0.5-0.8% decrease in sales. Tax increases that raise the real price of cigarettes by 10% are considered to reduce smoking by about 4% in high-income countries and by about 8% in other countries. Furthermore, increasing taxes on tobacco products is easy to implement. However, this measure can be seen as a "tax on the poor", in view of the increasing prevalence of smoking with lower social class (Fig. 4.2). Reducing subsidies for tobacco growing is an approach complementary to

increasing taxes. Subsidies for tobacco growing are very important: for example, in 1990, the European Union spent more than 700 million pounds sterling for this purpose, as compared to slightly more than 5 million pounds for tobacco control initiatives. In many developing countries, tobacco yields a higher net income for the producer than most food crops.
Restrictions in sales of tobacco products concern mainly the youth. The rationale for this is that most smokers take up their habit before age 18. Restrictions may include a complete ban of sales, a ban of automatic vending machines, and banning free distribution of tobacco products. Promotion of a tobacco-free environment has focused on hospitals and other health services, schools, workplaces, as well as different public settings. Separate spaces for smokers are often provided; sometimes a workplace ban only concerns areas where clients or the public are present. The strongest resistance against any restriction often comes from owners and managers of settings receiving the public,

such as bars and restaurants, who fear a decrease in business. In fact, the limited evidence from cities in the USA where this measure has been implemented speaks against a negative economic impact. In general, however, there has been little assessment of the effectiveness of promotion of tobacco-free environments. It should be stressed that fire prevention is an important positive side-effect of promotion of tobacco-free workplaces and public settings.

Various forms of restrictions on advertising of tobacco products have been implemented in many countries. A recent survey of 22 countries with policies of either complete or partial ban on direct advertising concluded that a comprehensive set of tobacco advertising bans can reduce tobacco consumption, but that a limited set of advertising bans will have little or no effect [12]. However, tobacco companies have developed sophisticated forms of indirect advertising through subsidiaries. Sponsorship of cultural and sporting events can be seen as part of the same strategy of indirect advertising: several countries are currently discussing regulation of such sponsorship. Moreover, organizations involved in tobacco control (e.g. cancer societies) have developed a proactive advertising strategy, often using icons of tobacco advertisements such as cowboys and camels.

A final form of tobacco control through health protection is the requirement that warnings are printed on tobacco products. Such health warnings are now widespread (a 1991 survey listed 77 countries where they were requested, although in most cases they consisted of "mild" statements about health without requirement of rotation [11]). In almost every respect, residents in developing countries are receiving inferior information about the hazards of smoking than residents of more developed countries [13]. There is no formal evidence that health warnings on cigarette boxes contribute to a decrease in tobacco consumption.

Health promotion
Discouraging smoking
The epidemic of smoking-induced cancer and other disease, both present and antic-

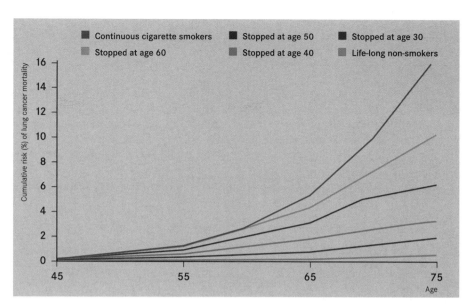

Fig. 4.3 Cessation of smoking greatly reduces the risk of death from lung cancer, and is even effective at age 60 (UK men, 1990) From: R. Peto et al. (2000) *BMJ* 321: 323-329.

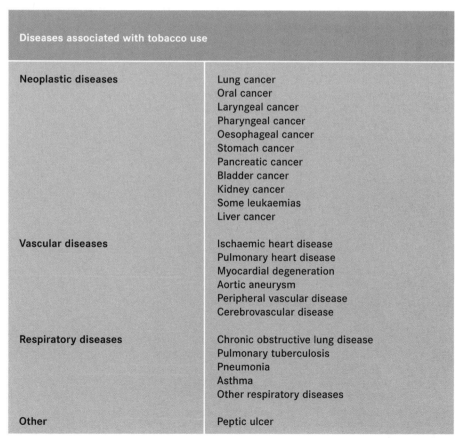

Diseases associated with tobacco use	
Neoplastic diseases	Lung cancer
	Oral cancer
	Laryngeal cancer
	Pharyngeal cancer
	Oesophageal cancer
	Stomach cancer
	Pancreatic cancer
	Bladder cancer
	Kidney cancer
	Some leukaemias
	Liver cancer
Vascular diseases	Ischaemic heart disease
	Pulmonary heart disease
	Myocardial degeneration
	Aortic aneurysm
	Peripheral vascular disease
	Cerebrovascular disease
Respiratory diseases	Chronic obstructive lung disease
	Pulmonary tuberculosis
	Pneumonia
	Asthma
	Other respiratory diseases
Other	Peptic ulcer

Table 4.3 Diseases associated with tobacco use.

ipated, is primarily attributable to young people taking up the habit. Factors that lead youngsters to start smoking include smoking by parents and siblings and, most significantly, peer pressure. Thus, smoking by a best friend, or belonging to a group where a majority smoke has a strong influence [14]. The task of promoting non-smoking as a healthy lifestyle choice may be accorded to teachers in general or to specialist educators. The goal must be to prevent schoolchildren from starting to smoke. Therefore, programmes must be initiated early (before the age at which experimentation is likely to start) and to achieve a positive impact, an intensive programme over several years should be integrated into the school curriculum. Limited interventions by health professionals from outside the school setting cannot be expected to have a lasting impact. Unless interventions are strengthened with inclusion of booster sessions, the positive effects of most programmes will wear off. However, even under the best conditions, there seems little room for optimism. Under real life conditions, it has proved impossible to replicate the encouraging results from pilot trials [15]. While effort continues to be directed at health promotion campaigns aimed at youth, there is abundant recognition of the worth and need for development of campaigns directed towards women [16] and members of communities in the developing world [17].

Smoking cessation

Preventing young people from starting smoking would cut the number of deaths related to tobacco, but not until after 2050. Quitting by current smokers is the only way in which tobacco-related mortality can be reduced in the medium term. The risk of lung cancer decreases inversely with the time since quitting smoking (Fig. 4.3). About 20% of smokers are prepared to make an active attempt to quit in the immediate future (within 30 days) [18].

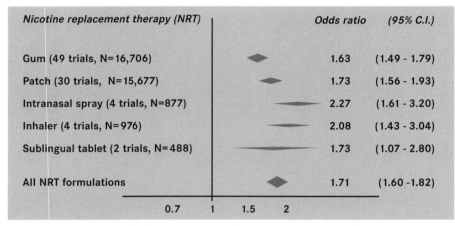

Fig. 4.4 Meta-analysis of nicotine replacement therapy trials; nicotine replacement therapy increases the chance of quitting smoking by more than one and a half times. T. Lancaster et al. (2000) *BMJ* 321, 355-358, with permission from the BMJ Publishing Group.

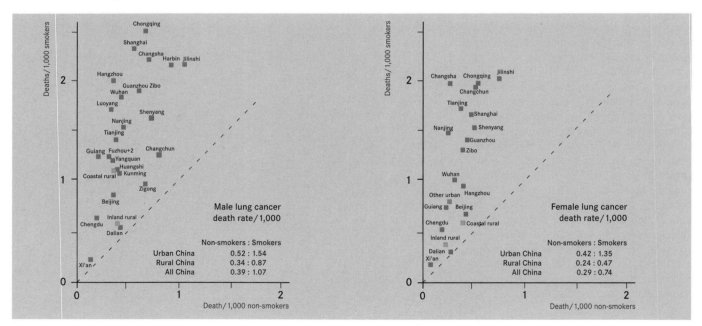

Fig. 4.5 Death rates at ages 35-69 from lung cancer in smokers versus non-smokers in various parts of China, 1986-88. Although lung cancer rates show wide variation between cities and between urban and rural areas, lung cancer mortality in smokers was consistently about three times higher in smokers than in non-smokers. Lung cancer mortality rates in some areas greatly exceed those found in the USA, which in 1990, similarly standardized for age, were 1.4 per 1,000 male and 0.6 per 1,000 female smokers, and 0.1 per 1,000 male or female non-smokers. R. Peto et al. (1999) *Nature Medicine* 5: 15-17.

However the challenge posed is daunting. Cigarette smoking is an addiction, as powerful in many respects as cocaine or opiate dependence. The rates of dependence for nicotine in the general population are higher than for alcohol, cocaine or marijuana. Among those who have ever tried even a single cigarette, almost one-third develop nicotine dependence. Although most smokers want to quit, they experience well-characterized barriers and withdrawal symptoms during their attempts and they are largely unsuccessful in quitting. In fact, spontaneous quit rates without any cessation intervention range from 2% to 5% [19]. The efficacy of a range of interventions calculated to increase the spontaneous quit rates have been evaluated, and for many options the results of ten or more trials have been published. Simple advice from doctors in the course of routine care in the context of primary care, hospital wards, outpatient consultations and industrial clinics increases the quit rate by a factor of 1.69. Nurses providing individual counselling, as distinct from general health promotion, are also effective. Likewise, counselling provided through quit clinics is effective whether provided on an individual or group basis. The relative efficacy of different psychological approaches that might be used in such a situation is poorly understood. In the absence of face-to-face contact, the efficacy of self-help material is not as great but is discernible. Increasingly, such self-help materials may be delivered through the Internet, though whether this will be more effective than publications, audiotapes or videotapes remains to be seen.

Nicotine replacement therapy is intended to provide the nicotine otherwise obtained from cigarettes, thereby reducing withdrawal symptoms associated with quitting. On the basis of more than 90 trials, this increases the chances of quitting up to two-fold (Fig. 4.4). The therapy is most effective if accompanied by at least some counselling. Nicotine may be delivered by various means (patch, inhaler, nasal spray, gum) and none has been identified as most effective; many protocols involve a combination of such products.

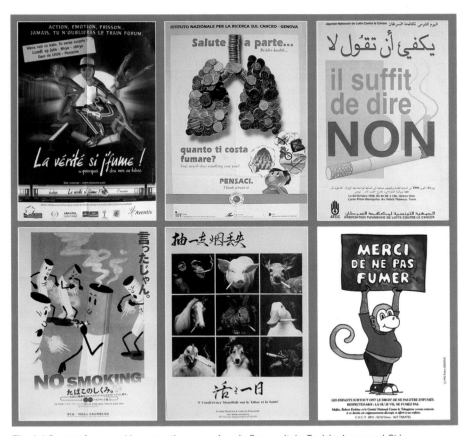

Fig. 4.6 Posters from smoking cessation campaigns in France, Italy, Tunisia, Japan and China.

Apart from nicotine, a range of pharmacological agents have been proposed as expediting smoking cessation. Anxiolytics are not effective, but some antidepressants, specifically including bupropion, are. The drug may be used alone, or in combination with nicotine, and quit rates are increased by a factor of approximately 2.75. In more limited investigations, similar results have been claimed for the tricyclic antidepressant nortriptyline. Relevant mechanisms have not been demonstrated. A range of other pharmacological interventions are under evaluation and, not surprisingly, the field is one of intense activity.

Reduced exposure to environmental tobacco smoke

A tangential benefit of smoking cessation is decreased exposure of individuals apart from the smoker to tobacco

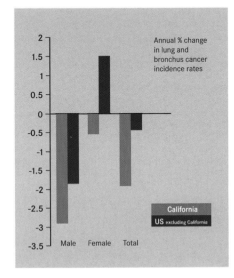

Fig. 4.7 Declining lung cancer rates in California by comparison with rates in other parts of the USA. Centers for Disease Control and Prevention (2000) *Mortality and Morbidity Weekly Report*, 49:1066-1069.

smoke. This may be achieved in part by health protection legislation which limits smoking indoors and the requirement to provide a safe workplace. In common with some other areas of tobacco control, it is possible that progress in this area may be influenced by the outcome of litigation and the associated financial risk incurred by those permitting or tolerating such exposure.

Outcome

The health benefits of smoking cessation are indisputable, and specifically include reduced risk of malignant disease. A classic example involves the impact of anti-smoking publicity and health education in California, where smoking rates declined more than twice as rapidly as in the rest of the USA. It is now evident that during the period 1988-1997, age-adjusted lung cancer incidence rates in California declined significantly compared with stable incidence rates in other parts of the USA (Fig. 4.7). Thus, California is one of the few regions in the developed world where lung cancer mortality among women is declining.

The efficacy of smoking cessation, as a means of decreasing the risk of malignant disease, is not an issue requiring further investigation. Hence, the immediate issue confronting governmental and other authorities is the amount and type of resources that should be allocated to this established means of cancer prevention. An important consideration is the limitation of those factors which tend to promote adoption of the smoking habit by the community in question.

REFERENCES

1. Wald NJ, Hackshaw AK (1996) Cigarette smoking: an epidemiological overview. *Br Med Bull*, 52: 3-11.

2. Doll R, Peto R, Wheatley K, Gray R, Sutherland I (1994) Mortality in relation to smoking: 40 years' observations on male British doctors. *BMJ*, 309: 901-911.

3. Doll R (1998) Uncovering the effects of smoking: historical perspective. *Stat Methods Med Res*, 7: 87-117.

4. Thun MJ, Heath CW, Jr. (1997) Changes in mortality from smoking in two American Cancer Society prospective studies since 1959. *Prev Med*, 26: 422-4 26

5. Murray CJL, Lopez AD (1996) Quantifying the burden of disease and injury attributable to ten major risk factors. In: Murray CJL, Lopez AD, eds, *The Global Burden of Disease*, Geneva, World Health Organization, 295-324.

6. Peto R, Lopez AD, Boreham J, Thun M, Health CJ, eds (1994) *Mortality from Smoking in Developed Countries 1950-2000: Indirect Estimates from National Vital Statistics*, Oxford, Oxford University Press.

7. Niu SR, Yang GH, Chen ZM, Wang JL, Wang GH, He XZ, Schoepff H, Boreham J, Pan HC, Peto R (1998) Emerging tobacco hazards in China: 2. Early mortality results from a prospective study. *BMJ*, 317: 1423-1424.

8. Chen ZM, Xu Z, Collins R, Li WX, Peto R (1997) Early health effects of the emerging tobacco epidemic in China. A 16-year prospective study. *JAMA*, 278: 1500-1504.

9. Sasco AJ (1992) Tobacco and cancer: how to react to the evidence. *Eur J Cancer Prev*, 1: 367-373.

10. WHO (1992) *Framework Convention on Tobacco Control. Technical Briefing Series Paper 2*. Improving Public Health through an International Framework Convention on Tobacco Control (Tobacco-Free Initiative), Geneva, World Health Organization.

11. Roemer R, ed. (1987) *Legislative Strategies for a Smoke-Free Europe*, Copenhagen, World Health Organization, Regional Office for Europe.

12. Saffer H, Chaloupka F (2000) The effect of tobacco advertising bans on tobacco consumption. *J Health Econ*, 19: 1117-1137.

13. Aftab M, Kolben D, Lurie P (1999) International cigarette labelling practices. *Tob Control*, 8: 368-372.

14. Sasco AJ, Kleihues P (1999) Why can't we convince the young not to smoke? *Eur J Cancer*, 35: 1933-1940.

15. Reid D (1996) Tobacco control: overview. *Br Med Bull*, 52: 108-120.

16. Greaves L ed. (1996) *Smoke Screen. Women's Smoking and Social Control*, Halifax, Fernwood Publishing.

17. The World Bank (1999) *Development in Practice. Curbing the Epidemic*. Governments and the Economics of Tobacco Control, Washington DC, The World Bank.

18. Curry SJ (2001) Bridging the clinical and public health perspectives in tobacco treatment research: scenes from a tobacco treatment research career. *Cancer Epidemiol Biomarkers Prev*, 10: 281-285.

19. Law M, Tang JL (1995) An analysis of the effectiveness of interventions intended to help people stop smoking. *Arch Intern Med*, 155: 1933-1941.

WEBSITES

GLOBALink, the International Tobacco Control Network, UICC:
http://www.globalink.org

Florida Tobacco Control Clearinghouse:
http://www.ftcc.fsu.edu

CDC's Tobacco Information and Prevention Source:
http://www.cdc.gov/tobacco/

List of smoking and tobacco control monographs from the National Cancer Institute:
http://rex.nci.nih.gov/NCI_MONOGRAPHS/LIST.HTM

Tobacco Control Research Branch (NCI), information on spit tobacco:
http://dccps.nci.nih.gov/TCRB/less_default.html

Tobacco Free Initiative, WHO:
http://tobacco.who.int/

11th World Conference on Tobacco or Health (August 2000):
http://www.wctoh.org/

Smoking Cessation, "Live Smoke Free", Health Canada:
http://www.hc-sc.gc.ca/hppb/cessation/

Framework Convention on Tobacco Control :
http://www.who.int/gb/fctc/

Quit: the National Tobacco Initiative (Australia):
http://www.quitnow.info.au

REDUCTION OF OCCUPATIONAL AND ENVIRONMENTAL EXPOSURES

SUMMARY

> The prevention of cancer attributable to occupational and environmental exposures is primarily achieved by regulatory action.

> Relevant measures include replacement of carcinogens with alternative chemicals or processes, improved ventilation, re-engineered manufacturing processes and, if this fails, use of protective clothing and equipment.

> A significant reduction in occupational cancer attributable to implementation of preventive measures has been demonstrated in many instances. However, there remains a burden of past exposure, particularly to asbestos.

In developed countries, it has been estimated that about 5% of all cancers are attributable to occupational exposures and about 1% to pollution [1] (*Occupational exposure*, p33; *Environmental pollution*, p39). These minor proportions might not command immediate attention. However, the cancers in question are immediately preventable, particularly those resulting from occupational exposures. In principle, an individual should not have to accept an increased risk of cancer which has been recognized as being caused by doing a particular job. It is notable that exposure to occupational carcinogens and to environmental pollutants is largely involuntary, as distinct from "lifestyle" exposures, such as active smoking, alcohol drinking and sun exposure, the extent of which are largely a matter of personal choice.

Prevention of cancers attributable to occupational exposures and environmental pollution involves at least two stages: firstly, identification of the specific agent or situation responsible for an increased cancer incidence and secondly, the imposition of appropriate regulatory controls. However, regulatory control of exposure to carcinogens or hazardous environments must vary according to the situation being addressed. Even in relation to the same agent, there may be several options and hence the procedures adopted by different countries may vary.

Occupational cancer

Prevention of exposure

The primary strategy for prevention of occupationally induced cancer involves preventing exposure to the recognized carcinogen in question. One option is to cease production, exemplified by the phasing out of 4-aminobiphenyl in the United Kingdom, following reports of increased risk of bladder cancer among exposed American workers [2]. Another approach is the adoption of protective measures, including those involving building design and ventilation systems. Consideration may be given to altered means of production (e.g. the use of "closed" rather than "open" engineering). As a general rule, reduced emissions and/or improved ventilation are more efficient than the use of protective equipment in achieving a durable reduction in exposure. Reduction of emission can often be achieved for chemicals generated incidentally in the course of production, such as intermediates formed during chemical manufacturing processes. However, reduction of exposure at source may be difficult to achieve when the hazardous material is the final manufactured product.

Adoption of protective clothing and "safe" handling procedures may be perceived as the last resort in a general assessment of preventive measures, but is recognized as being necessary and appropriate to particular situations. Safety equipment must be properly related to the hazard and be comfortable. Such equipment may include gloves, gowns, masks and/or respirators depending on the situation. Related measures include use of proper warning labels and secure storage arrangements.

Activities of the International Labour Organization (ILO) aimed specifically at the prevention of occupational cancer include the adoption and promotion of the Occupational Cancer Convention and Recommendation (ILO, 1974) and the production of a publication concerning prevention and control of occupational cancer (ILO, 1988). The Occupational Cancer Convention specifies the principles to be adopted and had, in 2001, been signed by 35 Member States. Article 3 states that "Each Member which ratifies this Convention shall prescribe the measures to be taken to protect workers against the risks of exposure to carcinogenic substances or agents and shall ensure the establishment of an appropriate system of records."

Screening

Screening of occupationally exposed workers for physical or biological indicators of exposure has been proposed, but

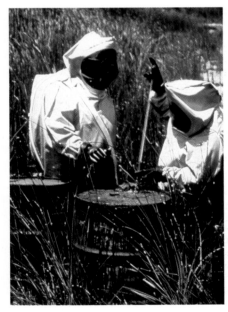

Fig. 4.8 Clothing to prevent contamination with chemical waste.

there is no evidence for the efficacy of this approach. This is specifically the case for lung cancer and mesothelioma among asbestos-exposed workers (screened using chest X-rays or cytological examination of sputum) and bladder cancer among workers exposed to aromatic amines (screened using cytological or mutagenicity analysis of urothelial cells in the urine). Education programmes directed at reducing any delay in examination and diagnosis of workers developing symptoms of disease are an option. These programmes not only require awareness and information campaigns, but also require appropriate facilities for diagnosis and treatment

[3]. In Finland, there is a policy of increasing awareness about carcinogens in the workplace and employers are required to maintain files on all employees, recording all exposures.

Actions and outcomes
Prompt regulatory action may be seen to have followed the identification of vinyl chloride as an occupational carcinogen. An occupational exposure limit of 500 parts per million (ppm) for vinyl chloride monomer was common during the 1960s, and was based on the explosive properties of the chemical. However, in 1974, several cases of an otherwise very rare cancer,

angiosarcoma of the liver, were described among workers exposed to vinyl chloride, and this was followed soon after by the results of animal experiments, confirming the carcinogenicity of this compound. These findings led to a rapid reduction in recommended exposure levels for vinyl chloride monomer to 10 ppm or less. However, a similar quick response to accumulating evidence of an unacceptable hazard has not occurred for other occupational carcinogens. The history of occupational exposure to asbestos is illustrative of an unacceptable time-lag between identification of risk and regulatory action. Epidemiological results indi-

Country	Year	Butadiene concentration (mg/m³)	Interpretation
Australia	1991	22 (Probable human carcinogen)	Time-weighted average
Belgium	1991	22 (Probable human carcinogen)	Time-weighted average
Czechoslovakia	1991	20	Time-weighted average
		40	Ceiling
Denmark	1993	22 (Potential occupational carcinogen)	Time-weighted average
Finland	1998	2.2	Time-weighted average
France	1993	36	Time-weighted average
Germany	1998	34 (Human carcinogen)	Technical exposure limit
		11	
Hungary	1993	10 (Potential occupational carcinogen)	Short-term exposure limit
The Netherlands	1996	46	Time-weighted average
The Philippines	1993	2200	Time-weighted average
Poland	1991	100	Time-weighted average
Russia	1991	100	Short-term exposure limit
Sweden	1991	20 (Suspected of having a carcinogenic potential)	Time-weighted average
		40 (Suspected of having a carcinogenic potential)	Ceiling
Switzerland	1991	11 (Suspected of being a carcinogen)	Time-weighted average
Turkey	1993	2200	Time-weighted average
United Kingdom	1991	22	Time-weighted average
United States:			
ACGIH (Threshold Limit Value)[a]	1997	4.4 (Suspected human carcinogen)	Time-weighted average
NIOSH (Recommended Exposure Limit)	1997	(Potential occupational carcinogen: lowest feasible concentration)	Time-weighted average
OSHA (Permissible Exposure Limit)	1996	2.2	Time-weighted average

Limits and guidelines from International Labour Office (1991); United States Occupational Safety and Health Administration (OSHA, 1996); American Conference of Governmental Industrial Hygienists (ACGIH, 1997); United States National Library of Medicine (1997); Deutsche Forschungsgemeinschaft (1998); Ministry of Social Affairs and Health (1998). [a] Countries that follow the ACGIH recommendations for threshold limit values include Bulgaria, Colombia, Jordan, Republic of Korea, New Zealand, Singapore and Viet Nam.

Table 4.4 International occupational exposure limits and guidelines for butadiene (which is classed by IARC as a probable human carcinogen, Group 2A).

cating that exposure to asbestos caused lung cancer accumulated from the 1930s and the evidence became conclusive during the 1950s and 1960s. However, only during the late 1970s were effective steps for limiting exposure initiated in some countries [4]. Even so, relatively little action concerning asbestos-induced cancer has been taken in many countries (notably in the developing world, see below) until recently.

After introduction of preventive measures, a progressive decrease in the risk of cancer among relevant workers may be evident. This may be seen by comparing groups of workers who were employed in different time periods. For example, the risk of lung cancer decreased among cohorts of American workers who were potentially exposed to chloromethyl ethers. This hazard was reduced after 1971, when a closed manufacturing system was introduced [5]. Among relevant workers, lung cancer incidence was greatest in the 1960s, and decreased after 1974. Change in risk of cancer is also evident amongst Norwegian workers employed in a nickel refinery smelter from the beginning of operation in the 1910s until the 1960s [6] (Fig. 4.9). Major changes in the process occurred during this time, particularly after 1950. [7]. Risk of nasal cancer has decreased; excess risk of lung cancer has also decreased but to a lesser degree, which may be attributable to the effects of increased smoking.

The situation in developing countries

Most documented examples of successful prevention of occupational cancer involve developed countries. To some extent, these examples have also led to improvement in conditions of occupational hygiene in developing countries. The quality of industrial hygiene in the Chinese chemical industry improved markedly during the 1970s such that by 1981, air concentrations of vinyl chloride monomer were similar to those in industries in Europe and North America [8]. However, lack of economic resources and health services may limit the adoption of preventive measures. Often, exposure levels in the informal employment sector and in small workshops, where a large propor-

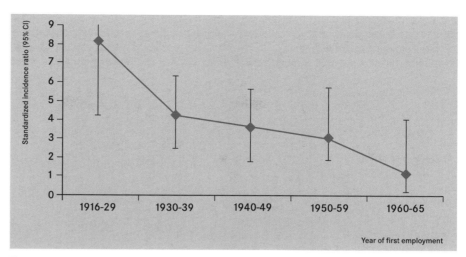

Fig. 4.9 Risk of lung cancer among nickel refinery workers, by year of first employment.

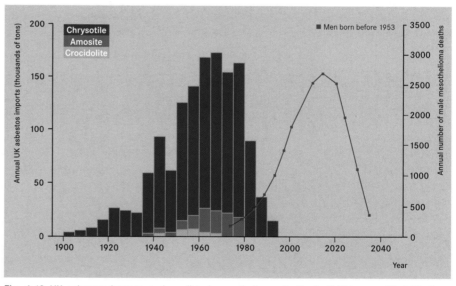

Fig. 4.10 UK asbestos imports and predicted mesothelioma deaths in British men. Mortality from mesothelioma reflects past exposure to asbestos. Despite the ban on the use of asbestos in the early 1990s, mesothelioma cases will continue to increase, with approximately 250,000 expected deaths in Europe over the next 35 years.

tion of workers are located in developing countries, are high compared to "best practice" adopted in large facilities [9]. Protective clothing may have limited effectiveness in some developing countries because of discomfort arising from its use in hot, humid climates. Exposure to asbestos, crystalline silica and pesticides are recognized priorities for control of occupational cancer hazards in developing countries. The greatest impact in terms of pre-

vention of disease is likely to come from the establishment and enforcement of national and international regulatory controls.

Child labour is another cause for concern. Even where regulations to protect workers from exposures to carcinogens are adopted, such regulations may not apply to children, who are often not employed legally [8]. Some nations have established legislation that applies specifically to the employment of children: for example, a detailed list of industries, processes and occupations that are deemed to be dangerous for children has been set out by the Philippines. Prevention of occupational cancer may positively affect general environmental conditions. A study of conditions at the Huannan coal mine, China, established that from 1953 to the 1980s underground dust levels decreased from 266 mg/m³ to 1.3 mg/m³, and this coincided with marked improvement in housing conditions, water quality, nutrition and sanitation [8].

Environmental pollution

The prevention of cancer caused by environmental pollution might be expected to follow the same principles and approaches adopted for prevention of occupational cancer. However, control of carcinogenic hazards in the general environment is usually more complex than at the workplace. Among other things, environmental pollution usually derives from many sources. Moreover, exposure levels vary greatly over space and time. Measures to reduce pollution can rarely be correlated with reduced cancer incidence. A decreased incidence of lung cancer, for example, cannot be attributed to reduced air pollution against a high background of tobac-

Pollutant	Decrease
Carbon monoxide (CO)	37%
Lead	78%
Nitrogen dioxide (NO₂)	14%
Ozone	6%
Particles of ≤10 μm diameter (PM-10) PM-10 measurements began in 1988	22%
Sulfur dioxide (SO₂)	37%

Table 4.5 Percent decrease in air concentrations of six key air pollutants, USA (1986-1995).

Compound	Average ambient air concentration [mg/m³]	Cancer associated	IARC classification
Acetaldehyde	5	Nasal tumours in rats	2B
Acrylonitrile	0.01 - 10	Lung cancer in workers	2A
Arsenic	$(1 - 30) \times 10^{-3}$	Lung cancer in humans	1
Benzo[a]pyrene	No data	Lung cancer in humans	1
Bis(chloromethyl)ether	No data	Epitheliomas in rats	1
Chloroform	0.3-10	Kidney tumours in rats	2B
Chromium VI	$(5 - 200) \times 10^{-3}$	Lung cancer in workers	1
1,2-Dichloroethane	0.07 – 4	Tumour formation in rodents	2B
Diesel exhaust	1.0 - 10.0	Lung cancer	2A
Nickel	1 - 180	Lung cancer in humans	1
Polycyclic aromatic hydrocarbons (benzo[a]pyrene)	$(1 - 10) \times 10^{-3}$	Lung cancer in humans	1
1,1,2,2-Tetrachloroethane	0.1 - 0.7	Hepatocellular carcinomas in mice	3
Trichloroethylene	1 – 10	Cell tumours in testes of rats	2A
Vinyl chloride	0.1 – 10	Haemangiosarcoma in workers Liver cancer in workers	1

Table 4.6 WHO guidelines (1999) for air pollutants with carcinogenic health end-points. These substances have been classified by IARC as either human carcinogens (Group 1), probable human carcinogens (Group 2A) or possible human carcinogens (Group 2B).

co-induced disease, including the impact of environmental tobacco smoke. However, such limitations do not detract from the value of initiatives to reduce environmental pollution. Such measures may reasonably be presumed to contribute to prevention of cancer, even in the absence of definitive data.

Air pollution
Air pollution has decreased in most developed countries during recent decades. In some Central and Eastern European countries, such as Poland, there has been a significant reduction in emissions of air pollutants as a result of the implementation of environmental protection programmes [10]. However, even when an increased risk of cancer is attributable to environmental pollution, appropriate preventive measures may not be adopted. People living in villages in Cappadocia, Central Turkey, where the local stone used for house construction was contaminated with the carcinogenic fibre, erionite, were burdened with a very high incidence of pleural mesothelioma [11]. Attempts to relocate exposed individuals away from contaminated houses were hampered by economic constraints and there is anecdotal evidence that migrants from poorer parts of the country moved into some of the houses left empty.

Regulation is the primary approach to preventing pollution-induced cancer. Improvements in air quality have been achieved by means of adopting guidelines and legislation, examples of which include the *WHO Air Quality Guidelines for Europe*, the *National Ambient Air Quality Standards* (US Environmental Protection Agency) and *Council Directives on Air Quality* (European Union). The Environmental Health Criteria series of the International Programme on Chemical Safety currently assesses the health risks of some 120 chemical compounds and mixtures. Limits have been set on motor vehicle exhaust emissions in many parts of the world. The Council of the European Communities has adopted a phased programme for the implementation of emission standards for carbon monoxide, hydrocarbons and nitrogen oxides from gasoline and diesel-powered vehicles [12]. One aspect of the control of atmospheric pollution in relation to cancer concerns the limiting of ozone depletion. The 1987 Montreal Protocol (mediated by United Nations Environment Programme and signed by 150 countries) has resulted in the cessation of production and consumption of a significant proportion of all ozone-depleting substances in industrialized countries. The worldwide consumption of ozone-depleting substances decreased by nearly 75% in the seven years to 1996. As a result of the subsequent decline in the rate at which global ultraviolet radiation is increasing, it has been estimated that 1.5 million cases of melanoma may be prevented in the next 60 years [13].

Indoor air pollution is a major public health challenge, which demands action in terms of research and policy-making [14]. The greatest burden of disease resulting from exposure to smoke from cooking

Standard (mg/L)	Countries (concentration and date standard was established, if known)
< 0.01	Australia (0.007, 1996), European Union (1998), Japan (1993), Jordan (1991), Laos (1999), Mongolia (1999), Namibia, Syria (1994)
0.01 -0.05	Canada (0.025, 1999)
0.05	United States (considering lowering standard from 0.05, 1986), Mexico (considering lowering standard, 1994) Bahrain, Bangladesh, Bolivia (1997), China, Egypt (1995), Indonesia (1990), Oman, Philippines (1978), Saudi Arabia, Sri Lanka (1983), Viet Nam (1989), Zimbabwe

Table 4.7 Currently accepted national standards for arsenic in drinking water.

Operative measure	Examples
Preventing exposure Use of gloves and face mask Full respirator	Pharmacists handling cytotoxic drugs Specified emergency procedure for spillage of hazardous material
Controlling exposure Environmental monitoring	Measurement of asbestos fibre level in breathing zone Film badge to assess radiation exposure
Assessing uptake and excretion	Urinary measurement of metabolite, e.g. dimethylphosphate in workers exposed to dichlorvos Urine analysis for haematuria Determination of protein adducts and screening for preneoplastic lesions in MOCA {4,4'-methylenebis(2-chloroaniline)}-exposed workers Determination of DNA adducts in coke oven workers exposed to polycyclic aromatic hydrocarbons

Table 4.8 Means to either prevent or determine the level of exposure to occupational carcinogens.

stoves arises in rural areas of developing countries. Exposure may be reduced by introducing improved stoves, better housing and cleaner fuels. Environmental exposure to tobacco smoke is a key aspect of atmospheric pollution and reducing this hazard is discussed elsewhere (*Tobacco control*, p128).

Soil and water pollution
The United Nations Environment Programme establishes warning systems for countries in which the environment and human health may be affected by the export of hazardous substances and pesticides from where they are manufactured. The Rotterdam Convention, 1998, which replaced various voluntary systems, obliges an importing country to give explicit informed consent before specific chemicals (such as DDT and polychlorinated biphenyls) can cross its borders. This measure is particularly important to countries with limited scientific expertise or equipment to deal with hazardous materials.

REFERENCES

1. Harvard Center for Cancer Prevention (1996) Harvard Report on Cancer Prevention. Volume 1: Causes of human cancer. *Cancer Causes Control*, 7 Suppl 1: S3-59.

2. Swerdlow AJ (1990) Effectiveness of primary prevention of occupational exposures on cancer risk. *Evaluating Effectiveness of Primary Prevention of Cancer (IARC Scientific Publications, No. 103)*, 23-56, Lyon, IARCPress.

3. Alderson M (1986) *Occupational cancer*, Butterworths.

4. Tomatis L, Aitio A, Day NE, Heseltine E, Kaldor J, Miller AB, Parkin DM, Riboli E, eds (1990) *Cancer: Causes, Occurrence and Control (IARC Scientific Publications, No. 100)*, Lyon, IARCPress.

5. Maher KV, DeFonso LR (1987) Respiratory cancer among chloromethyl ether workers. *J Natl Cancer Inst*, 78: 839-843.

6. Magnus K, Andersen A, Hogetveit AC (1982) Cancer of respiratory organs among workers at a nickel refinery in Norway. *Int J Cancer*, 30: 681-685.

7. Grimsrud TK, Berge SR, Resmann F, Norseth T, Andersen A (2000) Assessment of historical exposures in a nickel refinery in Norway. *Scand J Work Environ Health*, 26: 338-345.

8. Wu W (1988) Occupational cancer epidemiology in the People's Republic of China. *J Occup Med*, 30: 968-974.

9. Pearce N, Matos E, Vainio H, Boffetta P, Kogevinas M, eds (1994) *Occupational Cancer in Developing Countries (IARC Scientific Publications, No. 129)*, Lyon, IARCPress.

10. Jedrychowski W (1999) Ambient air pollution and respiratory health in the east Baltic region. *Scand J Work Environ Health*, 25 Suppl 3: 5-16.

11. Selcuk ZT, Emri S, Sahin AA, Baris YI, Coplu L, Kalyoncu F, Artvinli M (1999) Malignant mesothelioma and erionite exposure. *Eur Respir J*, 14: 480-481.

12. IARC (1989) *Diesel and Gasoline Engine Exhausts and Some Nitroarenes (IARC Monographs on the Evaluation of Carcinogenic Risks to Humans, Vol. 46)*, Lyon, IARCPress.

13. UNEP (2000) *UNEP Achievements. 2000*. United Nations Environment Programme http://www.unep.org/Documents/Default.asp?DocumentID=43&ArticleID=250

14. Bruce N, Perez-Padilla R, Albalak R (2000) Indoor air pollution in developing countries: a major environmental and public health challenge. *Bull World Health Organ*, 78: 1078-1092.

WEBSITES

International Labour Office:
http://www.ilo.org/

UK Health and Safety Directorate: Preventing or controlling exposure to substances which can cause occupational cancer:
http://www.hse.gov.uk/hthdir/noframes/cancers.htm

The Air Management Information System, WHO's Healthy Cities Programme:
http://www.who.int/peh/air/amis.html

EPA National Center for Environmental Assessment, Cancer Guidelines:
http://www.epa.gov/ncea/cancer.htm

United Nation Environment Programme:
http://www.unep.org

National Institute for Occupational Safety and Health (USA):
http://www.cdc.gov/niosh/homepage.html

REDUCTION OF EXPOSURE TO ULTRAVIOLET RADIATION

SUMMARY

> Encouragement of sun-protective behaviour is the most effective public health measure to reduce incidence of skin cancer, particularly in highly susceptible white populations, and especially in children.

> Available options include sun avoidance by using shade, wearing protective clothing and using sunscreens.

> Often, the protective effect of sunscreens is counteracted intentionally-extended periods of sun exposure, notably during vacations.

> Downward trends in melanoma incidence in some countries reflect a successful implementation of prevention policies.

Skin cancer is the most common cancer worldwide, although only one form, melanoma, is comprehensively documented (*Melanoma*, p253). Over 100,000 cases of melanoma occurred worldwide in 1990. It is estimated that 2.75 million basal and squamous cell carcinomas were diagnosed in 1985, which may be equated with 30% of all newly diagnosed cancer [1]. Such non-melanocytic cancers are usually not life-threatening, but are cause for the provision of medical services, including hospital admissions.

Solar radiation is established as a cause of skin cancer and may account for 80-90% of such disease [2]. The incidence of skin cancer in different communities varies according to skin type and distance from the equator. The highest rates occur in Australia, where cancer incidence is dominated by skin cancer that, in terms of incident cases, outnumbers all other forms of cancer by more than three to one [3].

The scope of sun-protection strategy

The extent of individual exposure to sunlight is, in the first instance, determined by personal behaviour. Two types of exposure can be distinguished: intentional exposure (usually in the context of achieving a tan) and unintentional exposure in the course of daily life. The immediate goal of sun protection programmes is to affect individual behaviour, specifically in relation to intentional exposure. Programmes may be targeted to particular population groups or to the community as a whole. Epidemiological evidence indicates that sun exposure during childhood and adolescence contributes markedly to lifelong risk of skin cancer [4]. The intensity and duration of targeted intervention largely determines the impact of such programmes. Individual sun-related behaviour may be influenced by mass media campaigns and the provision of educative material. Thus the "Sun Awareness" programme in Canada used strategies for improving community knowledge about skin cancer and sun protection, which included mass media, distribution of educational brochures and development of a school curriculum to promote sun protection [5].

Prevention programmes may appropriately focus on young people, parents, caregivers and the settings in which young people spend time outdoors. In relation to children and adolescents, relevant agencies to be engaged in sun protection programmes include early childhood services, schools and those involved in providing sport and recreational activity. Attention should also be paid to adults with high intermittent or cumulative sun exposure, specifically including workplace exposure for those involved in agricultural, forestry, fishery, construction and outdoor electricity transmission and similar work [6]. General practitioners and community health nurses may be encouraged to play a role in educating specific sections of the community to adopt improved sun protective behaviour.

Provision of structural and environmental support to reduce sun exposure necessitates an infrastructure that is responsive and well resourced to steer relevant programmes and strategies [7].

Means of intervention

Public health programmes developed to reduce skin cancer focus on a range of means to reduce sun exposure. The means to be used may vary between areas of high and low sunlight. Relevant strategies may include dissemination of knowledge about the intensity of sunlight in the local environment, scheduling activity or work to be indoors around solar noon, minimizing the time spent outdoors in sunny seasons, and advice as to how to avoid direct sunlight exposure during times when the ambient intensity is high. Protection when in direct sunlight may be achieved by wearing protective clothing, hats or sunglasses and using sunscreens [8].

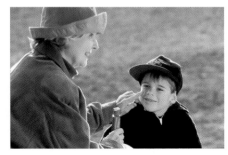

Fig. 4.11 Sun-protective behaviour can be taught at a young age.

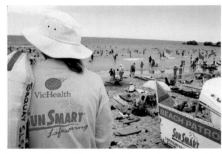

Fig. 4.12 T-shirt and sign advertising the "SunSmart Campaign" on a beach in Australia.

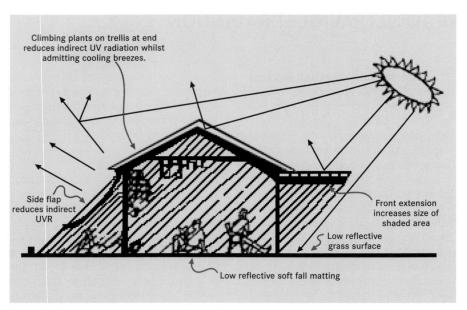

Fig. 4.13 Structural and other design features of a garden shelter designed to provide protection from exposure to the sun.

Means of sun protection include the provision of shade that falls in the right place at the right time of day (Fig. 4.13). Shade barriers, which may be either structures or trees, need to be of sufficient size, and provide at least 94% protection against direct ultraviolet radiation [9]. Natural shade is attractive because of its aesthetic appeal, cooling effect and fewer disposal problems than with built shade. Advantages of the latter include the precision with which shade needs can be met and other uses including rainwater collection and solar power generation. Provision of adequate and appropriate shade requires planning, an aspect of which is a "shade audit" to determine the adequacy of existing shade. Planning additional shade requires consideration of safety, site usage patterns, climatic conditions, aesthetics, sightlines and the possibility of vandalism.

Most summer clothing provides protection factors against sunburn of greater than 10; more than 85% of fabrics tested have protection factors of 20 or more. Factors that affect the protection offered by fabrics against sunlight include weave, colour, weight, stretch and wetness [10]. By comparison with other options, scant attention is given to sun-protective clothing in relevant groups [11].

Sunscreens are available worldwide as consumer products; the European Union and USA account for 75% of the world market. Sunscreens are regulated either as cosmetics (European Union, Japan, South Africa and South America) or as drugs (USA, Canada and Australia). Investigations of sunscreen usage have included determination of who uses them, in what circumstances are they used, why sunscreens are used, and what has been the experience of users. It is evident that sunscreen usage affects other sun-related behaviour, such as deliberate engagement in sun exposure, the duration of such exposure, and the duration of incidental or intentional sun exposure [12].

Sunscreens absorb ultraviolet radiation across the 290-400 nm spectrum. Efficacy is expressed through the "sunscreen protection factor" (SPF) which is the ratio of the least amount of ultraviolet energy required to produce minimal erythema on skin protected by the sunscreen in question to the energy required for the same effect on unprotected skin. Most commercial preparations are presented as having SPF values of up to 15-20. "Active" ingredients of sunscreens are the chemicals included to reduce the amount of ultraviolet radiation that reaches viable cells of the skin. Sunscreen formulations typically contain UVA absorbers (examples being cinnamates and derivatives of para-aminobenzoic acid) and UVB absorbers (such as the benzophenones) together with solvents, wetting and suspending agents and preservatives [13].

Outcome

A range of end-points may be employed to assess the efficacy of sun-protective activity as a means of preventing skin cancer. A high proportion of sun protection campaigns incorporate some measure of outcome, although few studies of large-scale community interventions have been reported. In assessing the results of particular campaigns, it is important to consider whether people change their behaviour in ways that counteract the benefits of a sun protection campaign [13].

The efficacy of particular interventions in reducing risk of cancer has been most comprehensively studied in relation to sunscreens. Sunscreens undoubtedly prevent sunburn. In experimental studies, sunscreens have been definitively shown to prevent squamous cell carcinoma induced by solar-simulated radiation in mice. The prevention of skin cancer in humans is less clearly established, determination of the issue being complicated by a number of factors. These include the consideration that use of the sunscreen may determine (and perhaps even encourage) sun exposure. Approximately half the relevant case-control studies recently reviewed by IARC (8/15) recorded significantly higher risks for melanoma in users of sunscreens than in non-users, while a minority of such studies showed lower risk for melanoma in users compared to non-users [13]. Some findings imply that sunscreen use may encourage prolonged sun exposure, a scenario which obviously complicates attempts to demonstrate protective effects of sunscreens. In contrast to the data concerning risk of melanoma, corresponding studies in relation to squamous cell carcinoma constituted "limited" evidence for the preventive effect of topical use of sunscreens [14].

In respect of the efficacy of all sun protection behaviour, the high incidence of skin cancer in Australia may constitute a sensitive indicator. In this regard, some positive results are already available. The incidence of basal cell carcinoma and melanoma in younger people (under 55), especially among women, is no longer increasing and, in some age groups, has begun to decline [15].

REFERENCES

1. Armstrong BK, Kricker A (1995) Skin cancer. *Dermatol Clin*, 13: 583-594.

2. IARC (1992) *Solar and Ultraviolet Radiation (IARC Monographs on the Evaluation of Carcinogenic Risks to Humans, Vol. 55)*, Lyon, IARCPress.

3. Giles GG, Marks R, Foley P (1988) Incidence of non-melanocytic skin cancer treated in Australia. *Br Med J (Clin Res Ed)*, 296: 13-17.

4. Elwood JM, Jopson J (1997) Melanoma and sun exposure: an overview of published studies. *Int J Cancer*, 73: 198-203.

5. Rivers JK, Gallagher RP (1995) Public education projects in skin cancer. Experience of the Canadian Dermatology Association. *Cancer*, 75: 661-666.

6. Cummings SR, Tripp MK, Herrmann NB (1997) Approaches to the prevention and control of skin cancer. *Cancer Metastasis Rev*, 16: 309-327.

7. Baum A, Cohen L (1998) Successful behavioral interventions to prevent cancer: the example of skin cancer. *Annu Rev Public Health*, 19: 319-333.

8. Diffey BL (1998) Human exposure to ultraviolet radiation. In: Hawk JLM, ed., *Photodermatology*, London, Chapman and Hall, 5-24.

9. The Cancer Council NSW and NSW Health Department (1998) *Under Cover: Guidelines for Shade Planning and Design*, Sydney, Australia.

10. Gies HP, Roy CR, Elliott G, Zongli W (1994) Ultraviolet radiation protection factors for clothing. *Health Phys* , 67: 131-139.

11. Horsley L, Charlton A, Wiggett C (2000) Current action for skin cancer risk reduction in English schools: a report on a survey carried out for the Department of Health. *Health Educ Res*, 15: 249-259.

12. McLean DI, Gallagher R (1998) Sunscreens. Use and misuse. *Dermatol Clin*, 16: 219-226.

13. IARC (2001) *Sunscreens (IARC Handbooks of Cancer Prevention, Vol. 5)*, Lyon, IARCPress.

14. Green A, Williams G, Neale R, Hart V, Leslie D, Parsons P, Marks GC, Gaffney P, Battistutta D, Frost C, Lang C, Russell A (1999) Daily sunscreen application and betacarotene supplementation in prevention of basal-cell and squamous-cell carcinomas of the skin: a randomised controlled trial. *Lancet*, 354: 723-729.

15. Australian Institute of Health and Welfare (1998) *Cancer in Australia 1995: Incidence and Mortality Data for 1995 and Selected Data for 1996*. Canberra, Australian Institute of Health and Welfare.

WEBSITE

Anticancer Council of Victoria SunSmart programme: http://www.sunsmart.com.au/

HEPATITIS B VACCINATION

SUMMARY

> Persons chronically infected with hepatitis B virus are at high risk of developing chronic liver disease (cirrhosis) and hepatocellular carcinoma.

> The likelihood of infection is greatest for infants and decreases with age.

> Childhood vaccination against hepatitis B is a cost-effective measure to prevent adult morbidity and has been shown to prevent the development of chronic carrier status in more than 95% of vaccinated children.

> Hepatitis B vaccine is the first and at present the only cancer-preventive vaccine It has already been demonstrated to reduce the risk of hepatocellular carcinoma in some high-incidence areas.

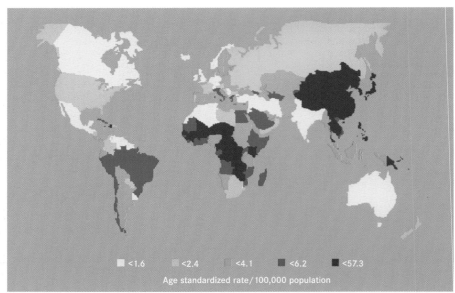

Fig. 4.14 Global incidence of liver cancer in women.

Hepatocellular carcinoma is one of the most common and most lethal cancers worldwide. The disease more commonly affects males, and generally those in their most economically productive years. There is striking geographical variation in incidence, with very high rates in South-East and East Asia, the Pacific rim and sub-Saharan Africa and much lower rates in North America and Europe (*Liver cancer*, p203).

The geographical distribution of chronic hepatitis B virus (HBV) infection and hepatocellular carcinoma is very similar (Figs. 4.14, 4.15). First discovered as a cause of acute fulminant hepatitis in 1969, HBV has since been identified as the major etiologic agent in hepatocellular carcinoma (Fig. 4.18). Subsequent research has documented variations in disease outcomes based on age of exposure, defined differences in HBV transmission patterns between high- and low-prevalence regions and provided estimates of the risk for chronic liver disease and hepatocellular carcinoma associated with long-term HBV

infection. It is estimated that 20-25% of all chronic carriers will die from liver disease associated with HBV infection (*Chronic infections*, p56).

Most individuals infected with HBV will develop no symptoms and subsequently will demonstrate complete resolution and lifelong immunity to the virus. A small portion of exposed persons will have an acute symptomatic infection with jaundice, malaise and flu-like symptoms, with a small subset of these individuals developing fulminant hepatic failure with significant mortality. The other possible outcome from HBV infection is chronic persistence of the virus and the development of the carrier state, defined by the expression of hepatitis B surface antigen (HBsAg) in the blood. The age of exposure to the virus is the primary determinant of infection outcome (Fig. 4.21). Younger children are extremely unlikely to develop any acute symptoms but have much higher rates of chronic persistent infection. The converse is true of adolescents and adults with more frequent symptomatic

acute infection but lower rates of chronic HBV infection. Children born to an HBV-infected mother have a 90% or greater chance of chronic infection. With increasing age of exposure, the risk of chronic HBV infection decreases markedly from a risk of up to 90% for infants to around a 30% risk for children around 5 years of age, decreasing to <5% for young adults [1].

The high HBV carriage rates in endemic regions result in a large pool of infectious individuals, which perpetuates horizontal and vertical transmission and ensures that children are exposed to the virus at a young age. Consequently, the age of infection is lower with resulting higher rates of chronic HBV infection, higher hepatocellular carcinoma incidence and a younger median age of cases. Unfortunately, the resources required to identify, treat and palliate affected individuals in many of these highly endemic regions are largely unavailable. In regions of low and intermediate endemicity, parenteral transmission is more common, through contaminated

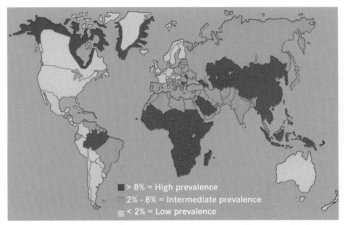

Fig. 4.15 Global prevalence of chronic hepatitis B virus (HBV) infection 1997, based on HB surface antigen serology.

Legend:
- > 8% = High prevalence
- 2% - 8% = Intermediate prevalence
- < 2% = Low prevalence

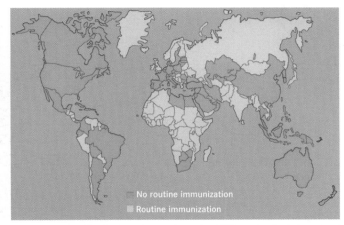

Fig. 4.16 Global distribution of countries using HBV vaccine in their national immunization programme, 2000.

Legend:
- No routine immunization
- Routine immunization

blood products, sharing contaminated needles during intravenous drug use and through sexual transmission.

Currently, there are around 350 million chronic carriers of HBV worldwide and, based on conservative assumptions, an estimated 70 million of these individuals are likely to die from HBV-related liver disease. Because of the relatively low cost of the hepatitis B vaccine and the uniformly fatal outcome of hepatocellular carcinoma, childhood hepatitis B vaccination in highly HBV endemic areas is one of the most cost-effective measures available for prevention of early mortality in adults [2].

Nature of the intervention

Vaccination efforts have historically concentrated on preventing acute infectious diseases, particularly those of childhood. Hepatitis B vaccine is the first vaccine designed to prevent a major human cancer and currently the only one in widespread use. The vaccine was initially developed by purifying the viral envelope component of the surface antigen particle (HBsAg) of the virus from the blood of individuals with chronic HBV infection. This plasma-derived vaccine undergoes intensive treatment to destroy any live virus, as well as to remove any other potential contaminants, and is then combined with an alum adjuvant to stimulate the immune system. Second-generation vaccines involved production of HBsAg particles through yeast or mammalian cells using recombinant DNA technology. Both plasma-derived and DNA recombinant vaccines are equally safe and effective. Since the early 1980s, hundreds of millions of doses of hepatitis B vaccine have been administered worldwide. Adverse reactions are uncommon and generally mild in nature, with this vaccine considered among the safest of vaccines. Hepatitis B vaccine is generally administered in sequential doses with at least four weeks between doses. An appropriate response to the vaccine is the development of antibodies to the surface antigen and is termed seroconversion. Three doses of vaccine will generally produce seroconversion rates in excess of 90%.

Vaccination campaigns aimed at reducing HBV-related hepatocellular carcinoma must take into consideration the patterns of HBV transmission. Because the highest risk for development of chronic HBV carriage occurs at the youngest ages, hepatitis B vaccine is most efficacious when given as close to birth as possible. This early vaccination benefit will be most pronounced in those high-endemicity countries with significant mother-to-child and early horizontal transmission. Hepatitis B vaccine does not interfere with other vaccines and can be administered simultaneously with many of the other routine childhood immunizations, including diphtheria, tetanus and whole-cell pertussis vaccine, oral attenuated poliomyelitis vaccine and BCG (bacille Calmette-Guérin). Integration of hepatitis B vaccine into the routine "Expanded Programme on Immunization" (EPI) efforts of individual countries provides the most appropriate strategy for global hepatitis B vaccination.

In addition to the focus on hepatitis B vaccination to prevent primary infection with HBV, new therapeutic vaccines have been designed to treat chronic HBV carriers and hopefully prevent progression to cirrhosis or cancer. Several novel vaccines, including DNA-based vaccines which incorporate the hepatitis B surface antigen gene, have been designed to stimulate the immune system of HBV-infected individuals, through induction of either a T-cell response or production of neutralizing antibodies [3]. Although therapeutic vaccines demonstrate potential, these trials are in the earliest stages and it remains to be seen what level of efficacy in reducing or stopping HBV replication and preventing progression can be achieved. The frequency and degree of serious adverse effects from these vaccines must also be demonstrated to be acceptably low.

Implementation of preventive measures

In the early 1990s, WHO/EPI recommended integration of hepatitis B vaccination into the routine EPI and this was subsequently endorsed by the World Health Assembly. Earlier, hepatitis B vaccine was utilized sporadically, with fewer than 20 countries routinely administering the vac-

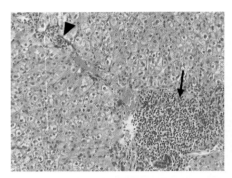

Fig. 4.17 Chronic active HBV-associated hepatitis is associated with risk of hepatocellular cancer. Inflammatory infiltrates are present in the parenchyma (arrowhead) and in the periportal space (arrow).

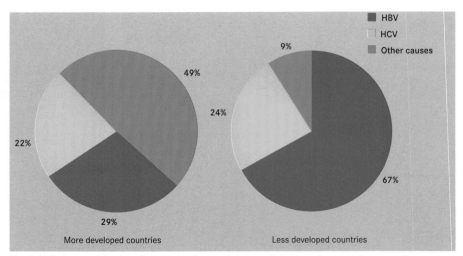

Fig. 4.18 Estimate of the risk of hepatocellular carcinoma attributable to hepatitis viruses and other causes (e.g. alcohol cirrhosis).

cine. Initial implementation strategies varied based on the local epidemiology. Routine childhood immunization was the recommendation for high-endemicity countries, having over 8% of the population with chronic HBsAg carriage. Low-endemicity regions (<2% HBsAg carriage) with delayed patterns of transmission may focus on vaccinating adolescents before their likely exposure through sexual contact or needle-sharing. Alternative "high-risk" strategies were also employed, focused on vaccinating individuals with behaviour (needle-sharing, multiple sexual partners) or occupations (health care workers) which put them at significant risk for HBV exposure. Although these targeted approaches were beneficial in some risk groups, they did not lead to any measurable reduction in HBV infection rates at a regional or national level.

The most effective preventive strategy worldwide is routine immunization as part of the regular EPI programme. Timing of doses of hepatitis B vaccine can be adjusted to conform to the childhood immunization schedule of the individual country with little decrease in seroconversion rates. Countries with limited maternal-child health services and low vaccine coverage for the other EPI vaccines may be hard-pressed to add any additional vaccines. The cost of the hepatitis B vaccine compared to other childhood vaccines is also a significant impediment to global implementation. However, over the last decade a dramatic decline in cost from over US$ 100 to as little as US$ 0.50 per paediatric dose in developing countries has greatly increased the feasibility of large-scale HBV control efforts.

Evidence of outcome

Protection against both acute and chronic HBV infection is related to the development of protective levels of antibody in response to vaccination. Hepatitis B vaccine has been used in numerous field trials throughout the world with documented immunogenicity in the 90-95% range. Despite rapidly declining levels of antibody following immunization, protection among vaccine responders is almost universal. Long-term protection against acute and chronic infection has been demonstrated in a variety of settings with follow-up ten years after vaccination [3]. One of the largest on-going cohort studies has shown that 80-90% of all HBV infections and 90-95% of chronic HBV infections can be prevented through immunization [4]. Similar rates of vaccine efficacy have been demonstrated in studies from other populations.

Prevention of chronic HBV carriage should lead to subsequent decreases in the rates of hepatocellular carcinoma after several decades – the period of time generally required for chronic persistent HBV infection to develop to hepatocellular carcinoma [5]. Validation of this premise is under way in the Gambia, West Africa, where both vaccinated and unvaccinated individuals will be followed for 25-35 years to document the effectiveness of the vaccine

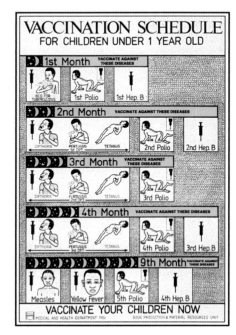

Fig. 4.19 Public health poster publicizing vaccination against HBV for children under one year old in the Gambia.

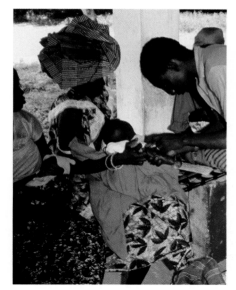

Fig. 4.20 HBV vaccination of infants in the Gambia.

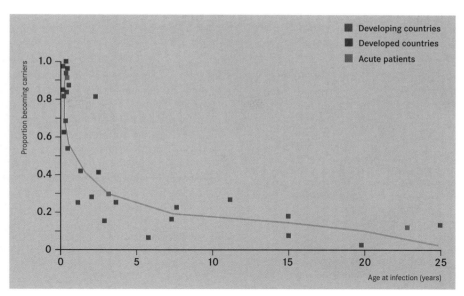

Fig. 4.21 Risk of becoming a chronic carrier of HBV based on age at infection. Risk is highest in very young children.[1]

in preventing chronic liver disease and hepatocellular carcinoma at the individual level. Taiwan, which has high HBV carriage rates and a high hepatocellular carcinoma incidence, was one of the first countries to introduce routine vaccination in 1984. A nationwide statistically significant reduction in childhood hepatocellular carcinoma has already been observed in Taiwan among the vaccinated cohort of children aged 6-14 compared to the cohort of children born before implementation of the vaccination programme [6].

Over 80 countries have now integrated hepatitis B vaccine into their routine immunization programme, with varying levels of coverage (Fig. 4.16). Hepatitis B vaccine may now be available to around half the world's children. However, children from countries with the highest risk of HBV infection are frequently the same countries with limited resources or infrastructure to provide the vaccination. Despite the decline in vaccine cost, limited health budgets in poorer countries make ability to purchase vaccine a primary obstacle to global immunization. WHO and other donor and non-profit agencies have focused on developing a vaccine support strategy to aid those needy countries with an adequate vaccination infrastructure to purchase and provide hepatitis B vaccine to the world's children.

REFERENCES

1. Edmunds WJ, Medley GF, Nokes DJ, Hall AJ, Whittle HC (1993) The influence of age on the development of the hepatitis B carrier state. *Proc R Soc Lond B Biol Sci*, 253: 197-201.

2. Hall AJ, Smith PG (1999) Prevention of hepatocellular cancer: one of the most cost-effective ways to reduce adult mortality? *Br J Cancer*, 81: 1097-1098.

3. Coursaget P, Muñoz N (1999) Vaccination against infectious agents associated with human cancer. In: Newton R, Beral V, Weiss RA eds, *Infection and Human Cancer, Vol. 33*, New York, Cold Spring Harbor Laboratory Press, 355-381.

4. Viviani S, Jack A, Hall AJ, Maine N, Mendy M, Montesano R, Whittle HC (1999) Hepatitis B vaccination in infancy in The Gambia: protection against carriage at 9 years of age. *Vaccine*, 17: 2946-2950.

5. Montesano R, Hainaut P, Wild CP (1997) Hepatocellular carcinoma: from gene to public health. *J Natl Cancer Inst*, 89: 1844-1851.

6. Chang MH, Chen CJ, Lai MS, Hsu HM, Wu TC, Kong MS, Liang DC, Shau WY, Chen DS (1997) Universal hepatitis B vaccination in Taiwan and the incidence of hepatocellular carcinoma in children. Taiwan Childhood Hepatoma Study Group. *N Engl J Med*, 336: 1855-1859.

WEBSITES

WHO fact sheets on vaccination against HBV and HCV: http://www.who.int/health-topics/hepatitis.htm

CDC National Center for Infectious Diseases: http://www.cdc.gov/ncidod/diseases/hepatitis/b/index.htm

HUMAN PAPILLOMAVIRUS VACCINATION

SUMMARY

> Infection with human papillomaviruses is common and causes some benign lesions as well as cervical and other cancers.

> Vaccines based on human papillomaviruses may be prophylactic, therapeutic or a combination of both, and are potentially a safe and effective means of preventing or controlling disease.

> Technical difficulties associated with the development of such vaccines are considerable, but several phase I, II and III trials are under way.

From a public health perspective, there is an overwhelming case to justify the development of human papillomavirus (HPV) vaccines. At least 50% of sexually active adults have had a genital HPV infection. So-called "low-risk" HPV types cause benign lesions or genital warts, while others, called "high-risk" or "oncogenic" types, are the principal cause of cervical cancer and are also associated with other cancers of the anogenital region, and possibly with cancers of the upper aerodigestive tract and of the skin (*Chronic infections*, p56; *Cancers of the female reproductive tract*, p215). Since both genital warts and cervical cancer rates are rising in young women in some populations, the burden of HPV-associated disease is likely to increase in coming decades.

HPV-associated lesions can regress spontaneously due to cell-mediated immunity. This is indicated by an increased risk of HPV infection and of HPV-associated lesions in immunosuppressed patients, and the observation that neutralizing antibodies can block HPV infection *in vivo* and *in vitro* [1]. On the other hand, the occurrence of chronic HPV infections and reinfections suggests that in some individuals natural immunity is not effective in controlling HPV infection. Although the exact mechanisms of immune evasion are not fully understood, the development of effective vaccines for papillomaviruses in various animal models [2-4] has stimulated the development of similar vaccines for humans.

Three main types of HPV vaccine are being developed: prophylactic vaccines, therapeutic vaccines and combined or chimeric vaccines which have both effects.

Prophylactic vaccines

Vaccines based on the induction of neutralizing antibodies against the HPV structural proteins L1 and L2 are termed "prophylactic". The generation of virus-like particles (VLPs), which are morphologically indistinguishable from authentic virions, apart from lacking the viral genome [5], has greatly accelerated the development of these vaccines (Table 4.9).

VLPs for HPV 6, 11, 16, 18, 31, 33, 39, 45 and 58 have been produced in various laboratories. At least five HPV VLP-based vaccines have been developed and have gone through pre-clinical evaluation. Phase I-II clinical trials to assess safety, immunogenicity, dose, schedule, route of administration and adjuvants for these vaccines are being planned or have been initiated. The US National Cancer Institute (NCI) vaccine has been shown, in a phase I study of 58 women and 14 men, to be able to induce serum antibody titres that are approximately 40-fold higher than that observed during natural infection [6]. However, certain basic issues need to be solved before the mass use of these vaccines can commence [7,8]. Such issues include the HPV types to be included (HPV 16 accounts for 50% and HPV 18, 31 and 45 for a further 30% of cervical cancers), the route of administration, the target population (ideally infants) and the cost (Table 4.10). The ideal HPV vaccine will have to be polyvalent (i.e. contain the VLPs of the HPV types most commonly associated with cancer in a given population, Fig. 4.22), inexpensive, and able to confer a long-lasting protection for infants of both sexes. Although HPV-associated genital tumours are much more frequent in women than men, men act as vectors of the virus.

While the problems already outlined are being solved, phase III trials to assess the efficacy of available VLP-based vaccines to prevent HPV infection and cervical intraepithelial neoplasia are being planned. For example, the NCI vaccine will be used in a phase III trial in Costa Rica in the context of a large cohort study on the natural history of HPV in Guanacaste province.

Therapeutic and combined vaccines

Vaccines based on the induction of cellular immunity directed against cells expressing viral proteins are termed "therapeutic" and are intended to induce

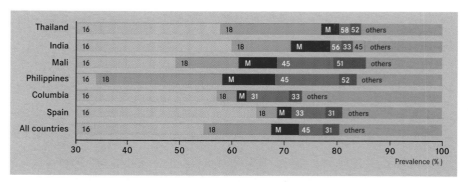

Fig. 4.22 The most common HPV types found in cervical carcinoma biopsies, by country. M = multiple infections with HPV 16 and/or 18.

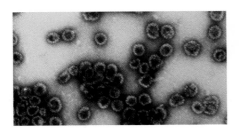

Fig. 4.23 Proteins which make up the HPV particle are used in the manufacture of a vaccine.

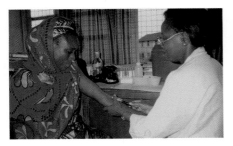

Fig. 4.24 Collecting blood from a participant in an HPV prevalence study, Ibadan, Nigeria.

Organization (vaccine name)	HPV type and antigen	Vaccine type	Current status
Medimmune SmithKline Beecham (MEDI-501)	HPV-11 L1	VLP	Phase II trials under way; safety and immune response proven in Phase I trials
Medimmune SmithKline Beecham (MEDI-503, 504)	HPV-16, 18 L1	VLP	Phase II trials under way
Merck, CSL Limited	HPV-16 L1	VLP	Phase II trials under way in USA, UK and Australia; Phase III to begin soon
National Cancer Institute, NIAID	HPV-16 L1	VLP	Phase II trials under way; large-scale efficacy trial planned to begin in Costa Rica in 2002
Medigene	HPV16 L1, E7	VLP	Phase I/II trial

Table 4.9 Prophylactic HPV vaccines under development in clinical trials. VLP = virus-like particles

regression of HPV-associated lesions. The E6 and E7 proteins (*Oncogenes and tumour suppressor genes*, p96) are the natural targets for these vaccines because such proteins are consistently expressed in cervical cancer cells. Since neither protein is located on the cell surface, the most effective mechanism for the destruction of cancer cells is likely to be through the action of cytotoxic T cells which recognize intracellular processed peptides in complex with major histocompatibility complex (MHC) class I molecules. Candidate therapeutic vaccines are constituted using either synthetic peptides, recombinant proteins or live vectors coding for HPV proteins [8].

Several vaccines that target the E6 and E7 oncoproteins of HPV 16 and 18 are now available and are being used in phase I-II trials (Table 4.11). These trials have been, or are being carried out in patients with advanced cervical cancer or in patients with genital precancerous lesions. Some of the vaccines are peptide-based while others are based on a recombinant vaccinia vector expressing E6 and E7 from both HPV 16 and 18 [9]. Results from only one of these trials have been published in full [10]. As is the case for prophylactic HPV vaccines, in order to develop safe and effective therapeutic vaccines, serious technical difficulties must be overcome. Such vaccines must be tailored to the MHC antigens of the recipients and must elicit a stronger anti-tumour response than that produced without vaccination.

Combined or chimeric vaccines are designed to have the ability to both protect against HPV infection and induce regression of HPV-associated lesions [8]. The first approach considered was to develop an L1 or L1-L2 VLP-based vaccine capable of inducing a cytotoxic T-cell response. Another approach being used is the production of chimeric VLPs that contains both L1 or L1-L2 and E6 or E7 proteins [9]. Such vaccines should induce a protective response elicited by L1 or L2 proteins and a cytotoxic T cell-mediated response elicited by the E6 or E7 proteins. There are still many technical and practical problems to be solved before safe, effective and inexpensive HPV vaccines are produced for mass use in the general population. Although these problems appear to be greater for therapeutic vaccines, their production has moved into an industrial phase. Lessons learnt from the slow introduction of hepatitis B virus vaccine into routine immunization pro-

Issue	Comments
HPV types to be included	At least 30 oncogenic types exist, but HPV 16 accounts for 50% and HPV 18, 31, and 45 together for a further 30% of cervical cancers
Route of administration	Oral or nasal spray
Target population	Ideally infants, girls and boys
Cost	It should be low, perhaps using bacterial vectors or transgenic plants

Table 4.10 Open issues in the development of prophylactic HPV vaccines.

Vaccine	Site of trial	Number of patients	Condition of patients
Recombinant vaccinia HPV 16 and 18 E6 and E7 proteins (Cantab Pharmaceuticals, UK)	UK (University of Wales) UK (University of Wales) US (NCI) UK, The Netherlands, Belgium, Germany and Sweden	8 10 14 18	Advanced cervical cancer CIN III lesions Advanced cervical cancer Early invasive cervical cancer
HPV 6-L2 E7 fusion protein (Cantab Pharmaceuticals, UK)	UK (London)	36	Genital warts
HPV 16-E7 protein	Australia (Queensland)	5	Advanced cervical cancer
HPV 16-E7 peptide	The Netherlands (Leiden University)	15	Advanced cervical cancer
HPV 16-peptide	US (Norris Cancer Center, USC)	45 15	CIN II-III lesions VIN lesions
HPV 16-E7 peptide	US (NCI) (Cytel Co, US)	15	Recurrent or refractory cervical cancer

Table 4.11 Phase I-II clinical trials with HPV therapeutic vaccines.

grammes should help to reduce the period between availability of an appropriate HPV vaccine and its introduction for routine use. However, it is unlikely that this will happen within the next 15-20 years. Meanwhile efforts should continue to introduce or improve existing screening programmes for cervical cancer (*Screening for cervical cancer*, p 167).

REFERENCES

1. IARC (1995) *Human Papillomaviruses (IARC Monographs on the Evaluation of Carcinogenic Risks to Humans, Vol. 64)*, Lyon, IARCPress.

2. Kirnbauer R, Chandrachud L M, O'Neil B W, Wagner E R, Grindlay G J, Armstrong A, McGarvie G M, Schiller J T, Lowy D R, Campo M S (1996) Virus-like particles of bovine papillomavirus type 4 in prophylactic and therapeutic immunization. *Virology*, 219: 37-44.

3. Suzich J A, Ghi S J, Palmer-Hill F (1995) Systemic immunization with papillomavirus L1 protein completely prevents the development of viral mucosal papillomavirus. *Proc Natl Acad Sci*, 92: 11553-11557.

4. Jansen K U, Rosolowsky M, Schultz L D, Markus H Z, Cook J C, Donnelly J J, Martinez D, Ellis R W, Shaw A R (1995) Vaccination with yeast-expressed cottontail rabbit papillomavirus (CRPV) virus-like particles protects rabbits from CRPV-induced papilloma formation. *Vaccine*, 13: 1509-1514.

5. Schiller J T, Roden R B (1995) Papillomavirus-like particles. *Papillomavirus Rep*, 6: 121-128.

6. Harro CD, Pang YY, Roden RB, Hildesheim A, Wang Z, Reynolds MJ, Mast TC, Robinson R, Murphy BR, Karron RA, Dillner J, Schiller JT, Lowy DR (2001) Safety and immunogenicity trial in adult volunteers of a human papillomavirus 16 L1 virus-like particle vaccine. *J Natl Cancer Inst*, 93: 284-292.

7. Bosch F X, Manos M M, Muñoz N, Sherman M, Jansen A M, Peto J, Schiffman M H, Moreno V, Kurman R, Shah K V (1995) Prevalence of human papillomavirus in cervical cancer: a worldwide perspective. International biological study on cervical cancer (IBSCC) Study Group. *J Natl Cancer Inst*, 87: 796-802.

8. Coursaget P, Muñoz N (1999) Vaccination against infectious agents associated with human cancer. In: Newton R, Beral V, Weiss RA eds, *Infection and Human Cancer*, Vol. 33, New York, Cold Spring Harbor Laboratory Press, 355-381.

8. McNeil C (1997) HPV vaccine treatment trials proliferate, diversify. *J Natl Cancer Inst*, 89: 280-281.

10. Borysiewicz L K, Fiander A, Nimako M, Man S, Wilkinson G W, Westmoreland D, Evans A S, Adams M, Stacey S N, Boursnell M E, Rutherford E, Hickling J K, Inglis S C (1996) A recombinant vaccinia virus encoding human papillomavirus types 16 and 18, E6 and E7 proteins as immunotherapy for cervical cancer. *Lancet*, 347: 1523-1527.

WEBSITE

Vaccines, Immunization and Biologicals (WHO): http://www.who.int/vaccines/en/hpvrd.shtml

CHEMOPREVENTION

SUMMARY

> Chemoprevention is defined as reduction of the risk of cancer development through the use of pharmaceuticals or micronutrients.

> The breast cancer drug tamoxifen reduces the risk of developing a second cancer in the other breast.

> A lower risk of colon cancer has been observed following regular use of aspirin and related non-steroidal anti-inflammatory drugs which reduce the risk of recurrence of adenomas.

> Trials to establish chemopreventive activity by micronutrients, including carotenoids and retinoids, among people at high risk, have been inconclusive.

The goal of chemoprevention is to prevent or reverse the process of carcinogenesis, or to enhance regression of abnormal cells or tissue to normality with minimal or no side-effects. Relevant mechanisms vary, and in many cases have not been determined. Although the carcinogenic process is often characterized as being dependent on mutation, epigenetic changes are also involved. These may be perturbed during the 20-year (or longer) latent period before invasion and metastasis occur (*Multistage carcinogenesis*, p84) and appear to provide the basis for chemopreventive activity by a variety of agents. Chemoprevention may have great potential for control of cancer.

The scope of chemopreventive agents

Many studies have shown that people who consume more vegetables and fruit than persons at otherwise the same risk who consume less or none, have a reduced risk of cancer (*Diet and nutri-*

tion, p62). Although the results of intervention trials of dietary augmentation with fibre and fruit and vegetables to reduce the occurrence of colonic polyps have so far been negative, there is considerable evidence, particularly from experimental studies, that some chemicals present in the diet at low concentrations play an important role in protecting against cancer. Some examples include folate, curcumin, genistein, selenium and tea catechins. Micronutrients (defined as nutrients present in the body in amounts less than 0.005% of body weight) which appear to protect against cancer include β-carotene, α-tocopherol and ascorbic acid. The preventive activity of vegetables and fruit is partially credited to micronutrients. However, intake of these agents as vitamin pills or diet supplements is yet to be established (through trials) as preventing cancer in humans. So, although the evidence suggests that modification of diet can lower cancer risk, the same effect is not yet achievable using easy-to-take, pre-packaged natural or synthetic compounds. Putative chemopreventive agents include pharmaceutical drugs and hormonally active agents. There is conclusive evidence that tamoxifen reduces the risk for contralateral breast cancer in women with a previous diagnosis of breast cancer. Observational studies indicate a moderately reduced risk for colorectal cancer in people using aspirin regularly, and an indication of greater reduction in risk with

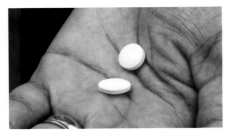

Fig. 4.25 The aim of chemoprevention is to prevent cancer by the administration of easy-to-take, pre-packaged natural or synthetic compounds typically in the form of a pill.

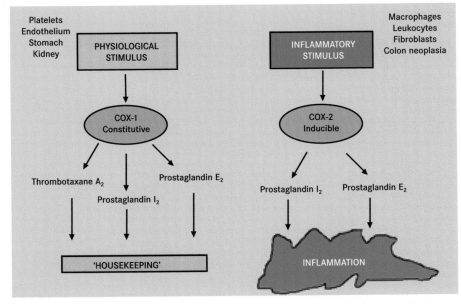

Fig. 4.26 COX-1 and COX-2 cyclooxygenases: COX-1 is constitutively expressed and regulates the homeostasis of various tissues, including the generation of cytoprotective prostaglandins. Inflammatory stimuli induce COX-2, which is also highly expressed in colorectal neoplasia in the absence of stimulation.

prolonged use. Similar drugs, that is other non-steroidal anti-inflammatory drugs, appear to have this effect, and cancers at sites apart from the bowel may be susceptible. In respect of these and similar agents, the IARC began a series of *Handbooks of Cancer Prevention* in 1997 by considering the cancer-preventive activity of non-steroidal anti-inflammatory drugs [1]. Subsequent volumes have been published on carotenoids [2], vitamin A [3], retinoids [4] and use of sunscreens [5], the latter being substances that reduce exposure to a carcinogenic agent (in this case, sunlight).

Relevant mechanisms

The appropriate use of a chemopreventive agent may depend on an understanding of the mechanism of action at all levels, in animals and humans. Without this knowledge, selection of preventive agents is intuitive or the product of chance. The

trend in the field of chemoprevention has therefore been to develop new agents based on known mechanisms of action.

COX-2 inhibition

One aspect of tumour development is the release of arachidonic acid and its metabolism to eicosanoids, including prostaglandins. Down-regulation of the cyclooxygenases (COX-1 and COX-2) by pharmacological means may result in reduced incidence of cancer, because cyclooxygenases catalyse the formation of prostaglandins, which have multiple effects that favour carcinogenesis [7] (Fig. 4.26). A number of prostaglandin synthesis inhibitors are effective in counteracting tumorigenesis. Compounds such as anti-inflammatory steroids (i.e. glucocorticoids) are potent inhibitors of experimental skin carcinogenesis [8]. These compounds are effective inhibitors of phospholipase A_2, which may explain their abil-

ity to decrease the amount of arachidonic acid available for metabolism to pro-inflammatory prostaglandins.

Aspirin and aspirin-like drugs can inhibit colorectal tumorigenesis and are among the few agents reported to be useful for chemoprevention of neoplasia [1]. The cyclooxygenase pathway is a major target for prevention by non-steroidal anti-inflammatory drugs, primarily because COX-2 plays a role in inflammation as well as in apoptosis and angiogenesis. From the perspective of chemoprevention, the recent finding that overexpression of the gene for COX-2, a key enzyme for the formation of prostaglandins from arachidonic acid, is an early and central event in colon carcinogenesis provides an important target for the development of chemopreventive agents [9]. Overexpression of COX-2 in epithelial cells inhibits apoptosis and increases the invasiveness of tumour cells [10]. Treatment of colon tumour cells

Agent	Humans	Animals
Non-steroidal anti-inflammatory drugs		
Aspirin	Limited	Sufficient
Sulindac	Limited	Sufficient
Piroxicam	Inadequate	Sufficient
Indomethacin	Inadequate	Sufficient
Carotenoids		
β-Carotene (high dose supplements)	Lack of activity	Sufficient
β-Carotene (usual dietary levels)	Inadequate	Sufficient
Canthaxanthin	Inadequate	Sufficient
α-Carotene	Inadequate	Limited
Lycopene	Inadequate	Limited
Lutein	Inadequate	Limited
Fucoxanthin	Inadequate	Limited
Retinoids		
all-*trans*-Retinoic acid	Inadequate	Inadequate
13-*cis*-Retinoic acid	Limited	Limited
9-*cis*-Retinoic acid	Inadequate	Limited
Fenretinide (4-HPR)	Inadequate	Sufficient
Etretinate	Inadequate	Limited
Acitretin	Inadequate	Inadequate
N-Ethylretinamide	Inadequate	Lack of activity
Targretin	Inadequate	Inadequate
LGD 1550	Inadequate	Inadequate
Preformed vitamin A	Lack of activity	Limited
Sunscreens	Limited (squamous cell carcinoma)	Sufficient
	Inadequate (basal cell carcinoma)	-
	Inadequate (malignant melanoma)	-

Table 4.12 Evidence of cancer preventive activity: evaluations from the *IARC Handbooks of Cancer Prevention* series.

with non-steroidal anti-inflammatory drugs results in a dramatic increase in arachidonic acid concentration, which, in turn, stimulates the conversion of sphingomyelin to ceramide, a known mediator of apoptosis. The activity of non-steroidal anti-inflammatory drugs to inhibit tumour growth may also be related to their induction of lipoxygenases [11].

New pharmacological agents, such as celecoxib, have recently been developed that are selective for inhibition of the enzymatic activity of COX-2, while not affecting the constitutive form of the enzyme, COX-1. Celecoxib has been shown to prevent colon carcinogenesis in a rodent model. In 2000, celecoxib was approved by the US Food and Drug Administration as an adjunct to standard care in patients with familial adenomatous polyposis, in whom *APC* gene defects result in a 100% chance of developing colorectal cancer. It is now in clinical trials in cohorts of patients at high risk of other cancers apart from the colorectum.

Estrogen receptor modulation

Through clinical trials, tamoxifen has been definitively shown to prevent contralateral breast cancer in women previously diagnosed with the disease [12], although an effect on survival has yet to be confirmed. Extensive trials are under way to determine whether a preventive effect may be achieved in women who have not had a previous breast cancer. Although tamoxifen and its derivatives have come into clinical use recently, they were synthesized well over 20 years ago, before the estrogen receptors were cloned. The mechanism of action of these drugs is now understood on the basis of the receptors. The demonstration of occurrence of the estrogen receptor-β, as contrasted with estrogen receptor-α, in the prostate, colon and ovary suggests that it may be useful to develop estrogen analogues that will selectively bind to this isoform of the receptor.

Retinoid receptors

Compounds related to vitamin A (retinoic acid and similar substances termed "retinoids") were initially shown to modu-

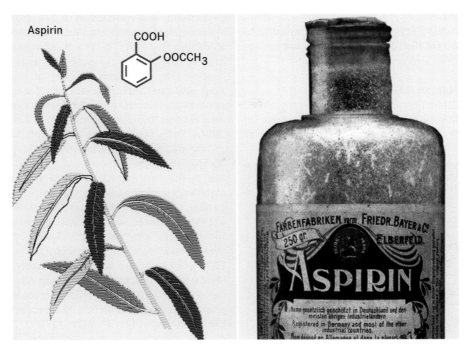

Fig. 4.27 The ancient Greeks chewed the bark of willow trees to alleviate pain and fever, but it was not until the last century that the active ingredient in willow bark, salicin, was isolated and commercially produced as aspirin. Observational studies have shown that regular use of aspirin reduces the risk of cancer of the colon and rectum.

late differentiation in many experimental systems [13]. Retinoids that are selective for binding to the three retinoid X receptors (RXRs), while not binding to the three retinoic acid receptors (RARs), may represent a specific class of chemopreventive agents. The retinoid X receptors are of particular importance in the nuclear receptor superfamily because of their ability to heterodimerize with many other members of this family, including retinoic acid receptors, the vitamin D receptor, the thyroid receptor, as well as with newly discovered "orphan" receptors, such as peroxisome-proliferator-activated receptor-γ.

Analytical epidemiology studies

Since 1970, the role of dietary fibre in colorectal cancer has been explored in many case-control studies, with relatively consistent results suggesting a reduced risk with higher consumption. A meta-analysis of these studies showed both an inverse association and a dose-response relationship [14]. The results of the cohort studies have been much less convincing.

In a recent prospective study of almost 90,000 female nurses who were followed up for more than 16 years, colorectal cancer developed in 787 women, and neither total dietary fibre nor dietary fibre from vegetables, fruit and cereals separately was associated with the risk for distal colonic or rectal adenomas. In fact, greater consumption of vegetable fibre was associated with a small increase in risk [15].

Both case-control and cohort studies have tended to show a reduced risk for colorectal cancer after prolonged use of aspirin [16]. Of 15 studies that specifically addressed the association between regular use of aspirin and/or other non-steroidal anti-inflammatory drugs and colorectal cancer, nine case-control and five out of six cohort studies recorded a lower risk for colorectal cancer; one cohort study showed an increased risk for colorectal cancer among users of non-steroidal anti-inflammatory drugs [1]. As observational epidemiological studies can be subject to bias, chemoprevention with aspirin and other non-steroidal anti-inflammatory drugs should only be considered established if there are appropriate results from a randomized trial.

Human intervention trials

A number of studies have been performed in which the serum concentrations of β-carotene or dietary intake of

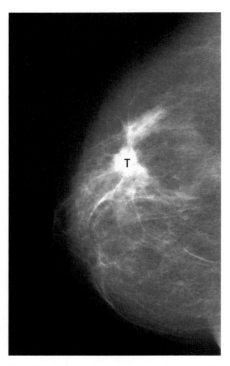

Fig. 4.28 Mammogram showing the location of a tumour (T). Treatment of invasive breast cancer with tamoxifen reduces the risk of a second tumour in the contralateral breast.

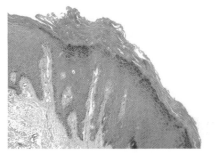

Fig. 4.29 Histopathology of oral leukoplakia which has been assayed in cancer chemopreventive trials with retinoids (see Box: *Precursor lesions in chemoprevention trials*, p87).

β-carotene were assessed in observational epidemiological studies in relation to cancer risk [17]. The results of these studies suggest that β-carotene has preventive effects against cancers of the lung, oral cavity and pharynx. In order to confirm this interpretation, three large intervention trials were started in the 1980s. Enthusiasm for use of β-carotene in chemoprevention was substantially dampened by the outcomes of these trials. In the two largest, β-carotene use significantly increased the risk for lung cancer among smokers and/or asbestos-exposed workers within three to six years after the start. The third trial, conducted among physicians in the USA who were primarily non-smokers, showed no increased risk for lung cancer [18]. In one of the trials, α-tocopherol supplementation had no effect on the occurrence of lung cancer [19].

A 32% reduction in the incidence of prostate cancer and a 41% reduction in deaths from this cancer were recorded among the smokers randomly assigned to a daily dose of α-tocopherol (vitamin E) in the Alpha-Tocopherol, Beta-Carotene Cancer Prevention Study. There was, however, a 50% increase in the occurrence of cerebral haemorrhage among those men taking vitamin E [19]. Thus, before use of vitamin E can be recommended for the prevention of prostate cancer, another trial should be conducted in an independent setting, with careful attention to possible side-effects. The chemoprevention of prostate cancer is otherwise under active evaluation. A number of ongoing randomized trials are comparing the effects of selenium, soy protein, finasteride and other agents. None of these trials have yet yielded unequivocal evidence for the efficacy of any particular agent. It is hoped, however, that dietary supplements will limit the progression of the ubiquitous latent prostate hyperplasia associated with the ageing male to aggressive, malignant disease.

Several combinations of vitamins and salt were tested in a large Chinese trial, and one of these combinations (β-carotene plus vitamins plus selenium)

led to a 13% reduction in total cancer mortality, significant 21% reduction in stomach cancer mortality, but no significant reduction in oesophageal cancer, which was the primary target of the study. Recently a clinical trial on men with a history of non-melanoma skin cancer found that the incidence of prostate cancer was 63% lower among those treated with selenium compared to men receiving a placebo [20].

The future of chemoprevention trials

An issue which is of primary concern for investigations on diet and cancer is to what extent the rather disappointing results from trials of cancer chemoprevention and antioxidants (with the possible exception of those on selenium) negate the results obtained in observational epidemiological studies on the same compounds and on fruit and vegetables. There are at least two important differences between these clinical trials and studies on diet. The first is the dose: the clinical trials used doses of β-carotene (15 to 25 mg per day) which led to blood concentrations 10 to 20 times higher than those achievable through high dietary intake of fruit and vegetables. The second is that clinical trials generally tested one or two compounds at a time, at high doses, while fruit and vegetables represent a complex mixture of hundreds of natural compounds.

The use of the double-blind, placebo-controlled randomized trial design for evaluating preventive actions is important. Many examples are now available of chemopreventive agents which appear to have a beneficial effect in observational studies, but which have failed in randomized trials. Regarding future research in this area, the contradictory results of clinical trials suggest that observational studies combining dietary data and biological markers of diet should be exploited more thoroughly to identify combinations of nutrients potentially associated with cancer prevention and which may be candidates for experimental studies on laboratory animals and, eventually, for chemoprevention trials in humans. We also need more knowledge of the concentrations of chemopreventive agents and their metabolites that prevent cancer in rodents and how such concentrations relate to those achievable in target human tissues. Finally, the selected intervention agents should be tested in pilot clinical studies before embarking on large-scale randomized efficacy trials.

REFERENCES

1. IARC (1997) *Non-Steroidal Anti-Inflammatory Drugs (IARC Handbooks of Cancer Prevention, Vol. 1)*, Lyon, IARCPress.

2. IARC (1998) *Carotenoids (IARC Handbooks of Cancer Prevention, Vol. 2)*, Lyon, IARCPress.

3. IARC (1998) *Vitamin A (IARC Handbooks of Cancer Prevention, Vol. 3)*, Lyon, IARCPress.

4. IARC (1999) *Retinoids (IARC Handbooks of Cancer Prevention, Vol. 4)*, Lyon, IARCPress.

5. IARC (2001) *Sunscreens (IARC Handbooks of Cancer Prevention, Vol. 5)*, Lyon, IARCPress.

6. IARC (2002) *Weight Control and Physical Activity (IARC Handbooks of Cancer Prevention, Vol. 6)*, Lyon, IARCPress.

7. Taketo MM (1998) Cyclooxygenase-2 inhibitors in tumorigenesis (Part I). *J Natl Cancer Inst*, 90: 1529-1536.

8. DiGiovanni J (1992) Multistage carcinogenesis in mouse skin. *Pharmacol Ther*, 54: 63-128.

9. Thun MJ, Henley SJ, Patrono C (2002) Nonsteroidal anti-inflammatory drugs as anticancer agents: mechanistic, pharmacologic, and clinical issues. *J Natl Cancer Inst*, 94: 252-266.

10. Gupta RA, DuBois RN (2001) Colorectal cancer prevention and treatment by inhibition of cyclooxygenase-2. *Nature Reviews Cancer*, 1: 11-21.

11. Shureiqi I, Lippman SM (2001) Lipoxygenase modulation to reverse carcinogenesis. *Cancer Res*, 61: 6307-6312.

12. IARC (1996) *Some Pharmaceutical Drugs (IARC Monographs on the Evaluation of Carcinogenic Risks to Humans, Vol. 66)*, Lyon, IARCPress.

13. Hansen LA, Sigman CC, Andreola F, Ross SA, Kelloff GJ, De Luca LM (2000) Retinoids in chemoprevention and differentiation therapy. *Carcinogenesis*, 21: 1271-1279.

14. Howe GR, Benito E, Castelleto R, Cornee J, Estève J, Gallagher RP, Iscovich JM, Deng-ao J, Kaaks R, Kune GA (1992) Dietary intake of fiber and decreased risk of cancers of the colon and rectum: evidence from the combined analysis of 13 case-control studies. *J Natl Cancer Inst*, 84: 1887-1896.

15. Fuchs CS, Giovannucci EL, Colditz GA, Hunter DJ, Stampfer MJ, Rosner B, Speizer FE, Willett WC (1999) Dietary fiber and the risk of colorectal cancer and adenoma in women. *N Engl J Med*, 340: 169-176.

16. Vainio H, Morgan G, Kleihues P (1997) An international evaluation of the cancer-preventive potential of non-steroidal anti-inflammatory drugs. *Cancer Epidemiol Biomarkers Prev*, 6: 749-753.

17. Vainio H, Rautalahti M (1998) An international evaluation of the cancer preventive potential of carotenoids. *Cancer Epidemiol Biomarkers Prev*, 7: 725-728.

18. Hennekens CH, Buring JE, Manson JE, Stampfer M, Rosner B, Cook NR, Belanger C, LaMotte F, Gaziano JM, Ridker PM, Willett W, Peto R (1996) Lack of effect of long-term supplementation with beta carotene on the incidence of malignant neoplasms and cardiovascular disease. *N Engl J Med*, 334: 1145-1149.

19. Heinonen OP, Albanes D, Virtamo J, Taylor PR, Huttunen JK, Hartman AM, Haapakoski J, Malila N, Rautalahti M, Ripatti S, Maenpaa H, Teerenhovi L, Koss L, Virolainen M, Edwards BK (1998) Prostate cancer and supplementation with alpha-tocopherol and beta-carotene: incidence and mortality in a controlled trial. *J Natl Cancer Inst*, 90: 440-446.

20. Clark LC, Dalkin B, Krongrad A, Combs GF, Jr., Turnbull BW, Slate EH, Witherington R, Herlong JH, Janosko E, Carpenter D, Borosso C, Falk S, Rounder J (1998) Decreased incidence of prostate cancer with selenium supplementation: results of a double-blind cancer prevention trial. *Br J Urol*, 81: 730-734.

WEBSITES

The NCI's Rapid Access to Preventive Intervention Development (RAPID) Program:
http://www.cancer.gov/prevention/rapid/#1

Medscape Drug Info (for information on aspirin, β-carotene, celecoxib, tamoxifen, vitamin A):
http://www.medscape.com/druginfo

SCREENING FOR BREAST CANCER

SUMMARY

> The epidemic increase in breast cancer incidence has led to the introduction of population-based mammography screening.

> The analysis of large randomized trials has shown that in women aged 50 to 69 years, mammography screening can reduce mortality from breast cancer by 25-30%. For women in the age group 40-49 years the screening efficacy is significantly less.

> The benefits of mammography in regional or national screening programmes is lower. Under optimal conditions with a high compliance rate, a mortality reduction of 20% appears achievable.

> There is only indirect evidence that screening by clinical breast examination will reduce the number of breast cancer deaths.

Cancer of the breast is the most common cancer in women worldwide and in many regions, including Europe and Australia, it is still the most common cause of death from cancer in women. Until recently, there has been little change in mortality rates in spite of the steady improvement in prognosis observed in recent years.

Breast cancer is characterized by early systemic dissemination. As a result, awareness of symptoms, and subsequent diagnosis, often occur when disease is advanced and metastatic. Mammography (an X-ray examination of the breasts) can detect preclinical cancer, that is, detect the tumour before it is palpable, or before it causes symptoms. Tumours detected and treated at an early stage, can be expected to be associated with a better survival rate than those detected symptomatically. Early diagnosis may permit breast-conserving surgery (stage I disease), reduce the need for adjuvant thera-

py or decrease complications related to intensive treatment and recurrence [1]. Population-based mammographic screening programmes were introduced in this context.

The impact of screening

Since the 1970s, the incidence of breast cancer has continued to increase. Only in 4 out of 70 populations assessed worldwide was there an average change between 1975 and 1990 of less than 0.5% per year [2,3]. Steep increases of the order of 3-5% per year have occurred in some Asian countries (e.g. Japan, Singapore), in Asian migrants to the USA (Japanese, Chinese and Filipino) and Southern Europe (Spain) (Fig. 4.31). In some developed countries (e.g. England and Wales, Finland, Denmark, The Netherlands, USA), a clear change in the speed of increase can be linked to the introduction of mass screening that occurred at different times in different countries, e.g. in the early 1980s in the USA, 1987-88 in England and Wales, early 1990s in The Netherlands. Some increase is attributable to reduced fertility and changing dietary habits. However, mam-

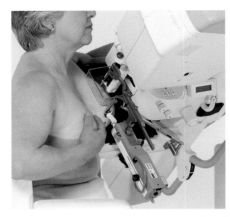

Fig. 4.30 Mammography, an X-ray examination of the breasts, is used to screen for breast cancer.
©GE Medical Systems

mography is the main determinant of these relatively recent increases as indicated by trends in the incidence of *in situ* cancers [4,5].

Mortality has not consistently paralleled incidence trends everywhere. In fact, in some developed countries rates have been rather stable, even with incidence on the increase. No clear overall decline in mortality had been observed in any place before the late 1980s, when a smooth downturn occurred in Europe, North America and Australia. Such changes before the era of mammography can be attributed to a progression towards early diagnosis that took place in the 1970s, particularly in young generations. More recently, in the early 1990s, a drastic fall in mortality was seen in the UK and North America [6,7]. However, the fall occurred too soon after the widespread availability of mammography to be a consequence of it; rather, the success of adjuvant therapy based on chemotherapy and tamoxifen is the likely major cause of this trend.

Protocols for screening

As currently practised, population-based screening for breast cancer is based on mammographic examination, at prescribed intervals, of all women within a

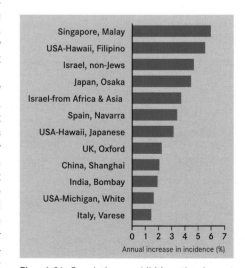

Fig. 4.31 Populations exhibiting the largest increases in the incidence of breast cancer between 1975 and 1990.

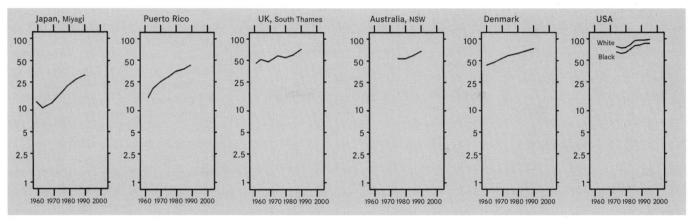

Fig. 4.32 Trends in breast cancer incidence. D.M. Parkin et al. (2001) *Eur J Cancer* 37, suppl. 8: S4-66.

specified age group. As of 1995, at least 22 countries had established national, sub-national or pilot population breast cancer screening programmes [8]. The specification of an eligible age range, and the "repeat interval", are matters for national (or other authoritative) policy and vary accordingly. All programmes screen women by age 50 and repeat intervals are between one and three years. Establishment of the programmes depends on national or other health policy. There is considerable variation between screening programmes in relation to factors such as sociopolitical status of the screened population, public health priorities and funding sources. Implementation of population-based screening necessitates the provision of technical resources and the availability of trained personnel, together with a media campaign to publicize the service. The latter may be directed in part toward particular groups, including the elderly and/or women of low socioeconomic status, or who are members of minorities, since such groups are known to undergo mammography less frequently than the general population [9].

The evaluation of individual mammograms requires appropriate expertise and quality assurance standardization. Independent double reading of mammograms is recommended, but not carried out in all screening programmes [8,10]. It is also essential to provide for adequate "follow-up" procedures in respect of initial mammographic results not categorized as satisfying the criteria for normality. Follow-up necessitates contact with the individuals concerned, repeat and more comprehensive mammography, physical examination, ultrasonography and potentially biopsy. Cancers diagnosed after a negative mammogram are known as "interval" cancers. Mammographic breast density appears to be a major risk factor for interval cancer, worst risk being associated with extremely dense breasts [11]. Clinical examination and self-examination, whilst not proven to show a benefit in terms of reduction in breast cancer mortality, may aid in the detection of interval cancers, and are being evaluated for screening in countries that cannot afford mammography programmes. The International Breast Cancer Screening Network provides a basis for international collaborative effort designed

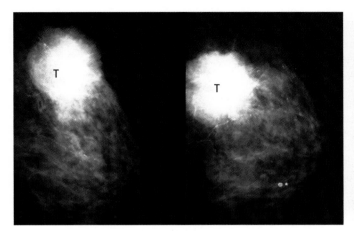

Fig. 4.33 Mammograms (2 views) from a patient displaying evidence of breast cancer. T = tumour.

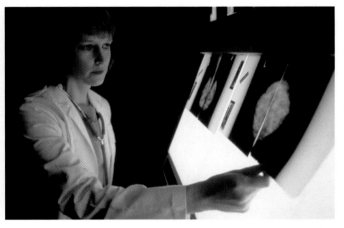

Fig. 4.34 The evaluation of mammograms requires appropriate expertise and standardization.

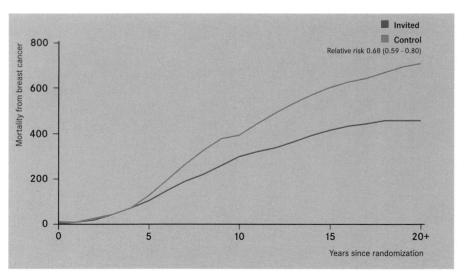

Fig. 4.35 Cumulative mortality from breast cancer in the Swedish Two-County screening trial. A reduction in mortality from breast cancer of 30% was found in the group of women that was invited for screening relative to the control group.

to document the varying breast cancer screening programmes, in order to produce international data on policies, administration and results of population-based breast cancer screening [7].

Evaluation of screening

Screening by mammography began to be widely adopted in the late 1980s following the publication of results of randomized trials. In fact, these studies gave heterogeneous results ranging from no reduction in mortality [12,13] to 30% of deaths prevented in women aged 50 or above [14]. In contrast, no significant reduction in mortality has been proven in younger women, which has led to differing recommendations and policies in various countries [15]. In most countries (e.g. United Kingdom,

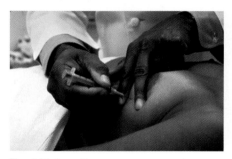

Fig. 4.36 A positive mammogram requires comprehensive follow-up, including fine needle biopsy.

Netherlands, Israel), screening is initiated in women of age 50 and above, whereas screening of women of ages 40-49 is performed in others (e.g. USA, Australia, Sweden). Several factors have been identified as possible sources of poorer performance in young women, including a lower sensitivity of the test due to greater density of the breast parenchyma (resulting in a higher risk of false positive and false negative results [16]) and faster tumour growth rate enhanced by circulating estrogen levels in premenopausal women [17]. Screening at more frequent intervals, every 12-18 months, may be required to obtain significant benefit in this age group [16].

Several countries have established organized screening programmes at the national or regional level, targeting women above the age of 50 [15]. These programmes were planned to reduce mortality by 25% and the effect was expected to become apparent about five years after implementation. So far, based on the results of randomized trials, the impact of screening interventions on older populations has been inferior to that expected, and the utility and justification of public financial support have been questioned [18,19]. IARC recently concluded that trials have provided sufficient evidence for the efficacy of

mammographic screening of women between 50 and 69 years old. Women who were invited to be screened showed a 25% reduction in breast cancer mortality. Since not all women accepted the invitation, the reduction among those who chose to participate in screening programmes is slightly higher, being estimated at 35%. For women aged 40-49, there is only limited evidence for a reduction [20].

By the time mammography was implemented for the general population, some benefit of early diagnosis was already being observed as an unplanned phenomenon, so the effect of the population-based programme was less than would have otherwise been expected. An impact of mammography is apparent from the increased relative frequency of *in situ* ductal carcinoma. If the lead time determined by modern mammography is significantly longer than that which characterized the test 20 years ago, a further reduction of mortality may be predicted. The natural history and biology of ductal carcinoma *in situ* is, however, poorly understood and the risk of over-treatment is at present of great concern [21]. Organized screening programmes should therefore be maintained and monitored until their full effect is clear.

REFERENCES

1. Leitch AM (1999) Breast cancer screening: success amid conflict. *Surg Oncol Clin N Am*, 8: 657-672, vi.

2. Parkin DM, Whelan SL, Ferlay J, Raymond L, Young J, eds (1997) *Cancer Incidence in Five Continents, Vol. VII (IARC Scientific Publications No. 143 and IARC Cancerbase No. 2)*, Lyon, IARCPress.

3. Waterhouse J, Muir C, Shanmugaratnam K, Powell J, Peacham D, Whelan S, eds (1982) *Cancer Incidence in Five Continents, Vol. IV (IARC Scientific Publications No. 42)*, Lyon, IARCPress.

4. Adams-Cameron M, Gilliland FD, Hunt WC, Key CR (1999) Trends in incidence and treatment for ductal carcinoma in situ in Hispanic, American Indian, and non-Hispanic white women in New Mexico, 1973-1994. *Cancer*, 85: 1084-1090.

5. Barchielli A, Paci E, Giorgi D (1999) Recent trends of in situ carcinoma of the breast and mammographic screening in the Florence area, Italy. *Cancer Causes Control*, 10: 313-317.

6. Quinn M, Allen E (1995) Changes in incidence of and mortality from breast cancer in England and Wales since introduction of screening. United Kingdom Association of Cancer Registries. *BMJ*, 311: 1391-1395.

7. Chu KC, Tarone RE, Kessler LG, Ries LA, Hankey BF, Miller BA, Edwards BK (1996) Recent trends in U.S. breast cancer incidence, survival, and mortality rates. *J Natl Cancer Inst*, 88: 1571-1579.

8. Ballard-Barbash R, Klabunde C, Paci E, Broeders M, Coleman EA, Fracheboud J, Bouchard F, Rennert G, Shapiro S (1999) Breast cancer screening in 21 countries: delivery of services, notification of results and outcomes ascertainment. *Eur J Cancer Prev*, 8: 417-426.

9. Whitman GJ (1999) The role of mammography in breast cancer prevention. *Curr Opin Oncol*, 11: 414-418.

10. Monsees BS (2000) The Mammography Quality Standards Act. An overview of the regulations and guidance. *Radiol Clin North Am*, 38: 759-772.

11. Mandelson MT, Oestreicher N, Porter PL, White D, Finder CA, Taplin SH, White E (2000) Breast density as a predictor of mammographic detection: comparison of interval- and screen-detected cancers. *J Natl Cancer Inst*, 92: 1081-1087.

12. Andersson I, Aspegren K, Janzon L, Landberg T, Lindholm K, Linell F, Ljungberg O, Ranstam J, Sigfusson B (1988) Mammographic screening and mortality from breast cancer: the Malmo mammographic screening trial. *BMJ*, 297: 943-948.

13. Miller AB, Baines CJ, To T, Wall C (1992) Canadian National Breast Screening Study: 1. Breast cancer detection and death rates among women aged 40 to 49 years. *CMAJ*, 147: 1459-1476.

14. Tabar L, Fagerberg G, Duffy SW, Day NE, Gad A, Grontoft O (1992) Update of the Swedish two-county program of mammographic screening for breast cancer. *Radiol Clin North Am*, 30: 187-210.

15. Moss S (1999) Breast cancer, In: Kramer BS, Gohagan JK, Prorok PC, eds, *Cancer Screening: Theory and Practice*, Marcel Dekker.

16. Primic-Zakelj M (1999) Screening mammography for early detection of breast cancer. *Ann Oncol*, 10 Suppl 6: 121-127.

17. Kerlikowske K, Barclay J (1997) Outcomes of modern screening mammography. *J Natl Cancer Inst Monogr*, 105-111.

18. De Koning HJ (2000) Breast cancer screening: cost-effective in practice? *Eur J Radiol*, 33: 32-37.

19. Olsen O, Gotzsche PC (2001) Cochrane review on screening for breast cancer with mammography. *Lancet*, 358: 1340-1342.

20. IARC (2002) *Breast Cancer Screening (IARC Handbooks of Cancer Prevention, Vol. 7)*, Lyon, IARCPress.

21. Ernster VL, Barclay J (1997) Increases in ductal carcinoma in situ (DCIS) of the breast in relation to mammography: a dilemma. *J Natl Cancer Inst Monogr*, 151-156.

WEBSITES

Information from the US NCI on testing for various cancers, including breast:
http://www.cancer.gov/cancerinfo/screening

NCI's Division of Cancer Prevention:
http://cancer.gov/prevention/

FDA's Mammography Programme:
http://www.fda.gov/cdrh/mammography/mqsa-rev.html

SCREENING FOR PROSTATE CANCER

SUMMARY

> Prostate-specific antigen (PSA) testing is widely used for the early detection of prostate cancer.

> Elevated levels of PSA are closely, but not definitively, associated with prostate cancer; false positive results may lead to unnecessary treatment.

> Assessment of population-based PSA screening suggests a reduction in mortality in countries with access to urological follow-up and treatment.

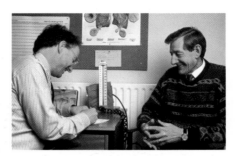

Fig. 4.37 A physician in discussion with a patient: informed consent is a prerequisite for PSA testing.

Secondary prevention of prostate cancer is feasible, but is subject to controversy, since the capacity to detect early disease must inevitably result in overtreatment for the individual patient, with substantial costs to society, in exchange for decreased mortality [1]. The lack of effective, appropriate markers of disease and any reasonable consensus on subsequent treatment necessitates extensive patient counselling as an important prerequisite, with some degree of prudence until the outcomes of the ongoing randomized trials in Europe and North America have been evaluated and audited [2].

Biological basis of secondary prevention

Prostate-specific antigen (PSA), a glycoprotein, is a proteinase that is responsible for the liquefaction of semen. PSA analysis has replaced prostatic acid phosphatase as the preferred serum marker of prostate cancer. The fact that PSA is highly tissue-specific and the consideration that few prostatic conditions result in a sustained, elevated level of serum PSA have made it the most efficacious marker currently available for the detection of prostate cancer. A serum "cut-off level" of 4 ng/ml for normality was used to demon-strate the efficacy of PSA as a diagnostic tool [3]. Unfortunately, 25% of patients diagnosed with prostate cancer have levels of serum PSA that are less than 4 ng/ml. Of men with PSA levels between 4-10 ng/ml, 25% have cancer, and 60% have cancer when PSA levels are greater than 10 ng/ml.

PSA analysis should be combined with a digital rectal examination, the latter providing an assessment of the volume of the gland, since PSA is also released into the bloodstream of patients with benign prostate hyperplasia and other prostatic diseases. To improve the sensitivity of the PSA analysis, a number of parameters may be assessed, most of which relate to concomitant benign prostate hyperplasia and also include age-specific reference ranges [4], typical values being: 40-49 years, <2.5 ng/ml; 50-59, <3.5 ng/ml, etc. A patient who proposes to have PSA assessed should be counselled about the relative risks and benefits that must be considered in relation to the procedure and its outcome (Table 4.13).

Other screening tests for prostate cancer focus on the different molecular forms of PSA, variously referred to as free PSA, total PSA, PSA-ACT complex assays and certain others. The ratio of free PSA to total PSA is reported to discriminate between cancer and benign prostate hyperplasia, thereby saving men from the prospect of intrusive biopsies, but always at the expense of missed cancers. For some of these newer forms of PSA analysis, the pre-analytical conditions for handling the blood sample should be closely monitored, since separation of the serum should be performed within three hours and the analyte then be determined within 24 hours. If this is difficult, the serum must be frozen for analysis at a later date. The efficacy of all these tests must be evaluated against prostatic biopsies that

Advantages	Disadvantages
Prostate cancer is an important public health problem	Available tests may detect innocuous and non-neoplastic lesions
Tests available are among the best screening tools in medicine	No consensus on optional early treatment
Advanced prostate cancer cannot be cured, early prostate cancer may be	Treatment morbidity may be high relative to benefit
Diagnosis at an earlier stage and lengthened survival are evident in many studies using PSA for early detection	Mortality reduction from screening has not yet been confirmed in prospective randomized trials

Table 4.13 A summary of the arguments in favour of, and against, prostate cancer screening.

Abnormal findings in digital rectal examination of the prostate
Induration of part of the gland
Asymmetry of the gland
A palpable nodule in the gland
Decreased mobility due to fixation of the gland

Table 4.14 Prostate characteristics indicative of abnormality in the context of digital rectal examination.

are positive, since the true prevalence of cancer in any cohort remains unknown (up to 20% of cancers can be missed). Continuous research to identify better markers is necessary, and in this regard studies of the kallikrein gene family are ongoing [5]. Prostate-specific membrane antigen has been seen to offer potential due to its consistent expression in prostate cancer, thereby opening possibilities for its use as a diagnostic, staging and predictive marker [6].

Development of screening protocols

The fate of patients with advanced stages of prostate cancer stands in sharp contrast to the outcome of treatment of patients with localized stages of the disease. The introduction of serum PSA analysis significantly changed the pattern of diagnosis of prostate cancer to include the non-palpable, non-visible tumours referred to as T1c tumours in the TNM classification (Box: *TNM classification of malignant tumours*, p124). In North America, Europe and other developed countries, evidence from the widespread application of digital rectal examination, serum PSA determination and subsequent transrectal ultrasound directed biopsy, has led to a significant shift in the time of diagnosis of prostate cancer to the earlier, confined stages of the disease. Recorded incidence rates have increased dramatically as an immediate result of earlier diagnosis of asymptomatic cancers through the introduction of PSA testing (Fig. 4.38). Subsequently, incidence rates have decreased in some populations, such as the USA, probably because the proportion of the population with latent tumours which can be detected by opportunistic screening has been exhausted [7].

Digital rectal examination is the simplest, safest and cheapest means of detecting prostate cancer provided that the tumour is localized in the gland. Although advanced local prostate cancer can be obvious, only one-third of suspicious abnormal findings on examination are actually confirmed as cancer (Table 4.14). Transrectal ultrasound was introduced as a possible refinement to digital rectal examination; prostate cancer may be detected as a hypo-echoic lesion. Wider adoption of the technique has revealed a false positive level comparable with that of digital examination, with only about one-third of all suspicious cases being confirmed as prostate cancer.

Evidence of outcome

A number of biases may complicate evaluation of any screening programme, and prostate cancer screening programmes in particular. These include lead-time bias, increasing survival as a consequence of earlier detection in the natural history of the disease and sampling that favours detection of less threatening cancers. Patient self-selection and overdiagnosis of preclinical cancers also tend to confuse outcome analysis. Even in the absence of trials, uncontrolled studies and the large numbers of specimens removed at radical prostatectomy have yielded important information about screening. These data indicate the extent to which diagnostic tests are performed and how such testing has led to a shift in disease stage at diagnosis and increased survival rates.

Some national authorities have recommended screening for the detection of prostate cancer by performing annual digital rectal examination and PSA tests, starting at the age of 50 (45 for high-risk patients), for men with at least a 10-year life expectancy [8]. These recommendations are generally being incorporated into men's health care programmes in many parts of the world. A slight but definite

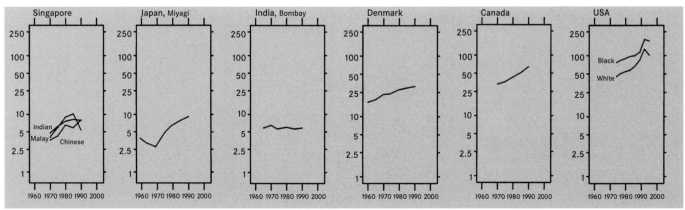

Fig. 4.38 Trends in the incidence of prostate cancer show a marked increase in many world regions, largely due to improved detection methods.
D.M. Parkin et al. (2001) *Eur J Cancer* 37, suppl. 8: S4-66.

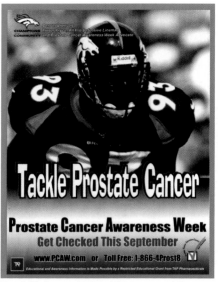

Fig. 4.39 Poster designed for an annual Prostate Cancer Awareness Week in the USA.

decrease in prostate cancer mortality has been recognized in countries where PSA was widely used in screening different cohorts of men. The decrease in mortality has become a major subject of discussion. A community-based randomized trial in Quebec suggested a mortality decrease of 69% in screened men, which provoked comment to the effect that a correct analysis by intention to treat showed no benefit [9]. There is a general expectation that the earlier detection of prostate cancer inevitably provides a unique chance for cure. The understanding of "cure", however, must include assessment of the quality of life experienced by the patient. Compli- cations currently inherent in the management of prostate cancer include those associated with procedures for diagnosis and treatment, the clear prevalence of over-diagnosis and the lack of any consensus on the appropriate treatment. Ultimately, resolution of many of these matters can only be achieved on the basis of the results of randomized controlled trials.

A multinational controlled trial in Europe has recruited 180,000 men randomized between diagnosis and treatment in screened men versus controls. In the USA, 74,000 men have been enrolled in a large controlled trial of screening for prostate, colorectal and other cancers. Collaboration between researchers concerned with these two trials has led to the development of the International Prostate Screening Trial Evaluation Group. The strength of the prospective planning and coordinated quality control will provide a sound basis for the scientific evidence required to answer the questions posed on the need for large population-based screening [10]. Currently, despite more than a decade of PSA-based screening, the impact of screening on mortality due to prostate cancer continues to be controversial, although some evidence of a decline in age-adjusted mortality rates for prostate cancer may be attributable, at least in part, to screening [11].

REFERENCES

1. Denis L, Mettlin C, Carter HB, De Koning HJ, Fourcade R, Fournier G, Hugosson J, Koroltchouk V, Moul J, Stephenson R (2000) Early detection and screening. In: Murphy GP, Khoury, S Partin, A Denis L, eds, *Prostate Cancer*, Paris, SCI, 221-233.

2. Standaert B, Denis L (1997) The European Randomized Study of Screening for Prostate Cancer: an update. *Cancer*, 80: 1830-1834.

3. Catalona WJ, Smith DS, Ratliff TL, Dodds KM, Coplen DE, Yuan JJ, Petros JA, Andriole GL (1991) Measurement of prostate-specific antigen in serum as a screening test for prostate cancer. *N Engl J Med*, 324: 1156-1161.

4. Morgan TO, Jacobsen SJ, McCarthy WF, Jacobson DJ, McLeod DG, Moul JW (1996) Age-specific reference ranges for prostate-specific antigen in black men. *N Engl J Med*, 335: 304-310.

5. Stephan C, Jung K, Lein M, Sinha P, Schnorr D, Loening SA (2000) Molecular forms of prostate-specific antigen and human kallikrein 2 as promising tools for early diagnosis of prostate cancer. *Cancer Epidemiol Biomarkers Prev*, 9: 1133-1147.

6. Chang SS, Gaudin PB, Reuter VE, Heston WD (2000) Prostate-specific membrane antigen: present and future applications. *Urology*, 55: 622-629.

7. Parkin DM, Bray FI, Devesa SS (2001) Cancer burden in the year 2000. The global picture. *Eur J Cancer*, 37 Suppl 8: S4-66.

8. von Eschenbach A, Ho R, Murphy GP, Cunningham M, Lins N (1997) American Cancer Society guidelines for the early detection of prostate cancer: update, June 10, 1997. *Cancer*, 80: 1805-1807.

9. Mettlin C (2000) Screening and early treatment of prostate cancer are accumulating strong evidence and support. *Prostate*, 43: 223-224.

10. The International Prostate Screening Trial Evaluation Group (1999) Rationale for randomised trials of prostate cancer screening. *Eur J Cancer*, 35: 262-271.

11. Cookson MM (2001) Prostate cancer: screening and early detection. *Cancer Control*, 8: 133-140.

WEBSITE

Preventing and detecting prostate cancer (NCI): http://www3.cancer.gov/prevention/spec_cancer.html#prostate

SCREENING FOR COLORECTAL CANCER

SUMMARY

> Faecal occult blood test (FOBT) is the most cost-effective and comprehensively-applicable screening method available, but its specificity and sensitivity are limited.

> Endoscopy provides the best method for detecting colorectal cancer and its precursor lesions, e.g. polyps. However, its application to population-based screening is limited by cost and availability of qualified specialists.

> For individuals at average risk in developed countries, screening may be recommended.

Registry	Number of cases (%)			
	Total	0-49 yrs	50-69 yrs	70-85+ yrs
Osaka Cancer Registry, 1987-89	8,051	1,016 (12.6%)	3,849 (47.8%)	3,185 (39.5%)
Denmark Cancer Registry, 1989	3,222	180 (5.5%)	1,146 (35.5%)	1,896 (58.8%)
Norway Cancer Registry, 1996	2,910	140 (4.8%)	954 (32.7%)	1,816 (62.4%)

Table 4.15 Age at diagnosis of colorectal cancer in Japan and Scandinavia, both sexes.

Colorectal cancer is one of the few internal cancers that are amenable to secondary prevention, that is, prevention by detection of preclinical lesions. A small proportion of colorectal cancers occurs among those with a family history of the disease. The main aim of screening is to detect the 90% of cases of colorectal cancer that occur sporadically, most of these in patients above the age of 50. The precursor of advanced colorectal cancer is either an adenomatous polyp or a flat neoplastic area (Fig. 4.40). In order to prevent premature deaths, people aged 50-69 years, among whom 35% of incident cases occur, are the main focus of attention (Table 4.15). Older age classes account for 60% of cases in developed countries, colorectal cancer being of relatively minor concern in developing countries. Simulation studies [1] conducted in the USA suggest small variations in cost and results with different strategies. The gain in life expectancy per person screened is small (1-4 weeks), but the benefit is great for the 5% destined to have cancer.

The faecal occult blood test

Screening by the faecal occult blood test (FOBT) is currently considered the optimal screening strategy in terms of cost-effectiveness. FOBT identifies persons at risk, though falling short of being definitive for cancer [2-7]. Guaiac resin-based slide tests indirectly measure haemoglobin levels in the faeces by the determination of peroxidase activity (Fig. 4.42). When a drop of water is added to the slide (i.e. the slide is rehydrated, as opposed to being non-hydrated) the test has been found to be more sensitive, although at the expense of a higher false positive rate. A false positive result to the guaiac resin reaction occurs after ingestion of dietary haemoglobin or peroxidase-containing foods. Between trials there is considerable variation in quantitative findings. Generally however, the test should be positive in no more than 2% of those screened. The sensitivity of the test is around 50% for cancer (of all screened persons who have cancer, 50% will be detected) but is low for polyps, at around 10%. The predictive value of a positive test

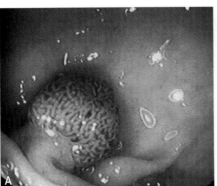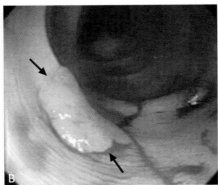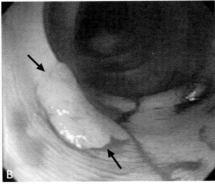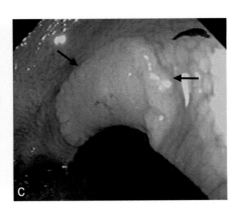

Fig. 4.40 Endoscopic features of (A) polypoid (B) slightly elevated and (C) flat adenoma of the colon.

is around 10% for cancer (out of every ten persons detected as positive, nine will not have cancer). An immunological FOBT for human haemoglobin is on trial; it is proving more specific, but also more costly. Screening procedures may be based on the malignant character of exfoliated cells. Genetic testing of stool samples for the *KRAS* oncogene and for p53 protein is not yet cost-effective.

Individuals at above average risk for colorectal cancer on the basis of family history may be stratified depending on the extent to which disease affects first-degree relatives. Having such a relative diagnosed at age 55 or over increases risk two-fold (by comparison with an individual with no family history), while one relative diagnosed under age 55, or two first degree relatives diagnosed at any age increases risk three- to six-fold. Persons at such increased risk should be monitored by annual FOBT. In some cases, familial predisposition may be dependent on a known gene defect. Genetic testing for adenomatous polyposis coli (*APC*) gene mutation diagnoses familial adenomatous polyposis. The test for microsatellite instability (replication error positive, RER, test), designed to establish a genetic basis for heritable nonpolyposis colon cancer, is also positive in 15% of sporadic cancers.

Endoscopy

Endoscopy [8], using either the flexible sigmoidoscope or the colonoscope [9-11], is the most definitive means of detection, but has limitations. The false negative rate for flat neoplastic lesions has been recognized and remains high [12]. Improved detection of flat neoplastic lesions is achieved using a high-resolution video-endoscope, with a contrast enhancement system and the use of chromoscopy (Fig. 4.40). A major advantage of endoscopy is in the potential for tissue sampling and interventional procedures. Population-based eradication of pedunculate or sessile adenomatous polyps may reduce cancer incidence.

With a depth of insertion varying from 48-55 cm, the limited reach of the flexible sigmoidoscope is its major weakness. In usual examinations, the instrument does not reach the splenic flexure and may not advance beyond the sigmoid colon. Accordingly, sigmoidoscopy may achieve 70% of the penetration that would be attained by colonoscopy. The colonoscope permits exploration of the colon with a low false negative rate for polypoid lesions of at least 10 mm in diameter. For this reason, the intervals allowed before re-examination are relatively long (up to ten years) after a negative assessment or up to five years after polypectomy. Patient compliance with such recommendations for re-examination after colonoscopy is poor, the cost of the procedure is high and the associated morbidity (perforation in about 0.3 examinations per 1000 performed by experienced gastroenterologists) may be of consequence in large series. To decrease costs, colonoscopy without sedation is being investigated. An imaging procedure which uses a camera system-on-a-chip (CMOS, which is cheaper than a closed-circuit display, CCD, camera) placed in a swallowed disposable capsule, is now suitable for exploration of the small intestinal lumen, but not that of the colon. Barium enema is rarely used in screening protocols; it is proposed when endoscopy is not available or has failed. "Virtual" endoscopy, a new imaging development, has not yet proved a reliable screening tool.

Mass screening protocols are generally recommended to be initiated in people of age 50 and above. Considerable uncertainty concerns the upper age limit, which has been recorded as high as 85 years for the first test. In general, screening may be stopped at age 70 after repeated negative tests. All protocols for follow-up of positive FOBT (Table 4.16) conclude with a colonoscopy, in a ratio varying from 4 to 100 % of those screened, depending on the strategy. Screening performed outside protocols is designated "opportunistic"; in this context endoscopy is the primary means of assessment.

Implementation of screening measures

Screening protocols have been evaluated through epidemiological studies. In respect of cost-effectiveness ratio (cost

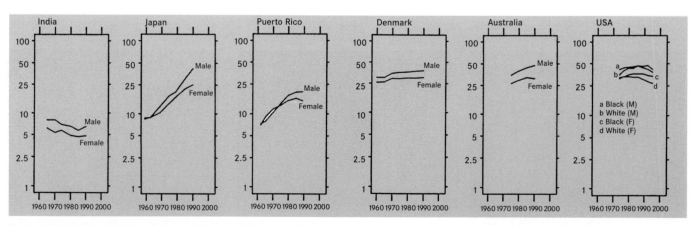

Fig. 4.41 Trends in the incidence of colorectal cancer. The increase is most prominent in countries which have most recently acquired the Western lifestyle.
D.M. Parkin et al. (2001) *Eur J Cancer* 37, suppl. 8: S4-66.

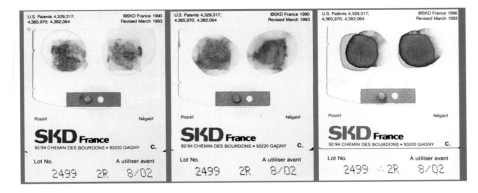

Fig. 4.42 The FOBT test for colorectal cancer (shown here is a Hemoccult II ® test). Three consecutive stools samples are applied to the test card. After addition of the reaction solution, a blue coloration indicates the presence of blood. A single positive result among the three samples indicates the need for a clinical examination of the colon.

Screening protocols
Annual faecal occult blood test
Biennial faecal occult blood test
Annual faecal occult blood test + fibrosigmoidoscopy every 5 years
Fibrosigmoidoscopy every 5 years
Colonoscopy every 10 years
Colonoscopy once in a lifetime

Table 4.16 Options for population-based screening protocols for colorectal cancer (in males and females, from the age of 50 years).

per year per life saved), screening for colorectal cancer in the USA has been evaluated as being below an arbitrary financial threshold adopted in screening (US$ 40,000 per year of life gained) and in this regard compares favourably with protocols for breast or cervical cancer screening. It has been estimated that screening 200,000 people in Australia using the FOBT would detect 250 colorectal cancers and prevent as many as 55 deaths. The FOBT gives the most cost-effective programme, but prevents fewer deaths than other programmes. A single colonoscopy has a greater impact on cancer mortality. Some health authorities in developed countries acknowledge the legitimacy of a screening protocol for colorectal cancer. However, the high cost of a generalized intervention and the limited acceptance of the tests by the population explain its limited application. It has been shown that nurses can perform sigmoidoscopy as competently as doctors, as indicated by the duration of the procedure, the ability to detect neoplasia and the risk of complications. When a lesion is detected in these circumstances, a colonoscopy is performed by a specialist.

Evidence of outcome

FOBT has been assessed in randomized trials. An American trial [2] was based on an annual rehydrated FOBT in volunteers.

The compliance was high (90.2%) and 38% of individuals screened underwent colonoscopy. There was a 33% reduction in specific mortality in the screened group (Table 4.17). Reduction in cancer incidence also occurred. In the two European, population-based, randomized trials [3,4] conducted in the UK and in Denmark with a biennial non-rehydrated FOBT, the compliance was lower (around 60%), only 4% of individuals tested had colonoscopy and the reduction in mortality was less (15%).

Screening by sigmoidoscopy has been evaluated in case-control studies. In the Kaiser study [13], rigid sigmoidoscopy was associated with a 59% reduction in mortality from cancer of the rectum and distal colon. Scandinavian trials have shown less compliance and a higher yield of detection with sigmoidoscopy than with the FOBT. A

cohort study in the USA has shown that screening by endoscopy reduces mortality from colorectal cancer by 50% and incidence by 40% [8]. Primary endoscopic screening is increasingly favoured as compared to the FOBT protocol [9].

There is indirect evidence that primary colonoscopy may reduce cancer mortality. The National Polyp Study in the USA has shown a 75% reduction in the risk of colorectal cancer after polypectomy [10,11]. Among persons of average risk, above age 50, screening by colonoscopy reveals cancer in 0-2.2% and large adenomas in 3-11%. The number of colonoscopies needed to detect one cancer in screening is estimated at 143 for individuals of either sex, aged at least 50, and 64 for males aged at least 60 years. The number of colonoscopies needed to detect one cancer in patients with a positive FOBT is

	Screened annually	Unscreened
Number of people	15,550	15,394
Number of colorectal cancers detected	323	356
Number of deaths from colorectal cancer	82	121
Mortality ratio (deaths in screened/deaths in unscreened)	0.67	1.00

Table 4.17 The efficacy of screening by FOBT as reflected by the reduced mortality due to colorectal cancers diagnosed in the group subject to annual screening in comparison with the unscreened group.

45 with one positive rehydrated FOBT, 9.8 with one positive non-rehydrated FOBT and only 2.7 if two positive non-rehydrated positive FOBT are required. The chance of finding a cancer in the five years after negative colonoscopy is very small. This justifies the tendency towards screening with primary endoscopy to explore at ten-year intervals or once in a lifetime. A recent comparative but non-randomized Finnish study on the endoscopic detection of neoplasia in families fulfilling the Amsterdam criteria for hereditary nonpolyposis colon cancer has suggested efficacy of colonoscopy in reducing the risk of and mortality from colorectal cancer.

International comparisons

In countries with a high rate of colorectal cancer, secondary prevention is justified. Mass screening with the FOBT is proposed and reimbursed in Japan, Germany and the Czech Republic for example, but implementation depends upon the accompanying awareness campaign. In the USA, an annual FOBT and/or sigmoidoscopy every five years is recommended. Screening with primary sigmoidoscopy is encouraged in Scandinavian countries and in the United Kingdom. Application of any large-scale endoscopic screening programme is hampered by a shortage of specialists and the high cost of their expertise.

REFERENCES

1. Winawer SJ, Fletcher RH, Miller L, Godlee F, Stolar MH, Mulrow CD, Woolf SH, Glick SN, Ganiats TG, Bond JH, Rosen L, Zapka JG, Olsen SJ, Giardiello FM, Sisk JE, Van Antwerp R, Brown-Davis C, Marciniak DA, Mayer RJ (1997) Colorectal cancer screening: clinical guidelines and rationale. *Gastroenterology*, 112: 594-642.

2. Mandel JS, Bond JH, Church TR, Snover DC, Bradley GM, Schuman LM, Ederer F (1993) Reducing mortality from colorectal cancer by screening for fecal occult blood. Minnesota Colon Cancer Control Study. *N Engl J Med*, 328: 1365-1371.

3. Hardcastle JD, Chamberlain JO, Robinson MH, Moss SM, Amar SS, Balfour TW, James PD, Mangham CM (1996) Randomised controlled trial of faecal-occult-blood screening for colorectal cancer. *Lancet*, 348: 1472-1477.

4. Kronborg O, Fenger C, Olsen J, Jorgensen OD, Sondergaard O (1996) Randomised study of screening for colorectal cancer with faecal-occult-blood test. *Lancet*, 348: 1467-1471.

5. Simon JB (1998) Should all people over the age of 50 have regular fecal occult-blood tests? Postpone population screening until problems are solved. *N Engl J Med*, 338: 1151-1152.

6. Fletcher RH (1998) Should all people over the age of 50 have regular fecal occult-blood tests? If it works, why not do it? *N Engl J Med*, 338: 1153-1154.

7. Rennert G, Rennert HS, Miron E, Peterburg Y (2001) Population colorectal cancer screening with fecal occult blood test. *Cancer Epidemiol Biomarkers Prev*, 10: 1165-1168.

8. Kavanagh AM, Giovannucci EL, Fuchs CS, Colditz GA (1998) Screening endoscopy and risk of colorectal cancer in United States men. *Cancer Causes Control*, 9: 455-462.

9. Lieberman DA (1997) Endoscopic screening for colorectal cancer. *Gastroenterol Clin N Am*, 26: 71-83.

10. Winawer SJ, Zauber AG, Ho MN, O'Brien MJ, Gottlieb LS, Sternberg SS, Waye JD, Schapiro M, Bond JH, Panish JF (1993) Prevention of colorectal cancer by colonoscopic polypectomy. The National Polyp Study Workgroup. *N Engl J Med*, 329: 1977-1981.

11. Winawer SJ, Zauber AG, O'Brien MJ, Ho MN, Gottlieb L, Sternberg SS, Waye JD, Bond J, Schapiro M, Stewart ET (1993) Randomized comparison of surveillance intervals after colonoscopic removal of newly diagnosed adenomatous polyps. The National Polyp Study Workgroup. *N Engl J Med*, 328: 901-906.

12. Kudo S, Kashida H, Tamura S, Nakajima T (1997) The problem of "flat" colonic adenoma. *Gastrointest Endosc Clin N Am*, 7: 87-98.

13. Friedman GD, Collen MF, Fireman BH (1986) Multiphasic Health Checkup Evaluation: a 16-year follow-up. *J Chronic Dis*, 39: 453-463.

WEBSITES

Colorectal cancer prevention and control initiatives CDC: http://www.cdc.gov/cancer/colorctl/colorect.htm

Colorectal cancer screening, the American Gastroenterological Association: http://www.gastro.org/public/brochures/cc_screening.html

SCREENING FOR CERVICAL CANCER

SUMMARY

> In most developed countries, cytological screening (Pap test) has led to a significant reduction in the incidence of and mortality from cervical cancer. In countries with lower participation compliance and a less developed health care system, screening has been much less or not at all effective in reducing mortality.

> In developing countries, the cost of infrastructure and initial investments for organized cytological screening may be prohibitive. The cost-effectiveness of screening programmes based on alternative tests, such as visual inspection following acetic acid application (VIA), are currently being investigated.

> Testing for HPV DNA is an alternative means of primary screening. Its accuracy and cost-effectiveness for the detection of precursor lesions (cervical intraepithelial neoplasia) are currently being investigated.

In many developed countries a decline in incidence and mortality of cervical cancer has been observed in the past 30 years (Fig. 4.43, 4.45). This shift suggests that the burden due to this form of cancer could be reduced worldwide by applying current knowledge [1]. Cancer of the cervix is related to sexual activity, and infection with human papillomavirus (HPV) is central to the etiology (*Chronic infections*, p56). While it has been established that HPV is responsible for 82% of cervical cancers occurring in developed countries and 91% in developing countries [2], cervical cancer is, like all other cancers of known infectious origin, a rare response to the relevant infection. Efforts are underway to develop and test vaccines against HPV infection (*Human papillomavirus vaccination*, p148). However, variation in sexual behaviour and HPV infection may not entirely account for the very high rate of cervical cancer in many countries and its declining trend over time in some others. This applies both in developing countries and in developed countries, where the disease is predominant in women of lower socioeconomic status. Accordingly, screening is the main strategy for prevention. Cervical intraepithelial neoplasia grades II and III represent a "preclinical" stage of squamous cell carcinoma that has high prevalence and is detectable in the course of population-based screening. The most commonly used screening test, the cytological smear, is acceptable to a substantial proportion of the population at risk, but the test has recognized limitations.

The efficacy of cytological screening

By far the best established screening method for cervical cancer is the Papanicolaou ("Pap") smear (Fig. 4.44). Population-based screening programmes using the Pap smear were initiated in British Columbia in 1949 and in regions of Norway in 1959 and Scotland in 1960. Since then, programmes based on the Pap smear have been introduced in many developed countries. The programmes vary in their organization, differing in the balance between public and private health care, whether the programme is systematic and population-based or opportunistic (based upon self-presentation), the age range of the women to whom screening is offered, the recommended interval between successive screens and the follow-up and management of women found to have cervical abnormalities. Pap smear programmes which have been implemented in developing countries are limited to offering the test to women attending primary health care, antenatal, gynaecology and family planning clinics in urban areas, with no organized efforts either to encourage testing for high-risk women, or to ensure that those found to have abnormal smears receive follow-up and treatment [3].

The main evidence for efficacy of screening based on the Pap smear is indirect,

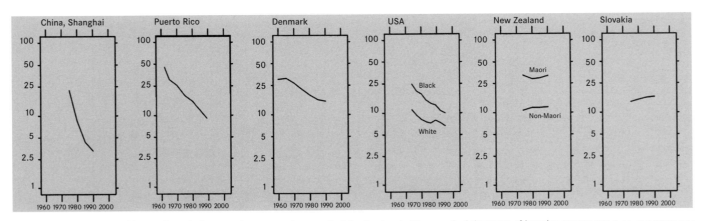

Fig. 4.43 Trends in the incidence of cervical cancer. In many regions, early detection has led to a marked decrease of invasive cancer. D.M. Parkin et al. (2001) *Eur J Cancer* 37, suppl. 8: S4-66.

Time since last negative smear (months)	Relative protection (no. of cases in brackets)		95% confidence interval
0-11	15.3	(25)	10.0-22.6
12-23	11.9	(23)	7.5-18.3
24-35	8.0	(25)	5.2-11.8
36-47	5.3	(30)	3.6-7.6
48-59	2.8	(30)	1.9-4.0
60-71	3.6	(16)	2.1-5.8
72-119	1.6	(6)	0.6-3.5
120+	0.8	(7)	0.3-1.6
Never screened	1.0		

Table 4.18 Screening offers protection against cervical cancer: combined analyses of cohort and case-control studies suggest that the shorter the time since the last negative smear result, the greater the protection a woman has against invasive cervical cancer.

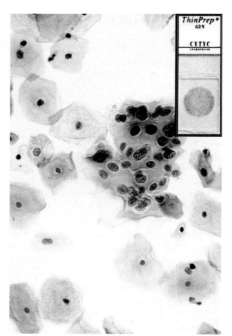

Fig. 4.44 Papanicolaou-stained cervical smear preparation showing a cluster of abnormal cells.

being based on (i) time trends in the incidence of, or mortality due to, cervical cancer in relation to screening intensity; (ii) risk of cervical cancer in individuals in relation to their screening history [1,4]. Nationwide programmes were established in Finland, Iceland and Sweden; in Denmark, programmes covered only 40% of the female population and in Norway only 5% [5]. In Iceland, cervical cancer mortality fell by 80% between 1965 and 1982, compared with 50% in Finland, 34% in Sweden, 25% in Denmark and 10% in Norway. More recently, the effect of cytologic screening on the incidence of cervical cancer has been examined in 17 populations covered by cancer registries between the early 1960s and late 1980s [6]. Compared with the time before the introduction of screening, the age standardized incidence rates decreased by at least 25% in 11 of the 17 populations, with the largest effect occurring in the 45-55 year age groups. The reduced efficacy of screening in older women is attributable to a lower screening coverage and possibly by lower test sensitivity. Where evident, apparently reduced efficacy in younger women may be the result of transfer of cases to younger ages, as a result of earlier detection in the women's lifetime due to cytological screening. This phenomenon in turn may obscure ineffec-

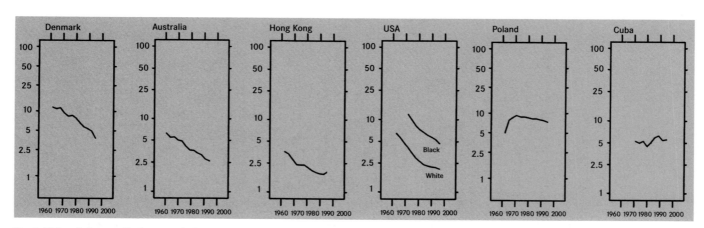

Fig. 4.45 Trends in mortality from cervical cancer. D.M. Parkin et al. (2001) *Eur J Cancer* 37, suppl. 8: S4-66.

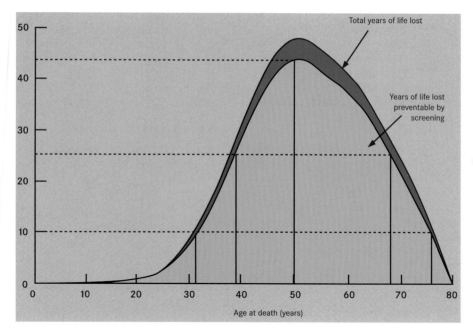

Fig. 4.46 Annual numbers of years of life lost as a result of deaths from cervical cancer per 10,000 women, at each year of age, up to age 80, in the absence of screening (dark blue plus light blue). If screening is implemented, many of these deaths can be prevented; at the peak (age 50), 44 years of life may be gained per 10,000 women screened (light blue).

tive screening at younger ages or, more controversially, the possibility that invasive cancers in young women might be a rapidly progressing subset of neoplasia [7].

In contrast to squamous cell carcinoma, adenocarcinoma of the cervix has no readily detectable pre-invasive stage. Therefore, cytological screening would not be expected to be effective in the control of this type of cervical cancer [7].

The application of cohort and case-control studies to the evaluation of screening effectiveness is complex. Self-selection for screening by individuals at lower risk of disease or mortality has been observed frequently. It is possible that signs or symptoms led to a cytological smear being performed, but this may have been misclassified as a screening test. If differential, this misclassification would bias the estimated effect of screening.

Implementation

The major barrier to prevention of cervical cancer is failure to be screened at all (Table 4.18). Organized screening is generally considered to be substantially more efficient than opportunistic screening. However, there have been few direct comparisons and the results of these have been inconsistent. Some reduction in incidence may be achieved by opportunistic screening [8].

An estimate of the years of life potentially saved as a result of screening on the basis of data has indicated that three-yearly cytological screening reduces mortality by 91% [9]. This may be an overestimate because of selection bias. At the age of 50, 44 years of life can be gained per 10,000 women screened. At the ages of 68 and 39, 25 years of life are gained per 10,000 women screened, and at ages 31 and 76, 10 years of life are gained (Fig. 4.46).

Selective screening has been considered. However, asking women about their sexual habits is at best difficult, and may be unacceptable in many societies. Moreover, it may be difficult to reduce screening coverage once a programme aimed at total population coverage is in place. Another proposal is to cease the offer of screening to women aged 50 or more who have had regular negative smears [10]. It has been suggested that if a combination of HPV and cytological testing were introduced in primary screening, screening could then be stopped at an earlier age in women negative on both tests [11].

Considerable variation in the sensitivity and specificity of cervical cytology smear tests has been reported [12]. A number of suggestions for methods to improve cervical specimen cytology have been made, with liquid-based cytology techniques currently receiving most attention. Overall,

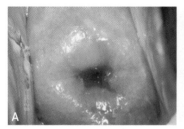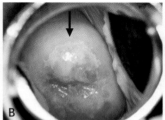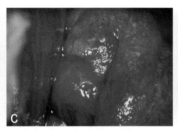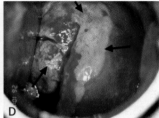

Fig. 4.47 Visual inspection of the cervix with 4% acetic acid. In the normal cervix, after the application of acetic acid, no definite acetowhite areas are seen (**A**). The visual inspection is declared positive (**B**) when, after the application of acetic acid, thick, dense, well-defined acetowhite areas develop (arrows). An invasive cancer is shown before (**C**) and after (**D**) the application of acetic acid.

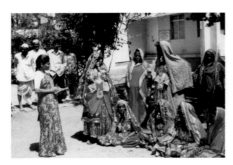

Fig. 4.48 Women at a clinic in India participating in a study of early detection of cervical cancer.

the liquid-based method seems to result in more slides being classified as having low-grade squamous epithelial lesions or higher, which were classified as having less severe disease by conventional smears, than the reverse situation. The difference in cost between liquid-based and conventional cytology is unclear because of substantial uncertainty about the relative effectiveness of these two approaches[13].

It has been suggested that improvements in the detection of dyskaryosis (abnormal changes in cell nuclei) using extended tip plastic spatulas instead of the traditional wooden Ayre's spatula would be of approximately similar magnitude to the improvements which might result from replacing conventional cytology with liquid-based methods [14]. Automated cytology reading systems are under development and some health economic evaluation has been carried out.

In view of the importance of HPV in the etiology of cervical cancer, HPV testing to allow women to be classified as high-risk HPV-positive (displaying HPV types associated with an increased risk of cervical neoplasia) or negative (otherwise) could be used as an adjunct to cytological smear tests. However, the possible value of HPV testing in the triage of women with low-grade abnormalities is uncertain.

Alternatives to the Pap smear
HPV testing
HPV testing may be used for primary screening. In developed countries, most attention has been focused on HPV testing as an adjunct to cytological screening (see above), in part because of ethical and medico-legal problems which might ensue in conducting a randomized trial which would involve withdrawal of the offer of cytological screening from the group assigned to be offered HPV testing. This would not be the case for populations in which Pap testing has not been introduced, notably in developing countries. The major issues in relation to such use of HPV testing have been the cost of the test itself and its relatively poor specificity [15,16]. Poor specificity results in follow-up for women without cervical disease, incurring costs which may be more than the society can afford. In both developed and developing countries, the development of primary screening based on HPV tests might be rendered obsolete by mass HPV vaccination (*Human papillomavirus vaccination*, p148).

Visual inspection
Unaided visual inspection of the cervix by nurses and other non-medical health workers, also known as "down-staging", has been proposed for developing countries which lack the laboratory facilities or resources to implement cytological screening [17]. Women with abnormal findings require further investigation, which entails a cytological test if appropriate facilities are available, or specialist medical examination if no cytology services are available.

In view of the unsatisfactory performance of unaided visual inspection, consideration has been given to aiding naked-eye visual inspection by impregnating the cervix with 3-4% freshly prepared acetic acid to detect acetowhite areas (Fig. 4.47). This screening approach is known as visual inspection with acetic acid (VIA) (synonyms are cervicoscopy and direct visual inspection). In studies in China, India, South Africa and Zimbabwe, visual inspection with acetic acid has emerged as a satisfactory screening test to detect cervical cancer precursor lesions, with a sensitivity ranging from 67 to 90% [14, 18-20]. This is similar to (or higher than) the sensitivity of cytological screening, but specificity is generally lower (range is 64-92%). Therefore, if screening based on visual inspection with acetic acid is instituted, a potential consequence would be high rates of referral for further investigation. Currently, randomized intervention trials are in progress in India to evaluate the cost-effectiveness of visual inspection with acetic acid in cervical cancer screening [21].

Addition of magnification to visual inspection with acetic acid has not further improved the test performance [14, 22]. Cervicography involves the taking of a photograph of the acetic acid-impregnated cervix to be reviewed by trained cervicographic interpreters. Cervicography has been found to have a lower sensitivity than cervical cytology [14, 23], and also reportedly suffers from high false positive rates [24].

REFERENCES

1. Pontén J, Adami HO, Bergstrom R, Dillner J, Friberg LG, Gustafsson L, Miller AB, Parkin DM, Sparen P, Trichopoulos D (1995) Strategies for global control of cervical cancer. *Int J Cancer*, 60: 1-26.

2. Pisani P, Parkin DM, Muñoz N, Ferlay J (1997) Cancer and infection: estimates of the attributable fraction in 1990. *Cancer Epidemiol Biomarkers Prev*, 6: 387-400.

3. Sankaranarayanan R, Pisani P (1997) Prevention Measures in the third world: are they practical? In: Franco E, Monsonego, J eds, *New Developments in Cervical Cancer Screening and Prevention*, Oxford, Blackwell Science, 70-83.

4. Coleman D, Day N, Douglas G, Farmery E, Lynge E, Philip J, Segnan N (1993) European Guidelines for Quality Assurance in Cervical Cancer Screening. Europe against cancer programme. *Eur J Cancer*, 29A Suppl 4: S1-38.

5. Läärä E, Day NE, Hakama M (1987) Trends in mortality from cervical cancer in the Nordic countries: association with organised screening programmes. *Lancet*, 1: 1247-1249.

6. Gustafsson L, Pontén J, Zack M, Adami HO (1997) International incidence rates of invasive cervical cancer after introduction of cytological screening. *Cancer Causes Control*, 8: 755-763.

7. Sparen P, Gustafsson L, Friberg LG, Ponten J, Bergstrom R, Adami HO (1995) Improved control of invasive cervical cancer in Sweden over six decades by earlier clinical detection and better treatment. *J Clin Oncol*, 13: 715-725.

8. Levi F, Lucchini F, Negri E, Franceschi S, La Vecchia C (2000) Cervical cancer mortality in young women in Europe: patterns and trends. *Eur J Cancer*, 36: 2266-2271.

9. Law MR, Morris JK, Wald NJ (1999) The importance of age in screening for cancer *J Med Screen*, 6: 16-20.

10. Sherlaw-Johnson C, Gallivan S, Jenkins D (1999) Withdrawing low risk women from cervical screening programmes: mathematical modelling study. *BMJ*, 318: 356-360.

11. Cuzick J, Beverley E, Ho L, Terry G, Sapper H, Mielzynska I, Lorincz A, Chan WK, Krausz T, Soutter P (1999) HPV testing in primary screening of older women. *Br J Cancer*, 81: 554-558.

12. Nanda K, McCrory DC, Myers ER, Bastian LA, Hasselblad V, Hickey JD, Matchar DB (2000) Accuracy of the Papanicolaou test in screening for and follow-up of cervical cytologic abnormalities: a systematic review. *Ann Intern Med*, 132: 810-819.

13. Bastian L, Datta S, Hasselblad V, Hickey J, Myers E and Nanda K (1999) *Evaluation of Cervical Cytology: Evidence Report Number 5. Publication No. 99-E010.* Rockville, Agency for Health Care Policy and Research.

14. Martin-Hirsch P, Lilford R, Jarvis G, Kitchener HC (1999) Efficacy of cervical-smear collection devices: a systematic review and meta-analysis. *Lancet*, 354: 1763-1770.

15. Denny L, Kuhn L, Pollack A, Wainwright H, Wright TC, Jr. (2000) Evaluation of alternative methods of cervical cancer screening for resource-poor settings. *Cancer*, 89: 826-833.

16. Kuhn L, Denny L, Pollack A, Lorincz A, Richart RM, Wright TC (2000) Human papillomavirus DNA testing for cervical cancer screening in low-resource settings. *J Natl Cancer Inst*, 92: 818-825.

17. Stjernswärd J, Eddy D, Luthra U, Stanley K (1987) Plotting a new course for cervical cancer screening in developing countries. *World Health Forum*, 8: 42-45.

18. Sankaranarayanan R, Wesley R, Somanathan T, Dhakad N, Skyamalakumary B, Amma NS, Parkin DM, Nair MK (1998) Visual inspection of the uterine cervix after the application of acetic acid in the detection of cervical carcinoma and its precursors. *Cancer*, 83: 2150-2156.

19. University of Zimbabwe/JHPIEGO Cervical Cancer Project (1999) Visual inspection with acetic acid for cervical-cancer screening: test qualities in a primary-care setting.

20. Belinson JL, Pretorius RG, Zhang WH, Wu LY, Qiao YL, Elson P (2001) Cervical cancer screening by simple visual inspection after acetic acid. *Obstet Gynecol*, 98: 441-444.

21. Sankaranarayanan R, Budukh AM, Rajkumar R (2001) Effective screening programmes for cervical cancer in low- and middle income developing countries. *Bull World Health Organ*, 79: 954-962.

22. Denny L, Kuhn L, Pollack A, Wright TC, Jr. (2002) Direct visual inspection for cervical cancer screening: an analysis of factors influencing test performance. *Cancer*, 94: 1699-1707.

23. Schneider DL, Herrero R, Bratti C, Greenberg MD, Hildesheim A, Sherman ME, Morales J, Hutchinson ML, Sedlacek TV, Lorincz A, Mango L, Wacholder S, Alfaro M, Schiffman M (1999) Cervicography screening for cervical cancer among 8460 women in a high-risk population, *Am J Obstet Gynecol*, 180: 290-298 .

24. Richart RM (1995) Screening. The next century. *Cancer*, 76: 1919-1927.

WEBSITES

CDC National breast and cervical cancer early detection program (USA) :
http://www.cdc.gov/cancer/nbccedp/about.htm

The NHS cervical screening programme (UK):
http://www.cancerscreening.nhs.uk/cervical/

National Cervical Cancer Coalition (Australia):
http://www.nccc-online.org

SCREENING FOR ORAL CANCER

SUMMARY

> Oral cancer and its precancerous lesions, including leukoplakia, can be readily detected by visual inspection of the oral cavity by trained health workers and doctors.

> Population screening for oral cancer results in the diagnosis of large numbers of oral precancers and an increased proportion of early stage tumours. However, a reduction in incidence of and mortality from oral cancer resulting from such interventions remains to be demonstrated.

Oral lesions such as leukoplakia, erythroplakia and oral submucous fibrosis are precancerous. A high risk of malignant transformation of such lesions has been established in follow-up studies. The proportion of oral cancers that arise from pre-existing precancerous lesions is variously reported in the range of 30-80%. The natural history of these lesions is not as extensively documented as that of the precursors to cervical cancer. Thus, for example, it is not known whether the different types of leukoplakia and erythroplakia constitute a continuum similar to the different stages evident during the development of cervical intraepithelial neoplasia.

Oral leukoplakia refers to uniform, flat, predominantly white lesions in the lining of the mouth that cannot be characterized as any other disease. White lesions with a smooth, corrugated or wrinkled surface are referred to as homogeneous leukoplakia, and those with irregularly flat or nodular or exophytic white or red and white lesions are referred to as non-homogeneous leukoplakia. Erythroplakia refers to velvety red, non-removable lesions in the oral mucosa. Oral submucous fibrosis is characterized by recur-rent inflammation and stiffness of the oral mucosa with progressive limitation in opening the mouth and protrusion of the tongue. In hospital-based studies, a malignant transformation rate of 44-17.5% for leukoplakia, and in population-based studies rates of 0.13-2.2% over several years have been reported [1]. The risk of malignant transformation varies with sex (higher in females), type and location of leukoplakia (higher with non-homogeneous types and those located on the tongue or the floor of the mouth), presence of *Candida albicans* and presence of epithelial dysplasia. The proportion of leukoplakias which regress has been reported to vary between 5 and 20% per year. In a subset of 159 individuals with oral leukoplakia in one oral cancer screening trial, after three years of follow-up the lesions could no longer be detected in 104 cases (71.2%). It is difficult to determine to what extent the above findings are due to variations in case selection or are a true reflection of the natural history.

Nature of the intervention

Early oral cancers mostly present as asymptomatic, small indurated nodules or thickening or ulceroproliferative growth (*Head and neck cancer*, p232). Auxiliary health care workers can identify the above early lesions after adequate training [2]. There are four methods available for the early detection of oral cancer: visual examination of the oral cavity by health professionals, visual examination after application of toluidine blue, mouth self-examination and oral cytology.

Visual inspection of the oral cavity by trained health workers and doctors is the most widely-evaluated early detection procedure for oral cancer. Except for an ongoing randomized intervention trial in India and the oral cancer screening programme in Cuba, all other studies are cross-sectional, mostly in selected clinical or industrial settings, with the exception of a few studies in specified general populations. Very limited information is available on intermediate and long-term end-points such as sensitivity and specificity, stage distribution, fatality rates, reduction in incidence and mortality.

Evidence of outcome

Oral visual inspection has been shown to be a sensitive and specific test to detect oral precancerous lesions and early asymptomatic oral cancers in several studies [1-7]. In the population-based studies, between 1.3 and 7.3% of screened subjects were referred for fur-

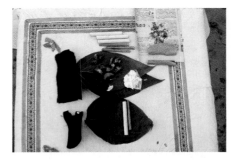

Fig. 4.49 The ingredients of betel-quid include betel leaf, slaked lime, areca nut and tobacco, with or without other condiments. Betel chewing is one of the major causative factors of oral cancer (together with bidi smoking and alcohol drinking) in the Indian subcontinent.

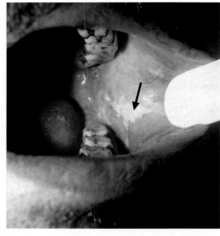

Fig. 4.50 Homogeneous oral leukoplakia. This precancerous lesion can be detected by visual inspection.

Stage	Intervention	Control
I (<2 cm)	24 (37.5%)	2 (6.9%)
II (2 - 4 cm)	14 (21.9%)	3 (10.3%)
III (>4 cm)	11 (17.2%)	7 (24.1%)
IV (adjacent structures involved)	8 (12.5%)	13 (44.8%)
Not known	7 (10.9%)	4 (13.9%)
Total	64 (100%)	29 (100%)

Table 4.19 Oral cancer cases according to stage (and percentage distribution), detected during an Indian screening trial (1995-1999), compared with an unscreened control population.

ther investigations although the compliance rates for referral were sub-optimal, ranging from 54 to 72%. The sensitivity of visual examination for detecting oral lesions varied from 58 to 94% and the specificity from 76 to 98%. In an on-going randomized controlled oral cancer

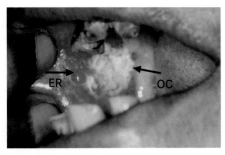

Fig. 4.51 Oral cancer (OC) arising from a pre-existing erythroplakia (ER).

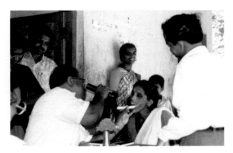

Fig. 4.52 Confirmatory examination by a dentist in a woman referred as "screen positive" after oral cancer screening in Trivandrum District, Kerala, India.

screening intervention trial during 1995-1999 in Trivandrum, South India, involving 115,000 subjects, 60% of oral cancers in the intervention group were detected in early stages as opposed to 17% in the control group (Table 4.19) [7].

An oral cancer screening programme in Cuba, which has been running since 1984, involves annual oral examination of subjects aged 15 and above by dentists. A descriptive evaluation in 1994 revealed that participation and compliance were sub-optimal [8]. There has been no decline in oral cancer incidence and mortality in Cuba since the initiation of the programme, though there is limited evidence for a shift in the stage of cancers detected, from advanced to early, after the introduction of screening. In summary, there is no evidence as yet to establish that screening with oral visual inspection can reduce incidence of and mortality from oral cancer.

Toluidine blue
Toluidine blue dye has been mostly used as an adjunct for early detection of oral cancer in selected subjects with precancerous lesions, in order to provide better demarcation of malignant and dysplastic changes so as to help select sites for biopsies [9]. This test has been evaluated only in a few specified clinical settings where the reported false negative and false positive rates ranged from 20 to

30%. There are no studies investigating its use in the context of screening. Thus, the value of visual examination after toluidine blue application in the early detection of oral cancer is not known.

Self-screening
There is very little information on self-screening for oral cancer or on health education to promote mouth self-examination, especially in high-risk population groups. In a study to evaluate the feasibility of mouth self-examination in India, 36% of 22,000 subjects who were taught mouth self-examination reportedly practised the test and in the 247 subjects visiting the clinic within two weeks of a promotion campaign, 89 precancers were detected and 7 oral cancers [10]. There is no information available on long-term feasibility of and detection rates with self-screening in oral cancer detection.

Oral cytology
Screening by oral cytology has never achieved the same recognition or efficacy as cervical cytology screening. There are major limitations for oral exfoliative cytology as a screening modality for oral cancer. Firstly, the lesion needs to be seen before a sample can be collected, to ensure adequate numbers of abnormal cells. Secondly, only a small number of cells are identifiable in a smear. Furthermore, interpretation is of a subjective nature and there are high false negative diagnosis rates with leukoplakia [11,12]. If a lesion can be seen, it may prove preferable to biopsy it rather than to take a cytological sample. Thus oral cytology has received only limited attention and no adequate information is available on the utility of this approach for oral cancer screening.

Implementation
Organization of oral cancer screening programmes based on visual inspection of the oral cavity is currently not recommended as a public health policy for high-risk countries due to lack of information on reduction in incidence and mortality, as well as cost-effectiveness of such an approach [13]. It is likely that the trial in

India will provide useful information in this regard in the future [7]. Meanwhile, in high-incidence regions, health education messages and information on self-examination may be regularly provided by mass media and by posters in health centres, dispensaries and other establishments, in order to prompt subjects at high risk and those who suspect that they may have an oral precancer to avail themselves of early detection services.

REFERENCES

1. Rodrigues VC, Moss SM, Tuomainen H (1998) Oral cancer in the UK: to screen or not to screen. *Oral Oncol*, 34: 454-465.

2. Sankaranarayanan R (1997) Health care auxiliaries in the detection and prevention of oral cancer. *Oral Oncol*, 33: 149-154.

3. Warnakulasuriya KA, Ekanayake AN, Sivayoham S, Stjernsward J, Pindborg JJ, Sobin LH, Perera KS (1984) Utilization of primary health care workers for early detection of oral cancer and precancer cases in Sri Lanka. *Bull World Health Organ*, 62: 243-250.

4. Mehta FS, Gupta PC, Bhonsle RB, Murti PR, Daftary DK, Pindborg JJ (1986) Detection of oral cancer using basic health workers in an area of high oral cancer incidence in India. *Cancer Detect Prev*, 9: 219-225.

5. Warnakulasuriya KA, Nanayakkara BG (1991) Reproducibility of an oral cancer and precancer detection program using a primary health care model in Sri Lanka. *Cancer Detect Prev*, 15: 331-334.

6. Mathew B, Sankaranarayanan R, Sunilkumar KB, Kuruvila B, Pisani P, Nair MK (1997) Reproducibility and validity of oral visual inspection by trained health workers in the detection of oral precancer and cancer. *Br J Cancer*, 76: 390-394.

7. Sankaranarayanan R, Mathew B, Binu J, Thomas G, Somanathan T, Pisani P, Pandey M, Ramadas K, Najeeb K, Abraham E (2000) Early findings from a community based cluster randomised oral cancer screening intervention trial in Kerala, India. *Cancer*, 88: 664-673.

8. Fernandez Garrote L, Sankaranarayanan R, Lence Anta JJ, Rodriguez Salva A, Parkin DM (1995) An evaluation of the oral cancer control programme in Cuba. *Epidemiology*, 6: 428-431.

9. Martin IC, Kerawala CJ, Reed M (1998) The application of toluidine blue as a diagnostic adjunct in the detection of epithelial dysplasia. *Oral Surg Oral Med Oral Pathol Oral Radiol Endod*, 85: 444-446.

10. Mathew B, Sankaranarayanan R, Wesley R, Nair MK (1995) Evaluation of mouth self-examination in the control of oral cancer. *Br J Cancer*, 71: 397-399.

11. Silverman S, Jr, Bilimoria KF, Bhargava K, Mani NJ, Shah RA (1977) Cytologic, histologic and clinical correlations of precancerous and cancerous oral lesions in 57,518 industrial workers of Gujarat, India. *Acta Cytol*, 21: 196-198.

12. Ogden GR, Cowpe JG, Wight AJ (1997) Oral exfoliative cytology: review of methods of assessment. *J Oral Pathol Med*, 26: 201-205.

13. Sankaranarayanan R (2000) Integration of cost-effective early detection programs into the health services of developing countries. *Cancer*, 89: 475-481.

STOMACH CANCER PREVENTION AND SCREENING

SUMMARY

> Prevention or eradication of *Helicobacter pylori* infection may contribute to reduced incidence of stomach cancer, in addition to other health benefits.

> Reduced intake of salted food and increased consumption of fresh fruit and vegetables has decreased the risk of this malignancy worldwide.

> Early detection of premalignant lesions by population-based screening, using photofluorography and/or endoscopy, improves the prognosis of stomach cancer patients.

Stomach cancer is a leading cause of cancer-related deaths worldwide that lends itself to primary and secondary prevention. Stomach cancer typically becomes clinically evident at an advanced stage and has a poor prognosis (*Stomach cancer*, p194). The natural history of gastric adenocarcinoma is characterized by the development of premalignant lesions that provide a basis for early detection and treatment which can improve the prognosis.

For decades, stomach cancer was known to be strongly associated with gastritis. The discovery that infection with a bacterium, *Helicobacter pylori* (*Chronic infections*, p56) causes gastritis and plays an etiological role in stomach cancer [1, 2] suggested that it might be possible to markedly reduce the incidence of stomach cancer, or even to eliminate it, on this basis. However, incidence varies among countries and regions with similar prevalence of *H. pylori* infection and incidence has declined rapidly in many countries and among specific ethnic groups (Fig. 4.54). These considerations suggest a role for additional environmental factors, such as diet, in causation and hence, potentially, in prevention.

Helicobacter pylori infection

The proportion of stomach cancers that can be attributed to *H. pylori* infection may be determined. "Attributable risk" refers to the proportion of stomach cancer cases that would be theoretically eliminated if *H. pylori* were to disappear and is mathematically dependent on the prevalence of *H. pylori* and the risk ratio (or odds ratio) linking *H. pylori* to stomach cancer. Accordingly, the calculated attributable risk of *H. pylori* is 40-70%. This estimate is considered likely to underestimate the true attributable risk associated with *H. pylori* (a study in Japanese patients indicated that stomach cancer developed in persons infected with *H. pylori*, but not in uninfected persons [3]). Moreover, a drawback of using "attributable risk" in this context is that, while not ever having an *H. pylori* infection probably reduces the risk of subsequent stomach cancer to a marked degree, it remains unclear whether curing an existing chronic *H. pylori* infection would have a similar effect.

Given the long lag period between acquisition of the infection and development of cancer in the small percentage of infected patients, it will be very difficult to demonstrate that cure of the infection prevents cancer. No study has yet accomplished this. In a small non-randomized Japanese study, patients underwent endoscopic resection for early stomach cancer followed by *H. pylori* treatment and cure. No new cancers developed after a follow-up of three years in those cured of infection (0/65) compared with a 9% rate of incidence of new intestinal-type stomach cancers in the (6/67) non-*H. pylori* treated group [4]. Small Japanese non-randomized trials have demonstrated reduced risk of malignant transformation of gastric adenomas after curing infection. Conversely, in other studies *H. pylori* eradication in patients with mild and moderate dysplasia did not result in a significant reduction in the progression of dysplasia into stomach cancer. Overall, neither dysplasia nor intestinal metaplasia is thought to regress significantly following cure of *H. pylori* infection and the problem of sampling error makes it unlikely that studies relying on endoscopic biopsies can ever answer this question.

There are other considerations relating to this issue. The major determinant of the cost-effectiveness of *H. pylori* screening and/or treatment is the reduction in can-

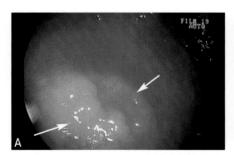 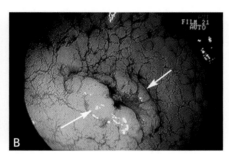 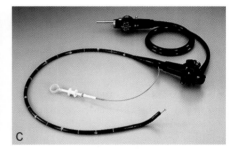

Fig. 4.53 Endoscopy showing early gastric carcinoma (superficial elevated type and superficial depressed type) in a 59-year-old male patient (**A**) and after methylene blue chromoendoscopy (**B**), obtained using a video gastroscope (**C**).

cer incidence following cure of infection; the higher the reduction, the more cost-effective screening becomes [5,6]. Factors that influence screening strategies are the prevalence of *H. pylori* in the population, and the need to focus upon older persons. The paradox is that the greatest benefit will be potentially gained by younger persons, in whom screening and treatment is less cost-effective. Due to associated comorbidity, the benefit in terms of life expectancy becomes negligible in older persons. Published analyses suggest favourable scenarios if screening and curing *H. pylori* among persons at a high risk of stomach cancer between the ages of 40 and 50 years were to reduce the risk of cancer by at least 30% [6]. However, in a high-risk population, most *H. pylori*-infected persons develop atrophic gastritis by age 40 and there is no evidence as to whether curing the infection at that stage will reduce the risk of cancer. Nonetheless, curing *H. pylori* infection gives the additional benefit of eliminating duodenal and gastric ulcer, a type of lymphoma associated with this condition, and up to 10% of cases of dyspepsia, as well as preventing transmission of the infection. There is considerable interest in the development of a vaccine to prevent *H. pylori* infection and possibly also to cure active infections [7,8]. Proof of concept has been obtained in animal experiments, candidate vaccines have been identified and clinical trials are poised to begin. An effective vaccine is the only practical method of eliminating *H. pylori* infection in developing countries where the incidence of the infection and the burden of disease are the greatest.

The role of dietary factors
Relevant dietary risk factors have been extensively investigated in observational epidemiological studies. Most studies of dietary factors in stomach cancer preceded the discovery of the role of *H. pylori*. Nevertheless, diet is thought to be a critical factor in the progression of superficial gastritis to chronic atrophic gastritis among persons infected with *H. pylori*. Several observations have been made that indicate a preventive role for

specific food items [9,10]. An inverse relationship between stomach cancer and regular dietary intake of fresh vegetables and fruits has been observed in many case-control studies as well as prospective studies conducted in several countries. Individuals eating 5-20 servings of fruits and 5-20 servings of raw vegetables every week reduce their risk of stomach cancer by almost half [11]. In addition, allium vegetables and onions have been negatively associated with stomach cancer in several countries. Fruits and vegetables are sources of many antioxidants, such as α-tocopherol, β-carotene, vitamin E, and vitamin C. However, a study in Finland found no impact of dietary supplementation with α-tocopherol and β-carotene for five years on the occurrence of neoplastic changes of the stomach in older male smokers with atrophic gastritis [12]. Intake of vitamin C is associated with an approximately 50% decrease in the risk of stomach cancer [11,13], although supplementation with vitamin C does not seem to reduce incidence among patients with pre-existing intestinal metaplasia.

Prolonged consumption of foods rich in salted, pickled, and smoked products increases the risk of stomach cancer. These foods have high salt content and nitrates and low levels of antioxidants due to storage for a long time at room temperature before consumption. Excessive dietary salt has been associated with gastric atrophy in animals and probably accelerates gastric atrophy in humans. In Japan, the correlation between salt intake and stomach cancer follows the gradient of salt intake. Similar correlations between salt intake and stomach cancer have been observed in other countries. Increase in the per capita consumption of fruits and vegetables and a concomitant decrease in salted foods have paralleled the decline in stomach cancer mortality in Japan. Foods rich in carbohydrates have been associated with an increased risk of stomach cancer. However, consumption of carbohydrate-rich foods overlaps with high dietary salt intake and reduced intake of fruits and vegetables. Despite the implications of certain animal studies, foods rich in nitrates, nitrites and secondary

amines have not been shown to be independent significant risks. The spread of refrigeration has been associated with the decrease in stomach cancer, which probably relates to the replacement of more traditional methods of food preservation such as salting and pickling and making fresh fruits and vegetables more available all year round. However, there have been no intervention trials showing that a specific dietary modification reduces the incidence of stomach cancer.

Secondary prevention: screening
Screening for stomach cancer has been practised in Japan since 1963. Annual screening using seven-film photofluorography examination or endoscopy (Box: *Screening for stomach cancer in Japan*, p177) has been recommended for people of age 50 and above, although this is a matter of some controversy. The false negative rate has been reported to be up to 19% for gastroscopy and up to 40% for photofluorography. Screening in Japan has increased the proportion of tumours detected at an early stage to approximately 50%. Prognosis for stomach cancer patients identified by screening may be better than for those identified by other means [14]. Certainly, detection of the cancer at an early stage improves chances of survival; the five-year survival rate following surgical treatment for early stomach cancer is higher (99.2%) than for non-early stomach cancer (48.5%). The overall five-year survival increased from 20% in 1965 to 40% in 1992. The five-year survival rate for stomach cancer in the USA and other Western countries remained stable at 20% during the same time period. Screening is the most likely explanation for the improved survival but a reduction in incidence is not attributable to screening. The Ministry of Health and Welfare of Japan determined that a programme of population-based screening by barium meal included only 7-13% of the population over 40. Therefore, it may be concluded that the official mass screening programme in Japan detects only a small proportion of stomach cancers (10-15%). The remaining cases are identified symptomatically. Screening for stomach cancer

SCREENING FOR STOMACH CANCER IN JAPAN

There has been a long history of screening for stomach cancer in Japan. Screening by indirect X-ray examination started in around 1960 and has been part of the "Health and Medical Service Law for the Aged" since 1983. The Ministry of Health and Welfare in Japan reported that in 1997 4,273,000 residents participated in screening programmes provided by local governments based on this law. Moreover, the Japanese system of annual health check-ups in the workplace has provided an opportunity for screening; about 16.7% of an estimated 6,759,000 employees were screened for stomach cancer in 1997. In addition, screening for stomach cancer is also undertaken during the so-called "Human Dry Dock", which incorporates multiple screening procedures, including measurement of blood pressure, urine analysis, blood tests, chest X-ray examination and stomach X-ray examination.

Consequently, at least 11,032,000 individuals (8.7% of the Japanese population) are estimated to have participated in screening for stomach cancer in 1997.

The main technique used to screen for stomach cancer in Japan is an indirect X-ray examination by the double contrast method, "double" referring to barium and air. When barium is swallowed, a small amount of air is also taken into the stomach. The barium makes the positive contrast and the air the negative contrast; this allows the detailed morphological patterns of the gastric surface to be visualized. This is usually conducted in a specially designed mobile unit equipped with a photofluorographic apparatus. This enables peo-

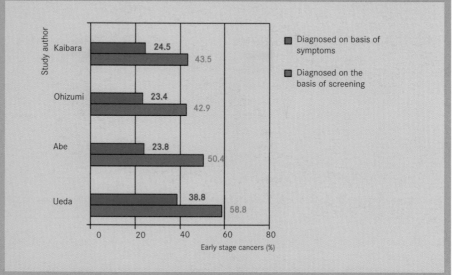

Fig. 4.55 Percentage of tumours detected at an early stage in Japanese patients diagnosed with stomach cancer, either during a screening programme or on the basis of presentation of symptoms.

ple to participate in screening near their homes or workplaces. Seven X-ray photographs are usually taken according to the standard method of the Japanese Society of Gastroenterology. Record linkage between participants in the screening and the lists of population-based cancer registry indicated that the sensitivity and the specificity of an indirect X-ray method by image intensifier were 88.5% and 92.0%, respectively (Murakami R et al., *Cancer* 65: 1255-1260, 1990).

Measurement of serum pepsinogen I and II levels has recently been introduced in Japan as a further method of screening for stomach cancer (Miki K, *Annual report 1997 of the research committee of studies on study of gastric cancer screening system using serum pepsinogen test*, 1998). However, a well-designed epidemiological evaluation of the efficacy of the pepsinogen method has not yet been conducted.
Randomized controlled trials to evaluate the effectiveness of screening for stom-

ach cancer have not been undertaken in Japan. There have however been many other types of studies, such as case-control studies, cohort studies, and time trend analyses to evaluate the effectiveness of screening for stomach cancer (Hisamichi S et al., Evaluation of mass screening programme for stomach cancer in Japan, in *UICC Cancer Screening*, eds. Miller AB et al., Cambridge University Press, 1991; Inaba S et al., Evaluation of a screening program on reduction of gastric cancer mortality in Japan: Preliminary results from a cohort study. *Prev Med*, 29: 102-106, 1999). There is an absolute confidence among most Japanese people that screening provides benefit. This confidence might be a product of the success of screening programmes for tuberculosis during the decades following the Second World War.

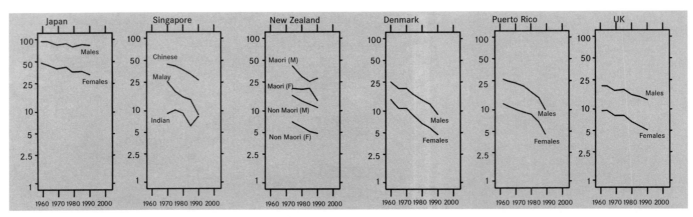

Fig. 4.54 The incidence of stomach cancer is decreasing worldwide. D.M. Parkin et al. (2001) *Eur J Cancer,* 37 Suppl. 8: S4-66.

has not been evaluated in a prospective, controlled study.

Outside Japan, there are conflicting data about the efficacy of screening. In the North-East of Italy, an area with an inter-mediate incidence rate, surveillance was employed for patients with dysplastic gas-tric lesions. Three-quarters of cancers detected during a secondary prevention surveillance programme were considered to be early stomach cancer. This contrasts with a case-control study in Venezuela which did not demonstrate a reduction in mortality among persons screened with radiography [15,16].

It is essential that in countries with a high incidence of stomach cancer, primary pre-vention should be promoted to reduce the disease burden. The pathogenesis of stomach cancer is multi-factorial and even if the most powerful risk factor is eradi-cated, this does not guarantee an immedi-ate or even rapid reduction in cancer risk. Testing and treatment for *H. pylori* in high-incidence areas should be complemented with dietary modifications. Population-based screening for stomach cancer is not appropriate in countries with low inci-dence rates.

REFERENCES

1. Asaka M, Kimura T, Kato M, Kudo M, Miki K, Ogoshi K, Kato T, Tatsuta M, Graham DY (1994) Possible role of *Helicobacter pylori* infection in early gastric cancer development. *Cancer*, 73: 2691-2694.

2. Graham DY (2000) *Helicobacter pylori* infection is the primary cause of gastric cancer. *J Gastroenterol*, 35 Suppl 12: 90-97.

3. Uemura N, Okamoto S, Yamamoto S, Matsumura N, Yamaguchi S, Yamakido M, Taniyama K, Sasaki N, Schlemper RJ (2001) *Helicobacter pylori* infection and the development of gastric cancer. *N Engl J Med*, 345: 784-789.

4. Uemura N, Mukai T, Okamoto S, Yamaguchi S, Mashiba H, Taniyama K, Sasaki N, Haruma K, Sumii K, Kajiyama G (1997) Effect of *Helicobacter pylori* eradication on subsequent development of cancer after endoscopic resection of early gastric cancer. *Cancer Epidemiol Biomarkers Prev*, 6: 639-642.

5. Parsonnet J, Harris RA, Hack HM, Owens DK (1996) Modelling cost-effectiveness of *Helicobacter pylori* screening to prevent gastric cancer: a mandate for clinical trials. *Lancet*, 348: 150-154.

6. Sonnenberg A, Inadomi JM (1998) Review article: Medical decision models of *Helicobacter pylori* therapy to prevent gastric cancer. *Aliment Pharmacol Ther*, 12 Suppl 1: 111-121.

7. Hatzifoti C, Wren BW, Morrow WJ (2000) *Helicobacter pylori* vaccine strategies—triggering a gut reaction. *Immunol Today*, 21: 615-619.

8. Corthesy-Theulaz I (2000) Vaccination against *Helicobacter pylori*. *Recent Results Cancer Res*, 156: 55-59.

9. Ogimoto I, Shibata A, Fukuda K (2000) World Cancer Research Fund/American Institute of Cancer Research 1997 recommendations: applicability to digestive tract cancer in Japan. *Cancer Causes Control*, 11: 9-23.

10. Berglund G, Hill MJ, Caygill CP, Farinati F, Giacosa A, De Koster E, Reed PI, Sobrinho-Simoes M, Stockbrugger R (1997) Consensus statement on diet and gastric cancer. Gastric Cancer Panel. *Eur J Cancer Prev*, 6: 404-407.

11. Correa P, Malcom G, Schmidt B, Fontham E, Ruiz B, Bravo JC, Bravo LE, Zarama G, Realpe JL (1998) Review article: Antioxidant micronutrients and gastric cancer. *Aliment Pharmacol Ther*, 12 Suppl 1: 73-82.

12. Varis K, Taylor PR, Sipponen P, Samloff IM, Heinonen OP, Albanes D, Harkonen M, Huttunen JK, Laxen F, Virtamo J (1998) Gastric cancer and premalignant lesions in atrophic gastritis: a controlled trial on the effect of supplementation with alpha-tocopherol and beta-carotene. The Helsinki Gastritis Study Group. *Scand J Gastroenterol*, 33: 294-300.

13. Youn HS, Ko GH, Chung MH, Lee WK, Cho MJ, Rhee KH (1996) Pathogenesis and prevention of stomach cancer. *J Korean Med Sci*, 11: 373-385.

14. Hanazaki K, Sodeyama H, Wakabayashi M, Miyazawa M, Yokoyama S, Sode Y, Kawamura N, Miyazaki T, Ohtsuka M (1997) Surgical treatment of gastric cancer detected by mass screening. *Hepatogastroenterology*, 44: 1126-1132.

15. Pisani P, Oliver WE, Parkin DM, Alvarez N, Vivas J (1994) Case-control study of gastric cancer screening in Venezuela. *Br J Cancer*, 69: 1102-1105.

16. Pisani P, Parkin DM (1996) Screening for gastric cancer. *Cancer Treat Res*, 86: 113-119.

5

Human cancers by organ site

Malignant tumours can develop in any organ from cell types still actively engaged in replication. The nomenclature refers to the tissue of origin: carcinoma (derived from epithelial tissues), sarcoma (soft tissues and bone), glioma (brain), leukaemia and lymphoma (haematopoietic and lymphatic tissues), carcinomas being by far the most frequent type. Irrespective of the site, malignant transformation is a multistep process involving the sequential accumulation of genetic alterations. However, the types of oncogene or suppressor genes involved and the sequence of amplification or mutation varies greatly in different organs and target cells. Susceptibility to carcinogenic factors may depend on the capacity to metabolize chemical carcinogens, to effectively repair DNA damage or to harbour chronic infections. There are also marked variations in response to therapy and overall clinical outcome.

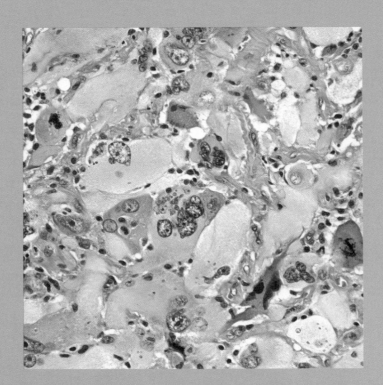

LUNG CANCER

SUMMARY

> Lung cancer is the most common tumour worldwide, with 900,000 new cases each year in men and 330,000 in women It is the leading cause of death from cancer.

> In men, more than 80% of lung cancer cases are caused by smoking; in women, the attributable risk is less (about 70% in Northern Europe; 45% worldwide).

> Some occupational exposures and air pollution (including environmental tobacco smoke) make a minor contribution to incidence.

> No population-based screening procedures have been established.

> No effective treatment is available; the five-year survival rate for lung cancer patients is less than 15%.

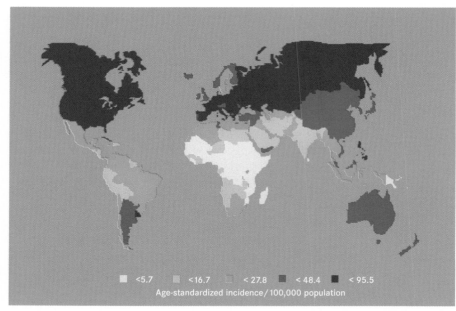

■ <5.7   ■ <16.7   □ < 27.8   ■ < 48.4   ■ < 95.5
Age-standardized incidence / 100,000 population

Fig. 5.1 The global incidence of lung cancer in men. Incidence is highest in Europe, especially Eastern Europe, and in North America and Australia.

Definition

Lung cancer almost exclusively involves carcinomas, these tumours arising from epithelia of the trachea, bronchi or lungs. There are several histological types, the most common being squamous cell carcinoma, adenocarcinoma and small (oat) cell carcinoma.

Epidemiology

Lung cancer is the most common malignant disease worldwide, and is the major cause of death from cancer, particularly amongst men. It was a rare disease until the beginning of the 20th century. Since then, the occurrence of lung cancer has increased rapidly and it now accounts for an estimated 901,746 new cases each year among men and 337,115 among women [1].

The highest incidence rates (>100 cases per 100,000 population) are recorded among Afro-Americans from New Orleans,

USA and Maoris from New Zealand and are followed by those in the United Kingdom and the Netherlands. The lowest incidence rates are reported from Africa and Southern Asia [2] (Fig. 5.1). Rates in women are high in the USA, Canada, Denmark and the UK, but are lower in countries such as France, Japan and Spain, in which the prevalence of smoking in women has increased only recently. The lowest rates (<3 cases per 100,000 population) are recorded in Africa and India. In most countries, lung cancer incidence is greater in lower socioeconomic classes; to a large extent, this pattern is explained by differences in the prevalence of smoking. Having risen dramatically since the turn of the century, lung cancer mortality amongst males is now abating in several countries, including the USA, the UK and Finland (Fig. 5.4).

Etiology

The geographical and temporal patterns of lung cancer incidence are overwhelmingly determined by consumption of tobacco.

The association between lung cancer and smoking is probably the most intensively investigated relationship in epidemiology. Smoking causes lung cancer. An increase in tobacco consumption is paralleled some 20 years later by an increase in the incidence of lung cancer, and a decrease in consumption (e.g. a large proportion of smokers who quit) is followed by a decrease in incidence. In both men and women, the incidence of lung cancer is low before age 40, and increases up to at least age 70. The situation in China appears to be different, given the relatively high rates of lung cancer (particularly adenocarcinoma) recorded among Chinese women, despite a low prevalence of smoking.

The association between lung cancer and smoking was demonstrated in the 1950s and has been recognized by public health and regulatory authorities since the mid-1960s. The risk of lung cancer among smokers relative to the risk among never-smokers is in the order of 8-15 in men and 2-10 in women. This overall risk reflects the contribution of the different aspects of tobacco smoking: age at start, average consumption, duration of smoking, time since quitting, type of tobacco product and inhalation pattern, with duration being the dominant factor. While lung cancer risks rise sharply with increasing numbers of cigarettes per day, the trends have been reported to be even stronger with duration of smoking. Such findings are essentially consistent in men from diverse communities, including those of the USA, UK and China. In populations with a long duration and heavy intensity of cigarette usage, the proportion of lung cancer attributable to smoking is of the order of 90% [3].

As compared to continuous smokers, the excess risk sharply decreases in ex-smokers approximately five years after quitting, but a small excess risk persists in long-term quitters throughout life. The risk of lung cancer is slightly lower among smokers of low-tar and low-nicotine cigarettes than among other smokers, although "low-tar smokers" tend to compensate for lower yields of nicotine by deeper inhalation or greater consumption. A relative reduction in risk has also been observed among long-term smokers of filtered cigarettes compared to smokers of unfiltered cigarettes. Smokers of black (air-cured) tobacco cigarettes are at a two to three-fold higher risk of lung cancer than smokers of blond (flue-cured) tobacco cigarettes. A causal association with lung cancer has also been shown for consumption of cigars, cigarillos, pipe, bidis and water pipe.

An association between exposure to passive smoke and lung cancer risk in non-smokers has been shown in a number of case-control and cohort studies (Fig. 5.9). In general, such studies involve exposure to environmental tobacco smoke in the home or the workplace or both. In many instances, the increased risk recorded is at the margin of statistical significance, and in some cases less than that. However, a causal relationship has been recognized on the basis of consistent findings and taking account of biological plausibility (that is, the established carcinogenic activity of tobacco smoke). The magnitude of the risk is in the order of 15-20% [4].

Occupational exposures have been associated with increased risk of lung cancer more than of any other tumour type (*Occupational exposures*, p33). For many workplace exposures associated with a high risk of lung cancer, the specific agent(s) responsible for the increased risk has been identified. Risk of lung cancer and mesothelioma (a malignant tumour of the pleura) is increased in a variety of occupations involving exposure to asbestos of various types. A characteristic of asbestos-related lung cancer is its synergistic relationship to cigarette smoking: risk is increased multiplicatively amongst persons who both smoke and are exposed to asbestos. Such a phenomenon has been recorded in relation to other occupational lung cancers.

Atomic bomb survivors and patients treated with radiotherapy are at increased risk

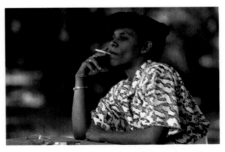

Fig. 5.2 The incidence of smoking-induced lung cancer in women is increasing in many countries at an alarming rate.

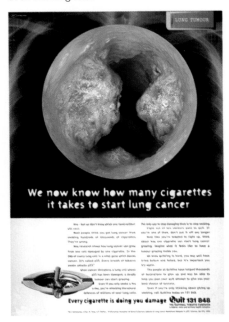

Fig. 5.3 Smoking is the primary cause of lung cancer. "Every cigarette is doing you damage" campaign, Australia.

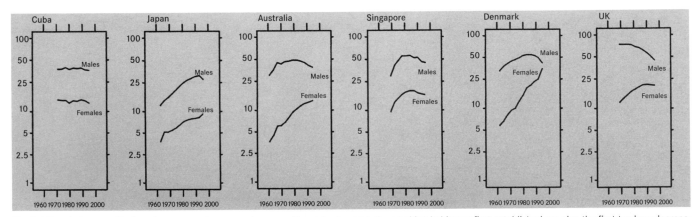

Fig. 5.4 Trends in mortality from lung cancer in men and women. Countries in which the smoking habit was first established are also the first to show decreases in mortality following reduction in the prevalence of smoking. D.M. Parkin et al. (2001) *Eur J Cancer* 37 Suppl. 8: S4 - 66.

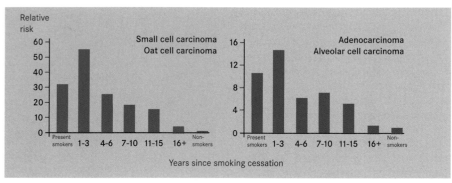

Fig. 5.5 The relative risk of lung cancer is markedly lower five years after quitting, and decreases further with time (by comparison with those who continue to smoke).

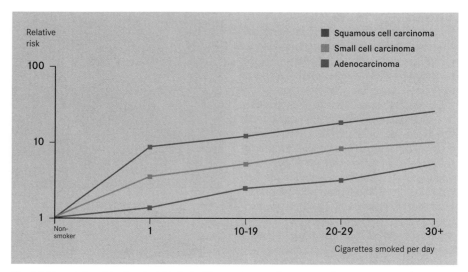

Fig. 5.6 The relative risk of major histological types of cancer by average cigarette consumption.

Detection

Sputum cytology and radiology (chest X-ray and computed tomography (CT)) scans are the only non-invasive methods of detecting early lung cancer. Sensitivity can be variable dependent on histological type (greater for small cell and squamous cell carcinomas), tumour size and location [10]. Sputum cytotology may be appropriate for certain clearly defined groups or individuals at risk of lung cancer. Currently, however, there are no practicable and effective procedures available to provide population-based screening for lung cancer.

The signs and symptoms of lung cancer depend on the location of the tumour, the spread and the effects of metastatic growth. Many patients are diagnosed on the basis of an asymptomatic lesion discovered incidentally on X-ray. Symptoms indicative of the primary tumour include fatigue, decreased activity, persistent cough, laboured breathing, chest pain, decreased appetite and weight loss. Hoarseness as a result of recurrent laryngeal nerve injury may be provoked by left-sided lesions, and superior vena cava syndrome by right-sided lesions. Wheeze or stridor may also develop in advanced stages. Continuous tumour growth may result in collapsed lung, pneumonia and abscess formation.

In some patients with lung cancer, metastatic deposits lead to the first symptoms; the majority of patients with lung cancer already have locally advanced disease or distant metastases at diagnosis; common metastatic sites are mediastinal and supraclavicular lymph nodes, liver, adrenal glands, brain, lungs, pleura and pericardium. Less commonly, a patient may be diagnosed on the basis of a paraneoplastic syndrome (signs and symptoms not produced by the direct effect of a tumour or its metastasis), such as the syndrome of inappropriate secretion of antidiuretic hormone in small cell lung cancers. Diagnostic procedures involve chest X-ray, bronchoscopy and sputum analysis, as well as CT and magnetic nuclear resonance. CT imaging is used for the detection of liver and adrenal gland metastases. Clinical and image-based

of lung cancer. Although the magnitude of the increased risk is moderate (relative risk, 1.5 to 2 for cumulative exposure in excess of 100 rads), the number of extra cases of lung cancer exceeds that of other neoplasms. Underground miners exposed to radioactive radon and its decay products have been found to be at an increased risk of lung cancer [5,6]. Indoor exposure to radon has been associated with a marginal increase in risk of lung cancer.

There is abundant evidence that lung cancer rates are higher in cities than in rural settings [7]. Urban air pollution is a risk factor for lung cancer and the excess risk may be in the order of 50% (*Environmental pollution*, p39). Two particular sources of indoor air pollution are the use of coal-burning heaters without proper exhaust emission (e.g. *kang* in North-Eastern China) and high-temperature cooking using unrefined vegetable oils, such as rapeseed oil (common in several parts of China). Indoor levels of benzo[a]pyrene have been reported to be very high in such circumstances [8]. Indoor air pollution is a major cause of lung cancer in Chinese women, who experience very high lung cancer rates despite a low prevalence of smoking.

There is convincing evidence that a diet rich in vegetables and fruits exerts a protective effect against lung cancer [9]. Subjects in the categories of highest consumption experience about 50% of the risk of lung cancer compared with subjects in the categories of lowest consumption.

diagnosis is usually confirmed by histological examination of biopsies obtained by fibre-optic endoscopy or surgical specimens. Percutaneous fine needle aspiration may be used to diagnose peripheral tumours, or in the event of inconclusive bronchoscopy results. The complementary use of spiral CT in screening may improve the robustness with which lung cancer of any cell type can be detected early [11]. However, many cases of lung cancer, especially at older ages and in low resource countries, are diagnosed only on the basis of clinical and X-ray evidence.

Pathology and genetics

Principal histological types of lung cancer are squamous cell carcinoma, adenocarcinoma, large cell carcinoma and small cell carcinoma. The first three are also referred to as "non-small cell" lung carcinomas. In North America and Europe over the last 20 years, the proportion of squamous cell carcinoma, previously the predominant type, has been decreasing, while an increase of adenocarcinoma has been recorded in both genders. Squamous cell carcinoma arises most frequently in proximal segmental bronchi and is associated with squamous metaplasia. This tumour type is very strongly associated with smoking and represents the most common type

of lung cancer in many populations. It tends to grow slowly, three to four years being required for development from an *in situ* lesion to a clinically apparent tumour. Adenocarcinoma is less strongly associated with smoking. This tumour is often peripheral in origin and may present as a solitary peripheral nodule, multifocal disease, or a rapidly progressive pneumonic form, spreading from lobe to lobe. These tumours form glands and produce mucin. Early metastasis is common, particularly to the brain, pleura and adrenal glands. Large cell carcinoma often appears in the distal bronchi and is generally undifferentiated. Small cell carcinoma typically arises in the central endobronchial location and is commonly aggressive and invasive; frequently metastases are present at diagnosis.

Although the histogenesis and the putative precursor lesions of lung cancer are largely unknown for the different histological types, the presence of putative precursor lesions (dysplasia, metaplasia and carcinoma *in situ*) are commonly reported in resection specimens and/or cytology for squamous cell carcinoma [12].

A positive familial history of lung cancer has been identified as a risk factor. Increased risk of lung cancer has been associated with certain polymorphisms of the cytochrome P450 genes and with defi-

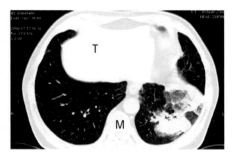

Fig. 5.7 A lung tumour viewed by computed tomography. T= tumour, M= mediastinum.

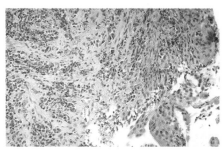

Fig. 5.8 Biopsy of a small cell lung carcinoma, showing a monomorphic proliferation of small tumour cells with dense nuclei and poorly-defined cytoplasm, invading the deep parts of the bronchial wall.

ciencies in DNA repair capacity [13]. Genetic changes associated with progression of premalignant lesions to malignant tumours have been identified [14] (Table 5.1). Mutations in the *p53* gene are frequent events in lung cancer, although adenocarcinoma shows a lower prevalence of *p53* mutations than other histological types. Among lung cancer cases, the proportion of *p53* mutations increases with duration and amount of tobacco smoking. A wide distribution and a variety of types of *p53* mutation have been observed following different environmental exposures; their analysis is likely to elucidate different mechanisms involved in lung carcinogenesis [15].

Activating point mutations in the *KRAS* oncogene (mainly at codon 12) occur in adenocarcinoma, with a prevalence ranging from 15% to 60%. This alteration, which is more prevalent in tumours from smokers than from non-smokers, may be a relatively early event in lung carcinogenesis. Frequent loss of heterozygosity and aber-

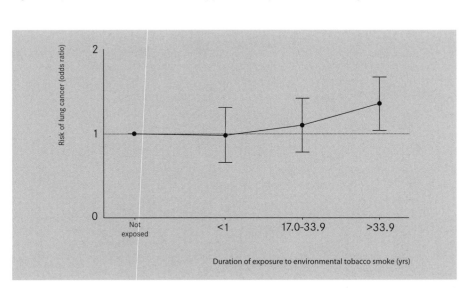

Fig. 5.9 Relative risk of lung cancer (odds ratio) among non-smokers by cumulative exposure to environmental tobacco smoke from the spouse and workplace. Pooled analysis of data from two studies in the USA and in Europe.

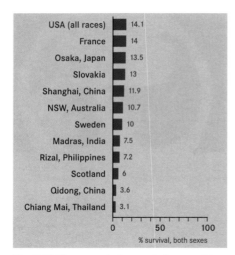

Fig. 5.10 Five-year relative survival rates of lung cancer patients after diagnosis.

rant transcripts of the Fragile Histidine Triad (*FHIT*) gene, located at chromosome 3p14.2, occur in pre-neoplastic and neoplastic lesions and such changes have been linked to smoking and asbestos exposure. Homozygous deletions and transcriptional silencing due to methylation in the locus of the cyclin-dependent kinase inhibitor p16^{INK4A} on chromosome 9p have been found in about 40% of lung cancer cases. Other oncogenes have also been implicated in lung carcinogenesis: in particular, *ERBB1* and *ERBB2*; *C-MYC*, *N-MYC* and *L-MYC*, and *BCL2* [16]. No clear correlations have been established as yet between particular genetic changes and histological type of tumour.

Management

Staging of lung cancer is based on an assessment of the presence of distant metastases and the condition of the chest and mediastinum (the tissues and organs separating the lungs), in accordance with the universally used TNM system (Box: *TNM*, p124). Although treatment protocols are subject to refinement and improvement, the outlook for patients diagnosed with lung cancer is poor by comparison with many other cancers. The main prognostic factors are stage of the tumour and performance status; other important factors include amount of weight loss, gender (men having a poorer prognosis than

women), serum concentration of lactate dehydrogenase and the detection of bone and liver metastases.

Non-small cell carcinomas are grouped together because of similarity in the response of the different subtypes to treatment. Early stage tumours are treated by surgical resection, if possible, with patients who refuse or who are deemed medically unfit for surgery being treated with radiotherapy. More advanced stage disease may be treated with a combination of surgery and radiotherapy. Radiotherapy can be effective for palliation of superior vena cava obstruction, haemoptysis (expectoration of blood), pain, dyspnoea (shortness of breath), brain metastases and atelectasis (partial or complete lung collapse) [17]. The introduction of cisplatin-containing drug combinations improves the rate of response to therapy, with accompanying moderate to severe toxicity. Combination chemotherapy (using cisplatin and etoposide, or mitomycin, vinblastine and cisplatin) with radiotherapy also seems to convey a survival advantage in patients with stage III disease. More recently, paclitaxel has shown significant activity when used as a single agent. Other drugs credited with response rates of at least 15% include gemcitabine, docetaxel and vinorelbine. The mainstay of treatment for small cell

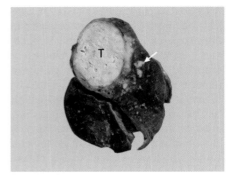

Fig. 5.11 A smoking-induced lung cancer. Autopsy specimen of a large-cell carcinoma of the left lung (T) with nearby metastases (arrow).

lung cancer is chemotherapy, with concomitant radiotherapy being used at an early point for patients with limited disease. Surgery may be considered in the case of a patient with a small isolated lesion [17]. Combinations of drugs, as a general rule, yield better results than the respective agents used alone and those commonly used include cisplatin and etoposide, cyclophosphamide, doxorubicin and vincristine, and cyclophosphamide, doxorubicin and etoposide. More recently, the taxanes paclitaxel and docetaxel and the camptothecins irinotecan and topotecan have shown promise as single agents and in combination. Despite good initial responses to therapy, relapse

Gene	Locus	Alteration	Frequency (% of tumours)		
			Small cell carcinoma	Adeno-carcinoma	Squamous cell carcinoma
p53	17p13	Deletion, mutation (G:C>T:A), (overexpression)	70-90	30	50
KRAS	12p21	Mutation (GGT>TGT)	<1	15-60	8-9
CDKN2A/ p16^{INK4}	9p21	Deletion, mutation, hypermethylation	<1	27-59	33-40
LOH 3p	3p	Deletion (loss of heterozygosity)	100	50-85	
FHIT	3p14.2	Deletion (loss of heterozygosity), transcriptional dysregulation	76	40-76	

Table 5.1 Genetic alterations in lung tumours.

is frequent and survival rates are poor (two-year survival of 20-30% for limited stage disease) although limited stage small cell cancer has a cure rate of about 10-15%. Treatment should be considered since good symptom control can be attained. Prophylactic cranial irradiation may reduce the risk of brain metastases, and has recently been shown in meta-analysis to prolong survival in limited small cell cancer.

Although survival for stage I cancers may reach about 65%, overall survival from lung cancer is poor (Fig. 5.10). In population-based series from high-income countries, the five-year relative survival barely exceeds 10%. However, survival is better among patients aged less than 55 at diagnosis (five-year relative survival in the order of 15%). There is evidence of a very modest improvement in survival during the last 20 years. In developing countries, survival rates are comparable to those in industrialized countries.

In the light of poor survival rates, prevention of lung cancer is a priority. However, the development of novel therapies remains important in view of the fact that most patients will die of disease progression and current treatments can be highly toxic. Trials of vaccination against tumour specific antigens such as carcinoembryonic antigen (CEA) and Fuc-GM1 are underway [18]. A further strategy under investigation is that of vaccination with tumour cells designed to have enhanced immunogenicity due to the expression of, for example, cytokine granulocyte-macrophage colony-stimulating factor (GM-CSF).

REFERENCES

1. Ferlay J, Bray F, Parkin DM, Pisani P (2001) *Globocan 2000: Cancer Incidence and Mortality Worldwide (IARC Cancer Bases No. 5)*, Lyon, IARCPress.

2. Parkin DM, Whelan SL, Ferlay J, Raymond L, Young J, eds (1997) *Cancer Incidence in Five Continents, Vol. VII (IARC Scientific Publication No. 143 and IARC Cancerbase No. 2)*, Lyon, IARCPress.

3. IARC (1986) Tobacco Smoking *(IARC Monographs on the Evaluation of the Carcinogenic Risk of Chemicals to Humans, Vol. 38)*, Lyon, IARCPress.

4. Hackshaw AK, Law MR, Wald NJ (1997) The accumulated evidence on lung cancer and environmental tobacco smoke. *BMJ*, 315: 980-988.

5. Samet JM (1989) Radon and lung cancer. *J Natl Cancer Inst*, 81: 745-757.

6. Lubin JH, Boice JD, Edling C, Hornung RW, Howe G, Kunz E (1994) Radon and lung cancer risk: a joint analysis of 11 underground miners studies. In: Public Health Service, National Institute of Health eds, *NIH Publication No. 94-3644*, Washington D.C., US Department of Health and Human Services.

7. Speizer FE, Samet JM (1994) Air pollution and lung cancer. In: Samet JM ed., *Epidemiology of Lung Cancer (Lung Biology in Health and Disease, Vol. 74)*, New York, Marcel Dekker, 131-150.

8. Smith KR, Liu Y (1994) Indoor air pollution in developing countries. In: Samet JM ed., *Epidemiology of Lung Cancer (Lung Biology in Health and Disease, Vol. 74)*, New York, Marcel Dekker, 151-184.

9. World Cancer Research Fund (1997) Lung. In: WCRF/AICR ed, *Food, Nutrition and the Prevention of Cancer: a Global Perspective*, Washington, DC, World Cancer Research Fund/American Institute of Cancer Research, 130-147.

10. Lam S, Shibuya H (1999) Early diagnosis of lung cancer. *Clin Chest Med*, 20: 53-61.

11. Mulshine JL, Henschke CI (2000) Prospects for lung-cancer screening. *Lancet*, 355: 592-593.

12. Montuenga LM, Mulshine JL (2000) New molecular strategies for early lung cancer detection. *Cancer Invest*, 18: 555-563.

13. Wright GS, Gruidl ME (2000) Early detection and prevention of lung cancer. *Curr Opin Oncol*, 12 : 143-148.

14. Bunn PA, Jr., Soriano A, Johnson G, Heasley L (2000) New therapeutic strategies for lung cancer: biology and molecular biology come of age. *Chest*, 117: 163S-168S.

15. Bennett WP, Hussain SP, Vahakangas KH, Khan MA, Shields PG, Harris CC (1999) Molecular epidemiology of human cancer risk: gene-environment interactions and p53 mutation spectrum in human lung cancer. *J Pathol*, 187: 8-18.

16. Minna JD, Sekido Y, Fong KM, Gazdar AF (1997) Molecular biology of lung cancer. In: DeVita VT, Hellman S, Rosenberg, SA eds, *Cancer: Principles and Practice of Oncology*, Philadelphia, Lippincott-Raven Publishers, 849-857.

17. Williams C (1998) Lung cancer. In: Morris D, Kearsley J, Williams C eds, *Cancer: a comprehensive clinical guide*, Harwood Academic Publishers, 141-152.

18. Antonia SJ, Sotomayor E (2000) Gene therapy for lung cancer. *Curr Opin Oncol*, 12: 138-142.

WEBSITE

NCI Lung Cancer Homepage:
http://www.cancer.gov/cancer_information/cancer_type/lung/

BREAST CANCER

SUMMARY

> Breast cancer is the most common malignancy affecting women, with more than one million cases occurring worldwide annually. Affluent societies carry the greatest risk, with incidence rates of >80 per 100,000 population per year.

> The worldwide breast cancer epidemic has many etiological factors, including reproductive history (early menarche, late or no pregnancy), and Western lifestyle (high caloric diet, lack of physical activity).

> In some regions, including North America, Western Europe and Australia, breast cancer mortality rates have started to decline, mainly due to improvements in early detection and treatment (chemotherapy and tamoxifen). Five-year survival rates are higher than 70% in most developed countries.

> Breast cancer screening trials of mammography have shown that mortality can be reduced by up to 30%. However, there is limited evidence that this can be achieved in population-based country-wide screening programmes.

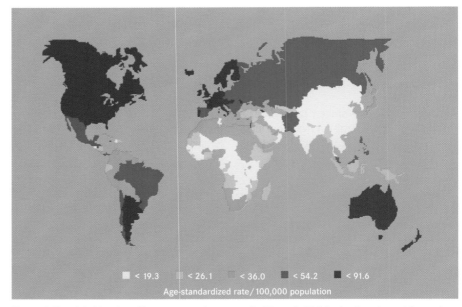

| ■ < 19.3 | ■ < 26.1 | □ < 36.0 | ■ < 54.2 | ■ < 91.6 |

Age-standardized rate / 100,000 population

Fig. 5.12 The global burden of breast cancer in women; incidence is high in developed countries such as the USA, UK and Australia.

Definition

Breast cancer generally refers to a malignancy in women that arises from the terminal ductal-lobular units of epithelial tissue, which in the mature breast represent 10% of the total volume.

Epidemiology

Latest estimates suggest that more than 1,050,000 new breast cancer cases occur worldwide annually, with nearly 580,000 cases occurring in developed countries and the remainder in developing countries [1]. Thus breast cancer now ranks first among cancers affecting women throughout the world and its marked impact is not restricted to Western industrialized societies (Fig. 5.12).

In 1998, there were 412,000 deaths attributed to breast cancer for women in the world, representing 1.6% of all female deaths. In terms of absolute numbers, the greatest contribution is now from developing countries, where 250,000 such deaths occurred, as compared to developed countries, which account for 160,000 deaths. However, the proportion of deaths due to breast cancer in women remains higher in the latter countries at 2.0% in comparison to 0.5% in the developing countries. Male breast cancer is about 100 times less frequent than the disease in women.

The Netherlands exemplifies the high incidence of breast cancer in developed countries, with an age-standardized incidence rate of 91.6 new cases per 100,000 woman-years, but there are sub-populations, such as white women in California, which exhibit age-adjusted incidence rates of 100 or more. Overall, the incidence rate in the USA is estimated at 91.4. Such high rates are also observed in Europe, Australia and New Zealand, and in

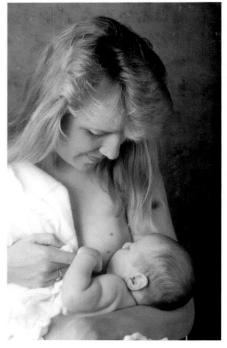

Fig. 5.13 Risk of breast cancer is decreased in women who have children early and who have breast-fed.

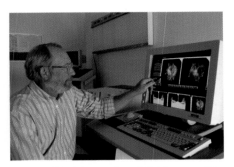
Fig. 5.14 Physician reading digital images of the breast in preparation for a computer-guided minimally invasive biopsy.

some parts of South America, especially Uruguay and Argentina. In contrast, low rates are found among African and Asian populations. Amongst population-based cancer registries (as distinct from national estimates), the 30 recording the highest rates include 20 registries from North America, one from South America (Montevideo), two from Israel and five from Europe. Amongst this group, the only one from Africa is for Europeans in Harare. By contrast, among population-based registries with the 30 lowest rates, five are from Africa, 18 from Asia and Israel, three from South America, two from Eastern Europe and two from the United States of America (American Indians in New Mexico and Koreans in Los Angeles, California) [2].

These large geographical differences are potentially explicable on the basis of genetics or the influences of lifestyle and environment. Studies of migrant populations have revealed that when women migrate from low-risk to high-risk regions, the migrant populations acquire the rates of the host country after two or three generations, indicating lifestyle as primarily determining the geographic variations in risk.

"Cumulative incidence" represents the probability of developing a particular disease over a life span. Given the uncertainties of breast cancer diagnosis in older women and the high likelihood of the disease not being reported in the oldest age groups, it is common practice to present cumulative incidence for the age span 0-74 years. In the world, cumulative inci-

dences for breast cancer vary from 0.76% for women in Kangwha, Korea to 11.9% for non-Hispanic whites in San Francisco, USA [2].

The absolute number of new breast cancer cases worldwide increased from 572,100 in 1980 to 1,050,346 for the most recent period [3]. Comparison of rates rather than absolute figures excludes change attributable to ageing of the population as well as differences in age structures across countries. Even so, most cancer registries of the world have recorded an increase in the incidence of breast cancer over the past 20 years (*Screening for breast cancer*, p156). In the period 1975-1990, the largest increases, greater than 1% and sometimes 5% per year, are exhibited by registries previously having low rates of disease, mostly in Asia and Africa, as well as in some parts of Europe. In contrast, the smallest increases, in general inferior to 0.5% per year, are usually seen in places previously having high rates, mostly in North America and Europe. These changes are particularly obvious in relation to disease in younger women, that is below 45 years of age [2,4]. However, mortality rates are falling, probably due to better treatment (Fig. 5.19).

Etiology

Risk factors for breast cancer (Fig. 5.18) specifically concern the reproductive life of women. Increased risk is correlated with early menarche, nulliparity or late age at first birth, late menopause, as well as hormonal factors, be they endogenous or exogenous (e.g. long term use of oral contraceptives or menopausal hormonal replacement, *Reproductive factors and hormones*, p76). Genetic risk factors are discussed later (Pathology and genetics). Other risk factors that may also be mediated through a hormonal pathway include obesity and diet, characterized by a high caloric intake, not counterbalanced by sufficient physical activity, high total and saturated animal fat, as well as a diet poor in fruits and vegetables and rich in meat and alcohol [5,6]. The role of contaminants, such as xenoestrogens and certain pesticides, remains controversial. Radiation, in

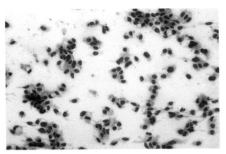
Fig. 5.15 Fine needle aspirate of cells from a breast tumour.

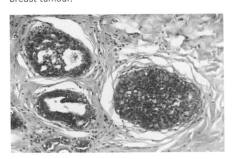
Fig. 5.16 An example of lobular carcinoma *in situ*, comprising a well-differentiated malignant proliferation without signs of invasion.

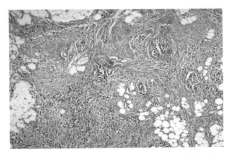
Fig. 5.17 Infiltrating ductal carcinoma. This is a poorly-differentiated adenocarcinoma infiltrating the adipose tissue.

particular at times of breast development, causes breast cancer. Women with epithelial proliferative lesions, particularly with atypical ductal or lobular hyperplasia by comparison with normal histology, have a four to five times increase in the risk of developing breast cancer [7].

Detection

The commonest presentation of breast cancer is of a painless lump; other symptoms may include dimpling of the overlying skin, nipple inversion, oedema or *peau d'orange* and blood-stained nipple discharge. In countries where no mammo-

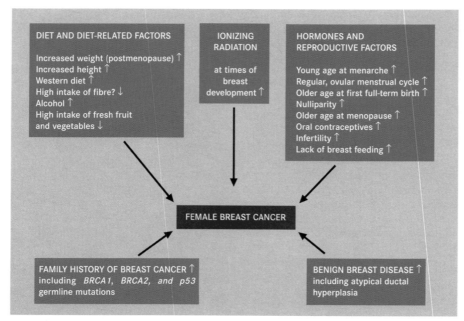

Fig. 5.18 Risk and protective factors for breast cancer. Factors associated with an increased (↑) or decreased (↓) risk of breast cancer.

A woman may be considered to be at a potentially high risk of breast cancer if there are three or more first or second degree relatives on the same side of the family with breast or ovarian cancer, or two or more first or second degree relatives on the same side of the family with breast or ovarian cancer which has been diagnosed at age 40 or younger, bilateral disease, both breast and ovarian cancer in the same individual or breast cancer in a male [11]. The currently available approaches to the management of the high-risk woman are close surveillance (involving regular self and clinical breast examination and annual mammography), genetic counselling or prophylactic mastectomy (a procedure which does not, however, guarantee complete prevention of subsequent breast cancer).

Pathology and genetics

Ductal carcinoma *in situ* is a proliferation of presumably malignant epithelial cells and is confined to the mammary ducts and lobules. It carries a 30% chance of developing into invasive disease, although the natural history of this progression remains uncertain. The rate of detection of ductal carcinoma *in situ* has increased significantly with the introduction of mammography and questions have been raised regarding the possible overtreatment of this condition. It can be classified into comedo and non-comedo subtypes based on growth pattern, the comedo

graphic screening exists, and in fact for women generally, health education should include recognition of breast cancer symptoms. Diagnosis of breast cancer is currently made by triple assessment of breast lumps – clinical history and examination, complemented by mammography and/or breast ultrasound plus fine needle aspiration cytology or biopsy [8]. Breast screening can have an impact on disease

mortality. Mammography is associated with a reduction of up to 30% in breast cancer mortality in the context of well-conducted trials [9]. Where adopted, population-based screening is commonly based on biennial examination from the age of 50 onwards. To realize the benefit of screening, prompt and adequate follow-up must be available to all women with a suspected malignancy [10].

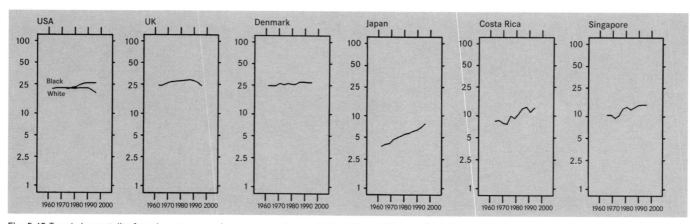

Fig. 5.19 Trends in mortality from breast cancer. In some countries, such the USA and UK mortality is decreasing; in almost all developing countries, mortality is increasing. D.M. Parkin et al. (2001) *Eur J Cancer* 37 Suppl 8: S4-66

Markers of prognosis in breast cancer

Commonly assessed markers:

Number of positive axillary lymph nodes
Tumour size
Tumour TNM stage
Lymphatic and vascular invasion
Histological tumour type
Steroid hormone receptors (estrogen receptors ER-α, ER-β; progesterone receptor)
Growth factor receptor genes (epidermal growth factor gene, *EGFR*)
DNA ploidy (DNA histogram)
Proliferative indices (fraction of cells in S-phase; thymidine labelling index; mitotic index)

Less commonly assessed markers:

Proliferative indices (Ki67, PCNA, cyclins, thymidylate synthetase, MIB1)
Topoisomerase II
Histone H3
Transforming growth factors (TGF-α, TGF-β)
Epidermal growth factor (EGF)
Insulin-like growth factors and their binding proteins (IGF-I, IGF-II)
Oncogene products (c-erbB2, ras, c-myc, int2)
Markers of apoptosis (mutations of p53, Bcl-2 proteins, caspases, survirin, p21, R6)
Markers of proteolysis (activation of urokinase-type plasminogen, cathepsin D, matrix metalloproteases)
Markers of cell adhesion (integrins, cadherins, CD-44 variants)
Markers of angiogenesis (endothelial markers: Factor VII, CD-31, CD34; angiogenic peptides e.g. VEGF)
Markers of cell mobility (cytokines)
Steroid hormones (estrogens, glucocorticoids, prolactin, progestins)
Tumour-associated antigens (carcinoembryogenic antigen, CEA; tissue polypeptide antigen, TPA; gross cystic disease fluid protein, GCDP; mucin-like molecules, CA 15.3, MAM-6, MSA, MC)
pS2
NM23
Heat shock proteins
MDR1

Table 5.2 Prognostic indicators in breast cancer.

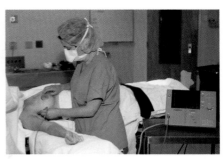

Fig. 5.20 Physician performing a sentinel lymph node biopsy. With this state-of-the-art radio-guided surgical equipment, the patient avoids complete resection of the axillary lymphatic nodes and the complications of lymphoedema.

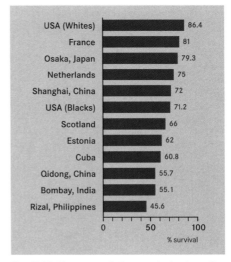

Fig. 5.21 Five-year relative survival rates after diagnosis of breast cancer.

type, having a higher rate of proliferation, being more aggressive and more likely to be associated with areas of microinvasion and with expression of markers such as aneuploidy and overexpression of p53, c-erbB2 and Bcl-2. Lobular carcinoma *in situ* (Fig. 5.16), unlike ductal carcinoma *in situ*, is not readily detected clinically or mammographically, is frequently multicentric and bilateral, and occurs more commonly in younger women. It is associated with an increased risk for development of cancer, but is not a precursor lesion. Lobular carcinoma *in situ* is characterized by a solid proliferation of small cells with small uniform, round or oval nuclei, which grow slowly, are usually estrogen receptor positive and rarely overexpress c-erbB2. The most frequent malignant lesion (80%) is invasive ductal carcinoma of no special type, with 20% of cancers

being lobular, tubular, medullary or other special types (Fig. 5.17).

The most important genes identified in the context of familial breast cancer are *BRCA1* and *BRCA2* [12]. Inherited mutations in these genes account for a very high relative risk of breast and sometimes ovarian cancer among carrier women [13], although such instances of breast cancer account for less than 5% of all cases (*Genetic susceptibility*, p71). Other genetic conditions suspected of playing a role include heterozygosity of the ataxia telangiectasia gene (Box: *ATM and breast cancer*, p192) and germline mutations of *p53* (the Li-Fraumeni syndrome) [14].

The most common genetic abnormality in breast carcinoma tissue appears to be a loss of heterogeneity at multiple loci. Such change may determine the influence of a mutated allele of a tumour suppressor gene (*Oncogenes and tumour suppressor*

genes, p96). Loss of heterogeneity on 13q and 17p may involve the *RB* or *p53* genes respectively. Gene amplification is also observed, the most studied gene in this context being that encoding the growth factor receptor c-erbB2. Although the estrogen receptor cannot be clearly classified as the product of an oncogene or tumour suppressor, expression of this gene mediates progression of breast cancer, and the responsiveness of tumours to hormone-based therapy.

Management

Successful management of a breast cancer implies a multidisciplinary approach to

ATM AND BREAST CANCER

Whilst mutations in the *BRCA1* and *BRCA2* genes contribute to familial breast cancer risk, their contribution to sporadic breast cancer is relatively minor. In the latter disease category, genes frequently altered in the general population, such as the gene mutated in ataxia telangiectasia, *ATM*, may be important risk factors. Studies of ataxia telangiectasia families initially revealed that ataxia telangiectasia heterozygotic women had an increased risk of breast cancer. Taken together with the estimation that 1% of the general population are *ATM* heterozygotes, up to 8% of breast cancer patients could thus be *ATM* heterozygotes. One of the identifying characteristics of ataxia telangiectasia patients is that they are extremely sensitive to ionizing radiation. Radiosensitivity, seen as exaggerated acute or late tissue reactions after radiotherapy, has been reported in a significant proportion of breast cancer patients. This suggests that ataxia telangiectasia heterozygosity plays a role in such radiosensitivity and in breast cancer development. Loss of heterozygosity in the region of the *ATM* gene on chromosome 11 has been found in about 40% of sporadic breast tumours. Screening for *ATM* mutations in sporadic breast cancer cases, regardless of adverse response to radiotherapy, has not

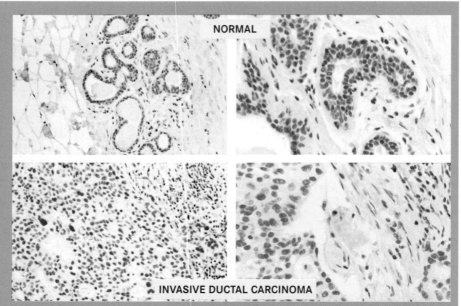

NORMAL

INVASIVE DUCTAL CARCINOMA

Fig. 5.22 Normal tissue showing a brown nuclear ATM staining in the inner epithelial cells of the breast ducts and no staining in the outer myoepithelial cells. Invasive ductal carcinoma shows no ATM staining in the tumour area, in contrast to lymphocytes in the same section.

revealed the magnitude of involvement of the *ATM* gene expected, based on the increased relative risk and mutation profile found in family studies (in terms of truncating mutations). However, the molecular approaches used in these studies have shown clearly that, in the general population, there are two groups of heterozygotes (Gatti RA et al., *Mol Genet Metab*, 68: 419-422, 1999). One group includes those who are heterozygous for a truncating allele and a second group comprises those who are heterozygous for a missense mutation; the latter group might predominantly include those individuals who are predisposed to developing sporadic cancers. Further research, in particular on the role and phenotype associated with these rare *ATM* sequence variants, is needed to clarify the understanding of *ATM* heterozygosity as a risk factor for breast cancer.

achieve local disease control (surgery and radiotherapy) and treat metastatic spread (chemotherapy) [15]. Optimal surgery may comprise a lumpectomy for a tumour of <4 cm, or mastectomy and excision of axillary lymph nodes for more advanced disease and depending on pathological findings [16]. Biopsy of the first lymph node to which a tumour drains ("sentinel node biopsy") is currently being investigated as an alternative to complete axillary lymph node dissection (which may be associated with post-surgical complications such as lymphœdema, numbness, a persistent burning sensation, infection, and limited movement of the shoulder) [17]. In early stage disease, lumpectomy

followed by radiotherapy will allow for breast conservation. For larger tumours, a primary mastectomy may be necessary. Immediate or delayed breast reconstruction will allow for an acceptable cosmetic result, many techniques for which exist, including insertion of subpectoral silicone implants or tissue expanders and myocutaneous latissimus dorsi or rectus abdominous flaps (*Rehabilitation*, p292). There is no evidence that immediate reconstructive surgery prevents the detection of local recurrence or affects survival. Surgical removal of a breast tumour should be followed by radiotherapy to the breast. There is no difference in long-term disease control between mastectomy and

complete local resection plus radiotherapy to reduce the incidence of local recurrence. In addition to local therapy, systemic adjuvant therapy, which may involve hormonal manipulation, including ovarian ablation and cytotoxic agents, is employed to treat undetectable remaining malignant cells. Ovarian ablation, whether achieved surgically or pharmacologically, is appropriate only for premenopausal women. The non-steroidal anti-estrogen drug tamoxifen is probably the single mostly widely-used agent for all stages of breast cancer, though it is more effective in women whose tumours exhibit estrogen receptors. Tamoxifen also substantially reduces the risk of a new primary breast cancer in the contralateral breast (*Chemoprevention*, p151), a property not seen with cytotoxic adjuvant therapy. In postmenopausal women who have had breast cancer, tamoxifen can reduce the annual rate of death by 17%. However, long-term use has been associated with endometrial thickening and endometrial carcinoma. A new-generation hormonal drug, anastrozole, has recently been reported to be just as, if not more, effective than tamoxifen in treating advanced breast cancer and as adjuvant therapy.

The strongest predictive factor for survival after diagnosis of breast cancer is the extent of cancer as defined in the TNM classification (Box: *TNM*, p124). If the tumour is large, diffuse or multicentric, mastectomy may be appropriate. Involvement of axillary lymph nodes is an indicator of high risk of relapse from metastatic disease. An increasing number of molecular markers of prognosis are also becoming commonly assessed (Table 5.2) [14]. Metastatic disease is incurable; once detected, average survival time is two years. However, at least half the patients with breast cancer will survive for five years, including those living in the developing world. Because of this relatively good prognosis, there are an estimated 3.46 million women alive who have had breast cancer diagnosed within the last five years. In Europe for example, survival is an average of 72.5% at five years (Fig. 5.21).

Patient follow-up involves the diagnosis and treatment of recurrent disease, evaluation of treatment effectiveness, monitoring for long-term complications, patient rehabilitation and psychological support. The combination of various treatment modalities has led to an improvement in survival for the last 20 years. The challenge remains of also providing adequate treatment in the developing world.

CLASSIFYING CANCERS: EPIDEMIOLOGICAL AND CLINICAL NEEDS

To monitor the impact of cancer within populations, epidemiological records are based on organ site (topography), liver cancer, breast cancer, colon cancer etc, using established codes (*International Classification of Disease*, see http://www.cdc.gov/nchs/about/otheract/icd9/abticd10.htm). Accordingly, this terminology applies to Chapters 1 and 2 of this Report.

To describe the type of cancer (or tumour) affecting an individual in terms which will indicate the prognosis and appropriate treatment, reference to organ site alone is inadequate. For clinical purposes, tumours are identified by a naming system based on the tissue or cell of origin. All organs involve multiple tissue types including glandular or secretory tissue, connective tissue of various types (muscle, fat), blood and immunological elements and nervous tissue. "Carcinoma" indicates a malignant tumour of surface or glandular tissue, "sarcoma" indicates connective tissue, "blastoma" indicates embryonic tissue, "leukaemia" involves elements of blood and there are other specialist terms. Of necessity, Chapters 5 and 6 of this Report use this terminology. The existence of a standardized classsification system is of key importance (*WHO Classification of Tumours*).

In practice, particularly in the context of broad generalizations about cancer, the complexity implicit in comprehensive tumour nomenclature is greatly reduced by the practical consideration that over 90% of the tumours afflicting humans are carcinomas. As a result, for many purposes (and often in common practice) "lung cancer" may be equated with "carcinoma of the lung".

REFERENCES

1. Ferlay J, Bray F, Parkin DM, Pisani P, eds (2001) *Globocan 2000: Cancer Incidence and Mortality Worldwide (IARC Cancer Bases No. 5)*, Lyon, IARCPress.

2. Parkin DM, Whelan SL, Ferlay J, Raymond L, Young J, eds (1997) *Cancer Incidence in Five Continents, Vol. VII (IARC Scientific Publication No. 143 and IARC Cancerbase No. 2)*, Lyon, IARCPress.

3. Parkin DM, Pisani P, Ferlay J (1999) Estimates of the worldwide incidence of 25 major cancers in 1990. *Int J Cancer*, 80: 827-841.

4. Peto R, Boreham J, Clarke M, Davies C, Beral V (2000) UK and USA breast cancer deaths down 25% in year 2000 at ages 20-69 years. *Lancet*, 355: 1822.

5. COMA Working Group on Diet and Cancer (1998) *Nutritional Aspects of the Development of Cancer (UK Department of Health Report on Health and Social Subjects No. 48)*, Norwich, HMSO.

6. Potter JD. (1997) *Food, nutrition and the prevention of cancer: a global perspective*. Washington DC, American Institute for Cancer Research.

7. Harris J, Morrow M, Norton L (1997) Malignant tumors of the breast. In: DeVita VTJ, Hellman,S, Rosenberg, SA eds, *Cancer Principles and Practice of Oncology*, Philadelphia, Lippincott-Raven Publishers, 1557-1616.

8. Marsden J, Baum M (1998) Breast cancer. In: Morris D, Kearsley J, Williams C eds, *Cancer: a comprehensive clinical guide*, Harwood Academic Publishers, 131-139.

9. Kerlikowske K, Grady D, Rubin SM, Sandrock C, Ernster VL (1995) Efficacy of screening mammography. A meta-analysis. *JAMA*, 273: 149-154.

10. Fletcher SW, Black W, Harris R, Rimer BK, Shapiro S (1993) Report of the International Workshop on Screening for Breast Cancer. *J Natl Cancer Inst*, 85: 1644-1656.

11. South East Health Public Health Unit. (2000) *Information for GPs: Risk of Breast Cancer*. www.sesahs.nsw.gov.au/cancerbulletins/. NSW Cancer Control Program, Australia.

12. Eeles RA (1999) Screening for hereditary cancer and genetic testing, epitomized by breast cancer. *Eur J Cancer*, 35: 1954-1962.

13. Bishop DT (1999) BRCA1 and BRCA2 and breast cancer incidence: a review. *Ann Oncol*, 10 Suppl 6: 113-119.

14. Tavassoli FA, Stratton MR, eds (2003) *World Health Organization Classification of Tumours. Pathology and Genetics of Tumours of the Breast and Female Genital Organs*, Lyon, IARC Press. *In preparation*.

15. Reviews (2001) Breast cancer. *Curr Opin Oncol*, 13: 415-449.

16. Early Breast Cancer Trialists' Collaborative Group (2000) Favourable and unfavourable effects on long-term survival of radiotherapy for early breast cancer: an overview of the randomised trials. *Lancet*, 355: 1757-1770.

17. Mansel RE, Khonji NI, Clarke D (2000) History, present status and future of sentinel node biopsy in breast cancer. The Mary Beves Lecture. *Acta Oncol*, 39: 265-268.

STOMACH CANCER

SUMMARY

> Cancer of the stomach is amongst the most common malignancies worldwide, with some 870,000 new cases every year. Mortality from stomach cancer is second only to lung cancer.

> Incidence is declining worldwide. In most European countries it has fallen by more than 60% during the past 50 years. This trend is mainly due to markedly decreased consumption of salt-preserved food, increasing avoidance of a high-salt diet and availability, in many countries, of fresh fruit and vegetables throughout the year.

> Infection with *Helicobacter pylori* causes chronic atrophic gastritis and is considered a factor in the development of stomach cancer.

> Patients are often diagnosed with advanced disease and five-year survival rates are poor, usually less than 30%.

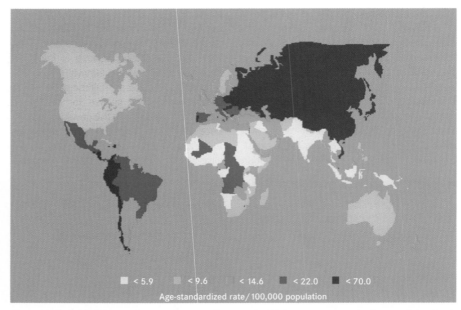

< 5.9   < 9.6   < 14.6   < 22.0   < 70.0
Age-standardized rate/100,000 population

Fig. 5.23 Global incidence of stomach cancer in men; the highest rates occur in Eastern Asia, South America and Eastern Europe.

Definition

The vast majority of stomach cancer cases are gastric carcinomas. Non-epithelial tumours predominantly include lymphomas and mesenchymal tumours.

Epidemiology

Stomach cancer was the fourth most common malignancy in the world in 2000, with an estimated 870,000 new cases and 650,000 deaths per year [1]. Approximately 60% of all stomach cancers occur in developing countries (Fig. 5.23). The areas with the highest incidence rates (>40/100,000 in males) are in Eastern Asia, the Andean regions of South America and Eastern Europe. Low rates (< 15/100,000) occur in North America, Northern Europe and most countries in Africa and in South Eastern Asia. There is marked geographical variation in incidence between countries and among different ethnic groups within the same locale. Migration studies show that the risk of cancer changes within two generations when people move from high-incidence to low-incidence areas. For example, Japanese immigrants to the USA retain their original risk of stomach cancer, whereas subsequent generations show the incidence of the host country. Incidence in men is twice that in women in both high- and low-risk countries.

The well-differentiated type of adenocarcinoma (which is showing the greatest decrease in incidence) occurs more predominantly in high-risk areas, while the diffuse poorly-differentiated type is relatively more frequent in low-risk areas [2]. In contrast to the overall decreasing trend, there has been an increase of cancers localized to the cardia, documented by data from the UK and USA. The reasons for this increase are not known. Over the last few decades, a steady decline in the incidence and mortality rates of gastric carcinoma has been observed worldwide and in particular in North America and Western Europe (Fig. 5.24 and *Stomach cancer prevention and screening*, p175). However, the absolute number of new cases per year is increasing mainly because of ageing of the population. Gastric carcinoma is extremely rare below age 30; thereafter incidence increases rapidly and steadily to reach the highest rates in the oldest age groups in both sexes.

Etiology

Dietary risk factors include inadequate intake of fresh fruits and vegetables, high salt intake and consumption of smoked or cured meats or fish. There is good evidence that refrigeration of food also protects against this cancer by facilitating year-round consumption of fruit and vegetables and probably by reducing the need for salt as a preservative. Vitamin C, contained in vegetables and fruits and other foods of plant origin, is probably protective, and so too are diets high in wholegrain cereals, carotenoids and allium compounds, and also green tea. Conversely,

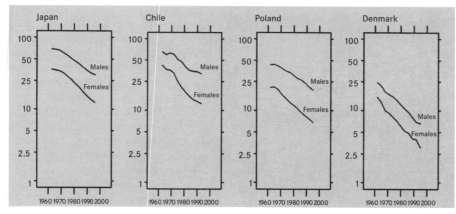

Fig. 5.24 The mortality from stomach cancer is decreasing worldwide, including in countries with a high disease burden. D.M. Parkin et al. (2001) *Eur J Cancer*, 37 Suppl. 8: S4-66.

monotonous diets which are rich in starchy food pose an increased risk, probably because they are deficient in the protective dietary constituents. Many studies suggest a small increase in risk (about two-fold) in smokers, but alcohol does not affect risk, other than at the gastric cardia. Conditions which cause an excessive rate of cell proliferation in the gastric epithelium, thus increasing the chance of fixation of replication errors induced by dietary and endogenous carcinogens, include *Helicobacter pylori* infection (*Chronic infections*, p56), gastric ulcer, atrophic gastritis and autoimmune gastritis associated with pernicious anaemia. Gastritis is associated with increased production of oxidants and reactive nitrogen intermediates, including nitric oxide. There is increased expression of the inducible isoform of nitric oxide synthase in gastritis. Gastritis and atrophy alter gastric acid secretion, elevating gastric pH, changing the gastric flora and allowing anaerobic bacteria to colonize the stomach.

Detection

Early stomach cancer is an adenocarcinoma limited to the mucosa, or the mucosa and submucosa. It often does not cause symptoms, although up to 50% of patients may have non-specific gastrointestinal complaints, such as dyspepsia. This often delays the diagnosis of stomach cancer. Approximately 80% of Western patients with stomach cancer present to the physician with advanced tumours, symptoms of which may include nausea, weight loss, back pain, epigastric pain, gastrointestinal bleeding or perforation [3]. Endoscopy and biopsy is considered to be the most sensitive and specific diagnostic test for stomach cancer. Endoscopic detection of early lesions may be improved with dye-endoscopy using indigo carmine, congored, truigine or methylene blue. Diagnosis may also be obtained by double-contrast barium X-ray. Screening for early disease by X-ray (photofluoroscopy), followed by gastroscopy and biopsy of suspicious findings, has been widely used in Japan since the 1960s. It is a costly approach to prevention, and the results have been controversial. Serum pepsinogen screening is a new and potentially useful method for detection of stomach cancer [4].

Tumour staging prior to treatment decision involves percutaneous ultrasound or computed tomography to detect liver metastases and distant lymph node metastases and laparoscopy (with or without laparoscopic ultrasound) to seek evidence for peritoneal spread or serosal involvement.

Pathology and genetics

Chronic atrophic gastritis, in particular *H. pylori*-associated chronic active gastritis,

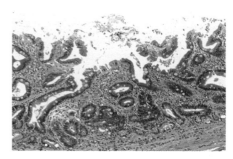

Fig. 5.25 Severe atrophic gastritis with intestinal metaplasia, a risk factor for gastric carcinoma.

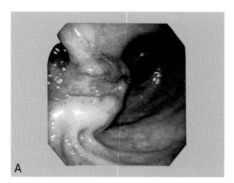

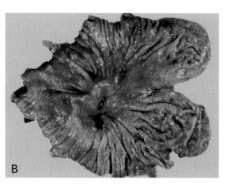

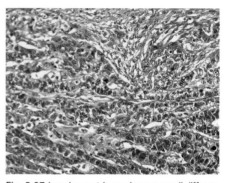

Fig. 5.27 Invasive gastric carcinoma: a well-differentiated trabecular invasive tubular adenocarcinoma.

Fig. 5.26 (A) Endoscopy showing advanced gastric carcinoma in an 80-year-old male patient (ulcerated tumour without definite limits, infiltrating into the surrounding stomach wall). (B) Corresponding gross feature of the resected stomach with advanced cancer located in the lesser curvature of the angulus.

Gene alterations	Histologic type	
	Poorly-differentiated (%)	Well-differentiated (%)
KRAS mutation	0	10-20
c-met Amplification 6.0 kb mRNA	≈ 40 ≈ 80	≈ 20 ≈ 50
K-sam amplification	20-30	0
c-erbB2 amplification	0	20-40
Cyclin E amplification	10	10
p53 LOH/mutation	≈ 80	≈ 60
APC LOH/mutation	-	40-60
DCC LOH	-	50
Cadherin, catenin deletion	50	-
CD44 abnormal transcript	100	100
Genetic instability	≈ 40	≈ 10

Table 5.3 Genetic alterations in gastric carcinomas, (≈ = approximately), [15, 16].

and intestinal metaplasia (Fig. 5.25), frequently precede and/or accompany intestinal type adenocarcinoma, especially in high incidence areas. Premalignant conditions include gastric polyps, Menetrier disease, gastric ulcer, pernicious anaemia (achlorydia) and previous gastric surgery to reduce acid output [3]. *H. pylori* strains containing a group of genes named *cag* induce a great degree of inflammation, and there is an association between infection with a *cag* positive *H. pylori* strain and the development of gastric carcinoma [5]. Gastric carcinomas are morphologically heterogeneous, resulting in various classifications based on histological appearance, degree of differentiation, growth pattern, and histogenesis [6]. The major histological types include tubular adenocarcinoma (Fig. 5.27), papillary adenocarcinoma, mucinous adenocarcinoma and signet-ring cell carcinoma. When more than one histological type is observed within the tumour, the diagnosis is based on the predominant histological pattern [7]. Based on their differentiation status, gastric carcinomas are also classified as

well-differentiated adenocarcinoma (composed of well-formed glands, often resembling metaplastic intestinal epithelium) and poorly-differentiated adenocarcinoma (composed of highly irregular glands or single cells that remain isolated). Moderately-differentiated adenocarcinomas show intermediate features between the two.

Gastric carcinomas may also be classified as diffuse and intestinal types (Laurén classification) [8]. Intestinal type carcinoma is composed of distinct glandular elements with well-defined lumina, sometimes accompanied by papillary structures or solid components. Diffuse gastric carcinoma is characterized by the lack of cell cohesion, and malignant cells infiltrate the surrounding tissue as single cells or small clusters of cells without glandular lumina [8]. Other classification systems are also in use.

Clinical and pathological staging of stomach cancer is based on the TNM system (Box: *TNM*, p124) in Western countries and the Japanese classification system in Japan [9]. Most gastric carcinomas occur sporadically, but up to 10% have an inherited familial

component [10]. Case-control studies also suggest a small but consistent increased risk in first-degree relatives of gastric carcinoma patients [11]. Germline E-cadherin (*CDH1*) mutations lead to an autosomal dominant predisposition to diffuse gastric carcinoma [12]. Gastric carcinomas may also develop as part of the hereditary nonpolyposis colon cancer (HNPCC) syndrome [13] (*Colorectal cancer*, p198). They exhibit intestinal type cancers and microsatellite instability.

Loss of heterozygosity studies and comparative genomic hybridization (CGH) studies have shown that frequent loss or gain occurs at chromosomal regions 1p, 1q, 3p, 4, 5q (*APC* locus), 6q, 7q, 9p, 17p (*p53* locus), 18q (*DCC* locus), and 20q [14]. Well- and poorly-differentiated adenocarcinomas frequently show different genetic alterations (Table 5.3), as do diffuse and intestinal types [15,16].

Management

Most patients diagnosed with stomach cancer have advanced disease and the prognosis is extremely poor with survival rates rarely exceeding 15%. Differences in classification of cancer lead to apparently much higher survival rates in Japan (Fig. 5.28). Management of stomach cancer

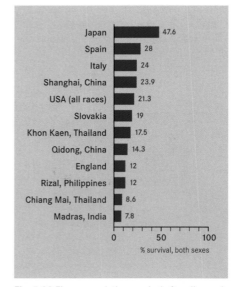

Fig. 5.28 Five-year relative survival after diagnosis of gastric carcinoma.

depends on staging. Small intramucosal cancers can be treated endoscopically by endoscopic mucosal resection [17]. For invasive cancer, standard treatment is gastrectomy with regional lymph node dissection [18]. For patients with advanced stage stomach cancer, neo-adjuvant (pre-operative) or adjuvant (post-operative) chemotherapy is currently being investigated in research protocols. Drugs most often employed are 5-fluorouracil, doxorubicin and cisplatin, and greatest success has been achieved on the basis of combination regimens rather than single agent treatments. Immunochemosurgery using *Corynebacterium parvum* is practised in Korea, but is still subject to scepticism in Western practice [3].

Annual surveillance endoscopy, post-gastrectomy, has been associated with a small beneficial outcome in terms of gain of life-years, but this may be inflated by the exaggerated assumptions of a high incidence rate of gastric stump cancer and a cure rate of 80% achieved by timely surgery after cancer detection.

In advanced stomach cancer, tumour stage, tumour size, histological tumour type, growth pattern, degree of cytological atypia, DNA-nuclear content, stromal reaction, lymphatic and vascular invasion all have prognostic value. Patients with cancers limited to the mucosa and sub-mucosa have a five-year survival of approximately 95%. Tumours that invade the muscularis propria have a 60% to 80% five-year survival, whereas tumours invading the subserosa and serosa have a less than 50% five-year survival on average [19]. There is recent evidence that the type of mucin and polymorphism of the gene encoding mucin may be an important factor determining susceptibility to stomach cancer [20].

REFERENCES

1. Ferlay J, Bray F, Parkin DM, Pisani P, eds (2001) *Globocan 2000: Cancer Incidence and Mortality Worldwide (IARC Cancer Bases No. 5)*, Lyon, IARCPress.

2. Muñoz N (1988) Descriptive epidemiology of stomach cancer. In: Reed PI, Hill, MJ eds, *Gastric Carcinogenesis*, Amsterdam, Excerpta Medica, 51-69.

3. Branicki FJ, Gotley DG (1998) Gastric cancer. In: Morris D, Kearsley J, Williams C, eds, *Cancer: a comprehensive clinical guide*, Harwood Academic Publishers, 165-169.

4. Miki K, Ichinose M, Ishikawa KB, Yahagi N, Matsushima M, Kakei N, Tsukada S, Kido M, Ishihama S, Shimizu Y (1993) Clinical application of serum pepsinogen I and II levels for mass screening to detect gastric cancer. *Jpn J Cancer Res*, 84: 1086-1090.

5. Queiroz DM, Mendes EN, Rocha GA, Oliveira AM, Oliveira CA, Cabral MM, Nogueira AM, Souza AF (1999) Serological and direct diagnosis of *Helicobacter pylori* in gastric carcinoma: a case-control study. *J Med Microbiol*, 48: 501-506.

6. Hamilton SR and Aaltonen LA, eds (2000) *World Health Organization Classification of Tumours. Pathology and Genetics of Tumours of the Digestive System*, Lyon, IARCPress.

7. Watanabe H, Jass JR, Sobin LH, eds (1990) *Histological Typing of Oesophageal and Gastric Tumours (International Histological Classification of Tumours, 2nd Ed.)*, Berlin, Springer-Verlag.

8. Laurén PA (1965) The two histological main types of gastric carcinoma: diffuse and so-called intestinal-type carcinoma. *Acta Pathol Microbiol Scand*, 64: 31-49.

9. Ichikura T, Tomimatsu S, Uefuji K, Kimura M, Uchida T, Morita D, Mochizuki H (1999) Evaluation of the New American Joint Committee on Cancer/International Union against cancer classification of lymph node metastasis from gastric carcinoma in comparison with the Japanese classification. *Cancer*, 86: 553-558.

10. La Vecchia C, Negri E, Franceschi S, Gentile A (1992) Family history and the risk of stomach and colorectal cancer. *Cancer*, 70: 50-55.

11. Zanghieri G, Di Gregorio C, Sacchetti C, Fante R, Sassatelli R, Cannizzo G, Carriero A, Ponz dL (1990) Familial occurrence of gastric cancer in the 2-year experience of a population-based registry. *Cancer*, 66: 2047-2051.

12. Guilford PJ, Hopkins JB, Grady WM, Markowitz SD, Willis J, Lynch H, Rajput A, Wiesner GL, Lindor NM, Burgart LJ, Toro TT, Lee D, Limacher JM, Shaw DW, Findlay MP, Reeve AE (1999) E-cadherin germline mutations define an inherited cancer syndrome dominated by diffuse gastric cancer. *Hum Mutat*, 14: 249-255.

13. Watson P, Lynch HT (1993) Extracolonic cancer in hereditary nonpolyposis colorectal cancer. *Cancer*, 71: 677-685.

14. Becker KF, Keller G, Hoefler H (2000) The use of molecular biology in diagnosis and prognosis of gastric cancer. *Surg Oncol*, 9: 5-11.

15. Tahara E (1995) Molecular biology of gastric cancer. *World J Surg*, 19: 484-488.

16. Hirohashi S, Sugimura T (1991) Genetic alterations in human gastric cancer. *Cancer Cells*, 3: 49-52.

17. Hiki Y, Sakakibara Y, Mieno H, Shimao H, Kobayashi N, Katada N (1991) Endoscopic treatment of gastric cancer. *Surg Endosc*, 5: 11-13.

18. Maruyama K, Sasako M, Kinoshita T, Okajima K (1993) Effectiveness of systemic lymph node dissection in gastric cancer surgery. In: Nishi M, Ichikawa H, Nakajima T, Maruyama K, Tahara E eds, *Gastric Cancer*, Tokyo, Springer-Verlag, 293-305.

19. Yoshikawa K, Maruyama K (1985) Characteristics of gastric cancer invading to the proper muscle layer—with special reference to mortality and cause of death. *Jpn J Clin Oncol*, 15: 499-503.

20. Utsunomiya T, Yonezawa S, Sakamoto H, Kitamura H, Hokita S, Aiko T, Tanaka S, Irimura T, Kim YS, Sato E (1998) Expression of MUC1 and MUC2 mucins in gastric carcinomas: its relationship with the prognosis of the patients. *Clin Cancer Res*, 4: 2605-2614.

WEBSITE

NCI Stomach (Gastric) Cancer Homepage:
http://www.cancer.gov/cancer_information/cancer_type/stomach/

COLORECTAL CANCER

SUMMARY

> Cancers of the colon and rectum are rare in developing countries, but are the second most frequent malignancy in affluent societies; over 940,000 cases occur annually worldwide.

> A major etiological factor is lifestyle involving a diet rich in fat, refined carbohydrates and animal protein, combined with low physical activity.

> Studies suggest that risk can be reduced by decreasing meat consumption and increasing intake of vegetables and fruit.

> Sequential genetic alterations mediate development of colon cancer, the earliest such change being mutation of the *APC* gene.

> Familial clustering has usually a genetic basis. Typical syndromes include familial adenomatosis polyposis (FAP) and hereditary non-polyposis colon cancer (HNPCC).

> Colonoscopy is the most reliable means for early detection. Progressively improved treatment has resulted in a five-year survival rate of about 50%.

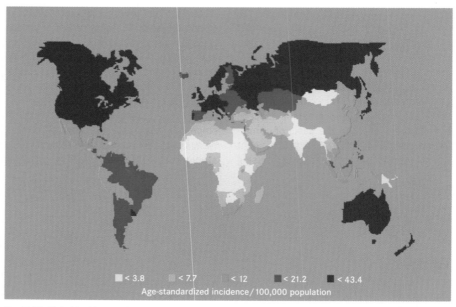

Age-standardized incidence/100,000 population

< 3.8   < 7.7   < 12   < 21.2   < 43.4

Fig. 5.29 Global incidence of colorectal cancer in women. Incidence rates are highest in North America, Western Europe and Australia/New Zealand.

Definition

The majority of cancers occurring in the colon and rectum are adenocarcinomas, which account for more than 90% of all large bowel tumours.

Epidemiology

Colorectal cancer ranks second in terms of both incidence and mortality in more developed countries. Nearly 945,000 new colorectal cancer cases are diagnosed worldwide each year and colorectal cancer is responsible for some 492,000 deaths. There is significant geographical variation in age-standardized incidence as well as in cumulative 0-74 year incidence, high rates occurring in countries of Europe, North America, in Australia and, more recently, in Japan (Fig. 5.29, Table 5.4). Migrant groups rapidly reach the higher level of risk of the adopted country, indicating that environmental factors play an important role in etiology. In North America, the trend towards increased incidence is now reversed [1] and a possible beneficial influence of dietary change and/or endoscopic polypectomy has been suggested. In Western Europe, this recent downward trend has not yet been observed. Most cases occur after the age of 60, except in individuals who carry a genetic predisposition.

Etiology

Colorectal cancer most commonly occurs sporadically and is inherited in only 5% of cases. Diet is by far the most important exogenous factor so far identified in the etiology of colorectal cancer [2]. It has been estimated that 70% of colorectal cancers could be prevented by nutritional intervention; various promoting and protective factors have been identified in cohort and case-control studies [3]. There is convincing evidence that a diet high in calories and rich in animal fats, most often as red meat, and

Country	Cumulative incidence (%)	
	Male	Female
Black, USA	5.60	4.22
White, USA	4.98	3.38
Denmark	4.48	3.53
Netherlands	4.25	3.25
Osaka, Japan	4.03	2.28
Qidong China	1.13	0.29
Khon Kaen, Thailand	1.06	0.64

Table 5.4 Cumulative incidence of colorectal cancer. The sum of incidence rates for all ages 0-74 provides a measure of the risk of developing colorectal cancer over a life span, in the absence of any other cause of death.

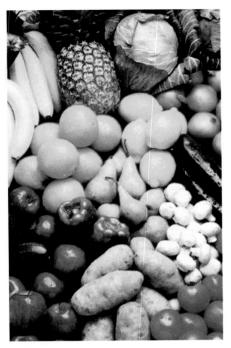

Fig. 5.30 A diet rich in fresh fruit and vegetables is associated with a lower risk of colorectal cancer.

poor in vegetables and fibre is associated with an increased risk of colorectal cancer. Alcohol intake and smoking (for polyps only) have also been suggested to increase risk. Conversely, a low fat, high vegetable and possibly high fibre diet has a protective effect. Persons with an increased intake of vitamin D and calcium have a reduced risk of colon cancer [4]. Physical activity is also protective. The chronic use of non-steroidal anti-inflammatory drugs (NSAIDs) and aspirin is associated with a significant risk reduction in certain groups [5] (*Chemoprevention*, p151). It has also been suggested that use of hormone replacement therapy in postmenopausal women may decrease the risk of colon cancer.

Conditions that predispose to the development of colorectal cancer include inflammatory bowel disease and Crohn disease [4]. Patients who have had previous malignant disease are also at a greater risk of developing a second colorectal tumour.

Detection

Bleeding is a common symptom of advanced cancer. Diarrhoea suggests a right-sided tumour and constipation or occlusion suggests a left-sided tumour. However, premalignant lesions (adenomatous polyps) and cancer limited to the mucosa and submucosa are asymptomatic as a rule. Thus screening is now proposed for healthy people, with a view to cancer prevention (*Screening for colorectal cancer*, p163). Appropriate populations for screening may be those at an average risk who are above the age of 50, or individuals selected by a risk factor questionnaire (which may also be used to search for other cases in the family of the person examined). Should the questionnaire findings be positive, the risk is increased 2.5 fold for that individual. The questionnaire is included in the assessment of patients with sporadic colorectal cancer. It also aims to detect genetic syndromes, transmitted in a dominant autosomal fashion, which are much less frequent than sporadic cancer.

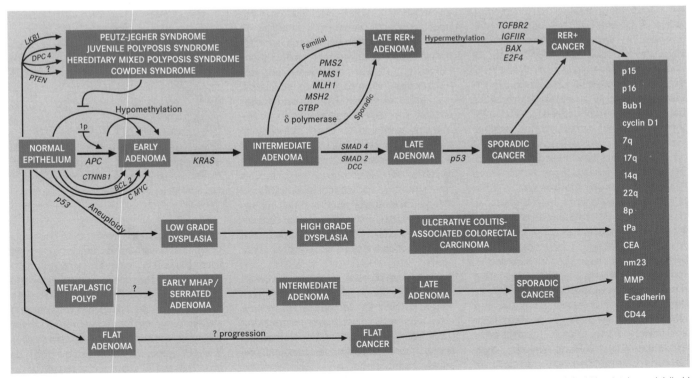

Fig. 5.31 Putative genetic pathways in colorectal cancer. It is thought that the majority of tumours develop according to the original Vogelstein model (bold arrows). See *Multistage carcinogenesis*, p 84. MHAP=Mixed hyperplastic adenomatous polyps.

Table 5.5 Criteria for hereditary nonpolyposis colorectal cancer syndrome.

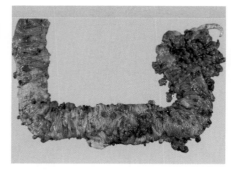

Fig. 5.32 Surgical specimen of the colon from a patient suffering from polyposis coli.

The occurrence of colorectal cancer in three successive generations and at a young age in at least one person is among the so-called Amsterdam criteria, which suggest the possibility of hereditary nonpolyposis colorectal cancer syndrome, and justifies colorectal exploration and genetic testing (Table 5.5). The detection of diffuse polyposis in the colon (Fig. 5.32) justifies genetic testing for familial adenomatous polyposis syndrome.

Occult bleeding in the stools of asymptomatic persons can be explored by the faecal occult blood test (FOBT). However, this test is reserved for mass screening interventions with assessment of its sensitivity and specificity. In other situations, endoscopy is the gold standard method of detection and should be preferred to the barium enema (Fig. 5.35), which while detecting large tumours is less reliable for the detection of small and flat lesions. Helical CT scan is proposed in most cases as a complementary investigation, helping to assess local tumour invasion and regional and distant metastases. In elderly persons with a poor health status, a colo-scanner with a water enema is a less aggressive procedure than colonoscopy.

A major advantage of endoscopy is the ease with which tissue can be sampled by forceps biopsy and the ability to detect small or flat neoplastic lesions, such as described by the Japanese school and classified as II type (IIa or elevated, IIb or completely flush, IIc or depressed). Detection of such lesions requires a high definition fibroscope with a contrast enhancement system and the use of chromoendoscopy (*Colorectal cancer screening*, p163). The depressed IIc type is a precursor of advanced cancer. Flexible sigmoidoscopy explores the distal colon; colonoscopy explores the whole of the colon. Another advantage of endoscopy is the potential for interventional procedures and the resection of adenomatous polyps.

Pathology and genetics

Abnormalities of the colonic epithelium, cell atypia and architectural disorders have been classified as premalignant (low-grade and high-grade dysplasia) or malignant (cancer). The current trend is to adopt a classification of tissue samples based upon the term "neoplasia" [6]. The following grades are considered: absence of neoplasia, indeterminate for neoplasia, certain for neoplasia with the two grades of light and severe cell atypia and intramucosal cancer. However, there is no invasion of lymph nodes when the lesion is limited to the mucosa. Therefore there is a tendency to use the term "cancer" only when there is a submucosal extension of the lesion. Epithelial abnormalities in polypoid neoplasia are usually called "adenoma" (Fig. 5.33). Only a small fraction of polypoid or flat lesions progress to carcinoma.

The major malignant histological type is adenocarcinoma (Fig. 5.34). Other less common epithelial tumour types include mucinous adenocarcinoma, signet-ring tumours, squamous cell carcinomas, adenosquamous carcinomas and undifferentiated carcinomas.

Genetic susceptibility to colorectal cancer may be attributable to either the polyposis

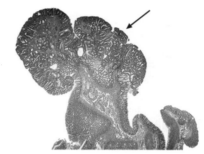

Fig. 5.33 A polypoid tubulovillus adenoma of the colon; the adenomatous proliferation (arrow) forms the head of the polyp, the stalk of which is lined by normal colonic mucosa.

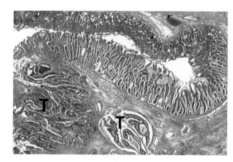

Fig. 5.34 Moderately differentiated adenocarcinoma of the colon (T), infiltrating the submucosa.

or the nonpolyposis syndromes. The major polyposis syndrome is familial adenomatous polyposis, caused by a germline mutation in the adenomatous polyposis coli (*APC*) gene. Familial adenomatous polyposis can be associated with nervous system tumours (Turcot syndrome) or with desmoid tumours (Gardner syndrome). The *APC* gene, on chromosome 5q21-22, produces the APC protein, a negative regulator that controls β-catenin concentration and interacts with E-cadherin, a membrane protein involved in cell adhesion. The following genotypic/phenotypic relationships have been demonstrated: *APC* mutations in the first or last third of the gene and attenuated polyposis; mutation after codon 1444 and desmoid tumours; mutations in the central region of the gene and a severe phenotype. Commercial genetic tests involve identification of the mutant *APC* allele by *in vitro* detection of truncated APC protein. Sigmoidoscopy is used to screen gene carriers from the age of 10-12 years.

Hereditary nonpolyposis colorectal cancer (often referred to as HNPCC) syndrome is associated with germline mutations in six DNA mismatch repair genes: *MSH2* and *MSH3*, *MLH1*, *PMS1*, *PMS2*, and *MSH6*. The protein products of these genes correct mismatches that arise during DNA replication (*Carcinogen activation and DNA repair*, p89). Mismatch repair deficiency gives rise to instability in microsatellite DNA and may aid in the diagnosis of this syndrome via the Replication Error positive (RER+) test. Surveillance of female hereditary nonpolyposis colorectal cancer syndrome patients includes exploration of endometrium and ovaries and other potential tumour sites by ultrasound. Kindreds with the Muir-Torre phenotype, as well as a subset of those with Turcot syndrome,

show mutations similar to those observed in classical hereditary nonpolyposis colorectal cancer.

Colon cancer has been the archetype for the correlation of tumour pathology and genetics since the publication of the first such correlative statement by Vogelstein et al. in 1988 (*Multistage carcinogenesis*, p84). As a result of extensive analysis of genetic alterations occurring during tumorigenesis [7-12], understanding of the complex and comprehensive nature of these relationships has since expanded (Fig. 5.31). Sporadic colorectal cancer arises mainly through two distinct pathways. In the first, chromosome instability, the initial mutation is inactivation of the *APC* tumour suppressor gene (*Oncogenes and tumour suppressor genes*, p96) (all tumours) followed by clonal accumulation of alterations in additional oncogenes (*KRAS*, 50% of tumours) and suppressor genes on chromosomes 18 and 17 (*DCC*; *p53* gene, found in 70% of tumours and associated with a shift to a malignant tumour). The second, associated with microsatellite instability, occurs in 15-20% of sporadic colorectal cancers. Alterations have been found to cluster in genes encoding enzymes involved in the repair of DNA mismatches (in particular *MLH1* and *MSH2*).

Histopathology related to poor prognosis includes deep infiltration of the layers of the bowel wall, poor differentiation, high levels of angiogenesis in the tumour and metastasis to numerous or distant lymph nodes. Evidence of host response such as intense inflammatory infiltrate is a favourable prognostic feature. Predictive factors relate to response to therapy [13]. The presence of wildtype *p53* is associated *in vitro* with a good response to many agents. In contrast, mutant *p53* is associated with lack of response to postoperative adjuvant chemotherapy with 5-FU-levamisole. In sporadic colorectal cancer, as well as in hereditary nonpolyposis colorectal cancer syndrome, microsatellite instability is a favourable indicator [12] and the tumour may respond to 5-FU-based chemotherapy. In the future, it is expected that information regarding the molecular biology of the tumour will give

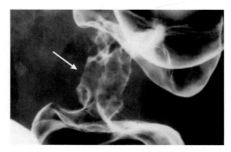

Fig. 5.35 Double contrast barium enema revealing an adenocarcinoma of the colon. Between the proximal (top) and distal (bottom) segment of the colon, the lumen is narrowed with an irregular surface (arrow), due to tumour infiltration.

valuable information regarding prognosis and response to treatment. For example, microarray technology is based on the simultaneous assay showing either deletion or overexpression of multiple gene fragments (around 20,000) and gives a characteristic "fingerprint" of the tumour [14].

Management

The management of familial colorectal cancer requires the systematic genetic and endoscopic screening of the proband (the person presenting with a disorder, whose case serves as a stimulus for a genetic/familial study). Total colo-proctectomy with ileo-anal anastomosis is performed when adenomatous polyps are detected in patients with familial adenomatous polyposis. With hereditary nonpolyposis colorectal cancer syndrome, total colectomy is the treatment for confirmed cancer, with a tendency to prophylactic colectomy in presence of multiple polyps. It has recently been shown that in probands of hereditary nonpolyposis colorectal cancer syndrome families carrying the mutation, surveillance colonoscopy at short (less than two years) intervals is a safe method to detect the first neoplastic lesions and prevents death from cancer.

Precursor adenomatous polyps are usually resected at endoscopy by snare polypectomy, when pedunculated, or by strip resection combined with saline submucosal injection, when sessile or flat. Endoscopic treatment is safe for flat or elevated lesions with intramucosal cancer up to 2 cm in diameter; however this

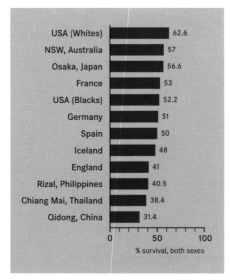

	% survival, both sexes
USA (Whites)	62.6
NSW, Australia	57
Osaka, Japan	56.6
France	53
USA (Blacks)	52.2
Germany	51
Spain	50
Iceland	48
England	41
Rizal, Philippines	40.5
Chiang Mai, Thailand	38.4
Qidong, China	31.4

Fig. 5.36 Five-year relative survival rates after diagnosis of colorectal cancer.

applies to depressed, flat neoplastic lesions (type IIc) only when the diameter does not exceed 1 cm.

Sporadic advanced colonic cancer is treated by segmental colectomy with a tendency to large resection. Adjuvant chemotherapy (5 FU-levamisole or 5 FU-leucovorine) is recommended if lymph node invasion is confirmed and some advocate a similar indication in B2 (subserosal) tumours. Recently introduced cytotoxic drugs, such as irinotecan and oxaliplatin, are beginning to become established in treatment regimes [15]. Advanced cancer located in the rectum is treated by neo-adjuvant radiotherapy if the tumour is either T3 (showing local invasion) or N+ (positive lymph nodes). Colorectal cancer is nowadays considered to be a chemosensitive tumour; in some patients, the occurrence of liver or pulmonary metastases does not exclude a curative management based upon combined resection and chemotherapy. The aggressive management of operable patients is based on initial segmental liver or lung resection followed by first line chemotherapy. In inoperable patients, first and second line chemotherapy protocols are proposed and a delayed surgical resection may be considered in some cases. The five-year survival following detection and treatment of colorectal cancer is around 50% (Fig. 5.36).

REFERENCES

1. Troisi RJ, Freedman AN, Devesa SS (1999) Incidence of colorectal carcinoma in the U.S.: an update of trends by gender, race, age, subsite, and stage, 1975-1994. *Cancer*, 85: 1670-1676.

2. Tomatis L, Aitio A, Day NE, Heseltine E, Kaldor J, Miller AB, Parkin DM, Riboli E, eds (1990) *Cancer: Causes, Occurrence and Control (IARC Scientific Publications, No. 100)*, Lyon, IARCPress.

3. Honda T, Kai I, Ohi G (1999) Fat and dietary fiber intake and colon cancer mortality: a chronological comparison between Japan and the United States. *Nutr Cancer*, 33: 95-99.

4. Cohen AM, Minsky BD, Schilsky RL (1997) Cancers of the Colon. In: DeVita VTJ, Hellman,S, Rosenberg,SA eds, *Cancer: Principles and Practice of Oncology*, Philadelphia-New York, Lippincott-Raven, 1144-1197.

5. Clapper ML, Chang WC, Meropol NJ (2001) Chemoprevention of colorectal cancer. *Curr Opin Oncol*, 13: 307-313.

6. Hamilton SR and Aaltonen LA, eds (2000) *World Health Organization Classification of Tumours. Pathology and Genetics of Tumours of the Digestive System*, Lyon, IARCPress.

7. Ilyas M, Straub J, Tomlinson IP, Bodmer WF (1999) Genetic pathways in colorectal and other cancers. *Eur J Cancer*, 35: 335-351.

8. Gryfe R, Swallow C, Bapat B, Redston M, Gallinger S, Couture J (1997) Molecular biology of colorectal cancer. *Curr Probl Cancer*, 21: 233-300.

9. Potter JD (1999) Colorectal cancer: molecules and populations. *J Natl Cancer Inst*, 91: 916-932.

10. Fujiwara T, Stolker JM, Watanabe T, Rashid A, Longo P, Eshleman JR, Booker S, Lynch HT, Jass JR, Green JS, Kim H, Jen J, Vogelstein B, Hamilton SR (1998) Accumulated clonal genetic alterations in familial and sporadic colorectal carcinomas with widespread instability in microsatellite sequences. *Am J Pathol*, 153: 1063-1078.

11. Boland CR, Thibodeau SN, Hamilton SR, Sidransky D, Eshleman JR, Burt RW, Meltzer SJ, Rodriguez-Bigas MA, Fodde R, Ranzani GN, Srivastava S (1998) A National Cancer Institute Workshop on Microsatellite Instability for cancer detection and familial predisposition: development of international criteria for the determination of microsatellite instability in colorectal cancer. *Cancer Res*, 58: 5248-5257.

12. Gryfe R, Kim H, Hsieh ET, Aronson MD, Holowaty EJ, Bull SB, Redston M, Gallinger S (2000) Tumor microsatellite instability and clinical outcome in young patients with colorectal cancer. *N Engl J Med*, 342: 69-77.

13. McLeod HL, Murray GI (1999) Tumour markers of prognosis in colorectal cancer. *Br J Cancer*, 79: 191-203.

14. Hegde P, Qi R, Gaspard R, Abernathy K, Dharap S, Earle-Hughes J, Gay C, Nwokekeh NU, Chen T, Saeed AI, Sharov V, Lee NH, Yeatman TJ, Quackenbush J (2001) Identification of tumor markers in models of human colorectal cancer using a 19,200-element complementary DNA microarray. *Cancer Res*, 61: 7792-7797.

15. Grothey A, Schmoll HJ (2001) New chemotherapy approaches in colorectal cancer. *Curr Opin Oncol*, 13: 275-286.

WEBSITES

Johns Hopkins Hereditary Colorectal Cancer Website: http://www.hopkins coloncancer.org/subspecialties/heredicolor_cancer/overview.htm

APC gene mutation database: http://perso.curie.fr/Thierry.Soussi/APC.html

LIVER CANCER

SUMMARY

> About 560,000 new cases of liver cancer, usually hepatocellular carcinoma, occur annually, and contribute significantly to cancer mortality worldwide. More than 80% of cases occur in Asia and Africa and irrespective of etiology, the incidence rate is more than twice as high in men as in women.

> In Africa and Asia, hepatocellular carcinoma is most frequently caused by hepatitis B virus infection; concomitant dietary exposure to aflatoxins multiplies the risk. In Japan, this cancer is predominantly caused by hepatitis C virus infection.

> In Western countries, liver cirrhosis due to chronic alcohol abuse is the major etiological factor.

> Hepatocellular carcinoma is almost always lethal, survival from time of diagnosis often being less than six months; only 10% of patients survive five years or more.

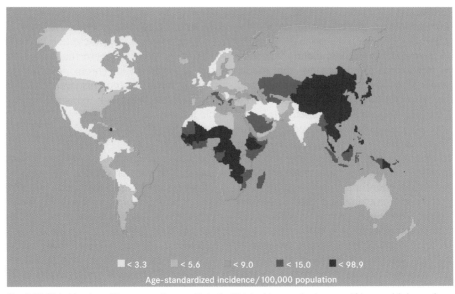

Age-standardized incidence/100,000 population

< 3.3   < 5.6   < 9.0   < 15.0   < 98.9

Fig. 5.37 Global burden of liver cancer in men. Note the high incidence rates in some African and Asian regions.

Definition

Hepatocellular carcinoma arises from hepatocytes and accounts for 80% of all primary cancers of the liver. Other tumour types include intrahepatic cholangiocarcinoma (tumours of that part of the bile duct epithelium located within the liver), hepatoblastoma (a malignant embryomal tumour of childhood) and angiosarcoma (arising from blood vessels) and are relatively rare.

Epidemiology

Liver cancer ranks third amongst the organ-specific causes of cancer-related deaths in men worldwide and accounts for almost 4% of all human cancers [1]. Globally, men are three times as likely as women to be afflicted; liver cancer is the fifth most common cancer among men worldwide, but is the eighth in women. Liver cancer is a major health problem in developing countries where more than 80% of the world total (457,000 new annual cases) occur. The highest incidence rates are recorded in China (55% of the world total), Japan, South East Asia and sub-Saharan Africa (Fig. 5.37). In both high and low incidence areas, there is great variability in incidence among ethnic groups [2].

Age-specific rates of incidence show marked geographical variation (Fig. 5.38). In the Gambia, age-specific rates peak in the 45-55 years age range, whereas in Europe and the USA, high risk is associated with old age.

Time trends in liver cancer are difficult to interpret due to changes in classification and variable inclusion of metastatic tumours [3]. However, the incidence of hepatocellular carcinoma in Japan, the UK, the USA and several Nordic countries has increased noticeably over the past two decades and has become progressively associated with younger age groups [4]. Mortality rates have increased in several regions, including France. Some of these increases may be the result of improved detection.

Etiology

Experimental evidence in a variety of *in vitro* and animal models has demonstrated the carcinogenic effects of hepatitis B virus (HBV) on hepatocytes through both direct and indirect mechanisms [5]. HBV viral DNA has been found to integrate into hepatocyte DNA and may serve as an insertional mutagen. Viral replication in infected cells and the concurrent host immune response results in persistent inflammation that may eventually progress to cirrhosis and also may dispose toward carcinogenesis; this is the mechanism most commonly exhibited by hepatitis C virus (HCV) (*Chronic infections*, p56). Consistent epidemiological data have associated a significant risk of hepatocellular carcinoma with chronic HBV infection, which accordingly has been categorized as causing cancer in the context of *IARC Monograph* evaluations [6]. Prevalence of carriers in developing countries is high (10-15%) and it can be estimated that two-thirds of liver cancer cases in developing countries are attributable to this virus [7]. HBV is particularly implicated in hepatocellular carcinoma in Africa and Asia, and HCV in Japan and the USA [4].

In developing countries, dietary ingestion of aflatoxins (produced by the mould *Aspergillus flavus*, which under hot and humid conditions contaminates stored grain), and specifically aflatoxin B₁, is causally associated with development of hepatocellular carcinoma, and exposure to aflatoxins may be synergistic with HBV infection (*Food contaminants*, p43). In developed countries, principal known risk factors are smoking and chronic alcohol abuse. The major clinical hepatocellular carcinoma risk factor is cirrhosis; 70-90% of hepatocellular carcinomas develop in patients with macronodular cirrhosis.

Iron overload caused by untreated haematochromatosis may provoke in some patient series a risk of death of as much as 45% from hepatocellular carcinoma [8]. Hepatocellular carcinoma may occur in 37% of patients with tyrosinaemia who survive to two years old and may occur in patients who have successfully undergone liver transplant. Other metabolic disorders

which may carry an increased risk of hepatocellular carcinoma or other liver cancers include alpha-1-trypsin deficiency, hypercitrullinaemia and glycogen storage disease (Table 5.6).

Hepatic cholangiocarcinoma is rare in most populations, the exception being in the population of Northern Thailand where it is associated with chronic infection by the liver fluke *Opisthorchis viverrini*, which is contracted through consumption of infected raw fish.

Detection

Screening programmes by ultrasound examination with or without pre-selection on the basis of raised levels of alpha-fetoprotein have not proved effective in reducing mortality. Recent observations indicate that free DNA originating from tumour cells is detectable in the plasma of liver cancer patients at an early stage. Detection of relevant genetic changes in the plasma (such as *p53* mutation at codon 249 in the inhabitants of high incidence areas and aberrant methylation of *CDKN2A* in most parts of the world) may soon become useful aids in screening tests for hepatocellular carcinoma. The availability of simple, genetic tests would be an important contribution to screening programmes.

Risk factors and predisposing conditions

Hepatocellular carcinoma
Chronic infection with hepatitis B virus
Infection with hepatitis C virus
Chronic liver cirrhosis
Untreated haemochromatosis
Tyrosinaemia
Alcohol abuse
Aflatoxins
Long-term use of oral contraceptives
High dose anabolic steroids
Agents causing peroxisome proliferation

Cholangiocarcinoma
Liver fluke (*Opisthorchis viverrini* and *Clonorchis sinensis*) infection (esp. certain areas of China and South East Asia)
Hepatolithiasis
Thorotrast (no-longer used X-ray contrast medium)
Inflammatory bowel disease
Nitrosamines

Angiosarcoma
Vinyl chloride (polymer industry)

Table 5.6 Risk factors and predisposing conditions for liver cancer.

Common symptoms of hepatocellular carcinoma are abdominal pain, weight loss, fatigue, abdominal swelling and anorexia. Most patients, particularly in sub-Saharan Africa, present with hepatomegaly; other common signs are ascites and jaundice. Hepatocellular carcinoma which infiltrates a cirrhotic liver often compromises the already impaired hepatic function and thus causes death before becoming very large, as is the case in most Japanese and American patients [8]. Intrahepatic cholangiocarcinoma is characterized by general malaise, mild abdominal pain and weight loss, and by jaundice and cholangitis at later stages [9]. The majority of cases can be diagnosed by computed tomography (CT) (Fig. 5.40) and ultrasonography. A definitive diagnosis may depend on histological analysis via fine needle biopsy. Endoscopic retrograde, transhepatic or magnetic resonance cholangiography can identify the level of biliary obstruction in the case of intrahepatic cholangiocarcinoma.

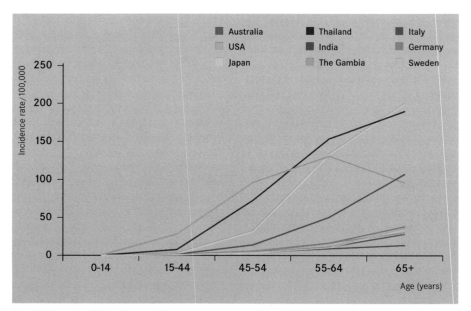

Fig. 5.38 Age-specific incidence of liver cancer in men; rates are higher in young men in areas where viral hepatitis is endemic.

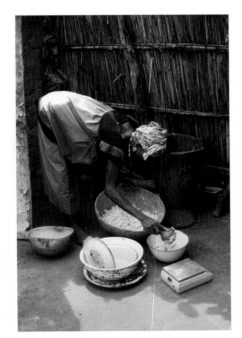

Fig. 5.39 A woman in the Gambia preparing food which is potentially contaminated by aflatoxin. The combination of aflatoxin ingestion and chronic hepatitis B poses a high risk of hepatocellular carcinoma (*Chronic infections*, p56).

Pathology and genetics

Hepatocellular carcinoma is a malignant epithelial tumour derived from hepatocytes, and thus resembles normal liver both structurally and cytologically. Small early-stage hepatocellular carcinomas (<2 cm) are well-differentiated histologically and arranged in a thin trabecular pattern without a capsule (Fig. 5.42) [8]. Tumour cells grow in cords of variable thickness that are separated by sinusoid-like blood spaces. Hepatocellular carcinoma is believed to progress from adenomatous hyperplasia (or dysplastic nodules) through atypical hyperplasia to early hepatocellular carcinoma. Trabeculae become thicker with de-differentiation. Larger cancer nodules may consist of more than two types of tissue of different histological grade [10]. Invasion into the blood vessels, especially the portal vein, is a characteristic of hepatocellular carcinoma. The malignant cells produce alpha-fetoprotein which may be detected in the serum of most patients.

Genetic change in hepatocellular carcinoma may be directly related to relevant environmental factors. In areas with high exposure to aflatoxin B$_1$, mutation of the third nucleotide in codon 249 of *p53* is frequent, compatible with mis-coding due to the binding of aflatoxin (adduct formation) to relevant nucleotides in DNA. There is evidence that mutation of *p53* is an early event in hepatocellular carcinomas in high-incidence areas, whereas it occurs as a late event in progression in industrialized countries. In hepatocellular carcinomas associated with low aflatoxin exposure, mutation of various other sites in *p53* may be detected. Sections of the HBV genome are frequently integrated into tumour DNA and expressed.

Mutational activation of known oncogenes is rare [10]. Point mutations of *KRAS* and co-amplification of the cyclin D1 gene are detected in only a minority of hepatocellular carcinomas. Mutations of the β-catenin gene are evident in about a third of tumours examined. Accordingly, the sequence of genetic events (Table 5.7) that leads to hepatocellular carcinoma is poorly known and may vary from one tumour to another.

Intrahepatic cholangiocarcinoma (Fig. 5.43) comprises cells resembling those of bile ducts, which is the site parasitized by liver flukes [9]. Most intrahepatic cholangiocarcinomas are adenocarcinomas showing tubular and/or papillary structures with a variable fibrous stroma. Mutations of the *KRAS* and *p53* genes are the most common genetic abnormalities identified.

Management

The treatment of primary and malignant liver tumours depends on the extent of the disease and the underlying liver function [11]. The most frequently used staging system is that in which the patient is evaluated according to the adverse criteria of ascites, serum albumin and bilirubin concentration and tumour size. The TNM system (Box: *TNM*, p124) is less useful as it does not take into account underlying liver disease. Liver cancer follows a rapid, progressive course: only about 10% of patients survive at least five years in the

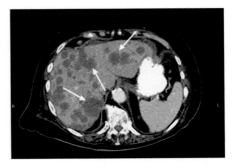

Fig. 5.40 CT image of a multifocal hepatocellular carcinoma (arrows).

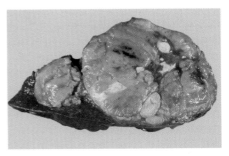

Fig. 5.41 Macroscopic appearance of hepatocellular carcinoma.

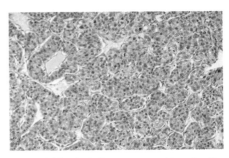

Fig. 5.42 Histological appearance of hepatocellular carcinoma: a well-differentiated, trabecular carcinoma containing numerous sinusoid-like capillary vessels.

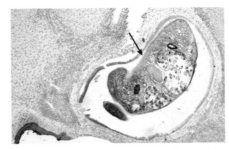

Fig. 5.43 Infection with the liver fluke *Opisthorchis viverrini* (arrow) is typically associated with cholangiocarcinoma in parts of Asia.

USA and the percentage is much lower in developing countries (Fig. 5.44).

In the absence of extrahepatic disease, resection with negative pathologic margins is the mainstay of treatment for malignant liver neoplasms. In patients in whom a small liver remnant is anticipated, portal vein embolization is used to increase the size of the future liver remnant [11]. The fact that most hepatocellular carcinomas occur in a cirrhotic liver excludes many patients from consideration for surgical resection, due to the risk of liver failure. Other techniques used alone or as an adjuvant to resection include radiofrequency ablation and cryoablation. Liver transplantation has been performed in non-resectable patients, although use of this procedure has declined due to a number of factors, including the frequency of death from tumour recurrence, especially in the transplanted liver, and organ shortages. Hepatocellular carcinoma is largely radiotherapy resistant [10]. Nonsurgical treatments include hepatic artery infusion of drugs or thrombotic agents (port or pump), chemoembolization and percutaneous alcohol or acetic acid injection, although side-effects are many and benefit to the unresectable patient is doubtful [4,11]. Hepatic intra-arterial iodine 131-labelled lipiodol (iodized poppy seed oil) shows promise for the future [4,12]. Recent results suggest that a chemother-apy regimen combining cisplatin, doxorubicin, interferon and 5-fluorouracil may elicit a response, although previously no agent, either singly or in combination, has been found to improve survival. Hormone therapy is also disappointing, although results with octreotide are more hopeful than with tamoxifen. Metastatic hepatocellular cancer commonly spreads to the lungs and bones. Response to chemother-apy and local regional therapy is poor [12]. The liver is also a frequent site of metastases from cancers at other sites, of which the most common is colorectal cancer.

The poor prognosis and lack of effective therapies for hepatocellular cancer suggest that the development of prevention programmes is of critical importance (*Hepatitis B vaccination*, p144).

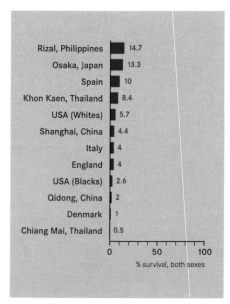

Fig. 5.44 Five-year relative survival after diagnosis of liver cancer.

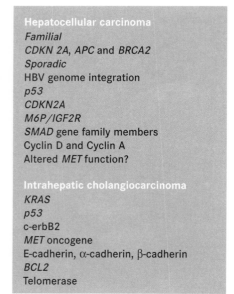

Table 5.7 Genes involved in the development of liver cancer.

REFERENCES

1. Ferlay J, Bray F, Parkin DM, Pisani P, eds (2001) *Globocan 2000: Cancer Incidence and Mortality Worldwide (IARC Cancer Bases No. 5)*, Lyon, IARCPress.

2. Engstrom PF, McGlynn K, Hoffman JP (1997) Primary neoplasms of the liver. In: Holland JF, Bast RC, Morton DL, Frei E, Kufe DW, Weichselbaum RR eds, *Cancer Medicine*, Williams and Wilkins, 1923-1938.

3. Parkin DM, Bray FI, Devesa SS (2001) Cancer burden in the year 2000. The global picture. *Eur J Cancer*, 37 Suppl 8: S4-66.

4. Bergsland EK, Venook AP (2000) Hepatocellular carcinoma. *Curr Opin Oncol*, 12: 357-361.

5. Okuda K (2000) Hepatocellular carcinoma. *J Hepatol*, 32: 225-237.

6. IARC (1994) *Hepatitis Viruses (IARC Monographs on the Evaluation of Carcinogenic Risks to Humans, Vol. 59)*, Lyon, IARCPress.

7. Pisani P, Parkin DM, Muñoz N, Ferlay J (1997) Cancer and infection: estimates of the attributable fraction in 1990. *Cancer Epidemiol Biomarkers Prev*, 6: 387-400.

8. Schafer DF, Sorrell MF (1999) Hepatocellular carcinoma. *Lancet*, 353: 1253-1257.

9. Nakanuma Y, Sripa B, Vatanasapt V, Leong AS-Y, Ponchon T, Ishak KG (2000) Intrahepatic cholangiocarcinoma. In: Hamilton SR, Aaltonen, LA eds, *World Health Organization Classification of Tumours. Pathology and Genetics of Tumours of the Digestive System,* Lyon, IARCPress, 173-180.

10. Hirohashi S, Ishak KG, Kojiro M, Wanless IR, Theise ND, Tsukuma H, Blum HE, Deugnier Y, Laurent Puig P, Fischer HP, Sakamoto M (2000) Hepatocellular carcinoma. In: Hamilton SR, Aaltonen, LA eds, *World Health Organization Classification of Tumours. Pathology and Genetics of Tumours of the Digestive System*, Lyon, IARCPress, 159-172.

11. Vauthey NJ (1999) *Multidisciplinary approaches to primary and metastatic liver cancer*, 2nd UICC Cancer Management Meeting: The Team Approach to Cancer Management, 14-18 April 1999, Antwerp, Belgium. http://www.uicc.org/publ/antwerp/landmarks4.htm

12. Clingan PR (1998) Hepatobiliary carcinoma. In: Morris D, Kearsley J, Williams C eds, *Cancer: a comprehensive clinical guide*, Harwood Academic Publishers.

WEBSITES

NCI Liver Cancer Homepage:
http://www.cancer.gov/cancer_information/cancer_type/liver/

American Association for the Study of Liver Diseases:
http://www.aasld.org/

CANCERS OF THE MALE REPRODUCTIVE TRACT

SUMMARY

> Prostate cancer accounts for about 200,000 deaths annually worldwide, predominantly afflicting older men in developed countries.

> Risk factors include high caloric intake and low physical activity. Black men have the highest, white men an intermediate, and Asian men a lower risk. Recorded incidence is increasing in many countries, partly as a result of screening for elevated serum levels of prostate-specific antigen.

> Testicular cancer mainly affects young men, with close to 50,000 new cases each year worldwide. Incidence is increasing in many developed countries; its etiology is largely unknown.

> The mean five-year survival rate is higher than 95% mainly due to the efficacy of chemotherapy using cisplatin; long-term disease-free survival can even be achieved in cases of metastatic testicular cancer.

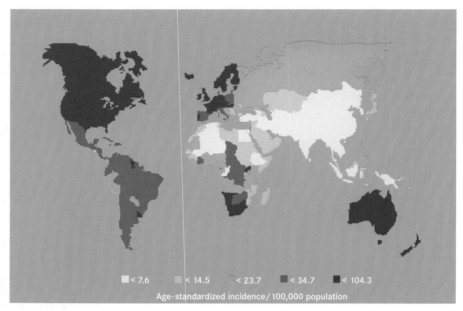

< 7.6   < 14.5   < 23.7   < 34.7   < 104.3

Age-standardized incidence / 100,000 population

Fig. 5.45 The global incidence of prostate cancer. Rates are highest in developed countries and in some parts of Africa.

PROSTATE CANCER

Definition

The majority of prostate cancers are adenocarcinomas of a heterogeneous nature, which develop primarily in the peripheral zone of the prostate gland.

Epidemiology

Prostate cancer is the third most common cancer in men in the world, with 543,000 new cases each year. In the majority of more developed and developing countries, prostate cancer is the most commonly diagnosed neoplasm affecting men beyond middle age.

In recent times, incidence rates (Fig. 5.45) of prostate cancer have been influenced by the diagnosis of latent cancers (whose presence has been suggested by screening of asymptomatic individuals) and also by detection of latent cancer in tissue removed during prostatectomy operations, or at autopsy. Thus, especially where screening examinations are prevalent, recorded incidence may be very high by comparison with earlier levels. In the USA, for example, the introduction of screening using prostate-specific antigen (PSA) testing has led to an enormous increase in the diagnosis of prostate cancer, recorded incidence now reaching 104 cases per 100,000 population, making it by far the most commonly diagnosed cancer in men (*Screening for prostate cancer*, p160). Similar changes have been observed in Australia, Finland and Sweden. However, incidence rates and, to a lesser extent, mortality rates are rising in many other countries where a possible impact of screening may be excluded. There is even a recognized increase in those Asian countries where risk is low, e.g. in Japan and China, as well as in Africa. Such changes suggest the influence of lifestyle or environmental factors in etiology.

The prevalence of latent prostate cancer shows much less geographic and ethnographic variation than clinical prostate cancer, where the ethnicity-specific rankings are much the same as for incidence [1]. The lifetime risk for microfocal cancer is estimated to be at least 30% of the male population, with progression to clinical cancer occurring in about 10%, while the lifetime risk of dying from prostate cancer is approximately 3%.

Incidence and mortality increase with ageing, with peaks somewhere within the seventh decade, depending on the degree of awareness and the establishment of population screening programmes in different populations. The low fatality rate means that many men are alive following a diagnosis of prostate cancer – an estimated 1.37 million at five years in 2000 - making this the most prevalent form of cancer in men. More than any other, this is a cancer of the elderly. Thus, about three-quarters of cases worldwide occur in men aged 65 or above.

Certain	Possible	Uncertain
Age	Androgens	Body size
High fat diet	Race	Sexual activity
Family history	*Estrogens*	Vasectomy
	Selenium	*Vitamin A*
	Vitamin E/D	*Calcium*
	Phyto-estrogens	*Lycopene*

Table 5.8 Risk and protective (in italics) factors for prostate cancer.

The distribution of mortality rates is less affected than incidence by the effects of early diagnosis of asymptomatic cancers (whether through screening, or by detection of latent cancer in tissue removed during prostatectomy operations). Mortality rates are comparatively high in North America, Northern and Western Europe, Australia/New Zealand, parts of South America (Brazil) and the Caribbean, and in much of sub-Saharan Africa and low in Asian populations, and in North Africa (Fig. 5.46). The difference in mortality between China and the USA is 26-fold (while it is almost 90-fold for incidence). Racially based differences are evident within the United States, where the black population has the highest incidence (and mortality) rates, those rates being some 35% higher than in whites, who in turn have rates considerably higher than populations of Asian origin (Chinese, Japanese, Korean).

Etiology

Age is the strongest risk factor for prostate cancer. Development of this malignancy is a multi-step process associated with a long natural history [2]. It can be inferred that the initiation of preneoplastic lesions and microscopic cancer is influenced by environmental factors which, in turn, implies a case for lifestyle causes and primary prevention.

Although many of the risk factors for adenocarcinoma of the prostate (Table 5.8) are weakly linked, the strong association of race, familial and geographic patterns with mortality directs attention to a significant role for genetic-environmental interactions as determining patterns of disease. Dietary patterns suggest that saturated fat is a significant risk factor, while micronutrients such as the vitamins A, E and D, selenium, lycopene and calcium may exercise a protective effect against cancer.

The role of hormones, especially androgens, is obviously important, granted the impact of orchidectomy (excision of the testes) on progression. However, an endocrine basis for carcinogenesis is still not well understood. Genetic polymorphisms in the androgen receptor may be more important than any imbalance of hormones in the circulation. Studies of body size, vasectomy, sexual activity and cigarette smoking as risk factors have produced inconclusive, equivocal results.

A diet characteristic of Asian countries such as Japan and China, essentially a low fat intake with consequent low body weight, with an intake of relatively high levels of phyto-estrogens (Box: *Phyto-estrogens*, p78) may provide the means of restraining the growth and progression of prostate cancer. A strategy for prevention would be to increase the intake of phyto-estrogens, essentially isoflavonoids, lignans and possibly certain flavonoids [3]. The years of potential life saved by preventive measures for prostate cancer may be less than for cancers occurring earlier in life, but the number of men with the disease worldwide adequately justifies a focus on this effort (*Screening for prostate cancer*, p160).

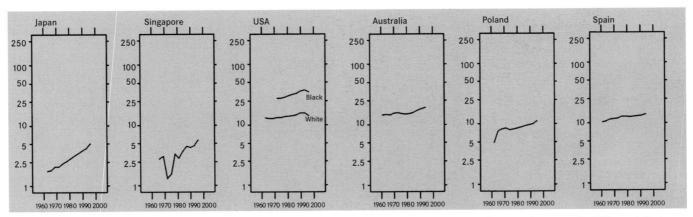

Fig. 5.46 Trends in prostate cancer mortality. Although mortality rates increased generally in the last 30 years, in some places, e.g. the USA, mortality is now falling. D.M. Parkin et al. (2001) *Eur J Cancer*, 37 Suppl.8: S4-66.

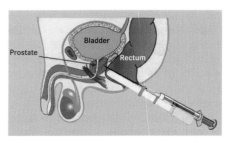

Fig. 5.47 Diagram describing patient configuration during transrectal ultrasound imaging of the prostate gland, which is an important technique used to measure prostate volume and to direct biopsies in prostatic tissue.

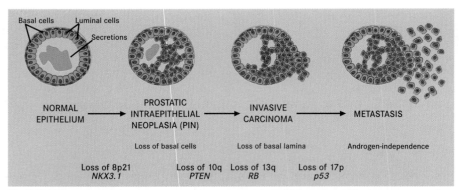

Fig. 5.50 Stages of prostate cancer progression are correlated with loss of specific chromosome regions and of candidate tumour suppressor genes.

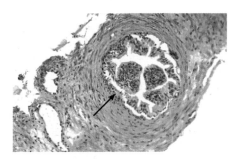

Fig. 5.48 A premalignant lesion of the prostate gland: this biopsy shows prostatic intraepithelial neoplasia (arrow) within a dilated gland.

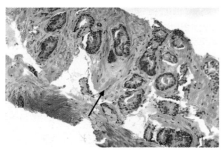

Fig. 5.49 A biopsy from the prostate gland showing a focus (arrow) of moderately differentiated adenocarcinoma with tubular architecture.

Detection

The presence of lower urinary tract symptoms (e.g. difficulty in urinating, frequent need) above age 50 are mostly due to concomitant benign prostatic hypertrophy. Latent cancer can progress to adenocarcinomas, which can infiltrate local urogenital organs and give rise to distant metastases, particularly to the bones. Digital rectal examination is the simplest way to detect anatomical abnormalities of the prostate gland, and asymmetry and induration are indicative of prostate cancer. Raised levels of PSA may confirm the suspicion and mandate an ultrasound-guided biopsy, after the patient has been informed of the consequences of both medical procedures [4]. Good clinical practice requires that symptomatic patients need a differential diagnosis (analysis of clinical data to determine specific nature of disease) whereas asymptomatic patients, especially those over 70 years of age, must be counselled as to the benefits and disadvantages of further investigation and treatment. Imaging provides no further support to confirm the suspicion of prostate cancer. Transrectal ultrasound guided biopsies establish the dimensions of the prostate gland and enable effective location of the usual six core biopsies (Fig. 5.47). Radiological examinations such as CT scans, MRI and especially bone scans, are performed only in order to stage a diagnosed cancer. Radiolabelled immunoproteins may well offer a potential imaging improvement.

Pathology and genetics

Cancer of the prostate is a slow but continuously growing form of neoplasia that is present in its preclinical form in men from the age of 30, remaining latent for up to 20 years before progressing to the aggressive, malignant clinical cancer that generally attains its peak incidence in the seventh decade. Prostatic intraepithelial neoplasia (Fig. 5.48) is thought to represent the precursor of prostate cancer. Microfocal, latent or incidental prostate cancer are terms used to describe small histological tumours found at autopsy, or in surgical specimens, the prevalence of which is correlated with age. The studies of Sakr [5] directed attention to the relatively high incidence of these microscopic cancers before the age of 50.

Most instances of prostate cancer are adenocarcinomas (Fig. 5.49), generally heterogeneous, that develop primarily in the peripheral zone of the prostate gland. A clinical cancer is recognized as having a volume over 0.5 cm^3 and is less well differentiated than the latent cancers. Slow growth with long doubling times, as well as de-differentiation over time, even in the advanced stages of the disease, are the hallmarks of prostate cancer [3]. The stages of progression are associated with specific genetic alterations.

It is estimated that up to 10% of all cases of prostate cancer may be inherited. Two familial genetic susceptibility loci have thus far been mapped to the X chromosome and to chromosome 1p [6]. Prostate cancer is genetically unstable and its genomic mutations can be divided into five major types: subtle sequence changes, alterations in chromosome number (aneuploidy), chromosome translocations, gene amplifications and allelic deletions. Tumour growth suppressor proteins such as p53 and bcl-2 are currently being evaluated as prognostic factors, together with an associated wide array of other genetic alterations [7-9].

Management

The dramatic division between localized curable prostate cancer versus the advanced incurable disease has provoked heated controversies regarding the impact of early diagnosis and appropriate management. For localized disease in patients with a reasonable life expectancy, cure is the ultimate goal [10]. Radical prostatectomy (retropubic, perineal or laparoscopic) is usually recommended for patients with a life expectancy of greater than ten years. Although the cure rate is very high, side effects may include incontinence (2-10%) and impotence (30-90%). Due to subsequent incapacity to produce semen, men who wish to father children may be advised concerning sperm-banking or retrieval. Radiotherapy is effective and may be recommended for patients who are not suitable for surgery. Proctitis (inflammation of the rectum) is, however, a common side effect of conventional external beam therapy (occurring severely in 3-5% of patients), as is erectile dysfunction (6-84%) [11]. Alternatives include conformal radiotherapy or brachytherapy. Locally advanced disease is frequently managed by a combination of endocrine therapy and radiotherapy, while endocrine treatment is the mainstay for metastatic disease. Such endocrine treatment may comprise luteinizing hormone-releasing hormone agonists, antiandrogens or orchidectomy. The initial choice of treatment is best done after counselling the patient and with access to a multidisciplinary team. Endocrine treatment almost invariably achieves a remission of the disease for a period, followed by a relapse and the development of endocrine unresponsive cancer. This type of disease needs aggressive but compassionate management, depending upon the general health status of the patient. More research is, however, essential to establish specific optimal treatment for the individual patient.

Stage and grade determine the outcome of the disease in both localized and advanced disease. The limiting factor to cure is the presence of extraprostatic extension of the disease, a frequent companion to surgical treatment due to the uncertainty of detecting extracapsular perforation before the operation. The TNM staging system (Box: *TNM*, p124) is universally recognized. The differentiation or grade of the tumour is a well-recognized dominant prognostic factor that predicts the outcome of disease in all stages and independently of the applied therapy. The Gleason grade scoring system is now widely accepted as a means to assess the histological degree of differentiation. Serum PSA values and tumour size are valuable indicators; other promising potential prognostic factors include kallikreins, microvessel density, epidermal growth factors and androgen receptors. Tuning or integrating the different prognostic factors into a nomogram, or an analysis by artificial neural net system may provide better probabilities for the individual patient in the future [12].

Survival time after diagnosis is significantly longer in high-risk countries (80% in the USA compared to 40% in developing countries), although this more favourable prognosis could well be due to the greater numbers of latent cancers being detected by screening procedures in these countries.

CANCER OF THE TESTIS

Definition

The most common malignant tumours of the testis (>90%) are germ cell tumours, which are classified as seminoma or nonseminoma. Less common testicular tumours are Leydig cell tumours, Sertoli tumours, rhabdomyosarcoma and, in the elderly, non-Hodgkin lymphoma.

Epidemiology

Cancer of the testis accounts for 1.5 % of all male cancers in most markedly affected populations and about 0.5% elsewhere. About 49,300 new cases are diagnosed each year. A rapid increase in incidence has been observed in most countries, such that in some populations testicular cancer is the most common malignancy among young men at age 15-34. The reasons for this trend are not well understood, although improved diagnostic procedures may be partially responsible. The highest incidence is in Central Europe (Denmark, Norway and Germany) and generally in Caucasian populations of developed countries (Fig. 5.51). In the USA and Western Europe, the lifetime incidence of germ cell tumours is one in 500 or 15-20 per 100,000 males per annum. Incidence is low in Africa and Asia, including Japan, with only Israel having an intermediate rate.

Cancer of the testis can occur at all ages, risk being maximal during the third and fourth decades of life and declining after age 50; the median age at diagnosis for testicular nonseminoma is 24 years and a

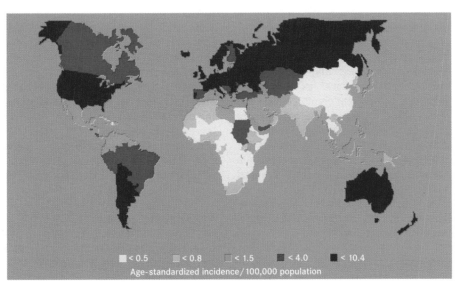

Fig. 5.51 Global incidence of testicular cancer. The highest rates are in affluent Caucasian populations.

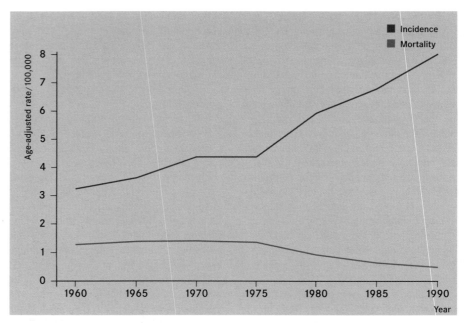

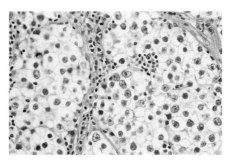

Fig. 5.53 Histology of a seminoma with uniform cells resembling primitive germ cells, large vesicular nuclei and a glycogen-rich clear cytoplasm. Note the scattered lymphocytic infiltrates.

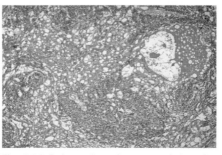

Fig. 5.54 Embryonal carcinoma consisting of a pleiomorphic proliferation containing glandular structures.

Fig. 5.52 Trends in incidence and mortality of testicular cancer in Norway, 1960-1990. Incidence has increased significantly while mortality has decreased, due to effective chemotherapy.

decade older for testicular seminoma. Mortality has declined markedly since the introduction of cisplatin as the basis of chemotherapy in the mid-1970s.

Etiology

Generally relevant environmental causes of testicular cancer have not been established. There is an increased incidence of the disease in individuals with a history of an undescended testicle, testicular feminization and those with a family history of testicular cancer. *In utero* exposure to exogenous estrogens may increase the risk of testicular cancer as a result of increased incidence of cryptorchidism and dysgenesis. A history of maternal exposure to diethylstilbestrol has been associated with an increased relative risk of up to 5.3 [13]. Testicular cancer is more common in higher socioeconomic groups. Hormonal and genetic factors seem likely to play an important, but currently unclear, role as risk factors; other factors may include the influence of heat [14].

Detection

Most patients with testicular germ cell tumours present with a painless swelling or a nodule in the testis. Other common presentations include back pain, (caused by retroperitoneal metastasis), haemoptysis (consequent upon pulmonary metastases) and gynecomastia (excessive development of male mammary glands). Diagnosis is based on physical examination, ultrasonography and biopsy. In patients with nonseminoma, serum tumour markers alpha-fetoprotein and/or human chorionic gonadotrophin are elevated in 80% of patients with disseminated disease and in 50% of patients with early stage disease. Patients with testicular seminoma may have modestly elevated levels of human chorionic gonadotrophin and of lactic dehydrogenase.

There are no reliable screening tests for testicular cancer. Due to low incidence and a high cure rate, advocacy of testicular self-examination and the impact of self-assessment are controversial.

Pathology and genetics

About 90% of testicular malignancies arise from germ cells and these tumours are classified as seminoma (40%) (Fig. 5.53) or nonseminoma, which includes embryonal tumours (20-25%) (Fig. 5.54),

teratoma (25-30%) and choriocarcinoma (1%). Germ cell tumours can also arise from extra-gonadal primary sites. Ovarian germ cell tumours of young women share clinical features and treatment approaches with male germ cell tumours. All germ cell tumours are commonly associated with the presence of isochromosome 12p (an abnormal chromosome 12 with two identical short arms), a region which contains the gene for cyclin D2 [15]. The initiation of a germ cell tumour is associated with various aberrations in the normal developmental pathway of the germ cell (Fig. 5.55).

Management

Current management of germ cell tumours should yield average cure rates in excess of 95%, and even 80% of patients with metastatic disease respond to chemotherapy, radiotherapy and surgery (Fig. 5.56). However, survival in develop-

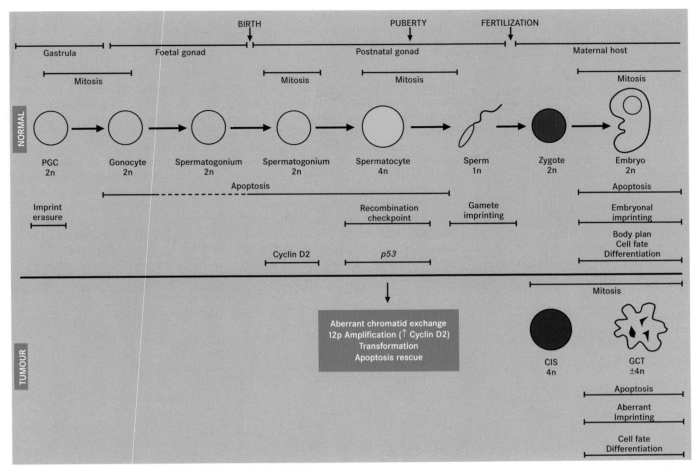

Fig. 5.55 Normal and neoplastic male germ cell development. The division of a precursor cell, the spermatocyte (4n), produces 4 sperm cells each with one set of chromosomes (1n). The fusion of egg and sperm to form the zygote doubles the number of chromosomes to the normal complement (2n). Aberrant development may produce a cell which has twice the normal chromosomal complement (4n). CIS = carcinoma *in situ*, GCT = germ cell tumour, PGC = primordial germ cell.

ing countries is only 42% to 61%, an indication of limited access to appropriate therapy [13].

Seminoma
Stage I disease, confined to the testis, is managed by post-operative radiotherapy to the retroperitoneal nodes which reduces risk of recurrence from about 20% to 2%. Patients who relapse either during surveillance or after radiation are reliably cured with chemotherapy or radiation at the time of relapse. Normal levels of alpha-fetoprotein, the presence of any human chorionic gonadotrophin or any lactic dehydrogenase are good prognostic factors. Patients with abdominal involve-ment from seminoma should receive either radiation therapy (<5 cm bulk disease) or primary chemotherapy (>5 cm bulk disease).

Nonseminoma
Patients with local nonseminoma confined to the testis should be offered either aggressive surveillance or nerve-sparing retroperitoneal lymph node dissection. Surveillance requires monthly chest X-rays and assay of markers and two-monthly abdominal CT scans for one year. In the second year following diagnosis, chest X-ray and assay of tumour markers should be carried out every six months and CT performed every three months. Good prognostic factors include low levels of alpha-fetoprotein (<1000 ng/ml), human chorionic gonadotrophin (<5000 iu/L) and lactic dehydrogenase (<1.5 times the upper limit of normal). Approximately 30% of patients under surveillance will relapse and are reliably cured with chemotherapy. Retroperitoneal lymph node dissection is both diagnostic and therapeutic. It also eliminates the need for abdominal imaging in follow-up.

Patients with abdominal involvement of nonseminoma should receive retroperitoneal lymph node dissection (<2 cm disease) or primary chemotherapy (>2 cm disease). Those who undergo retroperitoneal lymph node dissection and are

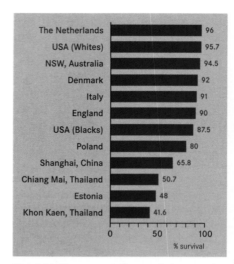

	% survival
The Netherlands	96
USA (Whites)	95.7
NSW, Australia	94.5
Denmark	92
Italy	91
England	90
USA (Blacks)	87.5
Poland	80
Shanghai, China	65.8
Chiang Mai, Thailand	50.7
Estonia	48
Khon Kaen, Thailand	41.6

Fig. 5.56 Five-year relative survival rates after diagnosis of testicular cancer.

found to have positive nodes can consider two cycles of adjuvant chemotherapy (100% cure rate).

Disseminated germ cell tumours
Guidelines for treatment of disseminated germ cell tumours (both seminoma and nonseminoma) are driven by the International Germ Cell Consensus (IGCC) prognostic index. Patients with low-risk nonseminoma (56% of cases) or seminoma (90% of cases) should receive three cycles of bleomycin, etoposide and cisplatin (BEP). Cure rate is approximately 90-95%. Patients with intermediate-risk disease or high-risk disease should receive four cycles of BEP, with an expected cure rate of 75% or 50% of patients respectively.

Patients with nonseminoma who have normalized serum tumour markers and residual radiographic abnormalities should be considered for post-chemotherapy resection of residual disease. Teratoma (a malignant tumour that contains a variety of embryo-derived tissues, such as bone, muscle, cartilage, nerve, tooth buds) and persistent cancer are common findings in this setting. In contrast, patients with seminoma and residual masses after chemotherapy should be simply observed, as teratoma and residual cancer are not common findings in this situation.
Patients with recurrent disease after chemotherapy still have the potential for cure. Salvage chemotherapy with vinblastine, ifosamide and cisplatin cures approximately 25% of these patients.

REFERENCES

1. Stanford JL, Damber JE, Fair WR, Sancho-Garnier H, Griffiths K, Gu FL, Kiemeney LA (2000) Epidemiology of prostate cancer. In: Murphy G, Khoury S, Partin A, Denis L eds, *Prostate cancer,* Health Publication Ltd, UK, 21-55.

2. von Eschenbach AC (1996) The biologic dilemma of early carcinoma of the prostate. *Cancer*, 78: 326-329.

3. Griffiths K, Denis LJ, Turkes A (2001) *Oestrogens, phyto-oestrogens and the pathogenesis of prostatic disease.* London, Martin Dunitz Publishers.

4. Dunn IB, Kirk D (2000) Legal pitfalls in the diagnosis of prostate cancer. *BJU Int*, 86: 304-307.

5. Sakr WA (1999) Prostatic intraepithelial neoplasia: A marker for high-risk groups and a potential target for chemoprevention. *Eur Urol*, 35: 474-478.

6. Abate-Shen C, Shen MM (2000) Molecular genetics of prostate cancer. *Genes Dev*, 14: 2410-2434.

7. Ozen M, Hopwood VL, Johnston DA, Babaian RJ, Logothetis CJ, von Eschenbach AC, Pathak S (1999) Aneuploidy index in blood: a potential marker for early onset, androgen response, and metastasis in human prostate cancer. *Urology*, 53: 381-385.

8. Navone NM, Labate ME, Troncoso P, Pisters LL, Conti CJ, von Eschenbach AC, Logothetis CJ (1999) *p53* mutations in prostate cancer bone metastases suggest that selected *p53* mutants in the primary site define foci with metastatic potential. *J Urol*, 161: 304-308.

9. Ozen M, Hopwood VL, Balbay MD, Johnston DA, Babaian RJ, Logothetis CJ, von Eschenbach AC, Pathak S (2000) Correlation of non-random chromosomal aberrations in lymphocytes of prostate cancer patients with specific clinical parameters. *Int J Oncol*, 17: 113-117.

10. Lu-Yao GL, Yao SL (1997) Population-based study of long-term survival in patients with clinically localised prostate cancer. *Lancet*, 349: 906-910.

11. Incrocci L, Slob AK, Levendag PC (2002) Sexual (dys)function after radiotherapy for prostate cancer: a review. *Int J Radiat Oncol Biol Phys*, 52: 681-693.

12. Denis L, Murphy GP (2000) Cancer of the Prostate. In: Pollock RE ed., *UICC Manual of Clinical Oncology,* New York, Wiley-Liss, 563-574.

13. Noss M, Klotz L (1998) Male urogenital cancer. In: Morris D, Kearsley J, Williams C eds, *Cancer: a comprehensive clinical guide*, Harwood Academic Publishers, 213-222.

14. Oliver RT (2001) Testicular cancer. *Curr Opin Oncol*, 13: 191-198.

15. Chaganti RS, Houldsworth J (2000) Genetics and biology of adult human male germ cell tumors. *Cancer Res*, 60: 1475-1482.

WEBSITES

Information for GPs: Screening for Prostate Cancer:
http://www.sesahs.nsw.gov.au/cancerbulletins/

The Prostate Cancer Research Institute (USA):
http://www.prostate-cancer.org/

NCI Prostate Cancer Homepage :
http://www.cancer.gov/cancer_type/prostate/

CANCERS OF THE FEMALE REPRODUCTIVE TRACT

SUMMARY

> Cervical cancer is the second most common cancer of women worldwide with more than 470,000 new cases per year. Of about 230,000 deaths every year, more than 80% occur in developing countries. Five-year survival rates are up to 70%.

> Sexually transmitted infection with human papillomavirus is fundamental to development of carcinoma of the cervix.

> Population-based screening has greatly reduced mortality in developed countries

> Endometrial cancer mainly affects post-menopausal women in developed countries; 188,000 new cases are diagnosed annually and obesity is a major risk factor.

> About 190,000 cases of ovarian cancer occur each year, predominantly among postmenopausal women in developed countries; five-year survival rates are about 40%.

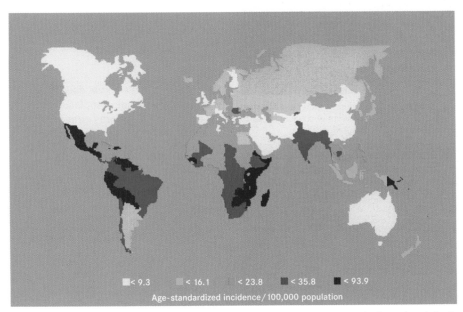

Age-standardized incidence/100,000 population

■ < 9.3   ■ < 16.1   < 23.8   ■ < 35.8   ■ < 93.9

Fig. 5.57 The global burden of cervical cancer. Note the high incidence rates in Central and South America, Southern Africa and India. Today, more than 80% of all cervical cancers occur in developing countries.

CERVICAL CANCER

Definition

The majority of epithelial tumours of the cervix are squamous cell carcinomas (85%). Adenocarcinomas are less common. Most cervical carcinomas arise at the junction between the columnar epithelium of the endocervix and the squamous epithelium of the ectocervix, a site of continuous metaplastic change, especially *in utero*, at puberty and during a first pregnancy.

Epidemiology

Cancer of the cervix is the second most common cancer among women worldwide, second only to breast cancer; about 470,000 new cases are diagnosed each year. 80% of cases of cervical cancer occur in developing countries where, in many regions, it is the most common cancer of women. The highest incidence rates are in South America and the Caribbean, sub-Saharan Africa, and South and South-Eastern Asia (Fig. 5.57). However, very low rates are observed in China, and in Western Asia. In developed countries, the incidence rates are generally low, with age-standardized rates of less than 15 per 100,000, with the exception of Eastern Europe, where incidence rates range from 18-35 per 100,000. The incidence of cancer of the cervix begins to rise at ages 20-29, and then increases rapidly to reach a peak at around ages 45-49 in European populations, but often rather later in developing countries.

Incidence and mortality have declined markedly in the last 40 years in Western Europe, USA, Canada, Australia and New Zealand, mainly in relation to extensive screening programmes based on exfoliative cervical cytology, typically by means of the Pap smear (*Screening for cervical cancer*, p167). Nevertheless, in several countries, notably the UK, Australia, New Zealand, and in central Europe, there have been increases in risk in younger women, probably the result of changes in exposure to risk factors. These changes are most evident for adenocarcinomas, which share to some extent the etiological agents of squamous cell carcinomas, but for which cytological screening is ineffective in countering the increase in risk. In developing countries the situation is more mixed, with high rates persisting in some areas (Latin America, India, Africa), and declines elsewhere, most notably in China.

Etiology

Risk factors for cancer of the cervix are primarily indicators of sexual behaviour. An increased risk of cervical cancer is associated with having multiple sexual partners, or a partner who has multiple

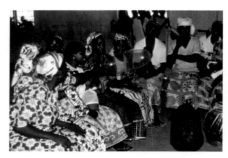

Fig. 5.58 A "Healthy Women" group in a Nigerian village discusses the benefits of condom usage to prevent sexually transmitted diseases.

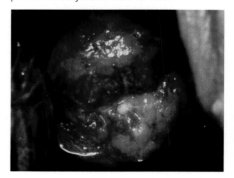

Fig. 5.59 An invasive cancer of the cervix, seen by unaided visual inspection.

partners, and with early age at initiation of sexual activity. Risk is also related to number of pregnancies, the presence of other sexually transmitted diseases and the use of oral contraceptives. In addition, low socioeconomic status, smoking, diet and immunosuppression may be implicated.

More than 90% of cervical cancers exhibit human papillomavirus (HPV) infection [1]. About 40 viral types have been found to infect the anogenital tract [2]. The high oncogenic risk group includes HPV 16, 18, 45 and 56, the intermediate group includes HPV 31, 33, 35, 52, 58 and a low-risk group includes 6, 11, 42, 43, 44 [3]. High-risk type HPV-16 can be detected in about 50% of precursor lesions and cancers of the cervix. Although HPV infection is a major risk factor for cervical cancer, not all infected women develop cervical cancer. Only a very small proportion of carcinomas appear to be HPV-negative.

Use by pregnant women of diethylstilbestrol, a drug once employed to prevent miscarriage, has been linked to clear cell carcinomas in their daughters. Being positive for antibodies to the human immunodeficiency virus (HIV) has been associated with a high incidence of cervical intraepithelial neoplasia and invasive cancer (Box: *Tumours associated with HIV/AIDS*, p60).

Detection

Early changes in the cervix, specifically cervical intraepithelial neoplasia, can be detected years before invasive cancer develops, and this is the basis for the effectiveness of cytological screening in secondary prevention. The diagnosis of cervical cancer is made on examination of cytological samples taken from the endocervix with a cytobrush and from the ectocervix with an Ayre's spatula (an ectocervical or a Papanicolaou smear) [4]. A tissue specimen may also be obtained by colposcopy and biopsy, which may be the loop electrosurgical excision procedure. In the course of screening, false negatives are common so all suspicious lesions are biopsied. If clinical cancer is apparent, a punch biopsy specimen is evaluated. Patients with abnormal Pap smear and no visible lesion require colposcopy and biopsy. The diagnosis of microinvasive carcinoma is made from cone biopsy or hysterectomy specimen pathology.

Cervical cancer does not tend to produce any symptoms in the early stages. Only when invasive disease is established do symptoms such as vaginal bleeding, discharge and pain become manifest. Advanced carcinoma is suggested by backpain, oedema of the lower extremity, a nonfunctioning kidney (due to ureteral obstruction), invasion of sacral nerve branches or extranodal extension and encroachment of the pelvic wall veins and lymphatics [3].

In the event of invasive disease, investigations are undertaken to determine whether metastatic disease is present, i.e. chest radiography, blood cell count and serum chemistry. Intravenous pyelography is used to investigate the possibility of uretic obstruction; abdominal CT and MRI are used to indicate spread and to take tumour measurements, respectively. Cytoscopy and sigmoidoscopy are necessary in the event of anterior or posterior spread.

Pathology and genetics

Precursor lesions of the cervix are commonly classified using terminology for histological diagnosis, thus mild dysplasia is categorized as cervical intraepithelial neoplasia CIN I, moderate dysplasia is CIN II, and severe dysplasia, CIN III. However, newer terminology for precursor lesions of the cervix classifies them as squamous intraepithelial lesions, which are graded from low (mild dysplasia, usually diploid or polyploid, associated with various HPV types) to high (associated with intermediate or high-risk HPV type, typically aneuploid, moderate or severe dysplasia or carcinoma *in situ*) [3]. One of the precursors of invasive adenocarcinoma is recognized as adenocarcinoma *in situ*. This is sometimes difficult to diagnose, often not being detected by Pap smear [5].

Squamous cell carcinomas may be either large cell non-keratinizing or large cell ker-

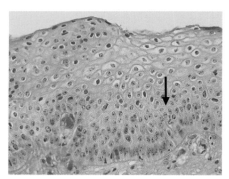

Fig. 5.60 Histology of cervical intraepithelial neoplasia stage I (CIN1). Note that dysplastic cells (arrow) are confined to the lower third of the epithelium.

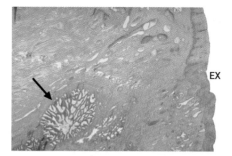

Fig. 5.61 A well-differentiated mucinous adenocarcinoma (arrow) with a papillary architecture developing from the endocervical mucosa, deep under the normal squamous epithelium of the exocervical mucosa (EX).

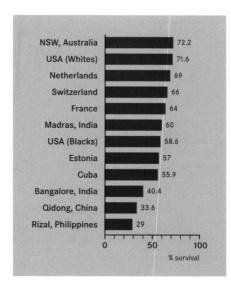

NSW, Australia	72.2
USA (Whites)	71.6
Netherlands	69
Switzerland	66
France	64
Madras, India	60
USA (Blacks)	58.6
Estonia	57
Cuba	55.9
Bangalore, India	40.4
Qidong, China	33.6
Rizal, Philippines	29

0   50   100
% survival

Fig. 5.62 Five-year relative survival rates after diagnosis of cervical cancer.

atinizing, or a less common variant, such as the well-differentiated verrucous carcinoma. The worldwide prevalence of adenocarcinomas of the cervix has increased from 5% in 1950-60 to 20-25% of all cervical tumours [3]. The most common type is mucinous adenocarcinoma, which may be intestinal, endocervical or signet-ring, followed by endometrioid adenocarcinoma. Another epithelial tumour type consists of a mixture of squamous cell carcinomas and adenocarcinomas.

Subsequent to infection, the HPV genome of high-risk types becomes stably integrated into the host DNA, commonly near cellular oncogenes such as C-MYC and N-MYC, or into regulatory sequences, such as the genes encoding transcription factors Erg and Ets-2 [6]. The observation that low frequencies of p53 gene mutations are found in tumours associated with HPV is probably a reflection of the fact that the viral protein E6 is able to functionally inactivate p53 protein. A variety of molecular markers for cervical cancer are under preliminary investigation, including telomerase (Box: Telomeres and Telomerase, p108), which appears to be expressed in most cervical epithelial neoplasias and KRAS (mutations having been detected in DNA extracted from cervical aspirates) [7]. Loss of heterozygosity on

chromosome 3p has been observed in invasive and pre-invasive lesions [8] suggesting the presence of a tumour suppressor gene; the FHIT gene (fragile histidine triad) has been mapped to 3p14.2 (a suspected HPV integration site which is commonly altered in cervical cancer).

Management

Cervical intraepithelial neoplasms may be treated by local excision (wire loop electrode, conisation with laser or scalpel) or destruction (laser vapourisation, radical diathermy or cryocautery). Methods which do not produce a tissue specimen for histology may ablate an undetected adenocarcinoma in situ or microinvasive carcinoma [9]. Recurrences or persistent residual disease may occur.

For early stage invasive carcinoma, where the cancer is confined to the cervix or spread to the upper vagina, surgery and radiotherapy are the primary treatment options. Radiotherapy is usually employed for patients with advanced disease and external beam therapy is used initially for patients with bulky tumours. The use of an intracavity radium source is being replaced with caesium-137, which is considered safer. Radiotherapy may be given post-operatively to patients at a high risk of recurrence (although benefits are not proven) [10].

Unresectable lymph node metastases are a risk factor for persistent disease. Invasive carcinoma of the cervix may follow a more rapidly progressive course in HIV-positive women. Despite initial treatment and even hysterectomy, cervical intraepithelial neoplasia and even invasive cancer may still recur, or residual disease may persist. Common sites of recurrence are the paraortic lymph nodes, liver, lungs, abdomen, bones, the central nervous system and supraclavicular lymph nodes. Recent treatment advances include high dose rate brachytherapy, refinement of treatment dose to minimize failure rate, and addition of chemotherapy concurrently with radiotherapy to minimize local and distant failures. Palliative treatment of those with advanced or metastatic disease may consist of combination platinum-based chemotherapy [11].

Survival from cancer of the cervix depends on stage of disease, with 70-85% of localized cancer cases surviving five years compared to less than 10% of cases with distant spread. Important differences are present in relation to age and ethnic or socioeconomic characteristics, probably as a consequence of differential access to medical care. Survival rates for all stages also vary between regions; even in developing countries, where many cases present at relatively advanced stage, survival rates reach 49% on average (Fig. 5.62). The poorest survival is estimated for Eastern Europe.

UTERINE CANCER

Definition

Tumours of the uterine corpus are predominantly adenocarcinomas, arising from the endometrium, or lining, of the uterus.

Epidemiology

Cancer of the uterus is the seventh most common cancer of women with 189,000 new cases and 45,000 deaths occurring worldwide each year; about 60% of these occur in more developed countries. The highest incidence rates are in the USA and Canada, while other regions with age-standardized rates in excess of 10 per 100,000 include Europe, Australia and New Zealand, the southern part of South America, and the Pacific Island nations. Low rates occur in Africa and Asia (Fig. 5.63).

Some countries, such as the USA and Canada, are experiencing a clear decline in incidence and mortality from cancer of the uterus, particularly among young women. In Europe, rates appear stable in the south and to be decreasing in the north. Uterine cancer occurs primarily in elderly women, the median age of onset being around 60 years old; only 5% of cases develop before age 40.

Etiology

Cancer of the endometrium is linked to reproductive life with increased risk among nulliparous women and women undergoing late menopause (Reproductive factors and hormones, p76). The

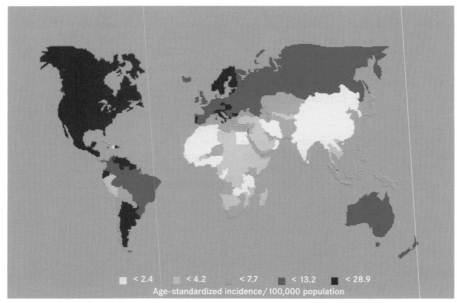

Age-standardized incidence/100,000 population

| < 2.4 | < 4.2 | < 7.7 | < 13.2 | < 28.9 |

Fig. 5.63 The global incidence of endometrial cancer. Affluent populations are predominantly affected.

endometrium is normally a hormonally responsive tissue, responding to estrogens with growth and glandular proliferation and to progesterones with maturation. Exogenous estrogens, as in unopposed estrogen therapy for menopause or prior oophorectomy, increase the risk of cancer whereas oral contraceptives containing an estrogen-progesterone combination decrease it. Syndromes of increased endogenous estrogen exposure, such as granulosa-theca cell tumours of ovary and polycystic ovary, are also associated with an increased risk. Other risk factors include a history of colon or breast carcinoma. Use of tamoxifen as a therapeutic or chemopreventive agent is a risk factor [12]. The disease is clearly associated with obesity, diabetes and hypertension.

Detection

The most common sign is metrorragia (uterine bleeding), especially after menopause. Irregular or postmenopausal bleeding is the presenting symptom in at least 75% of patients. At the time of diagnosis, 75% of patients have disease confined to the uterus although up to 20% of patients have no symptoms [13, 4].

Other signs include those linked to a mass in the lower abdomen, such as dysuria (difficult urination), constipation or bloating. Histological sampling of the endometrium and cervix, either through biopsy or dilation and curettage, should be undertaken in the event of symptoms. Endovaginal echography and hysteroscopy are useful adjuncts in the diagnosis of endometrial pathology.

Pathology and genetics

Endometrioid adenocarcinoma (Fig. 5.64) is the most common histology (60-65%). This tumour type is characterized by the disappearance of stroma between abnormal glands that have infoldings of their linings into the lumens, disordered nuclear chromatin distribution, nuclear enlargement, a variable degree of mitosis and is associated with necrosis and haemorrhage [13]. Adenosquamous carcinoma, which comprises 7% or less of cases, has a poor prognosis. 5-10% of endometrial carcinomas are uterine papillary serous carcinomas, a very virulent type. Clear cell carcinoma is more frequent in older women.

Endometrial cancer is a significant risk for women affected by the dominantly inherited hereditary nonpolyposis colorectal carcinoma (HNPCC) syndrome and by Li-Fraumeni syndrome, due to germline mutations in mismatch repair genes and p53 respectively [14]. An enhanced susceptibility to endometrial cancer has also been linked with an insertional p53 mutation, a rare mutant in the methylenetetrahydrofolate reductase gene and certain germline variants of the CYP1A1 gene.

Endometrial tumours which occur in pre- and perimenopausal women and are estrogen-related, with hyperplasia antecedent (adenomatous and atypical adenomatous hyperplasias) are of stable behaviour (Type II). Non-endometrioid tumours which appear in postmenopausal women tend to have a virulent behaviour (Type I). A model for the genetic alterations involved in endometrial tumorigenesis is becoming characterized (Fig. 5.66).

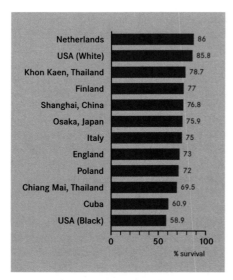

Netherlands	86
USA (White)	85.8
Khon Kaen, Thailand	78.7
Finland	77
Shanghai, China	76.8
Osaka, Japan	75.9
Italy	75
England	73
Poland	72
Chiang Mai, Thailand	69.5
Cuba	60.9
USA (Black)	58.9

% survival

Fig. 5.65 Five-year relative survival rates after diagnosis of cancer of the uterus.

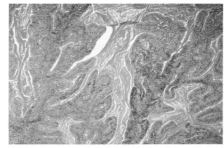

Fig. 5.64 A well-differentiated mucus-secreting endometrial adenocarcinoma with a glandular architecture.

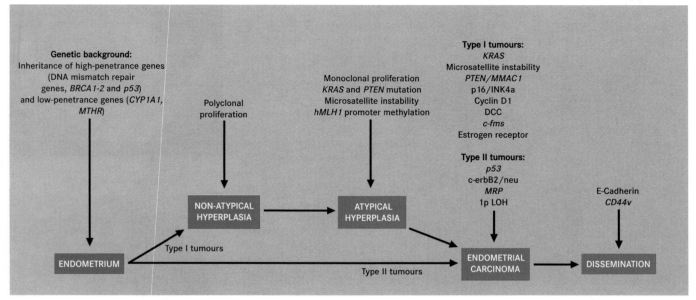

Fig. 5.66 A genetic model for endometrial tumorigenesis.

Patients with lesions which are positive for cytoplasmic estrogen and progesterone receptors have a better rate of disease-free survival than those with no identifiable receptors [13]. *PTEN* mutations are associated with a more favourable prognosis; tumours with *PTEN* mutations tend to be of endometrioid histology as opposed to clear cell serous cell types and have fewer *p53* mutations. Aneuploidy is associated with poor prognosis, as is the overexpression of c-erbB2/neu and p53 and mutations of codon 12 or 13 of the *KRAS* gene. Decreased expression of CD44 and E-cadherin are associated with metastasis and depth of myometrial invasion.

Management

Pre-cancerous lesions of the endometrium and *in situ* tumours are treated by simple hysterectomy. For frank carcinoma, total abdominal hysterectomy and bilateral salpingo-oophorectomy (removal of the fallopian tubes and ovaries) are the definitive treatment, although tailoring of therapy to meet individual needs is important. More than 50% of recurrences occur in the first two years post-surgery. Thus regular and frequent follow-up is recommended. Post-operative radiation therapy is cur-rently given to patients at a high risk of relapse following surgery. In inoperable cases, pelvic radiation therapy, usually external beam and intracavity irradiation, may be the sole treatment [13].

High levels of expression of MDR1 protein (multi-drug resistance) or associated proteins in a large number of endometrial tumours and normal endometrial tissues suggest there is a neoplasm which is intrinsically resistant to chemotherapy [15] (Box: *Resistance to cancer chemotherapy*, p285). In fact, use of chemotherapy is restricted to those with advanced or recurrent metastatic disease, although cisplatin, doxorubicin and cyclophosphamide or a combination of methotrexate, vinblastine, doxorubicin and cisplatin can produce high response rates and prolonged remissions. Response to high dose progesterone therapy in receptor-positive patients is about 70%. Estrogen-replacement therapy is recommended initially only in patients with *in situ* disease or with low risk stage I tumours.

Survival is usually good, overall around 75-85% and for localized disease up to 90% (Fig. 5.65), although there is some evidence to suggest that black women have a poorer prognosis for survival from endometrial carcinoma than their white counterparts.

OVARIAN CANCER

Definition

The majority of ovarian cancers are carcinomas, which arise from the surface epithelium of the ovary.

Epidemiology

About 190,000 new cases and 114,000 deaths from ovarian cancer are estimated to occur annually. The highest rates are reported in Scandinavia and Eastern Europe, the USA, and Canada. Low rates are found in Africa and Asia (Fig. 5.67).

The risk of epithelial tumours increases with age, occurring predominantly in peri- and postmenopausal women. Tumours of germinal or embryonic origin are more frequent in young adults.

Etiology

Although most ovarian cancers are sporadic, a family history is the single most important risk factor for ovarian cancer (5-10% of cases), risk being increased four-fold in women with an affected first-degree relative. Cancer of the ovary is influenced by hor-

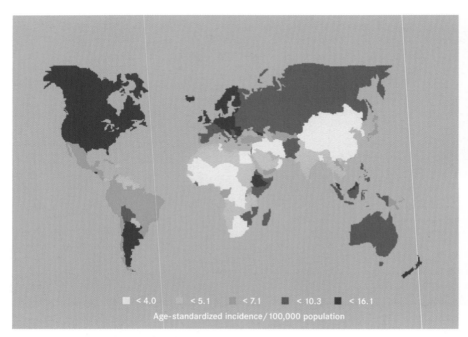

Fig. 5.67 The global incidence of ovarian cancer. This cancer occurs predominantly in developed countries.

< 4.0   < 5.1   < 7.1   < 10.3   < 16.1
Age-standardized incidence/100,000 population

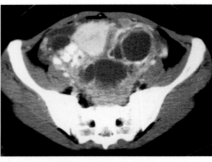

Fig. 5.68 Magnetic resonance image (MRI) of a large, partly cystic ovarian carcinoma.

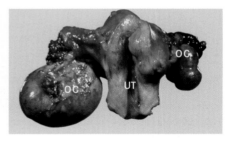

Fig. 5.69 Surgical specimen of a bilateral ovarian carcinoma (OC). UT = uterus.

mones and reproductive factors (*Reproductive factors and hormones*, p76). Risk is slightly increased with nulliparity and a personal history of breast cancer. Decreased risk follows the use of oral contraceptives. In contrast, hormonal treatment for infertility entails an increased risk, whereas treatment at the menopause is only associated with a small risk. Early menarche or late menopause may also entail a slightly increased risk [15]. Diet plays a role, with increased risk linked to obesity and height, as well as some nutritional factors (e.g. lactose). A history of pelvic inflammatory disease, polycystic ovary syndrome and endometriosis have also been associated with increased risk, whilst tubal ligation and hysterectomy may decrease risk.

Detection

The great majority of patients with epithelial ovarian cancer present with disease that has spread outside of the ovary and even the pelvis [16]. Symptoms may include abdominal discomfort, bloating, abnormal vaginal bleeding and gastrointestinal or urinary tract abnormalities. Abdominal and vaginal ultrasonography may suggest the presence of an ovarian tumour, but definitive diagnosis requires laparotomy and biopsy. Pelvic ultrasonography, tumour markers and clinical examination have proved ineffective in mass screening [4] and are employed only for patients having a high familial risk of ovarian cancer. The comparison of molecular profiles generated by laser capture microdissection is hoped to identify patterns of proteins which are uniquely expressed in early disease in order to generate valuable markers for early detection [17].

Pathology and genetics

Most ovarian tumours are of epithelial origin and include serous (45% of epithelial tumours), mucinous, endometrioid (Fig. 5.70) and clear cell adenocarcinomas, as well as the rare Brenner tumour. Non-epithelial tumours, including germ cell tumours, gonadal-stromal tumours and tumours which have metastasized to the ovary, are less common. Three categories of lesions are recognized: benign, low malignancy potential or invasive malignant. Malignant germ cell tumours are uncommon.

A majority of familial ovarian cancer seems to be due to mutations in the *BRCA1* and *BRCA2* genes, which are also associated with a predisposition for breast cancer (*Genetic susceptibility*, p71), (although *BRCA1* is also mutated in a minority of sporadic tumours [15]). Familial syndromes linked to increased risk of ovarian cancer include breast-ovarian cancer syndrome, rare families who present with ovarian cancers only and Lynch type II syndrome, which is characterized by inheritance of nonpolyposis colorectal cancer (*Colorectal cancer*, p198), endometrial cancer and ovarian cancer and is linked to mutations in DNA mismatch repair genes *MSH2, MLH1, PMS1* and *PMS2* (*Carcinogen activation and DNA repair*, p89)[15,16]. Prophylactic oophorectomy is a potential option for genetically high-risk women.

The *ERBB2 (HER-2/neu)* oncogene is overexpressed in about 30% of ovarian tumours, as is *C-MYC* [18]. *KRAS* mutational activation is also implicated in ovarian cancer. *p53* mutations have been found in 50% of cases.

Management

Surgery is most often the first recourse in diagnosis and treatment. Treatment of early disease includes bilateral salpingo-oophorectomy and total abdominal hysterectomy, total omentectomy, appendectomy, collecting samples of peritoneal washings for cytological analysis and possibly removal of pelvic retroperitoneal and aortic lymph nodes. Reproductive function and fertility may be conserved in patients with a unilateral, low-grade, unruptured epithelial ovarian tumour. Advanced stage ovarian cancer requires cytoreductive surgery to remove all gross tumour, followed by chemotherapy. External beam radiotherapy may play a limited role in selected patients with minimal residual disease. Intraperitoneal implants may be used as adjuvant treatment for high-risk patients with early disease.

A standard chemotherapy for advanced stage ovarian cancer using cisplatin and paclitaxel achieves response rates of up to 60-80%. Germ cell tumours are very sensitive to chemotherapy and may be treat-

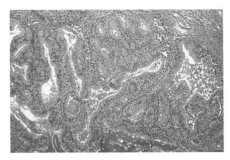

Fig. 5.70 Histopathology of a well-differentiated, mucus-secreting, endometrial-like adenocarcinoma of the ovary.

MULTICULTURAL ISSUES

Although incidence of cancer is often recorded with reference to national or otherwise large populations, the disease burden is rarely distributed uniformly across such groupings. This becomes apparent when consideration is given to specific minority groups within a wider community. A number of variables may contribute to such an outcome. One such variable, genetic make-up, is not amenable to intervention but nonetheless may have an impact. For example, there are large racial/ethnic differences in prostate cancer risk, with high rates of incidence in African-Americans, which may be partly related to genetic differences in hormone metabolism (Farkas A et al., *Ethn Dis*, 10: 69-75, 2000). However, mutations which confer susceptibility to cancer may be carried by individuals from any and all ethnic groups (Neuhausen SL, *Cancer*, 86: 2575-82, 1999).

In many instances, there are clear indications that in some ethnic minorities, immigrant populations and the poor and disadvantaged, the burden of cancer is greater than that of the general population (e.g. Kogevinas M et al., *Social inequalities and cancer*, Lyon, IARCPress, 1997). In the USA, for example, whilst incidence and mortality rates for some cancers have decreased in the population overall, rates have increased in some ethnic minority groups. The mortality rate for cancer at all

sites in white people in 1990-96 was 167.5 per 100,000 whilst in the black population it was 223.4. The reasons for such differences are likely to be complex and multifactorial.

Environmental/behavioural factors may differ between ethnic/cultural groups. For instance, the diet to which some migrant populations are accustomed (e.g. small quantities of red meat, large quantities of fruit and vegetables) may be protective in relation to risk of colorectal cancer, but risk increases with the adoption of a Western diet (e.g. Santani DL, *J Assoc Acad Minor Phys*, 10: 68-76, 1999).

Timely visits to a medical practitioner and participation in screening programmes are critical for early detection and initiation of treatment. Language may be a barrier to understanding health issues. Women from certain ethnic and racial minorities are less likely to take up invitations to participate in breast or cervical screening programmes. This may be partly attributable to the novelty of the concept of preventive health, unfamiliarity with the disease, or with the health system, as well as modesty and religious/cultural barriers. Women of lower socioeconomic status tend to present with a more advanced stage of breast cancer than women of higher socioeconomic status. African-American, Hispanic, American Indian and Hawaiian women also tend to present with a more advanced stage of breast cancer than white women (e.g. Hunter CP, *Cancer*, 88: 1193-202, 2000). In

the USA, women who do not subscribe to private health insurance are less likely to undergo screening for breast, cervical and colorectal cancers (Hsia J et al., *Prev Med*, 31: 261-70, 2000). Such differences involving increased incidence provide an opportunity for strategic action.

Treatment and its outcome may also be affected by ethnic and social differences. For example, the way that pain is perceived and dealt with is influenced by the ethnocultural background of the patient (Gordon C, *Nurse Pract Forum*, 8: 5-13, 1997). Ethical dilemmas can develop in multicultural settings due to differing cultural beliefs and practices. More research into the relationship between ethnicity and accessibility of medical care, patient support, survival, and quality of life is needed (Meyerowitz BE, *Psychol Bull*, 123: 47-70, 1998).

Recognition of multicultural issues is becoming more widespread. The NCI has launched an initiative to investigate the reasons for disparities in cancer in minority populations (the "Special Populations Networks for Cancer Awareness Research and Training", Mitka M, *JAMA*, 283: 2092-3, 2000). Many areas have units designed to improve equality of access to health care (e.g. NSW Health Multicultural Health Communication Service, http://www.health.nsw.gov.au).

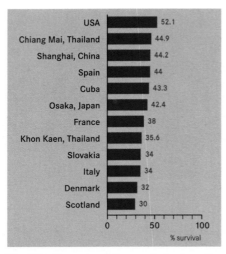

USA	52.1
Chiang Mai, Thailand	44.9
Shanghai, China	44.2
Spain	44
Cuba	43.3
Osaka, Japan	42.4
France	38
Khon Kaen, Thailand	35.6
Slovakia	34
Italy	34
Denmark	32
Scotland	30

% survival

Fig. 5.71 Five-year relative survival rates after diagnosis of ovarian cancer.

ed with vincristine, actinomycin and cyclophosphamide; cisplatin, vinblastine and bleomycin; or cisplatin, etoposide and bleomycin. Recurrent ovarian cancer may be treated with cytoreductive surgery plus chemotherapy and palliative radiotherapy. Hormonal therapy may include progestational agents and anti-estrogens.

Tumour stage (determined surgically) is the most important prognostic factor. Clear cell and small cell carcinomas are associated with a worse prognosis than other histological types. Aneuploidy has been linked to poor survival. In the assessment of response to treatment, decrease in serum CA-125 measurements indicates a more favourable prognosis. Early stage disease has a very good prognosis. Overal five-year survival rates for all stages combined (Fig. 5.71) range from 30-50%. Most women, however, present with late stage disease which is associated with a five-year survival rate of about 20%.

REFERENCES

1. IARC (1995) *Human Papillomaviruses (IARC Monographs on the Evaluation of Carcinogenic Risks to Humans, Vol. 64)*, Lyon, IARCPress.

2. zur Hausen H (1999) Viruses in human cancers. *Eur J Cancer*, 35: 1174-1181.

3. Webb MJ (1998) Female Genital Cancers. In: Morris D, Kearsley J, Williams C eds, *Cancer: a comprehensive clinical guide*, Harwood Academic Publishers.

4. Wharton JT (1997) Neoplasms of the cervix. In: Holland JF, Bast, RC, Morton, DL, Frei, E, Kufe, DW, Weichselbaum, RR eds, *Cancer Medicine*, Williams and Wilkins.

5. Shipman SD, Bristow RE (2001) Adenocarcinoma in situ and early invasive adenocarcinoma of the uterine cervix. *Curr Opin Oncol*, 13: 394-398.

6. Duggan BD, Dubeau L (1998) Genetics and biology of gynecologic cancer. *Curr Opin Oncol*, 10: 439-446.

7. Rosenthal AN (1998) Screening for gynecologic cancers. *Curr Opin Oncol*, 10: 447-451.

8. Larson AA, Liao SY, Stanbridge EJ, Cavenee WK, Hampton GM (1997) Genetic alterations accumulate during cervical tumorigenesis and indicate a common origin for multifocal lesions. *Cancer Res*, 57: 4171-4176.

9. Cox JT (1999) Management of cervical intraepithelial neoplasia. *Lancet*, 353: 857-859.

10. Brooks SE, Wakeley KE (1999) Current trends in the management of carcinoma of the cervix, vulva, and vagina. *Curr Opin Oncol*, 11: 383-387.

11. Sabbatini P, Aghajanian C, Spriggs D (1998) Chemotherapy in gynecologic cancer. *Curr Opin Oncol*, 10: 429-433.

12. IARC (1996) *Some Pharmaceutical Drugs (IARC Monographs on the Evaluation of Carcinogenic Risks to Humans, Vol. 66)*, Lyon, IARCPress.

13. Cohen CJ, Thomas GM (1997) Endometrial cancer. In: Holland JF, Bast, RC, Morton, DL, Frei, E, Kufe, DW, Weichselbaum, RR eds, *Cancer Medicine*, Williams and Wilkins.

14. Esteller M, Xercavins J, Reventos J (1999) Advances in the molecular genetics of endometrial cancer. *Oncol Rep*, 6: 1377-1382.

15. Holschneider CH, Berek JS (2000) Ovarian cancer: epidemiology, biology, and prognostic factors. *Semin Surg Oncol*, 19: 3-10.

16. Ozols RF, Schwartz PE, Eifel PA (1997) Ovarian cancer, fallopian tube carcinoma and peritoneal carcinoma. In: DeVita VTJ, Hellman S, Rosenberg SA eds, *Cancer Principles and Practice of Oncology*, Philadelphia, Lippincott-Raven Publishers, 1502-1539.

17. Jones MB, Krutzsch H, Shu H, Zhao Y, Liotta LA, Kohn EC, Petricoin EF, III (2002) Proteomic analysis and identification of new biomarkers and therapeutic targets for invasive ovarian cancer. *Proteomics*, 2: 76-84.

18. Aunoble B, Sanches R, Didier E, Bignon YJ (2000) Major oncogenes and tumor suppressor genes involved in epithelial ovarian cancer. *Int J Oncol*, 16: 567-576.

WEBSITES

NCI Homepages for Cervical Cancer, Endometrial Cancer and Ovarian Cancer:
http://www.cancer.gov/cancer_information/cancer_type/

The Alliance for Cervical Cancer Prevention:
http://www.alliance-cxca.org/

National Ovarian Cancer Coalition (USA):
http://www.ovarian.org/

OESOPHAGEAL CANCER

SUMMARY

> Cancer of the oesophagus is the sixth most common cancer worldwide (more than 400,00 cases per year). Incidence varies markedly, and is highest in Western and South Central Asia.

> Squamous cell carcinoma is most common in developing countries, and is typically associated with tobacco smoking and alcohol abuse. Other risk factors include consumption of very hot beverages and malnutrition.

> Adenocarcinoma occurs predominantly in white men from developed countries, the most important etiological factors being obesity and chronic gastro-oesophageal reflux.

> Most cancers of the oesophagus are detected at an advanced stage; five-year survival rates are less than 15%.

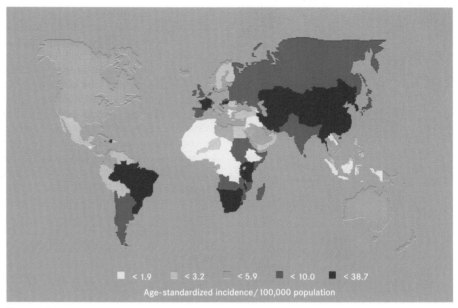

< 1.9   < 3.2   < 5.9   < 10.0   < 38.7

Age-standardized incidence/100,000 population

Fig. 5.72 The global burden of oesophageal cancer in men. High incidence rates occur in Northern Iran, the Central Asian republics, North-Central China, parts of South America and in Southern and Eastern Africa.

Definition

The great majority of oesophageal cancers (over 95%) are either squamous cell carcinomas or adenocarcinomas. Tumours of the cardia, which arise within the gastro-oesophageal junction, are sometimes classified in the same group as adenocarcinomas of the oesophagus.

Epidemiology

Cancers of the oesophagus are the sixth most frequent cancers worldwide. In 2000, the number of deaths due to oesophageal cancer amounted to some 337,500 out of a total of 6.2 million cancer deaths worldwide. About 412,000 cases of cancer of the oesophagus occur each year, of which over 80% are in developing countries. While squamous cell carcinoma occurs at high frequency in many developing countries, adenocarci-

noma is essentially a tumour of more developed, industrialized countries.

The differences between incidence of oesophageal cancer in distinct geographical areas are more extreme than observed for any other cancer. Regions of high incidence of squamous cell carcinoma in Asia [1] stretch from the Turkoman plain in northern Iran through the central Asian republics to Henan province in North-Central China, characterized as the "oesophageal cancer belt" (Fig. 5.72). Incidence rates are as high as 200 per 100,000 and in some areas there is a female predominance. Other high-incidence areas are found in parts of South America and in Southern and Eastern Africa. Even within these high-risk areas, there are striking local variations in risk. Studies of migrant populations suggest that when they move to areas of low-risk, they lose their high rates, confirming the importance of local environmental factors in causation.

In Europe and the USA, the age-standardized annual mortality from squa-

mous cell carcinoma is up to five in males and one in females per 100,000 population. However, in particular areas, such as Normandy and Brittany in France and in the north-east of Italy, the incidence rates are much higher in males (up to 30 per 100,000), while remaining relatively low in females. The incidence of adenocarcinoma is steadily increasing in Europe and the USA at a rate of 5-10% per year. This type of cancer now accounts for more than 50% of all oesophageal cancers in the USA and in some European countries [2]. Trends in incidence of all oesophageal cancers vary greatly (Fig. 5.75).

Etiology

Consumption of tobacco and alcohol, associated with low intake of fresh fruit, vegetables and meat, is causally associated with squamous cell carcinoma of the oesophagus worldwide. However, the relative contribution of these risk factors varies from one geographic area to another. In more developed countries, it is esti-

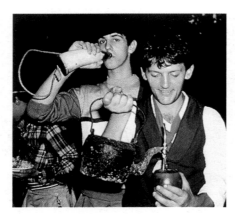

Fig. 5.73 Drinking the scalding beverage *maté* is associated with an increased risk of oesophageal cancer.

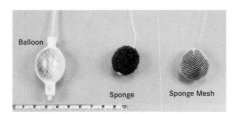

Fig. 5.74 Devices used to collect histological samples from the oesophagus, used for screening in Iran.

mated that 90% of squamous cell carcinomas are attributable to tobacco and alcohol, with a multiplicative increase in risk when individuals are exposed to both factors [3]. The consumption of scalding hot beverages, such as *maté* in South America (Fig. 5.73), is a risk factor [4], malignancy being the outcome of chronic mucosal injury. Other risk factors include consumption of pickled vegetables, betel chewing in South East Asia, and oral consumption of opium by-products in the Caspian Sea area. Conflicting reports have proposed a role for human papillomaviruses in squamous cell carcinoma [5]. Other environmental risk factors include nitrosamines, food contamination with fungi such as *Geotrichum candidum* and *Fusarium sp.* (*Food contaminants*, p43) and deficiency of vitamins A and C, molybdenum, copper and zinc.

Adenocarcinoma of the oesophagus has been associated with chronic gastro-oesophageal reflux, which most often underlies repetitive mucosal injury and predisposes to metaplasia [6]. This tumour type is directly associated with Barrett oesophagus, a premalignant lesion.

Detection

Although endoscopic or cytologic screening may be useful for early diagnosis in regions of high incidence, there are no widely accepted protocols for such interventions. Cytologic screening of high-risk asymptomatic populations is carried out in China with a swallowed balloon catheter and in Japan with a swallowed encapsulated brush (Fig. 5.74). Endoscopic dye-staining with Lugol's iodine or toluidine blue aids detection of early lesions.

The vast majority of patients initially complain of progressive dysphagia, which may not become apparent until some two-thirds of the lumen has been obstructed, especially in the case of squamous cell carcinoma [7]. Regurgitation and pain on swallowing are frequent, as is weight loss. Laryngeal nerve involvement may be indicated by hoarseness. Patients with adenocarcinomas of the cardia may also suffer from gastrointestinal bleeding [8]. A barium swallow (ingestion of liquid containing barium prior to X-ray) (Fig. 5.76) may indicate narrowing or mucosal irregularity, whereas a chest X-ray may reveal late signs such as the presence of a mass, tracheal compression, aspiration pneumonia or metastases. Endoscopic ultrasonography is currently the most accurate staging method, but is not widely available. CT scanning remains the mainstay of staging prior to resection, supplemented by laparoscopy (for lower one-third cancers) or bronchoscopy (for upper one-third cancers).

Pathology and genetics

Squamous cell carcinoma (Fig. 5.77) develops from squamous epithelium according to a classical dysplasia-carcinoma sequence (*Multistage carcinogenesis*, p84). The most common site of squamous cell carcinoma is the middle third of the oesophagus. Microscopically, most squamous tumours contain islands of

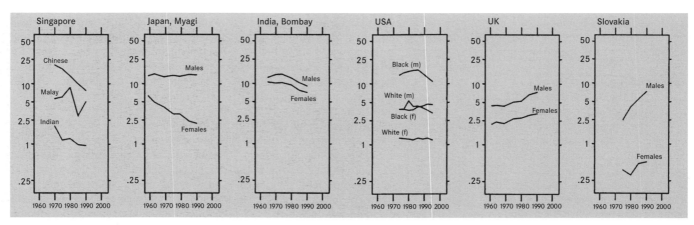

Fig. 5.75 Trends in incidence of oesophageal cancer differ considerably according to geography and reflect differences in prevalence of the two main histological types. D.M. Parkin et al. (2001) *Eur J Cancer*, 37 Suppl. 8: S4-66.

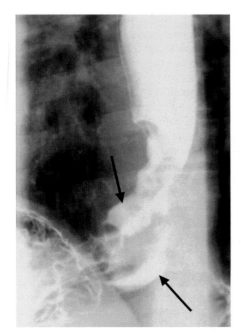

Fig. 5.76 A radiographic view of an oesophageal cancer taken following a barium swallow. Arrows indicate a filling defect caused by obstruction by the tumour.

atypical squamous cells which infiltrate the underlying normal tissue and contain keratin pearl formation and intercellular bridges [9].

The sequence of genetic events leading to squamous cell carcinoma is only partially understood (Fig. 5.78). Mutation of the *p53* gene is an early event, detected in 35-70% of tumours, depending on geographic origin. Tumours from high-incidence areas of Western Europe show a high proportion of mutations at A:T base pairs. These mutations may reflect a contribution of metabolites of alcohol. In East Asia, mutations at A:T base pairs are less common, but transversions at G:C base pairs occur at a higher rate than in Western Europe [10]. Mutations in *p53* have been observed in dysplasia, and in normal mucosa adjacent to cancer lesions [11].

In squamous cell carcinoma, other commonly mutated genes are those encoding proteins involved in the control of the G1/S cell-cycle checkpoint, such as cyclin D1 and p16^{INK4A} (*Cell cycle*, p104). Amplification of the cyclin D1 gene *CCDN1* (11q13) occurs in 20-40% of tumours. The gene encoding p16^{INK4A} is often subject to hypermethylation of the promoter region, resulting in down-regulation of expression. Amplification of a number of proto-oncogenes (*HST-1, HST-2, EGFR, MYC*) has also been reported [12]. In the Japanese population, a polymorphism in the gene encoding aldehyde dehydrogenase 2 (*ALDH2*), which plays a role in ethanol metabolism, is significantly associated with squamous cell carcinoma [13].

Adenocarcinoma of the oesophagus mostly occurs within the distal third of the oesophagus and is preceded by a

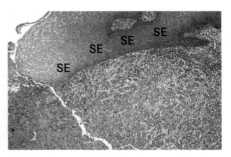

Fig. 5.77 Moderately differentiated squamous cell carcinoma of the oesophagus, ulcerated, deeply invasive and extending below the normal squamous epithelium (SE).

well-defined preneoplastic lesion called Barrett mucosa (or Barrett oesophagus) (Fig. 5.79). Barrett mucosa is a glandular, metaplastic mucosa of the normal squamous epithelium. It is often associated with chronic gastro-oesophageal acid reflux. However, it also occurs in the context of chronic biliary alkaline reflux, as well as, in some cases, the absence of a detectable reflux. Men are seven times more commonly affected than women [14].

The estimated risk of developing an adenocarcinoma for patients with Barrett mucosa is 30-125 times greater than in the general population. There are three subtypes: fundic (base of oesophagus), cardiac (the region between the oesophagus and the stomach), and intestinal.

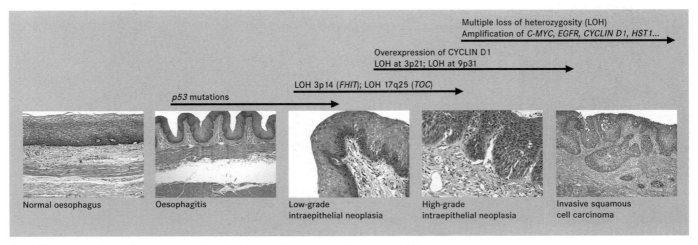

Fig. 5.78 Sequence of genetic alterations in the development of squamous cell carcinoma of the oesophagus.

Factor	Alteration
Tumour suppressor genes	
p53	60% mutation – high-grade intraepithelial neoplasia and carcinoma
APC	Late in intraepithelial neoplasia-carcinoma sequence
FHIT	Common, early abnormalities
CDKN2A (p16^{INK4A})	Hypermethylation common in intraepithelial neoplasia
Growth factor receptors	
CD95/APO/Fas	Shift to cytoplasm in carcinoma
EGFR	Expressed in 60% of carcinomas, gene amplification
c-erbB2	Late in dysplasia-carcinoma sequence, gene amplification
Cell adhesion	
E-cadherin	Loss of expression in intraepithelial and invasive carcinoma
Catenins	Similar loss of expression to E-cadherin
Proteases	
UPA	Prognostic factor in carcinoma
Proliferation	
Ki-67	Abnormal distribution in high-grade intraepithelial neoplasia
Membrane trafficking	
rab11	High expression in low-grade intraepithelial neoplasia

Table 5.9 Genes and proteins involved in the development of adenocarcinoma from Barrett oesophagus.

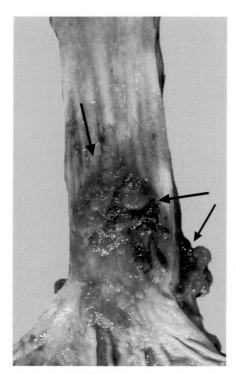

Fig. 5.79 A highly infiltrative adenocarcinoma in a Barrett oesophagus.

Mutation of the *p53* gene is common in the early stages of adenocarcinoma of the oesophagus (Table 5.9). The presence of a *p53* mutation in Barrett mucosa and in dysplasia may precede the development of adenocarcinoma. In high-grade dysplasia, a prevalence of *p53* mutations of approximately 60% is found, similar to that found in adenocarcinoma. Almost half of these are C to T transitions at dipyrimidine sites (CpG islands).

Alteration in transcription of *FHIT* and of p16^{INK4A} may be early events in adenocarcinoma. In contrast, a number of other loci are altered at a relatively late stage with no obligate sequence of events. Prevalent changes (>50%) include loss of heterozygosity on chromosomes 4q, 5q (several loci including *APC*), 17p and amplification of the gene encoding c-erbB2. Molecules involved in membrane traffic, such as rab11, have been reported to be specific for the loss of polarity (rounding-up of cell nuclei) seen in low-grade dysplasia. In invasive oesophageal adenocarcinoma, reduced expression of the cadherin/catenin complex and increased expression of various proteases is detectable [15].

Management

Endoscopic ultrasonography is used to evaluate both depth of tumour infiltration and para-oesophageal lymph node involvement. In advanced carcinomas, CT and MRI give information about local and systemic spread. Tumour growth is characterized as swelling of the oesophageal wall, with or without direct invasion to surrounding organs. The primary treatment for local disease is oesophagectomy. This surgical approach is rarely curative (eventually 85 to 90% of the patients die of recurrent disease) but palliation of dysphagia is an important secondary objective. Placement of a prosthetic tube or stent across the tumour stenosis (narrowing) may be indicated to restore swallowing in patients not suitable for surgery. Radiotherapy (external beam or brachytherapy) as well as multiple chemotherapeutic protocols have also been proposed (alone or combined with surgery), but these approaches are rarely curative. Palliation with radiation alone is an alternative to surgery, particularly if combined

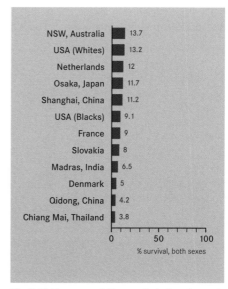

NSW, Australia	13.7
USA (Whites)	13.2
Netherlands	12
Osaka, Japan	11.7
Shanghai, China	11.2
USA (Blacks)	9.1
France	9
Slovakia	8
Madras, India	6.5
Denmark	5
Qidong, China	4.2
Chiang Mai, Thailand	3.8

% survival, both sexes

Fig. 5.80 Five-year relative survival after diagnosis of oesophageal cancer.

with a stent; laser recannulation, alcohol injection and dilation may be used to maintain the oesophageal lumen [8]. Prognostic factors include stage at diagnosis, patient's general health, morphological and molecular features of the tumour, for squamous cell carcinoma the depth of invasion and for adenocarcinoma presence of lymphatic metastases. Overall five-year relative survival rates are poor (Fig. 5.80), survival ranging from about 10% in patients with squamous cell carcinoma to 20% in patients with adenocarcinoma.

REFERENCES

1. Muñoz N, Day NE (1996) Esophageal cancer. In: Scottenfeld D, Fraumeni FJ eds, *Cancer Epidemiology and Prevention*, Oxford, New York, Oxford University Press, 681-706.

2. Parkin DM, Whelan SL, Ferlay J, Raymond L, Young J, eds (1997) *Cancer Incidence in Five Continents, Vol. VII (IARC Scientific Publications No. 143 and IARC Cancerbase No. 2)*, Lyon, IARCPress.

3. Launoy G, Milan CH, Faivre J, Pienkowski P, Milan CI, Gignoux M (1997) Alcohol, tobacco and oesophageal cancer: effects of the duration of consumption, mean intake and current and former consumption. *Br J Cancer*, 75: 1389-1396.

4. De Stefani E, Muñoz N, Esteve J, Vasallo A, Victora CG, Teuchmann S (1990) Mate drinking, alcohol, tobacco, diet, and esophageal cancer in Uruguay. *Cancer Res*, 50: 426-431.

5. de Villiers EM, Lavergne D, Chang F, Syrjanen K, Tosi P, Cintorino M, Santopietro R, Syrjanen S (1999) An interlaboratory study to determine the presence of human papillomavirus DNA in esophageal carcinoma from China. *Int J Cancer*, 81: 225-228.

6. Spechler SJ, Goyal RK (1986) Barrett's esophagus. *N Engl J Med*, 315: 362-371.

7. Goodnight J, Venook A, Ames M, Taylor C, Gilden R, Figlin RA (1996) Practice Guidelines for Esophageal Cancer. *Cancer J Sci Am*, 2: S37.

8. Law S, Wong J (1998) Cancer of the Esophagus. In: Morris D, Kearsley J, Williams C eds, *Cancer: A comprehensive clinical guide*, Harwood Academic Publishers, 155-162.

9. Gabbert HE, Shimoda T, Hainaut P, Nakamura Y, Field JK, Inoue H (2000) Squamous cell carcinoma of the oesophagus. In: Hamilton SR, Aaltonen LA, eds, *World Health Organization Classification of Tumours. Pathology and Genetics of Tumours of the Digestive System*, Lyon, IARCPress, 11-19.

10. Taniere P, Martel-Planche G, Puttawibul P, Casson A, Montesano R, Chanvitan A, Hainaut P (2000) TP53 mutations and MDM2 gene amplification in squamous-cell carcinomas of the esophagus in south Thailand. *Int J Cancer*, 88: 223-227.

11. Mandard AM, Hainaut P, Hollstein M (2000) Genetic steps in the development of squamous cell carcinoma of the esophagus. *Mutat Res,* 462: 335-342.

12. Montesano R, Hollstein M, Hainaut P (1996) Genetic alterations in esophageal cancer and their relevance to etiology and pathogenesis: a review. *Int J Cancer*, 69: 225-235.

13. Yokoyama A, Muramatsu T, Ohmori T, Yokoyama T, Okuyama K, Takahashi H, Hasegawa Y, Higuchi S, Maruyama K, Shirakura K, Ishii H (1998) Alcohol-related cancers and aldehyde dehydrogenase 2 in Japanese alcoholics. *Carcinogenesis*, 19: 1383-1387.

14. Werner M, Flejou JF, Hainaut P, Höfler H, Lambert R, Keller G, Stein HJ (2000) Adenocarcinoma of the oesophagus. In: Hamilton SR, Aaltonen LA eds, *World Health Organization Classification of Tumours. Pathology and Genetics of Tumours of the Digestive System*, Lyon, IARCPress, 20-26.

15. Tselepis C, Perry I, Jankowski J (2000) Barrett's esophagus: disregulation of cell cycling and intercellular adhesion in the metaplasia-dysplasia-carcinoma sequence. *Digestion*, 61: 1-5.

WEBSITE

NCI Esophageal Cancer Homepage:
http://www.cancer.gov/cancer_information/cancer_type/esophageal/

BLADDER CANCER

SUMMARY

> Bladder cancer is the ninth most common cancer worldwide, with 330,000 new cases and more than 130,000 deaths per year.

> Bladder cancer is primarily attributable to smoking, which accounts for 65% of male and 30% of female cases in some developed countries. Other less important causes include analgesic abuse (phenacetin), some types of cancer chemotherapy and, historically, occupational exposure to chemicals such as 2-naphthylamine. In Egypt and some Asian regions, chronic cystitis caused by *Schistosoma haematodium* infection is a major risk factor.

> Treatment based on endoscopy, surgery, radiotherapy and cytotoxic drugs often permits long-term survival in developed countries, where 65% of patients live for at least five years after diagnosis.

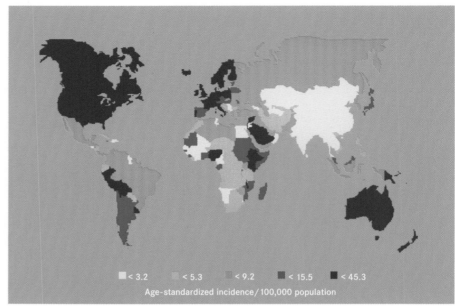

| < 3.2 | < 5.3 | < 9.2 | < 15.5 | < 45.3 |

Age-standardized incidence/100,000 population

Fig. 5.81 The global incidence of bladder cancer in men. Although the majority of cases occur in developed countries, bladder cancer also occurs at high rates in some developing countries, including parts of Northern Africa and South America.

Definition

More than 90% of bladder cancers are transitional cell carcinomas. Much less common are adenocarcinoma (6%), squamous cell carcinoma (2%) and small cell carcinoma (less than 1%).

Epidemiology

Bladder cancer accounts for approximately two-thirds of all urinary tract cancers. By incidence, bladder cancer is the ninth most common cancer worldwide, although in the USA, for example, bladder cancer is the fourth most frequent tumour among men. Approximately 336,000 new cases occurred in 2000, two-thirds of which were in developed countries [1]. Incidence and mortality rise sharply with age and about two-thirds of cases occur in people over the age of 65. The male:female ratio is approximately 3:1. High incidence rates (>12 per 100,000 men and >3 per 100,000 women)

are observed throughout Southern, Western and Northern Europe, North America, Australia, Western Asia, Northern Africa and Uruguay (Fig. 5.81) Bladder cancer incidence is either rising moderately or is steady in most developed countries. About 132,000 people each year die from bladder cancer, men throughout the world having a mortality rate of 10 per 100,000 population, and women 2.4, although these values nearly double for developed countries.

Etiology

The most important risk factor for bladder cancer is cigarette smoking, which accounts for approximately 65% of male cases and 30% of female cases in populations of developed countries [2]. It is likely that smokers of black (air-cured) tobacco are at a greater risk than smokers of blond (flue-cured) tobacco and this may explain some of the disparity observed in European incidence rates and also the high incidence observed in Uruguay. The

risk associated with tobacco smoking, and in particular with black tobacco smoking, is likely to be due to the presence in the smoke of aromatic amines including benzidine, 4-aminobiphenyl, 2-naphthylamine and 4-chloro-*ortho*-toluidine. Bladder cancer risk increases approximately linearly with duration of smoking, reaching a fivefold risk after 40 years (Fig. 5.82). The risk also increases with the number of cigarettes smoked, up to approximately 20 cigarettes per day; above that level, no further increase in risk is observed. Upon smoking cessation, a substantial decrease in risk of bladder cancer is observed within several years, implying an effect in late stages of the carcinogenic process.

Work in the rubber and dyestuff industries and specifically occupational exposure to aromatic amines, particularly including 2-naphthylamine and benzidine, are correlated with a high risk of bladder cancer [3]. Exposure to polycyclic aromatic hydrocarbons, polychlorinated biphenyls, formaldehyde, asbestos and solvents, and work in

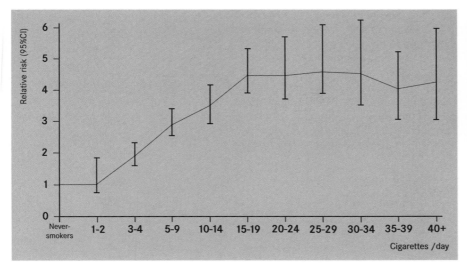

Fig. 5.82 Risk of bladder cancer among men who smoke relative to never-smokers, according to daily cigarette consumption.

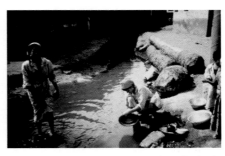

Fig. 5.83 A canal in a poor housing district in Egypt. Such canals may provide a habitat for the snails which are host to *Schistosoma* parasites. Chronic infection with *Schistosoma haematobium* causes cystitis and often bladder cancer.

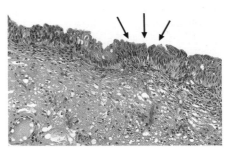

Fig. 5.84 Carcinoma *in situ* of the bladder; the normal transitional epithelium has been replaced by a disorganized, poorly-differentiated cell layer (arrows).

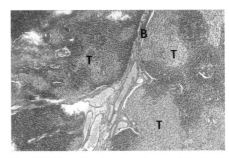

Fig. 5.85 Transitional cell carcinoma of the bladder, moderately differentiated, with a papillary architecture. B = blood vessel, T = tumour.

leather manufacturing, as a painter and as a barber or hairdresser have been variously associated with increased risk. The uncertainty surrounding these associations is partly due to difficulty in measuring past exposure to specific chemical agents.

In common with cancer of the renal pelvis, a consistent relationship has been observed between use of phenacetin-containing analgesics and bladder cancer, with relative risks varying from 2.4 to over 6-fold. Use of the anticancer drug cyclophosphamide, an alkylating agent, has been strongly and consistently linked to bladder cancer. Non-Hodgkin lymphoma patients treated with cyclophosphamide therapy have a dose-dependent increased risk of bladder cancer.

Infection by the trematode worm, *Schistosoma haematobium,* is associated with an up to five-fold increased risk. In endemic areas, which include most of Africa and in several West Asian countries, infection as a result of ingestion of contaminated water occurs from childhood (Fig. 5.83), and risk of bladder cancer, especially of the squamous cell type, increases as from the third decade of life. The infection is responsible for about 10% of bladder cancer cases in the developing world and about 3% of cases overall [4].

Decreased risk of bladder cancer is associated with consumption of foods rich in vitamin A and carotenoids; evidence concerning a risk associated with coffee consumption is inconsistent.

Detection

Detection of neoplastic alterations in exfoliated bladder cells collected in the urine has been proposed as a screening approach for bladder cancer, in particular among industrial workers potentially exposed to aromatic amines, but there is no evidence in favour of its effectiveness. Other methods are also under investigation [5].

Haematuria, usually painless, is the presenting symptom for the majority of patients with bladder cancer. Patients may also present with bladder irritability, including urinary frequency, urgency and dysuria. Diagnosis is made by urine analysis and after visualization of the bladder by ultrasound and cystoscopy. Tissue for histopathological analysis may be obtained through transurethral resection.

Pathology and genetics

Approximately 90% of bladder cancers are classified as transitional cell carcinoma and are believed to originate in intraepithelial neoplastic transformation of the bladder transitional epithelium. The localized proliferation of transformed cells can give rise to a carcinoma *in situ*, which may take several clinical forms, not necessarily associated with high grade or high risk of progression (Fig. 5.84) [6]. Spread can occur by growth into the submucosa and muscularis of the bladder wall (25% of cases). About 70% of transitional cell carcinomas are of the papillary type (Fig. 5.85) and do not invade the muscularis propria of the bladder wall, 10% are described as nodular and 20% as mixed.

Infection with *S. haematobium* is associated with the development of squamous cell carcinoma and in endemic areas, such as Egypt, this type constitutes 90% of bladder tumours [7].

A number of genes which regulate enzymes involved in the metabolism of bladder carcinogens have been identified and it has been hypothesized that subjects carrying specific genotypes could be at an increased risk of bladder cancer [8]. For example, a dominant mutation in the *NAT2* gene causes slow metabolism of aromatic amines, favouring their transformation into active carcinogens; slow metabolizers may be at a 40% increased risk of bladder cancer. Similarly, individuals who are null for the *GSTM1* gene, which encodes an enzyme involved in the detoxification of polycyclic aromatic hydrocarbons, have been reported to be at increased risk of bladder cancer. There is no evidence for high-penetrance gene mutations that carry an elevated risk of bladder cancer. The oncogene *HRAS* is mutated at codon 12 in about 40% of bladder tumours. Overexpression of the epidermal growth factor receptor is associated with invasive disease. The gene encoding c-erbB2 (*ERBB2*) is amplified in a small proportion of bladder tumours. Cytogenetic and molecular techniques have implicated aberration/partial loss of chromosome 9 as a common feature in bladder cancer, and the cyclin-dependent kinase inhibitors p16^{INK4A} and p15 are also implicated in this context. Altered expression of the phosphorylated form of the retinoblastoma protein is common, and most often encountered in invasive tumours. Nuclear overexpression of p53 protein, essentially attributable to mutation of the gene, is common and is associated with disease progression (Fig. 5.86) [9].

Management

Most patients with carcinoma *in situ* progress to muscle invasion within 10 years, but can achieve good responses to intravesical therapy - the administration of a therapeutic agent directly into the bladder, thereby exposing the mucosa to high drug concentrations [10]. The most commonly used agent in intravesical therapy for superficial transitional cell carcinomas, to prevent recurrence, and possibly decrease progression and improve survival, is bacille Calmette-Guérin (BCG), an attenuated strain of the *Mycobacterium bovis* bacterium which causes tuberculosis. Cytotoxic drugs such as thiotepa, doxorubicin, mitomycin C and/or ethoglucid may be used for superficial tumours to prevent recurrence.

The currently preferred treatment for patients with invasive bladder cancer is radical cystectomy. This involves excision of the bladder, prostate and seminal vesicles in males or the bladder, ovaries, uterus, urethra and part of the vagina in females. Urinary diversion, and some restoration of bladder function, may be achieved through a range of reconstruction options that continue to be refined and improved. Adjuvant chemotherapy (e.g with cisplatin, methotrexate and vinblastine, or the latter combination plus doxorubicin) may be employed. Several new agents have been identified [11].

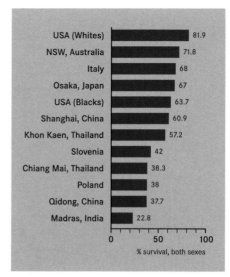

Fig. 5.87 Five-year relative survival rates after diagnosis of bladder cancer.

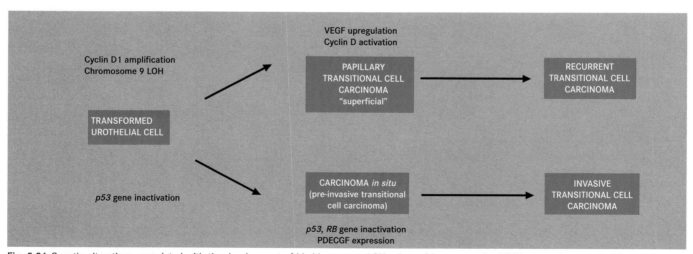

Fig. 5.86 Genetic alterations associated with the development of bladder cancer. LOH = loss of heterozygosity, VEGF = vascular endothelial growth factor, PDECGF = platelet derived endothelial cell growth factor.

Partial cystectomy is appropriate for only a minor proportion of patients with invasive bladder cancer. Radical radiation therapy as sole treatment has been evaluated, and criteria contributing to a favourable outcome (tumour size, stage, morphology, etc.) have been determined. Tumour staging is based on the degree to which the tumour has invaded the bladder wall.

In more developed countries, five-year relative survival is in the order of 65% (Fig. 5.87), and there has been a steady improvement during the last decades. Survival is poorer in developing countries, with five-year relative survival rates of 30-50%.

REFERENCES

1. Ferlay J, Bray F, Parkin DM, Pisani P, eds (2001) *Globocan 2000: Cancer Incidence and Mortality Worldwide (IARC Cancer Bases No. 5)*, Lyon, IARCPress.

2. Brennan P, Bogillot O, Cordier S, Greiser E, Schill W, Vineis P, Lopez-Abente G, Tzonou A, Chang-Claude J, Bolm-Audorff U, Jockel KH, Donato F, Serra C, Wahrendorf J, Hours M, T'Mannetje A, Kogevinas M, Boffetta P (2000) Cigarette smoking and bladder cancer in men: a pooled analysis of 11 case-control studies. *Int J Cancer*, 86: 289-294.

3. Silverman DT, Morrison AS, Devesa SS (1996) Bladder cancer. In: Scottenfeld D, Fraumeni, FJ eds, *Cancer Epidemiology and Prevention*, Oxford, New York, Oxford University Press, 1156-1179.

4. Pisani P, Parkin DM, Muñoz N, Ferlay J (1997) Cancer and infection: estimates of the attributable fraction in 1990. *Cancer Epidemiol Biomarkers Prev*, 6: 387-400.

5. Saad A, Hanbury DC, McNicholas TA, Boustead GB, Woodman AC (2001) The early detection and diagnosis of bladder cancer: a critical review of the options. *Eur Urol*, 39: 619-633.

6. Lee R, Droller MJ (2000) The natural history of bladder cancer. Implications for therapy. *Urol Clin North Am*, 27: 1-13, vii.

7. Noss M, Klotz L (1998) Male urogenital cancer. In: Morris D, Kearsley J, Williams C eds, *Cancer: a comprehensive clinical guide*, Harwood Academic Publishers, 213-222.

8. d'Errico A, Malats N, Vineis P, Boffetta P (1999) Review of studies of selected metabolic polymorphisms and cancer. In: Vineis P, Malats N, Lang M, d'Errico A, Caporaso N, Cuzick J, Boffetta P eds, *Metabolic Polymorphisms and Susceptibility to Cancer (IARC Scientific Publication No. 148)*, Lyon, IARCPress, 323-393.

9. Brandau S, Bohle A (2001) Bladder cancer. I. Molecular and genetic basis of carcinogenesis. *Eur Urol*, 39: 491-497.

10. Metts MC, Metts JC, Milito SJ, Thomas CR, Jr. (2000) Bladder cancer: a review of diagnosis and management. *J Natl Med Assoc*, 92: 285-294.

11. Maluf FC, Bajorin DF (2001) Chemotherapy agents in transitional cell carcinoma: the old and the new. *Semin Urol Oncol*, 19: 2-8.

WEBSITE

NCI Bladder Cancer Homepage.
http://www.cancer.gov/cancer_information/cancer_type/bladder/

HEAD AND NECK CANCER

SUMMARY

> The most common cancer of the head and neck, namely oral cancer, ranks eleventh worldwide (390,000 new cases per year), while cancers of the pharynx (65,000 cases) and larynx (160,000 cases) are less common.

> Head and neck cancers mainly afflict men, with sex ratios exceeding 10:1, and are typically caused by smoking, together with alcohol abuse. In some regions (e.g. India) oral cancer is mainly due to tobacco chewing. Multiple primary carcinomas are not uncommon.

> Early-stage tumours can be surgically resected, but many patients are diagnosed with advanced disease and prognosis is poor. Oral cancer patients have a five-year survival rate of less than 50%.

> Nasopharyngeal cancer is largely restricted to Southern Chinese populations and strongly associated with Epstein-Barr virus infection.

Definition

Head and neck cancers as described here will be restricted to squamous cell carcinomas of the upper aerodigestive tract (which extends from the surface of the lips to the neck region of the oesophagus) and include the oral cavity, larynx and pharynx (comprising the oropharynx, hypopharynx and nasopharynx). Other tumours which occur in this area, such as those of the brain and thyroid and melanoma, are conventionally dealt with separately (*Tumours of the nervous system*, p265; *Thyroid cancer*, p257; *Melanoma*, p253).

Epidemiology

Cancers of the oral mucosa and oro- and hypopharynx can be considered together, as there are similarities in their epidemiology, treatment and prognosis. The geographic

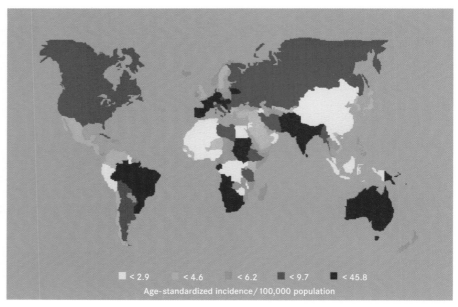

< 2.9   < 4.6   < 6.2   < 9.7   < 45.8
Age-standardized incidence / 100,000 population

Fig. 5.88 The global incidence of oral cancer in men. Oral cancer is common in India, Australia, Hungary, France, Brazil and Southern Africa.

patterns and trends in incidence for these cancers vary depending upon the anatomical sub-sites concerned, a phenomenon that is often explicable by the influence of risk factors, such as tobacco use and alcohol consumption. A high incidence of these cancers is observed in the Indian subcontinent, Australia, France, South America (Brazil) and Southern Africa (Fig. 5.88). Oral cancer is the 11th most common cancer in the world in terms of number of cases, while cancer of the pharynx (apart from nasopharynx) ranks as 20th. Worldwide, about 389,000 new cases occurred in 2000, two-thirds of which were in developing countries, and these cancers are responsible for some 200,000 deaths each year.

The male:female ratio of occurrence varies from 2-15:1 depending on the anatomical sub-site, with extreme ratios characteristic of tongue, floor of mouth and pharyngeal cancers. The highest incidence among males is reported in Bas-Rhin and Calvados in France, whereas among females the highest occurrence is observed in India. Cancers of the mouth and anterior two-thirds of the tongue

generally predominate in developing countries, whereas pharyngeal cancers are common in developed countries and in Central and Eastern Europe. In most countries, oral/pharyngeal cancer incidence and mortality rates have either been stable or increasing in the last four decades. Sharp increases in incidence have been reported in Germany, Denmark, Scotland, Central and Eastern Europe, and there are increases in Japan, Australia and New Zealand, and in the USA among non-whites.

New cases of cancer of the larynx occurring worldwide number about 160,000, i.e. about 2% of the total world cancer cases, making laryngeal cancer the 18th most common cancer. The disease is markedly more frequent in males than in females (male:female ratio of 12:1 and 6:1 in developing and developed countries respectively). There is a large geographic variability in disease frequency, high-risk countries being in Southern Europe (France, Italy, Spain), Eastern Europe (Russia, Ukraine), South America (Uruguay, Argentina), and Western Asia (Turkey, Iraq) (Fig. 5.89). Mortality from laryngeal cancer is poorly known since hypopharyngeal cancer deaths are often mis-certified as deaths from cancer of the larynx.

Carcinomas of the salivary glands and nasopharynx are distinguished from head and neck cancers at other sites both by epidemiology and by etiology. Nasopharyngeal cancer is relatively rare on a world scale (65,000 new cases per year, or 0.6% of all cancers), but it has a very distinctive geographic distribution. Age-standardized incidence rates are high for populations living in or originating from Southern China, whilst populations elsewhere in China, South East Asia, North Africa, and the Inuits (Eskimos) of Canada and Alaska, all have moderately elevated rates (Fig. 5.90). Males are more often affected than females (sex ratio 2–3:1), and in most populations, there is a progressive increase in risk with age. In moderate-risk populations, however, most notably in North Africa, there is a peak in incidence in adolescence. There appears to have been a decrease in incidence over time in some high-risk populations (e.g. Hong Kong).

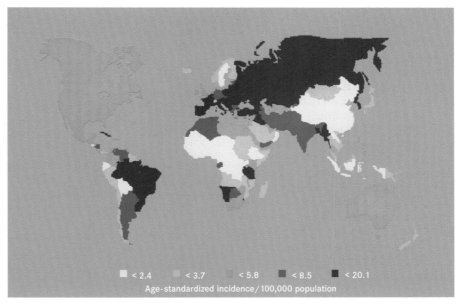

Age-standardized incidence/100,000 population

< 2.4   < 3.7   < 5.8   < 8.5   < 20.1

Fig. 5.89 The global incidence of cancer of the larynx in men. High-risk countries are found in Southern and Eastern Europe, Latin America and Western Asia.

Etiology

Smoking and drinking are the major risk factors for head and neck cancer in developed countries, in the Caribbean and in South American countries [1-3]. Smoking is estimated to be responsible for about 41% of laryngeal and oral/pharyngeal cancers in men, and 15% in women worldwide and these proportions vary amongst different populations. Tobacco smoking has also been found to be an important risk factor for nasopharyngeal cancer in otherwise low-risk populations. These risk factors have been shown, for laryngeal and oropharyngeal cancers, to have a joint "multiplicative" or synergistic effect.

In the Indian subcontinent, chewing tobacco in the form of betel quid (a combination of betel leaf, slaked lime, areca-nut and tobacco with or without other condiments), bidi (a locally hand-rolled cigarette of dried temburni leaf containing coarse tobacco) smoking and drinking locally brewed crude alcoholic drinks are the major causative factors. The role of betel quids without tobacco is not clear, though a recent case-control study from Pakistan reported a high risk of oral cancer [4]. Reverse smoking (in which the lit

end of the cigarette is placed in the mouth so that an intense heat is experienced) is a risk factor for cancer of the hard palate. Oral snuff use is an emerging risk factor for oral cancer, particularly among young males in the USA.

A generally impoverished diet, particularly lacking in vegetables and fruits, is another risk factor for oral cancer [5]. Consistently, studies also indicate a protective effect of a diet rich in vegetables and fruits (20-60% reduction in risk). A high intake of salted fish and meat and the release of nitrosamines on cooking such foods have been linked to nasopharyngeal cancer in endemic regions.

Oral human papillomavirus (HPV) infection (transmitted sexually or perinatally) is associated with an increased risk of head and neck squamous cell carcinoma development [6]. Overall estimates for HPV prevalence in head and neck squamous cell carcinoma are very variable, ranging from 8-100%, but an unusual laryngeal pathologic subtype, verrucous laryngeal carcinoma, has a 100% prevalence of HPV. Tumours of the oropharynx (and in particular, tonsillar tissue) have been found to be three times more likely to be HPV-positive than tumours at other head and neck sites. Women with a history of *in situ* or inva-

sive cervical carcinoma have a two to four-fold increased risk of oral or laryngeal cancer, in addition to increased risks of other cancers associated with HPV. Additional risk factors implicated in cancer of the larynx include chronic laryngitis, chronic gastric reflux and exposure to wood dust, asbestos or ionizing radiation.

Infection with Epstein-Barr virus is important in the etiology of nasopharyngeal cancer. This virus is not found in normal epithelial cells of the nasopharynx, but is present in all nasopharyngeal tumour cells, and even in dysplastic precursor lesions [7] (*Chronic infections*, p56).

Detection

Although many head and neck cancers arise in anatomically accessible areas, delayed diagnosis is common. Symptoms of oral cancer include pain, bleeding, difficulty in opening the mouth, chewing, swallowing and speech, and a swelling in the neck. Early lesions are often painless and present as slightly elevated, velvety red mucosal patches, as punctate lesions, or as indurated small ulcers or growths. In more advanced stages, a large ulceroproliferative mass, with areas of necrosis, and extension to neighbouring structures such as bone, muscles and skin may be evident. Cancers of the oral cavity may be preceded by, and present with, leukoplakias (Fig. 5.92) or with mucosal rigidity and fibrosis, restricted mouth opening and tongue mobility (oral submucus fibrosis). Some 5-15% of patients with cancer of the lip mucosa present with lymph node metastases, compared with more than 50-70% of those with tongue and floor of the mouth cancers. Distant metastases from oral cancer are uncommon. A careful oral examination and palpation of the neck leads to diagnosis, which is confirmed by biopsy.

Oral visual inspection in high-risk individuals leads to early diagnosis of oral precancer [8,9]. However, the effectiveness of organized screening in reducing incidence of and mortality from oral cancer remains to be established.

An asymptomatic high neck mass in an adult is frequently associated with a primary oropharyngeal (tongue base and tonsil) or hypopharyngeal primary tumour. Fine needle aspiration biopsy and careful direct laryn-

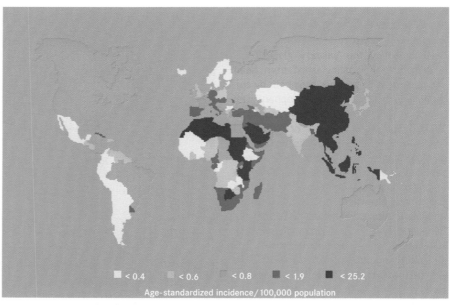

Fig. 5.90 The global incidence of nasopharyngeal cancer in men. This cancer is very common in Southern China.

goscopy in order to identify the primary tumour are mandatory. Frequently, a surgical panendoscopy with tonsillectomy is indicated. Patients with pharyngeal cancers may complain of difficulty in swallowing and hoarseness of voice, particularly in advanced stages. The early symptoms of laryngeal cancer are hoarseness with dysphagia, pain and a neck mass. In most cases, the first sign of nasopharyngeal cancer is a mass in the neck (due to lymph node metastasis). Because the tumour is close to the foramina through which several cranial nerves pass, there may be signs due to their compression, as well as pain, blocked Eustachian tubes and nasal stuffiness. Early detection of nasopharyngeal cancer by screening for elevated antibody titres to Epstein-Barr virus has been widely performed in populations of Southern China, although so far, it is not known whether this procedure can prevent deaths.

Pathology and genetics

Most cancers of the head and neck are squamous cell carcinoma, which may be poorly, moderately or well-differentiated, according to the degree of keratinization (Fig. 5.94). Other variants of squamous cell carcinoma include verrucous carcinoma, sarcamoid squamous cell carcinoma and lymphoepithe-

lioma [10]. The vast majority of nasopharyngeal cancers in endemic regions is comprised of non-keratinizing and undifferentiated histological types, whereas in non-endemic countries, some 30-50% are keratinizing squamous cell carcinomas [11].

Conditions carrying increased risk of head and neck cancer include epithelial differentiation disorders, such as dyskeratosis congenita, and DNA repair deficiency syndromes such as Blooms' syndrome, Fanconi anaemia, ataxia telangiectasia and xeroderma pigmentosum (*Carcinogen activation and DNA repair*, p89).

A strong genetic component to the risk of developing nasopharyngeal cancer is evident. Migrant populations of Chinese or North African origin appear to retain their elevated risk, as do their children, born in a new host country. An association between human leucocyte antigen (HLA) profile and risk of nasopharyngeal cancer has been reported, and a study of affected siblings in Singapore identified a gene locus close to HLA with a 20-fold increased risk for nasopharyngeal cancer.

Cytogenetic abnormalities have been reported in head and neck squamous cell carcinoma, including gain or loss of the Y chromosome and abnormalities at other loci; very

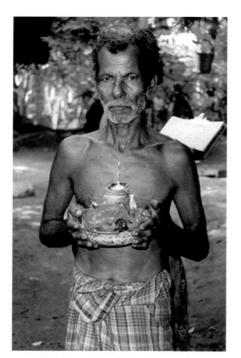

Fig. 5.91 A paan-tobacco chewer in Kerala, South India, with ingredients for betel quid (betel leaf, areca-nut, lime and tobacco). This habit is associated with a high risk of oral cancer.

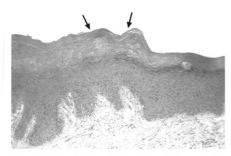

Fig. 5.92 Oral leukoplakia with mild dysplasia; leukoplakia is a precursor to oral cancer.

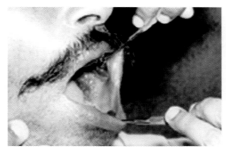

Fig. 5.93 A moderately advanced invasive cancer in the buccal mucosa.

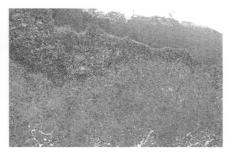

Fig. 5.94 A well-differentiated, invasive squamous cell carcinoma of the larynx.

complex karyotypes are frequent [12] (Fig. 5.96). The genetic alterations observed in oral cancer include activation of proto-oncogenes such as cyclin D1, *MYC*, *RAS*, *EGFR* and inactivation of tumour suppressor genes such as those encoding p16^{INK4A} and p53 and other putative suppressor loci [13]. Early changes include loss of tumour suppressor genes on chromosomes 13p and 9p, followed by 17p. *p53* mutations and overexpression are seen in the progression of preinvasive lesions to invasive lesions. *p53* mutations are more frequently reported in developed (40-50%) than in developing countries (5-25%). Tumours from India and South East Asia are characterized by the involvement of *RAS* oncogenes, including mutation, loss of heterozygosity (*HRAS*) and amplification (*KRAS* and *NRAS*). Various genetic polymorphisms in genes such as *GSTM1* or *CYP450A1* are associated with oral carcinogenesis.

Management

Surgery and radiotherapy have been the mainstay of treatment for oral cancer. Those with early or intermediate tumour stages are treated with curative intent with moderate morbidity while those with more advanced disease are treated with definitive radiation therapy and chemotherapy. Radical surgery aims for tumour-free surgical margins with the preservation of critical anatomical structures. However, a major challenge is reconstruction after resection to preserve function and cosmesis. Definitive radiotherapy is delivered either by external beams of radiation from a telecobalt machine or linear accelerator. The mainstay management of lymph node metastases is by radical neck dissection with or without post-operative radiotherapy. For patients with cancer of the larynx, very early tumours and cancer *in situ* can be managed with local surgery, while early invasive tumours can be managed with radiation therapy. More advanced tumours can be treated primarily with induction chemotherapy or chemoradiotherapy, reserving laryngectomy as a salvage procedure. Early nasopharynx cancer is treated with intensive radiotherapy while more advanced cancers should be treated with a combination of chemoradiotherapy and adjuvant chemotherapy.

Radiotherapy may also be used to sterilize microscopic residual cancer after surgery. In frail patients with accessible tumours (< 3 cm in size), brachytherapy over a 3-5 day period may be curative. Radiotherapy to the head and neck can lead to troublesome side-effects. Acute skin and mucosal inflammation and sometimes ulcerations, as well as superinfection with *Candida* (fungus), may make normal food intake impossible and necessitate use of a feeding tube. Later effects may include loss of taste, reduced and thick saliva production and a dry mouth [14]. Dental hygiene assessment and treatment prior to commencement of radiotherapy are extremely important.

Chemotherapy has not been demonstrated to elicit an overall improvement in survival, although combinations of cytotoxic drugs such as cisplatin, methotrexate, 5-fluorouracil and bleomycin can cause dramatic tumour reduction in 80-90% of cases. A combined approach, chemoradiotherapy, appears to improve overall survival [15].

The most important prognostic factors for oral cancer are regional lymph node involve-ment, size of the primary lesion, primary site of cancer within the oral cavity and age. The presence of a lymph node metastasis is the most important negative prognostic factor in squamous carcinoma of the mouth and pharynx. Aggressive histopathologic features include significant lymphovascular invasion, perineural infiltration or high grade. Overexpression of Bcl-2 is associated with improved survival in head and neck cancer patients undergoing radiation therapy, as well as with better local control and the absence of local lymph node involvement. Abnormalities of 11q13 are associated with a poor prognosis [12].

Overall population based five-year survival from oral cancer is mostly less than 50% (Fig. 5.95) [17]. Females, in general, have a higher

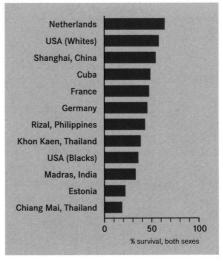

Fig. 5.95 Five-year relative survival after diagnosis of cancer of the oral cavity. USA data include both oral and pharyngeal cancers.

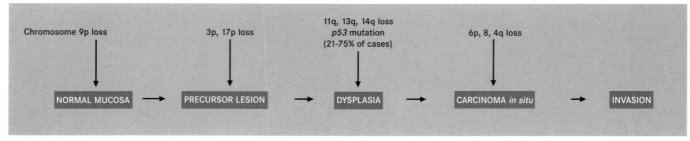

Fig. 5.96 Genetic alterations in squamous cell carcinoma of the head and neck. The accumulation and not necessarily the order of these genetic changes determines progression.

survival rate than males. There has been very little improvement in five-year survival from this cancer, or other head and neck cancers, over the last four decades [18]. Early-stage head and neck cancers have a good cure rate, but over 60% of patients present with advanced disease. Moreover, a significant percentage of patients with squamous cell carcinoma go on to develop a second primary tumour although initially cured. Patients may also face serious reductions in quality of life after definitive surgical therapy; despite improving rehabilitation and reconstructive surgery, residual cosmetic and functional debilities may be significant.

The overall relative survival of laryngeal cancer patients varies between 60 and 70% in Europe and North America, but is lower in developing countries. It is highly dependent on the sub-site of the disease which itself is dependent on the etiological factors involved. In countries with elevated alcohol consumption the prognosis is poorer because there are more tumours of the upper part of the larynx, which have a lower survival.

REFERENCES

1. IARC (1985) *Tobacco habits other than smoking; betel-quid and areca-nut chewing; and some related nitrosamines (IARC Monographs on the Evaluation of Carcinogenic Risks to Humans, Vol. 37)*, Lyon, IARCPress.

2. IARC (1986) *Tobacco Smoking (IARC Monographs on the Evaluation of the Carcinogenic Risk of Chemicals to Humans, Vol. 38)*, Lyon, IARCPress.

3. IARC (1988) *Alcohol drinking (IARC Monographs on the Evaluation of Carcinogenic risks to Humans, Vol. 44)*, Lyon, IARCPress.

4. Merchant A, Husain SS, Hosain M, Fikree FF, Pitiphat W, Siddiqui AR, Hayder SJ, Haider SM, Ikram M, Chuang SK, Saeed SA (2000) Paan without tobacco: an independent risk factor for oral cancer. *Int J Cancer*, 86: 128-131.

5. Steinmetz KA, Potter JD (1991) Vegetables, fruit, and cancer. I. Epidemiology. *Cancer Causes Control*, 2: 325-357.

6. Gillison ML, Koch WM, Shah KV (1999) Human papillomavirus in head and neck squamous cell carcinoma: are some head and neck cancers a sexually transmitted disease? *Curr Opin Oncol*, 11: 191-199.

7. IARC (1997) *Epstein-Barr Virus and Kaposi's Sarcoma Herpesvirus / Human Herpesvirus 8 (IARC Monographs on the Evaluation of Carcinogenic Risks to Humans, Vol. 70)*, Lyon, IARCPress.

8. Fernandez-Garrote L, Sankaranarayanan R, Lence anta JJ, Rodriguez-Salva A, Parkin DM (1995) An evaluation of the oral cancer control programme in Cuba. *Epidemiology*, 6: 428-431.

9. Sankaranarayanan R, Mathew B, Jacob Bj, Thomas G, Somanathan T, Pisani P, Pandey M, Ramadas K, Najeeb K, Abraham E (2000) Early findings from a community-based, cluster randomized, controlled oral cancer screening trial in Kerala, India. The Trivandrum Oral Cancer Screening Study Group. *Cancer*, 88: 664-673.

10. Schantz SP, Harrison LB, Forastiere AA (1997) Tumours of the nasal cavity and paranasal sinuses, nasopharynx, oral cavity and oropharynx. In: DeVita VTJ, Hellman S, Rosenberg SA eds, *Cancer: Principles and Practice of Oncology*, Philadelphia-New York, Lippincott-Raven, 741-799.

11. Chan AT, Teo PM, Johnson PJ (1998) Controversies in the management of locoregionally advanced nasopharyngeal carcinoma. *Curr Opin Oncol*, 10: 219-225.

12. Oh Y, Mao L (1997) Biomarkers in head and neck carcinoma. *Curr Opin Oncol*, 9: 247-256.

13. Schwartz JL (2000) Biomarkers and molecular epidemiology and chemoprevention of oral cancer. *Crit Rev Oral Biol Med*, 11: 92-122.

14. Norman JE de B (1998) Cancers of the head and neck. In: Morris D, Kearsley J, Williams C eds, *Cancer: a comprehensive clinical guide*, Harwood Academic Publishers.

15. Adelstein DJ (1998) Recent randomized trials of chemoradiation in the management of locally advanced head and neck cancer. *Curr Opin Oncol*, 10: 213-218.

16. Khuri FR, Nemunaitis J, Ganly I, Arseneau J, Tannock IF, Romel L, Gore M, Ironside J, MacDougall RH, Heise C, Randlev B, Gillenwater AM, Bruso P, Kaye SB, Hong WK, Kirn DH (2000) a controlled trial of intratumoral ONYX-015, a selectively-replicating adenovirus, in combination with cisplatin and 5-fluorouracil in patients with recurrent head and neck cancer. *Nat Med*, 6: 879-885.

17. Berrino F, Capocaccia J, Estève J, Gatta G, Hakulinen T, Micheli A, Sant M, Verdecchia A, eds (1999) *Survival of Cancer Patients in Europe: The EUROCARE-2 Study (IARC Scientific Publications, No. 151)*, Lyon, IARCPress.

18. Clayman GL, Lippma SM, Laramore GE, Hong WK (1997) Head and neck cancer. In: Holland JF, Bast RC, Morton DL, Frei E, Kufe DW, Weichselbaum RR eds, *Cancer Medicine*, Williams and Wilkins.

WEBSITE

NCI Head and Neck Cancer Homepage:
http://www.cancer.gov/cancer_information/cancer_type/head_and_neck/

LYMPHOMA

SUMMARY

> Malignant lymphomas are classified as either Hodgkin disease or non-Hodgkin lymphoma.

> Hodgkin disease afflicts mainly children and the elderly in developing countries and young adults in more developed countries; 62,000 new cases are diagnosed annually.

> The incidence of malignant non-Hodgkin lymphomas is increasing worldwide; more than 280,000 new cases occur annually, predominantly in more developed countries.

> Burkitt lymphoma is a subtype of malignant B-cell lymphoma common in Africa in regions with endemic malaria. B-cell lymphomas may also be caused by immunosuppression. Both are commonly associated with the Epstein-Barr virus.

> Advances in chemotherapy have led to a five-year survival rate for Hodgkin disease of more than 70% and that for non-Hodgkin lymphomas has increased to 60-70%.

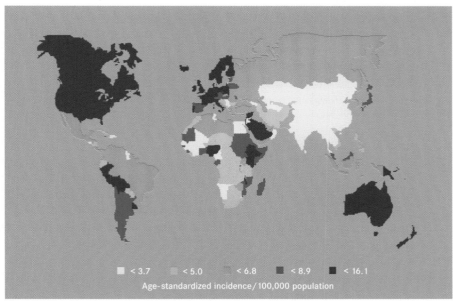

< 3.7   < 5.0   < 6.8   < 8.9   < 16.1

Age-standardized incidence/100,000 population

Fig. 5.97 Global incidence of non-Hodgkin lymphoma in men. The disease is most common in developed countries, although there are areas of moderate to high incidence in some Middle-Eastern countries and in parts of sub-Saharan Africa.

Definition

The term lymphoma covers a heterogeneous group of neoplasms of lymphoid tissue. Traditionally, lymphomas are categorized as either Hodgkin disease or non-Hodgkin lymphoma, these distinct entities having different patterns of behaviour and response to treatment. Within each of these two entities there is a range of diverse subtypes.

Epidemiology

Non-Hodgkin lymphomas are a very varied group of neoplasms. Excluding the types that generally manifest as leukaemias rather than single or multiple aggregates of cells, there are around 287,000 cases of non-Hodgkin lymphoma in the world

per year. More males than females are affected (17.1 cases per 100,000 males compared to 11.2 cases per 100,000 females in the USA) and incidence increases with age. Geographically, non-Hodgkin lymphoma is most common in developed countries (52% of the world total cases, and the seventh most common cancer in more developed countries), although in the developing world there are areas of moderate to high incidence in some Middle-Eastern countries (Saudi Arabia, Israel) and in parts of sub-Saharan Africa (Fig. 5.97). The latter is due to the high incidence of Burkitt lymphoma, an aggressive subtype of non-Hodgkin lymphoma, particularly in children in tropical Africa. Papua New Guinea also has high rates of Burkitt lymphoma.

The incidence rates of non-Hodgkin lymphoma have risen dramatically in the last 20 years, particularly in developed countries, including Western Europe, North America and Australia (Fig. 5.99). This may in part reflect better diagnosis, or

changing classification systems. However, these considerations together do not account for the extent of increase. Likewise, the fact that non-Hodgkin lymphoma is a complication of AIDS (occurring in up to 5-10% of AIDS cases in developed countries) does not completely account for the increasing trend. In contrast to incidence, mortality rates have, in general, been declining as a consequence of improvement in therapy.

Hodgkin disease comprises about 23% of malignant lymphomas worldwide (about 62,000 annual cases). There is a male predominance (sex ratio 1.6:1). In developing countries, Hodgkin disease (predominantly the mixed cellularity subtype) occurs mainly in children and in the elderly, while in developed countries there is a peak in young adults (mainly the nodular sclerosing subtype). The disease is rare in Eastern and South-Eastern Asian populations at any age (Fig. 5.100). The pattern of Hodgkin disease in black Americans more closely resembles that of white

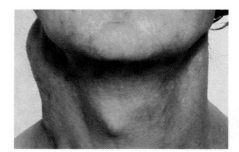

Fig. 5.98 Non-Hodgkin lymphoma in the neck of a patient suffering from AIDS.

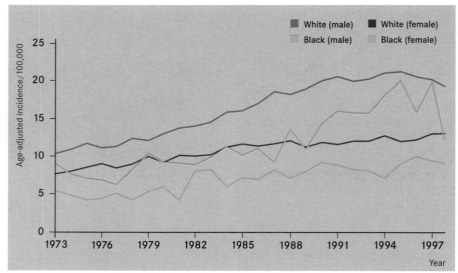

Fig. 5.99 Trends in incidence of non-Hodgkin lymphoma in the USA. Rates are increasing, as they are worldwide.

Americans than that of black Africans, suggesting that socioeconomic conditions may be more important than ethnicity in determining risk. In developed countries, incidence has fallen in the last 20 years [1]. Mortality rates are also decreasing, probably due to effective therapy.

Etiology

Non-Hodgkin lymphoma

Patients with HIV/AIDS (Box: *Tumours associated with HIV/AIDS*, p60), or who have received immunosuppressant therapy (*Immunosuppression*, p68), have a higher risk of developing non-Hodgkin lymphoma [2]. Viral infections such as HIV-1, HTLV-1 and EBV are also associated with non-Hodgkin lymphoma. Infection of the stomach with *Helicobacter pylori* is associated with gastric lymphoma. Agricultural work with possible exposure to pesticides (particularly chlorophenoxy herbicides) and occupational exposure to solvents or fertilizers have been implicated but have yet to be confirmed as causes of non-Hodgkin lymphoma.

There is an increased risk of non-Hodgkin lymphoma among persons with a family history of lymphoma or haematologic cancer [2].

Hodgkin disease

A subset of Hodgkin disease cases, particularly the mixed cellularity type, has been linked to the Epstein-Barr virus (EBV) [2]. Overall, around 45% of cases may be attributable to EBV. The presence of EBV in tumours seems also to be related to age and socioeconomic circumstances. EBV is involved in the etiology of Burkitt lymphoma,

especially in cases in tropical Africa, where over 95% of tumours contain the virus. The proportion of EBV-positive tumours is much less in the sporadic cases of Hodgkin disease occurring in Europe and North America. The singular geographic distribution of Burkitt lymphoma is not explicable on the basis of EBV alone, however, since infec-

tion by the virus is ubiquitous. Suspicion has fallen upon intense malaria infection as predisposing to Burkitt lymphoma in the presence of EBV infection. Chronic exposure to wood or wood products has also been associated with increased risk. The risk of Hodgkin disease is also increased in patients with HIV infection.

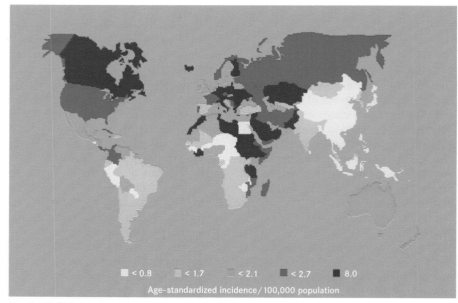

Fig. 5.100 Global incidence of Hodgkin disease in men. The disease is rare in Eastern and South-Eastern Asian populations.

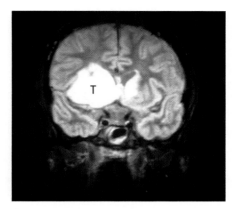

Fig. 5.101 Nuclear magnetic resonance imaging scan of the brain of an HIV-infected patient showing a large lymphoma (T) in the basal ganglia.

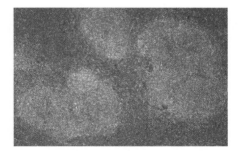

Fig. 5.102 Follicular non-Hodgkin lymphoma.

Detection

The most common presentation of non-Hodgkin lymphoma is painless swelling of the lymph nodes in the neck, armpit or groin. This may be associated with so called "B symptoms" of unexplained fever, night sweats and weight loss. Other related symptoms include fatigue, malaise, pruritus, or those related to organ involvement (e.g. indigestion caused by gastric lymphoma). Extranodal involvement is common. Diagnosis is dependent on obtaining a tissue biopsy, usually by excision of an enlarged node. Pathological review is crucial to identify the type of lymphoma.

Staging practice commonly involves full blood count, biochemical screen including tests of liver function and renal function, chest X-ray, CT scan of neck, chest, abdomen and pelvis, and bone marrow biopsy. In some instances, lumbar puncture may be required to assess central nervous system involvement, which can have important therapeutic implications. Hodgkin disease usually originates in lymph nodes (often in the neck), and only rarely spreads outside primary lymphoid tissues. Diagnosis requires a tissue biopsy, ideally a whole lymph node. Many of the staging techniques employed are the same as for non-Hodgkin lymphoma, and the Ann Arbor staging system is used to provide treatment planning information and aid response assessment.

Pathology and genetics

Lymphomas constitute a diverse range of diseases (Table 5.10). Advances in molecular biology, genetics and immunology have meant that there have been profound changes in the classification of neoplasms of lymphoid cells over the last 20 years. In the Revised European-American Lymphoma classification system, three broad categories are recognized: Hodgkin disease and T-cell and B-cell non-Hodgkin lymphomas. A WHO classification has recently been published [3]; prior to this the International Working Formulation (IWF) was the most widely used classification.

Non-Hodgkin lymphomas are derived from B or T lymphocytes. In Western countries, B-cell tumours are more common (about 75% of cases), whereas T-cell tumours are less common but are generally more biologically aggressive. T-cell tumours are relatively more common in East Asia. A follicular lymphoma is defined by the retention of the follicles within a lymph node (Fig. 5.102), whereas a diffuse lymphoma results from the infiltration of the node with effacement of the follicles by the malignant cells. The size of the malignant lymphocytes is also important.

In contrast, Hodgkin disease is characterized by the presence of multinucleate, giant so-called "Reed-Sternberg" cells, which may be rare in a particular biopsy specimen and the surrounding cell proliferation. The Revised European-American Lymphoma classification [4] also covers Hodgkin disease; four histological subtypes of Hodgkin disease are recognized: nodular sclerosing, mixed cellularity, lymphocyte predominance and lymphocyte depletion.

Many cytogenetic and molecular abnormalities in non-Hodgkin lymphoma, in particular Burkitt lymphoma, are caused by a translocation of the oncogene *C-MYC* from chromosome 8 to either the immunoglobulin heavy chain region on chromosome 14 or to one of the light chain loci on chromosomes 2 or 22 [5]. Technological innovations, such as microarrays, are revolutionizing diagnosis (Fig. 5.105).

Genetic abnormalities in Hodgkin disease are less frequently described, perhaps due to the paucity of malignant cells in the biopsy specimen.

Diagnosis	% of total cases
Diffuse large B-cell lymphoma	30.6
Follicular lymphoma	22.1
MALT lymphoma	7.6
Mature T-cell lymphomas (except ALCL)	7.6
Chronic lymphocytic leukaemia/small lymphocytic lymphoma	6.7
Mantle cell lymphoma	6.0
Mediastinal large B-cell lymphoma	2.4
Anaplastic large cell lymphoma (ALCL)	2.4
Burkitt lymphoma	2.5
Nodal marginal zone lymphoma	1.8
Precursor T lymphoblastic	1.7
Lymphoplasmacytic lymphoma	1.2
Other types	7.4

Table 5.10 Frequency of various types of non-Hodgkin lymphoma.

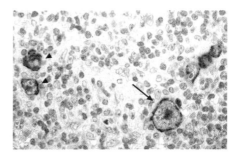

Fig. 5.103 Classical Hodgkin disease. Hodgkin (arrow) and Reed-Sternberg cells (arrowhead) infected by the Epstein-Barr virus strongly express the virus-encoded latent membrane protein LMP1.

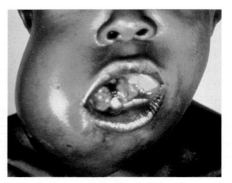

Fig. 5.104 Burkitt lymphoma presenting as a large tumour of the jaw in an African child.

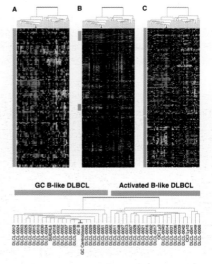

Fig. 5.105 Microarray technology can be used to identify two major patterns of gene expression among diffuse large B-cell lymphomas (DLBCL). One displays a germinal centre T-cell signature, the other an activated B-cell signature. The analysis is based on the expression of about 12,000 genes.

Management

The treatment of non-Hodgkin lymphomas depends on the pathological classification, the stage of the disease, the biological behaviour of the disease, the age of the patient and their general health [6,7]. In general, it is convenient to classify the pathological entities into indolent, aggressive or highly aggressive non-Hodgkin lymphomas, which parallels the IWF classification.

Indolent non-Hodgkin lymphomas

About two-thirds of indolent lymphomas in developed countries are follicular lymphomas and often present as advanced stage disease in patients over 50 years of age. This disease usually runs a prolonged course and is rarely cured (except in a few cases of early stage disease). The median survival is eight to ten years, and therapy is often palliative. Local radiotherapy is useful for early stage localized disease, and other options include alkylating agents, purine analogues, combination chemotherapy, interferon, monoclonal antibodies and high dose therapy with autologous stem cell support. Lymphoplasmacytoid lymphoma is often associated with a monoclonal paraprotein and, like small lymphocytic lymphoma/chronic lymphocytic leukaemia, will often respond to alkylating agent therapy. Marginal zone lymphomas can be divided into those at nodal sites (monocytoid B-cell lymphomas) and those at extra nodal sites, usually mucosal (gastrointestinal, lung, salivary gland etc.) when they are termed MALT (mucosa associated lymphoid tissue) lymphomas. Gastric MALT lymphomas are often associated with *H. pylori* infection and appropriate antibiotic treatment often results in resolution of the lymphoma, albeit over six to twelve months [8]. Splenic marginal zone lymphoma, often called splenic lymphoma with villous lymphocytes, presents with splenomegaly and usually responds to splenectomy.

Aggressive non-Hodgkin lymphomas

Diffuse large cell lymphoma is the most common of these types. Biologically these tumours are more aggressive than the indolent lymphomas, although remission and even cure may be obtained with appropriate therapy in a significant proportion of cases. The factors associated with prognosis in these patients are age, stage, performance status, the presence of extranodal disease, and lactic dehydrogenase levels, which can be summed to form the International Prognostic Index. Using this model, four risk groups can be identified with a predicted five-year survival of 73%, 51%, 43% and 26% when treated with conventional anthracycline based chemotherapy (e.g. cyclophosphamide, doxorubicin, vincristine, prednisone). Attempts to improve outcome with more aggressive chemo-

Histology	Translocations
Small cleaved cell, follicular	t(14;18)(q32;q21.3)
Small non-cleaved cell (Burkitt and non-Burkitt)	t(8;14)(q24;q32) t(2;8)(p12;q24) t(8;22)(q24;q11)
Centrocytic/mantle cell	t(11;14)(q13;q32)
Large cell, diffuse, B-cell	t(3;14)(q27;q32) t(3;22)(q27;q11) t(2;3)(p12;q27)
Small lymphocytic/extranodal (MALT)	t(11;18)(q21;q21.1)
Large cell, anaplastic	t(2;5)(p23;q35)

Table 5.11 Some common chromosomal translocations found in non-Hodgkin lymphomas.

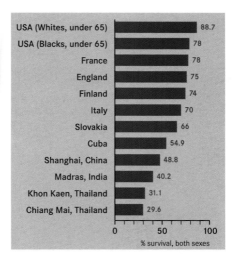

Fig. 5.106 Five-year relative survival rates after diagnosis of Hodgkin disease.

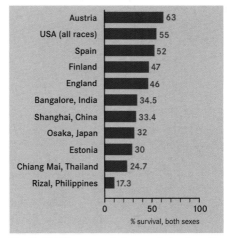

Fig. 5.107 Five-year relative survival rates after diagnosis of non-Hodgkin lymphoma.

therapy protocols, so-called "second and third generation regimens", have met with little success. However, the introduction of the International Prognostic Index may help to identify patients who will benefit from more aggressive strategies [9]. In patients who relapse after conventional therapy, and who still have "sensitive disease", high-dose chemotherapy with stem cell rescue appears to offer a reasonable salvage option.

Hodgkin disease
In contrast to non-Hodgkin lymphomas, the management of Hodgkin disease is usually dictated by the stage of disease rather than the histology [10,11]. Most centres would use radiotherapy for early stage (IA or IIA) disease, although there is a trend towards considering limited chemotherapy as an option. All other stages should have chemotherapy, and the traditional "gold standard" MOPP (mustine, vincristine, procarbazine and prednisone) therapy has been superseded by ABVD (adriamycin [doxorubicin], bleomycin, vinblastine and dacarbazine) which appears to be as efficacious without the adverse effects (particularly related to fertility and the development of second malignancies). The German Hodgkin Disease Study Group has proposed a prognostic model for advanced stage disease, and has identified seven factors which influence outcome. These are age, sex, histology, B symptoms, number of involved sites, bulk of disease and erythrocyte sedimentation rate. Using such models it may be possible to identify poor prognosis patients who will benefit from more aggressive high-dose therapies, such as Stanford V (doxorubicin, vinblastine, mustard, bleomycin, vincristine, etoposide and prednisone) or BEACOPP (bleomycin, etoposide, adriamycin [doxorubicin], cyclophosphamide, oncovin [vincristine], procarbazine and prednisone) from the outset (*Medical oncology*, p281).

Survival for both Hodgkin disease and non-Hodgkin lymphomas has improved markedly with time, in response to the development of more effective chemotherapy and bone marrow transplantation. Five-year survival after diagnosis of non-Hodgkin lymphoma patients in most developed countries is more than 50%, but only 17-35% in developing countries (Fig. 5.107). Currently, survival of Hodgkin disease patients is related to extent of disease at diagnosis; overall, at five years it is between 70% and 90% in North America and Europe, but only 30-55% in developing countries (Fig. 5.106).

REFERENCES

1. Cartwright RA, Gilman EA, Gurney KA (1999) Time trends in incidence of haematological malignancies and related conditions. *Br J Haematol*, 106: 281-295.

2. Baris D, Zahm SH (2000) Epidemiology of lymphomas. *Curr Opin Oncol*, 12: 383-394.

3. Jaffe ES, Lee Harris N, Stein H, Vardiman JW, eds (2001) *World Health Organization Classification of Tumours. Pathology and Genetics of Tumours of Haematopoietic and Lymphoid Tissues*, Lyon, IARCPress.

4. Harris NL, Jaffe ES, Stein H, Banks PM, Chan JK, Cleary ML, Delsol G, Wolf-Peeters C, Falini B, Gatter KC (1994) A revised European-American classification of lymphoid neoplasms: a proposal from the International Lymphoma Study Group. *Blood*, 84: 1361-1392.

5. Macintyre EA, Delabesse E (1999) Molecular approaches to the diagnosis and evaluation of lymphoid malignancies. *Semin Hematol*, 36: 373-389.

6. Bierman PJ, Armitage JO (1996) Non-Hodgkin's lymphoma. *Curr Opin Hematol*, 3: 266-272.

7. Pinkerton CR (1999) The continuing challenge of treatment for non-Hodgkin's lymphoma in children. *Br J Haematol*, 107: 220-234.

8. Zucca E, Bertoni F, Roggero E, Cavalli F (2000) The gastric marginal zone B-cell lymphoma of MALT type. *Blood*, 96: 410-419.

9. International Non-Hodgkin's Lymphoma Prognostic Factors Project (1993) A predictive model for aggressive non-Hodgkin's lymphoma. The International Non-Hodgkin's Lymphoma Prognostic Factors Project. *N Engl J Med*, 329: 987-994.

10. Horwitz SM, Horning SJ (2000) Advances in the treatment of Hodgkin's lymphoma. *Curr Opin Hematol*, 7: 235-240.

11. Aisenberg AC (1999) Problems in Hodgkin's disease management. *Blood*, 93: 761-779.

LEUKAEMIA

SUMMARY

> Leukaemia is the eleventh most common cancer worldwide with more than 250,000 new cases each year. It typicallyresults from malignant transformation of white blood cells or their precursors. Subtypes are identified on the basis of the cell of origin (lymphocytic or myeloid, etc.) and clinical course (acute or chronic).

> The etiology of leukaemia is largely unknown, although a small proportion of cases is attributable to treatment with anticancer drugs or exposure to ionizing radiation. The genetic characteristics of many leukaemias have been elucidated.

> Treatment of acute leukaemia has made muchg progress and helped to establish general principles of cancer chemotherapy and management.

> Survival varies greatly according to type, with acute lymphoblastic leukaemia patients having a five-year survival rate of up to 70%, whilst for those with acute myeloid leukaemia it is only 20-30%.

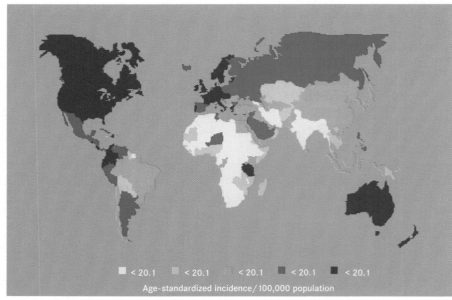

< 20.1   < 20.1   < 20.1   < 20.1   < 20.1
Age-standardized incidence/100,000 population

Fig. 5.108 Global incidence of leukaemia in women.

Definition

Leukaemias involve clonal, neoplastic proliferation of immature cells, or blasts, of the haematopoietic system. Principal subtypes are identified on the basis of malignancy involving either lymphoid (B-cells and T-cells) or myeloid (i.e. granulocytic, erythroid and megakaryocytic) cells, and upon whether disease is acute or chronic in onset [1].

Epidemiology

Leukaemias comprise about 3% of all incident cancers worldwide, with about 257,000 new cases occurring annually. Incidence rates for all types taken together vary from about 1 to 12 per 100,000 population. A relatively high incidence is evident in the USA, Canada, Western Europe, Australia and New Zealand, whilst rates are generally low in most African and Asian countries with rates less than half those in the former group (Fig. 5.108). The trends in overall incidence of leukaemia have generally been stable or slowly increasing. However, a substantial reduction in death rates from leukaemias, particularly in childhood, have been observed since the 1960s, thanks to advances in treatment and consequent improvement in survival.

Leukaemia has a peak in incidence in the first four years of life, which is predominantly due to acute lymphoblastic leukaemia (ALL), the most common paediatric malignancy, accounting for nearly 25% of all such disease. After infancy, there is a steep decline in rates of leukaemia with age, lowest incidence being at age 15 to 25, after which there is an exponential rise up to age 85 (Fig. 5.110). The frequency of leukaemia per 100,000 individuals at risk at age 85 is more than 300 times that for those in the second decade of life.

The overall incidence of acute leukaemia is 4 cases per 100,000 population, the usual form of the disease in adults being acute myeloid leukaemia (AML) accounting for 70% of all cases. The more differentiated, or chronic forms of leukaemia, are predominantly adult diseases, rarely occurring below the age of 30, then increasing progressively in incidence with age. Chronic myelogenous leukaemia (CML) accounts for 15-20% of all cases of leukaemia, with a worldwide incidence of 1-1.5 cases per 100,000 population. For patients over 50, chronic lymphocytic leukaemia (CLL) is the dominant type of leukaemia. All types of leukaemia combined cause some 195,000 deaths worldwide.

Etiology

The cause of most leukaemias is not known. A range of risk factors has been predominantly, although not exclusively, associated with particular leukaemia subtypes. Ionizing radiation (nuclear bombs, medical procedures, [e.g. 2, 3]) and occupational exposure to benzene are associated with acute myeloid leukaemia.

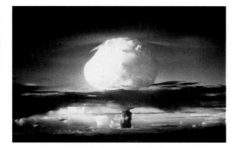

Fig. 5.109 The immediate aftermath of a nuclear explosion. An increased incidence of leukaemia and some other cancer types occurred amongst the survivors of the bombing of Hiroshima and Nagasaki.

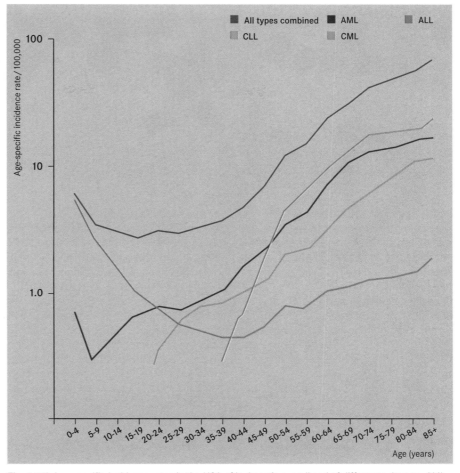

Fig. 5.110 Age-specific incidence rates in the USA of leukaemia overall and of different subtypes. AML = acute myeloid leukaemia, ALL = acute lymphoblastic leukaemia, CLL = chronic lymphocytic leukaemia, CML = chronic myelogenous leukaemia. Note the high incidence of ALL in children.

Leukaemia (mainly acute myeloid) may occur in a small proportion of cancer patients treated with chloroambucil, cyclophosphamide, melphalan, thiotepa, treosulphan or etoposide, as well as certain combination chemotherapy (*Medicinal drugs*, p48). Leukaemia has followed induction of aplastic anaemia by the antibiotic, chloramphenicol. Certain risk factors, such as Down's syndrome, have been identified for childhood leukaemia, but generally the causes of the disease are not known. Some studies have shown a risk of childhood leukaemia with exposure to high level residential extremely low frequency electromagnetic fields, but causality has not been established [4].

Infection with the virus HTLV-I has been established as a cause of leukaemia. This virus is responsible for adult T-cell leukaemia, a disease mainly observed in tropical countries and Japan, and rarely in the USA and Europe. In experimental animals, particularly in mice, there are many retroviruses which can cause a variety of leukaemias, but such retroviruses have not been identified in humans.

Detection

In the case of the myeloid leukaemias, the primary manifestations result from suppression of normal haematopoiesis. This causes anaemia, leading to weakness, leukopenia (decreased numbers of white blood cells) resulting in an increased frequency of infection, and thrombocytopenia (decreased numbers of platelets)

resulting in increased risk of haemorrhage. Patients with chronic myelogenous leukaemia, usually adults aged 30-50, present with slow onset of symptoms of anaemia, weight loss and massive enlargement of the spleen.

In the case of lymphoid malignancies, the primary effect is on the host immune response, with an increased susceptibility to infection and, in the advanced stages, interference with bone marrow function. Children with acute lymphoblastic leukaemia (or young adults with acute myeloid leukaemia) may present with anaemia, features of infection and bleeding, which are of rapid onset. Enlargement of the liver and spleen is common. Patients with

acute lymphoblastic leukaemia additionally present with bone and joint pain and multiple lymph node enlargement (lymphadenopathy). Chronic lymphocytic leukaemia presents with multiple lymph node enlargement, with or without splenic enlargement. As the disease progresses, anaemia sets in slowly. For leukaemia generally, diagnosis may be suspected from examination of peripheral blood and is confirmed by bone marrow examination.

Pathology and genetics

Leukaemias are clonal neoplastic proliferations of immature haematopoietic cells characterized by aberrant or arrested differentiation. Leukaemic cells rapid-

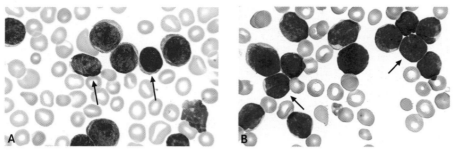

Fig. 5.111 (A) Bone marrow smear from a patient with acute lymphoblastic leukaemia. (B) Precursor B lymphoblastic leukaemia. This bone marrow smear shows several lymphoblasts with a high nuclear cytoplasmic ratio and variably condensed nuclear chromatin.

ly accumulate in the bone marrow, ultimately replacing most of the normal cells and circulate in the peripheral blood. As already noted, leukaemias are categorized in relation to clinical course and cell lineage. In addition, reference may be made to the morphology, degree of differentiation, immuno-phenotype and genetic character of the malignant cell population [5].

Acute lymphoblastic leukaemia (Fig. 5.111 A) is characterized by lymphoblasts, most often of B-cell phenotype (about 80% of both childhood and adult disease), and distinguished from lymphomas which involve more mature lymphoid cells and primarily inhabit lymph nodes and spleen. Precursor B-lineage blasts (Fig. 5.111B) exhibit a range of cytogenetic abnormalities. The t(9;22) translocation, which results in fusion of the "breakpoint cluster region" BCR on chromosome 22 and the cytoplasmic tyrosine kinase ABL on chromosome 9, is associated with poor prognosis. B-lineage blasts express surface antigens such as CD10, CD19 and CD22 [6]. Precursor

T-cell phenotypes, expressing CD2, CD3, CD5 and CD7 surface antigens, make up 15-20% of acute lymphoblastic leukaemia cases.

Acute myeloid leukaemia (Fig. 5.113) is a clonal expansion of myeloid blasts in bone marrow, blood or other tissue [5]. The disease is heterogeneous and consists of several subtypes, which can be identified by karyotype [7]. Approximately 20% of patients have favourable cytogenetic abnormalities, including t(8;21), inv(16) and t(15;17). These types are uniformly distributed across age groups, suggesting a distinct etiologic agent. Approximately 30% (predominantly patients over the age of 50, with a progressive increase in incidence with age) have unfavourable cytogenetic abnormalities, which include deletions of the long arm of chromosome 5 or 7 or trisomy of chromosome 8. Approximately half have diploid cytogenetics and an intermediate prognosis. A significant fraction of the favourable cytogenetic group and a small fraction of the diploid group can be cured with combination chemotherapy. One subtype, acute promyelocytic leukaemia, is characterized by t(15;17) (Fig. 5.114, 5.116). The break point on chromosome 17 occurs within the gene for an all-trans-retinoic acid receptor (RARα) and generates the fusion gene PML-RARα on the derivative chromosome 15 [8].

Chronic myelogenous leukaemia (Fig. 5.117) originates in an abnormal pluripotent bone marrow stem cell [5,9]. The disease has a cytogenetic hallmark, the Philadelphia chromosome, namely t(9;22) (Fig. 5.115). This translocation relocates the C-ABL proto-oncogene from chromosome 9 to the breakpoint cluster region on chromosome 22 to form a new hybrid BCR-ABL oncogene. The BCR-ABL transcript is present in over 95% of chronic myelogenous leukaemia cases, and encodes a novel tyrosine kinase that is involved in pathogenesis, possibly by perturbing apoptosis.

Chronic lymphocytic leukaemia is now recognized as being the same disease entity as small cell lymphoma, being a neoplasm of monomorphic small, round B-lymphocytes in the peripheral blood,

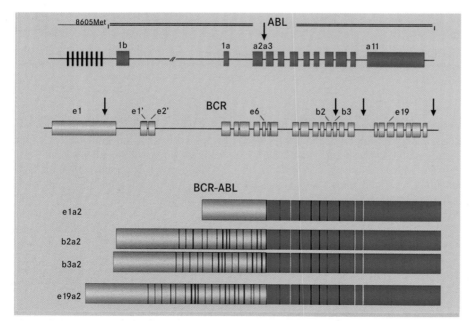

Fig. 5.112 Schematic representation of the disruption of the ABL and BCR genes in the t(9;22)(q34;21) chromosomal abnormality found in chronic myeloid leukaemia, which results in the formation of oncogenic BCR-ABL fusion genes. Segments of DNA which are transcribed to form the protein (exons) are labelled a, b and e. Arrows mark the breakage points.

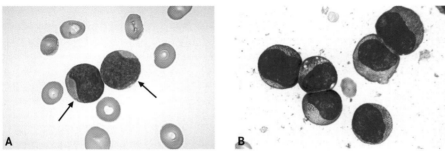

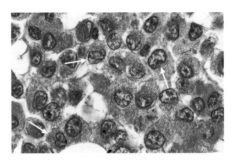

Fig. 5.113 Acute myeloid leukaemia; agranular myeloblasts **(A)** and granulated myeloblasts **(B)**.

Fig. 5.114 A bone marrow biopsy of acute promyelocytic leukaemia. Abnormal promyelocytes have abundant hypergranulated cytoplasm. The nuclei are generally round to oval, several being irregular and invaginated.

bone marrow and lymph nodes, admixed with prolymphocytes and paraimmunoblasts, usually expressing CD5 and CD23 surface antigen [5]. Chronic lymphocytic leukaemia [10] is a heterogeneous disease which can occur in an indolent form with very little progression, whilst at the other extreme it may present with severe bone marrow failure and a poor prognosis.

Management

Remarkable progress in the understanding and treatment of leukaemia has been made in the past century [11]. In the first instance, this generalization refers specifically to paediatric disease. Prior to 1960, leukaemia was the leading cause of death from malignancy in children under 15; currently, more than 80% of children with acute lymphoblastic leukaemia can be cured with chemotherapy [12]. Treatment involves induction of remission with combinations of agents (such as vincristine, daunorubicin, cytarabine [cytosine arabinoside], L-asparaginase, 6-thioguanine, and steroids) followed by consolidation, maintenance and post-remission intensification therapy to eradicate residual leukaemic blast cells, aiming at cure. Intensive supportive care throughout treatment is of major importance. Prophylactic treatment with intrathecal methotrexate injections, with or without craniospinal irradiation, is mandatory in the management of acute lymphoblastic leukaemia to prevent possible involvement of or relapse in the central nervous system. The use of radiotherapy is limited because of the potential long-term side-effects, particularly effects on the growth of the young child and the risk of second malignancies. The adult form of acute lymphoblastic leukaemia is also susceptible to therapy and can be cured, (although not as readily as childhood leukaemia), with intensive combination therapy [13].

For acute leukaemia in adults, the initial aim of management is to stabilize the patient with supportive measures to counteract bone marrow failure which leads to anaemia, neutropenia and thrombocytopenia. Most patients with leukaemia who die in the first three weeks of diagno-

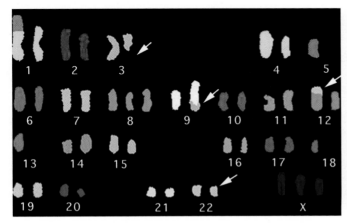

Fig. 5.115 Spectral karyotyping of a chronic myeloid leukaemia case reveals a variant Philadelphia chromosome involving translocations between chromosomes 3, 9, 12 and 22. Secondary changes involving chromosomes 1, 5, 8, 18 and X are also seen, indicating advanced disease.

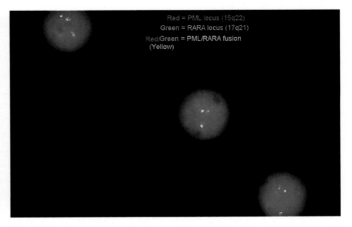

Fig. 5.116 Acute promyelocytic leukaemia cells with t(15;17)(q22;q12) translocation. Fluorescence *in situ* hybridization with probes for PML (red) and RARα (green) demonstrates the presence of a PML/RARα fusion protein (overlapping of red and green = yellow signal) resulting from the breakage and fusion of these chromosome bands.

THE MOLECULAR DETECTION OF MINIMAL RESIDUAL DISEASE

The accurate identification of submicroscopic numbers of residual cancer cells has important clinical implications for many malignancies. Treatment efficacy is frequently monitored by the disappearance of tumour cells from the blood or bone marrow, and while microscopic examination of marrow is extremely valuable, it is a relatively insensitive tool for the detection of this "minimal residual disease". Much effort has therefore been directed towards the development of sensitive and specific molecular assays of minimal residual disease with the main molecular strategy involving the use of the polymerase chain reaction (PCR) technique. Since its inception in 1985, this technique has been widely utilized as a means of amplifying (i.e. repeatedly copying) target DNA sequences up to a million-fold with great specificity, due to the use of oligonucleotide primers unique to the sequence of interest (Saiki RK et al., *Science*, 230: 1350-54, 1985). Numerous studies have reported the use of PCR-based techniques for detecting minimal residual disease in a range of cancers including leukaemia, lymphoma, breast cancer, prostate cancer and melanoma. Detection limits of one cancer cell amongst 10^4-10^6 normal cells can routinely be achieved, a level of sensitivity that is some 3 to 5 orders of magnitude more sensitive than conventional techniques. PCR can, therefore, serve as an ultrasensitive tool for accurately identifying small numbers of cancer cells in patient samples.

The potential clinical utility of minimal residual disease detection for both haematopoietic malignancies and solid tumours has been demonstrated in a range of studies. For example, there is now strong evidence that the level of minimal residual disease measured in the first few months of therapy in children undergoing treatment for acute lymphoblastic leukaemia is highly prognostic of outcome (Cave H et al., *New Engl J Med*, 339: 591-8, 1998; van Dongen JJM et al., *Lancet*, 352:1731-8, 1998). These studies have utilized clone-specific rearrangements of antigen receptor genes as the targets for PCR amplification of genomic DNA. Other studies, particularly those involving solid tumours, have relied on reverse transcriptase (RT-PCR) amplification of cancer-specific messenger RNA as an indicator of the presence of residual disease. While these RT-PCR techniques offer valuable clinical information, especially in tumour staging, there is currently enormous variability when comparing inter-laboratory assays. Such ultrasensitive methods can be plagued by false positivity of normal bone marrow and peripheral blood samples, particularly since it has been shown that by using RT-PCR it is possible to detect the expression of otherwise tissue-specific genes in any cell type. This process has been termed "illegitimate" transcription (Chelly J et al., *Proc Natl Acad Sci USA*, 86: 2617-21, 1989) and in order to avoid this it may be necessary to employ multiple markers for use in residual disease testing.

The molecular detection of minimal residual disease undoubtedly offers great potential as an aid in the management of cancer patients. However, there is also an urgent need to develop appropriate treatment strategies for use in conjunction with this new tool. It is at present unknown whether patients in whom persistent minimal residual disease is detected will benefit from adjuvant therapy, although a number of clinical trials have begun in order to address this question. Critical to their success will be the use of uniform and standardized minimal residual disease methods that provide accurate and reproducible results. The use of multiple molecular minimal residual disease markers and the development of "real-time" PCR assays (e.g. Kwan E et al., *Brit J Haem*, 109: 430-34, 2000) may be particularly helpful in this regard.

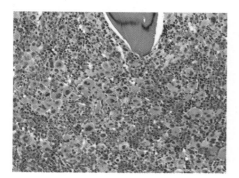

Fig. 5.117 A biopsy section from a patient with chronic myelogenous leukaemia, myeloid blast phase. Sheets of abnormal megakaryocytes, including micromegakaryocytes, are illustrated. Blasts infiltrate between the abnormal megakaryocytes.

sis die of infection or, less commonly, bleeding. Large gains in survival in acute myeloid leukaemia have come with the introduction of improved supportive care and combination chemotherapy. Effective drugs include cytarabine, anthracyclines, etoposide, mitoxantrone, amsacrine, 6-thioguanine and 5-azacytidine. Intensive therapy is applied until a complete remission is achieved with <5% blasts in the marrow. Typically, 50-70% of patients achieve complete remission. Bone marrow transplantation from an HLA-matched donor is one form of therapy for the late intensification of remission in younger patients with acute myeloid leukaemia.

Retinoic acid derivatives, particularly *all-trans*-retinoic acid, given by mouth can induce haematologic remissions of acute promyelocytic leukaemia without significant myelosuppression, although this therapy itself is not curative.

Treatment is essentially palliative in chronic leukaemias. The major risk to patients with chronic myelogenous leukaemia is transformation to an acute phase, which resembles acute leukaemia and is referred to as the blastic phase of the disease. This development is highly malignant and refractory to conventional treatment and results in a short survival. The anti-tyrosine kinase compound "Gleevec", or

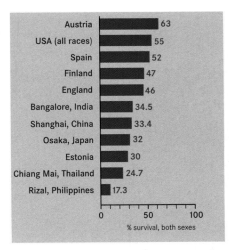

Fig. 5.118 Five-year relative survival rates after diagnosis of leukaemia.

ST-571, α-interferon and arabinosyl cytosine, a chemotherapeutic agent, can produce complete cytogenetic remissions, prevention of blastic transformation and significant prolongation of survival, with a small fraction of patients being cured. However, the development of resistance to ST-571 may cause patients to relapse within a few months [14]. Without treatment, the life span for the average individual with chronic lymphocytic leukaemia is under five years from diagnosis. The treatment for this disease historically was with alkylating agents. Recently the purine antimetabolite, fludarabine, has substantially increased the frequency and the quality of response to chemotherapy. A new monoclonal antibody directed against the T-cell antigen, CD52

("CAMPATH"), has been found to be highly effective in this disease. At the present time, combinations of antimetabolite, alkylating agents and monoclonal antibody in various combinations and sequences are being aggressively investigated and the prognosis for patients in this category of disease has substantially improved.

Generally, 60-70% of patients with acute lymphoblastic leukaemia, and 20-30% of patients with acute myeloid leukaemia (Fig. 5.118) survive in excess of five years. Approximately 30-50% of the patients diagnosed with chronic leukaemias survive five years. Survival is much poorer in developing countries (generally <20%) due to the cost and lack of access to these complex therapeutic regimes.

REFERENCES

1. Freireich EJ, Lemak N (1991) *Milestones in Leukemia Research and Therapy*, Baltimore, Maryland, Johns Hopkins University Press.

2. IARC (2000) *Ionizing Radiation, Part 1: X- and Gamma Radiation and Neutrons (IARC Monographs on the Evaluation of Carcinogenic Risks to Humans, Vol. 75)*, Lyon, IARCPress.

3. Noshchenko AG, Moysich KB, Bondar A, Zamostyan PV, Drosdova VD, Michalek AM (2001) Patterns of acute leukaemia occurrence among children in the Chernobyl region. *Int J Epidemiol*, 30: 125-129.

4. IARC (2002) *Non-ionizing Radiation, Part 1: Static and Extremely Low-Frequency Electric and Magnetic Fields (IARC Monographs on the Evaluation of Carcinogenic Risks to Humans, Vol. 80)*, Lyon, IARCPress.

5. Jaffe ES, Harris NL, Stein H, Vardiman JW, eds (2001) *World Health Organization Classification of Tumours. Pathology and Genetics of Tumours of Haematopoietic and Lymphoid Tissues*, Lyon, IARCPress.

6. Farhi DC, Rosenthal NS (2000) Acute lymphoblastic leukemia. *Clin Lab Med*, 20: 17-28, vii.

7. Estey EH (2001) Therapeutic options for acute myelogenous leukemia. *Cancer*, 92: 1059-1073.

8. Alcalay M, Orleth A, Sebastiani C, Meani N, Chiaradonna F, Casciari C, Sciurpi MT, Gelmetti V, Riganelli D, Minucci S, Fagioli M, Pelicci PG (2001) Common themes in the pathogenesis of acute myeloid leukemia. *Oncogene*, 20: 5680-5694.

9. Faderl S, Talpaz M, Estrov Z, Kantarjian HM (1999) Chronic myelogenous leukemia: biology and therapy. *Ann Intern Med*, 131: 207-219.

10. Keating MJ, O'Brien S (2000) Conventional management of chronic lymphocytic leukemia. In: Foa R, Hoffbrand, AV eds, *Reviews in Clinical and Experimental Haematology*, 118-133.

11. Brenner MK, Pinkel D (1999) Cure of leukemia. *Semin Hematol*, 36: 73-83.

12. Pui C-H, Campana D, Evans WE (2001) Childhood acute lymphoblastic leukaemia - current status and future perspectives. *Lancet Oncology*, 2: 597-607.

13. Kantarjian HM, O'Brien S, Smith TL, Cortes J, Giles FJ, Beran M, Pierce S, Huh Y, Andreeff M, Koller C, Ha CS, Keating MJ, Murphy S, Freireich EJ (2000) Results of treatment with hyper-CVAD, a dose-intensive regimen, in adult acute lymphocytic leukemia. *J Clin Oncol*, 18: 547-561.

14. McCormick F (2001) New-age drug meets resistance. *Nature*, 412: 281-282.

WEBSITE

NCI Leukemia Homepage:
http://www.cancer.gov/cancer_information/cancer_type/leukemia/

PANCREATIC CANCER

SUMMARY

> Pancreatic cancer is the 14th most common cancer worldwide, with approximately 216,000 new cases per year. Highest incidence rates occur in more developed countries.

> In countries with high smoking prevalence, more than 40% of cases is attributable to tobacco consumption. Familial risk, often involving hereditary pancreatitis, is evident in up to 10% of cases.

> No effective early diagnostic test or population-based screening procedure is available.

> KRAS and p53 gene mutations are implicated in the development of the most common type, ductal adenocarcinoma.

> Five-year survival rates are poor (less than 5%) and the vast majority of pancreatic cancer patients die within a year of clinical diagnosis.

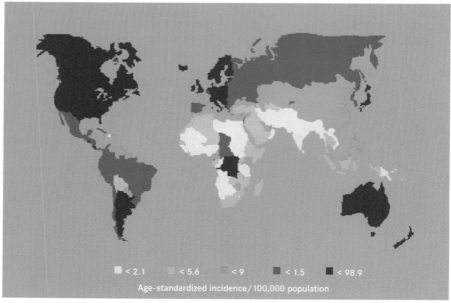

Age-standardized incidence/100,000 population

< 2.1   < 5.6   < 9   < 1.5   < 98.9

Fig. 5.119 Global burden of pancreatic cancer in women. Incidence rates are generally high in the Americas, Europe and Australia.

Definition

Most (90%) pancreatic tumours are adenocarcinomas arising from the ductal epithelium of the exocrine pancreas. Some 70% of these tumours develop in the head of the pancreas. Endocrine tumours of the pancreas, which are rare, arise from the islets of Langerhans.

Epidemiology

Pancreatic cancer is the 14th most common cancer worldwide, with more than 216,000 new cases occurring each year. Groups with the highest incidence include black male Americans, New Zealand Maoris, Korean Americans and native female Hawaiians, as well as the male population of Kazakhstan. The lowest rates are in Ahmedabad Indians and in the populations of some African countries such as Tanzania and Guinea, and in those of Papua New Guinea and Sri Lanka [1] (Fig. 5.119). In the developed world, incidence has risen three-fold since the 1920s, stabilizing in the late 1970s. Pancreatic cancer is significantly more common in younger men than in younger women, the sex ratio varying from between 1.25-1.75:1 [2]. However, the gender bias decreases with increasing age. Prognosis is very poor and pancreatic cancer causes some 213,000 deaths each year. In the USA, cancer of the pancreas is now the fourth leading cause of cancer-related death in both men and women.

Etiology

About 30% of cases of pancreatic cancer are attributable to smoking. Cigarette smokers develop this disease two to three times more often than non-smokers. A number of dietary factors have been putatively connected with pancreatic cancer, including a diet low in fibre and high in meat and fat, and a diet rich in the heterocyclic amines present in cooked meat and fish. Smoking and diet are believed to account for much of the increased incidence observed since the 1920s. Coffee consumption was once thought to be a risk factor, but recent studies have not established significant associations.

Working in mines, metalworks, sawmills, chemical plants, coke plants, rubber factories, and the petrochemical industry have been variously indicated as risk factors, as has exposure to solvents, napthylamine, benzidine, and polychlorinated biphenyl used in transformers. Other risk factors include chronic and hereditary pancreatitis, diabetes (although the significance of the latter is much weaker if cases of recent onset are excluded) and cirrhosis. The sex ratio of pancreatic cancer incidence has suggested a role for sex hormones in disease development [3].

Detection

The diagnosis of pancreatic cancer is rarely made at an early stage and the most frequently recognized clinical symptoms are usually portents of advanced dis-

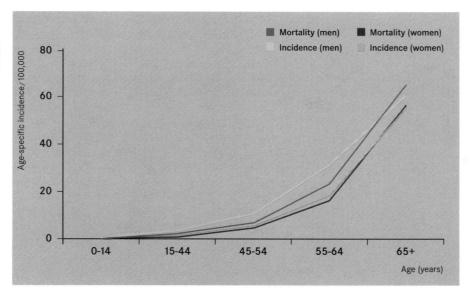

Fig. 5.120 Age-specific incidence and mortality of pancreatic cancer in men and women in North America. The small differences between incidence and mortality reflect the very poor prognosis of this disease. Men are somewhat more frequently affected than women.

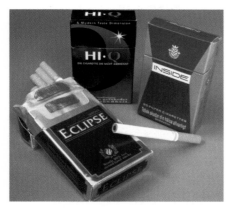

Fig. 5.121 Cigarette smoking is one of the main risk factors for pancreatic cancer.

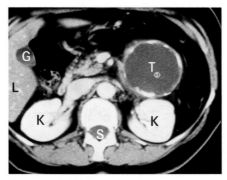

Fig. 5.122 A CT image of a mucinous cystic neoplasm in the pancreas. The thick wall shows focal calcification. T = tumour, K = kidney, L = liver, S = spinal cord, G = gallbladder.

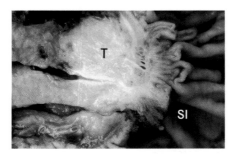

Fig. 5.123 Surgical specimen of a pancreatic ductal adenocarcinoma (T) in the head of the pancreas. SI = small intestine.

ease. These include unexplained weight loss, nausea, diarrhoea, weakness, jaundice (caused by compression of the intrapancreatic common bile duct) and upper abdominal and back pain. Mature onset diabetes in the absence of a family history may also indicate the possibility of pancreatic cancer. Insulin antagonism by tumour-produced factors (islet amyloid peptide, glucagon and somatostatin) is believed to be the cause [4]. Whilst 85% of patients have systemic disease or locally unresectable tumours on clinical evaluation, some 25% have symptoms compatible with upper abdominal disease up to six months prior to diagnosis and 15% of patients seek medical attention more than six months prior to diagnosis [5].

Ultrasonography is the initial diagnostic imaging system currently employed, although visualization of the body and tail of the pancreas is often unsatisfactory due to the presence of intestinal gas. Computed tomography (CT) scanning allows clearer imaging of the tail and body and can detect lesions of >1 cm with accuracy, as well as secondary signs of pancreatic cancer, such as dilation of common bile and main pancreatic ducts, invasion of surrounding structures, liver secondaries, lymphadenopathy and ascites (Fig. 5.122).

Cytological or histological confirmation is obtained from samples taken during endoscopic retrograde cholangiopancreatography, or by fine needle aspiration and core biopsy under radiological guidance. However, it is often difficult to obtain histological proof for small lesions, which have the best potential for curative surgery. Patients who are candidates for surgery undergo ultrasound and laparoscopy, which identify those with small peritoneal and liver nodules below the resolution of current imaging.

Pathology and genetics

The first stage of neoplasia (Fig. 5.124), flat hyperplasia, entails the columnarization of the ductal epithelium. It is estimated that as many as half the normal elderly population may exhibit flat hyperplasia [6]. This may advance to papillary hyperplasia, the presence of a crowded mucosa with a folded structure, which may possess varying degrees of cellular and nuclear abnormalities. True carcinoma is characterized by invasion of the ductal wall and a desmoplastic response, i.e. acollagenous, inflammatory reaction, such that the tumour may comprise less than 25% cancer cells. The major histological types include benign microcystic serous adeno-

ma, tumours of uncertain biological behaviour, including mucinous cystic tumour and solid cystic tumour, as well as malignant forms, such as adenocarcinoma, microcystic serous adenocarcinoma and mucinous cystadenocarcinoma.

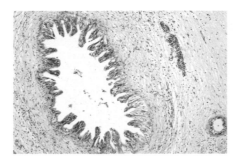

Fig. 5.124 Pancreatic duct showing high-grade intraepithelial neoplasia.

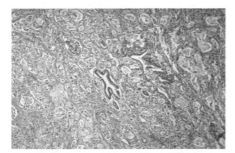

Fig. 5.125 Well-differentiated, mucus-secreting invasive ductal adenocarcinoma of the pancreas.

Gene	Chromosome	Mechanism of alteration	% of cancers
Oncogenes			
KRAS	12p	Point mutation	> 90
MYB, AKT2, AIB1	6q, 19q, 20q	Amplification[1]	10-20
ERBB2 (HER/2-neu)	17q	Overexpression	70
Tumour suppressor genes			
p16^{INK4A}	9p	Homozygous deletion	40
		Loss of heterozygosity and intragenic mutation	40
		Promoter hypermethylation	15
p53	17p	Loss of heterozygosity and intragenic mutation	50-70
DPC4	18q	Homozygous deletion	35
		Loss of heterozygosity and intragenic mutation	20
BRCA2	13q	Inherited intragenic mutation and loss of heterozygosity	7
MKK4	17p	Homozygous deletion, loss of heterozygosity and intragenic mutation	4
LKB1/STK11	19p	Loss of heterozygosity and intragenic mutation, homozygous deletion	5
ALK5 and TGF βR2	9q, 3p	Homozygous deletion	4
DNA mismatch repair			
MSH2, MLH1, others	2p, 3p, others	Unknown	<5

[1]In cases of amplification, it is generally not possible to identify the key oncogene unambiguously due to the involvement of multiple genes.

Table 5.12 Genetic alterations found in pancreatic ductal carcinoma.

Hereditary conditions

Around 10% of cases of pancreatic cancer exhibit some degree of familial risk, this fraction being the highest for any human organ site [6]. In this context, germline mutations have been identified in a number of oncogenes and tumour suppressors, including *BRCA2*, (predisposing to breast and pancreatic carcinoma) and p16^{INK4} (predisposing to melanoma and pancreatic cancer) (Table 5.13). The *STK11/LKB1* gene is mutated in Peutz-Jeghers syndrome patients, this group being predisposed to pancreatic cancer [7]. Sufferers from hereditary pancreatitis experience attacks of acute pancreatitis from an early age and face a 40% risk of cancer by age 70. Most families appear to possess one of two mutations in the cationic trypsinogen gene (chromosome 7q35) [8] which cause the production of a mutant protein. Consequently, associated enzymatic activity is not inactivated and is hypothesized to contribute to autodigestion of the pancreas and pancreatitis; cancer may then be a consequence of the prolonged inflammatory microenvironment in the pancreas. Other conditions which carry increased susceptibility to pancreatic cancer include intraductal papillary mucinous tumour, familial adenomatous polyposis, familial atypical multiple mole melanoma syndrome, cystic fibrosis, heritable nonpolyposis colon cancer and Li-Fraumeni syndrome [9].

Sporadic genetic alterations

Mutations of the *KRAS* oncogene, most frequently of codon 12, occur in 95% of sporadic pancreatic tumours and may represent an early molecular event in pancreatic carcinogenesis; they may also be present in some benign lesions [6]. Alterations in tumour suppressor genes such as *p53*, p16^{INK4}, *DCC* and *DPC4/SMAD4* have also been detailed, as has overexpression of some growth factors e.g. EGF, TGFα, TGFβ1-3, αFGF and their receptors [10, 11]. Mutation of the gene encoding c-erbB2 is associated with late stage pancreatic adenocarcinoma and that encoding c-erbB3 with shorter postoperative survival. (Table 5.12) [12].

Management

Currently, surgery offers the patient the only chance of cure. However, treatment can improve quality of life by controlling the symptoms and complications of this disease. Pancreaticoduodenectomy, the "Whipple procedure", involves the resection of all of the duodenum with a short section of the jejunum, the pancreatic head, cholecystectomy and excision of the common bile duct and a distal gastrectomy followed by reconstruction.

Hereditary condition	Mode of inheritance	Gene (chromosomal location)	Lifetime risk of pancreatic cancer
Early onset familial pancreatic adenocarcinoma associated with diabetes (Seattle family)	Autosomal dominant	Unknown	About 30%; 100-fold increased risk of pancreatic cancer; high risk of diabetes and pancreatitis
Hereditary pancreatitis	Autosomal dominant	Cationic trypsinogen (7q35)	30%; 50-fold increased risk of pancreatic cancer
FAMMM: familial atypical multiple mole melanoma	Autosomal dominant	$p16^{INK4A}/CMM2$ (9p21)	10%
Familial breast cancer	Autosomal dominant	BRCA2 (13q12-q13)	5-10%; 6174delT in Ashkenazi Jews, 999del5 in Iceland
Ataxia telangiectasia (heterozygote state)	Autosomal recessive	ATM, ATB, others (11q22-q23)	Unknown; somewhat increased
Peutz-Jeghers syndrome	Autosomal dominant	STK11/LKB1 (19p)	Unknown; somewhat increased
HNPCC: hereditary non-polyposis colorectal cancer	Autosomal dominant	MSH2 (2p), MLH1 (3p), others	Unknown; somewhat increased
Familial pancreatic cancer	Possibly autosomal dominant	Unknown	Unknown; 5-10 fold increased risk if a first-degree relative has pancreatic cancer

Table 5.13 Hereditary conditions predisposing to the development of pancreatic cancer.

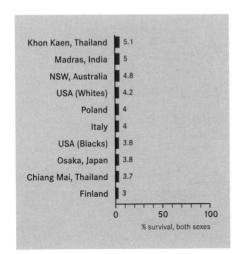

Fig. 5.126 Five-year relative survival rates after diagnosis of pancreatic cancer. Less than 5% of patients survive more than five years.

However, morbidity remains high at 30-40%, and complications are common. In a total pancreatectomy, the entire pancreas, as well as the duodenum, common bile duct, gallbladder, spleen, and nearby lymph nodes are removed. Symptoms of unresectable tumours may also be relieved by surgery.

In Western countries and Japan, different classification systems for staging of pancreatic cancer have evolved, resulting in difficulties in assessing the efficacy of different therapies. Both to overcome the barriers inherent in international classification systems and to achieve a universal prospective data acquisition, a uniform International Documentation System for Exocrine Pancreatic Cancer has been developed by an international group of pancreatologists [13].

Palliative treatment is required for the treatment of jaundice, gastric outlet obstruction and pain. Adjuvant chemotherapy (5-fluorouracil and folinic acid), but not adjuvant radiotherapy, appears to confer a slight survival benefit. Confirmatory trials with newer agents are ongoing. Despite substantial evidence for hormone-dependence of pancreatic cancer, there are no data currently confirming a role for estrogens, androgens, cholecystokinin or their antagonists in clinical treatment of exocrine pancreatic cancer [2].

Survival is poor and the majority of pancreatic cancer patients die within one year of diagnosis, although five-year survival rates can reach >30% for lesions of less than 2 cm, negative lymph nodes and clear surgical margins. In American males, for example, the overall five-year survival rate is 3.7%, and for females, 4.4% (Fig. 5.126).

REFERENCES

1. Jorgensen J, Imrie CW (1998) Pancreatic cancer. In: Morris D, Kearsley J., Williams C. eds, *Cancer: a comprehensive clinical guide*, Harwood Academic Publishers.

2. Andren-Sandberg A, Hoem D, Backman PL (1999) Other risk factors for pancreatic cancer: hormonal aspects. *Ann Oncol*, 10 Suppl 4: 131-135.

3. Gold EB, Goldin SB (1998) Epidemiology of and risk factors for pancreatic cancer. *Surg Oncol Clin N Am*, 7: 67-91.

4. Barkin JS, Goldstein JA (1999) Diagnostic approach to pancreatic cancer. *Gastroenterol Clin North Am*, 28: 709-22, xi.

5. DiMagno EP (1999) Pancreatic cancer: clinical presentation, pitfalls and early clues. *Ann Oncol*, 10 Suppl 4: 140-142.

6. Hilgers W, Kern SE (1999) Molecular genetic basis of pancreatic adenocarcinoma. *Genes Chromosomes Cancer*, 26: 1-12.

7. Hruban RH, Petersen GM, Goggins M, Tersmette AC, Offerhaus GJ, Falatko F, Yeo CJ, Kern SE (1999) Familial pancreatic cancer. *Ann Oncol*, 10 Suppl 4: 69-73.

8. Whitcomb DC (1999) The spectrum of complications of hereditary pancreatitis. Is this a model for future gene therapy? *Gastroenterol Clin North Am*, 28: 525-541.

9. Lowenfels AB, Maisonneuve P (1999) Pancreatic cancer: development of a unifying etiologic concept. *Ann N Y Acad Sci*, 880: 191-200.

10. Sakorafas GH, Tsiotou AG, Tsiotos GG (2000) Molecular biology of pancreatic cancer; oncogenes, tumour suppressor genes, growth factors, and their receptors from a clinical perspective. *Cancer Treat Rev*, 26: 29-52.

11. Schutte M (1999) DPC4/SMAD4 gene alterations in human cancer, and their functional implications. *Ann Oncol*, 10 Suppl 4: 56-59.

12. Klöppel G, Hruban RH, Longnecker MP, Adler G, Kern SE, Partanen TJ (2000) Ductal adenocarcinoma of the pancreas. In: Hamilton SR, Aaltonen LA eds, *World Health Organization Classification of Tumours. Pathology and Genetics of Tumours of the Digestive System*, Lyon, IARCPress, 221-230.

13. Birk D, Beger HG, Fortnagel G, Hermanek P (1997) International documentation system for pancreatic cancer (IDS). The future in pancreatic cancer evaluation. *Digestion*, 58: 578-579.

WEBSITES

NCI Pancreatic Cancer Homepage:
http://www.cancer.gov/cancer_information/cancer_type/pancreatic/

The Johns Hopkins Medical Institution, Pancreatic Cancer Homepage:
http://www.path.jhu.edu/pancreas/

MELANOMA

SUMMARY

> Approximately 133,000 new cases of malignant melanoma are diagnosed worldwide each year.

> The risk of developing this highly malignant skin tumour varies markedly according to racial background (skin pigmentation) and geography (sunlight-derived ultraviolet irradiation); highest incidence rates occur in white populations in Australia.

> In Nordic countries, a steep increase in melanoma incidence has been attributed to excessive sun exposure during vacations in Southern countries.

> Prognosis for patients with early-stage melanoma is very good, while metastatic melanoma is largely resistant to current therapies.

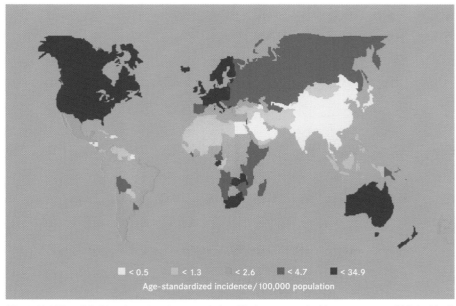

< 0.5   < 1.3   < 2.6   < 4.7   < 34.9
Age-standardized incidence/100,000 population

Fig. 5.127 The global burden of melanoma of the skin in women. Incidence rates are high in North America, Europe, Australia and New Zealand.

Definition

Melanoma is a malignant proliferation of melanocytes, the pigment-forming cells of the skin, which is the site of most (>95%) disease.

Epidemiology

There are about 133,000 new cases of melanoma worldwide each year, of which almost 80% are in North America, Europe, Australia and New Zealand. Incidence is similar in men and in women.

Malignant melanoma of the skin occurs predominantly in white-skinned populations ("Caucasians") living in countries where there is high intensity ultraviolet radiation but this malignancy afflicts to some degree all ethnic groups (Fig. 5.127). Assessed in relation to skin colour, melanoma incidence falls dramatically as skin pigmentation increases and the disease is very rare in dark skinned people. The highest incidence of melanoma occurs in Australia where the population is predominantly white, there is an average of six hours of bright sunlight every day of the year and there is an essentially outdoors lifestyle. The lifetime risk of developing melanoma in Australia is 4-5% in men and 3-4% in women.

Dark-skinned people have a low risk of melanoma. In Africa and South America, the sole of the foot, where the skin is not pigmented, is the most frequent site affected in the context of a low incidence. Asian peoples have a low risk of melanoma despite their paler skins; naevi in Asian people, though common, are predominantly of the acral-lentiginous type which have low malignant potential. Marked increases in incidence and mortality are being observed in both sexes in many countries (e.g. Fig. 5.128), even where rates were formerly low, such as Japan. In the Nordic countries, for example, this averages some 30% every five years. Mortality rates are slightly higher in men than in women, with Australia and New Zealand registering rates of 4.8 and 5.3 for men, and 2.5 and 3.2 for women, respectively [1].

Etiology

It is estimated that 80% of melanoma is caused by ultraviolet damage [2] to sensitive skin, i.e. skin that burns easily, fair or reddish skin, multiple freckles, skin that does not tan and develops naevi in response to early sunlight exposure. Prevention of melanoma is based on limitation of exposure to ultraviolet radiation, particularly in the first 20 years of life (*Reduction of exposure to UV radiation*, p141).

Ultraviolet radiation is particularly hazardous when it involves sporadic intense exposure and sunburn. Most damage caused by sunlight occurs in childhood and adolescence, making this the most important target group for prevention programmes. Established but rare risk factors include congenital naevi, immunosuppression and excessive use of solaria. While melanoma may occur anywhere on the skin, the majority of melanoma in men is

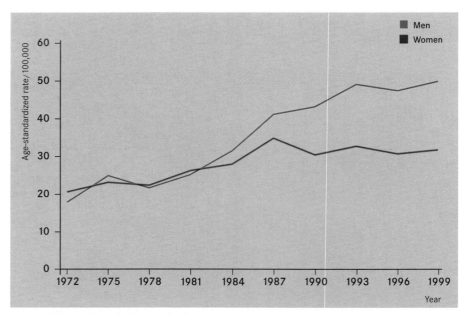

Fig. 5.128 Trends in the incidence of malignant melanoma in New South Wales, Australia.
New South Wales Central Cancer Registry, Australia

on the back, while in women the majority is on the legs. This difference in site incidence is not completely explained by differential exposure to ultraviolet light.

Detection

Melanoma is usually asymptomatic but a person with melanoma sometimes complains of an intermittent itch. Pain, bleeding and ulceration are rare in early melanoma. A melanoma often arises from a pre-existing pigmented lesion of the skin (a mole or "naevus") but these tumours can also develop in unblemished skin. The common predisposing skin lesions are dysplastic naevi, junctional and dermal naevi and blue naevi. However, the risk for melanoma development from mature dermal, junctional and blue naevi is quite small, estimated at approximately 1 in 200,000. Congenital naevi are also known precursors of melanoma but the risk for malignant change is related specifically to the size of the naevus. Naevi greater than 20 mm in diameter and, in particular, the large bathing trunk naevi have a high risk of malignant degeneration. The highest risk naevus is the dysplastic (atypical) naevus. These are naevi that are larger than six mm in diameter, have irregular pigmentation, an ill-defined margin and often exist in multiples. Of particular risk is the dysplastic naevus syndrome (familial atypical mole syndrome) (Fig. 5.130), in which the patient may have more than 100 of these irregular naevi; risk is highest in those patients with dysplastic naevus syndrome who have a near relative diagnosed with melanoma.

The clinical features of melanoma are asymmetry (A), a coastline border (B), multiple colours and quite often some areas of blue/black pigmentation (C), and a diameter greater than six mm (D). As the melanoma progresses, part or all of the lesion will become elevated (E) (Figs. 5.131, 5.132). This ABCDE system has been the basis for clinical diagnosis for melanoma for many years.

Surface microscopy [4] (dermoscopy, epiluminescence microscopy) has developed as an aid to the clinical diagnosis of melanoma. In this technique, the skin surface is rendered translucent by the application of oil and a hand-held instrument providing magnification of at least ten times is used to view the internal details of the tumour. Many additional characteristics, such as pseudopods, radial streaming, blue/grey veil, peripheral black dots and multiple colours are visible and have been used in diagnostic systems now readily accessible to the clinician with an interest in cutaneous diagnosis (Fig. 5.133).

Pathology and genetics

Melanocytes occur primarily in the skin (where more than 95% of cases of melanoma occurs) but are also found in the mucous membranes of the mouth, nose, anus and vagina and, to a lesser extent, the intestine; melanocytes are also present in the conjunctiva, the retina and the meninges. The morphological classification system for melanoma defines four types: superficial spreading melanoma, nodular melanoma, acral-lentiginous melanoma, and lentigo maligna melanoma. However, this classification has been superseded by a system based on the histopathological parameters of the excised lesion. Melanoma is now classified essentially on the vertical diameter of

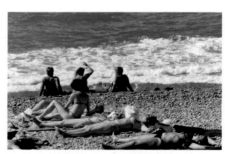

Fig. 5.129 Intentional sun exposure by holidaymakers on a beach in Nice, France. The majority of cases of melanoma is attributable to sporadic, excessive exposure to ultraviolet radiation which may clinically manifest as sunburn.

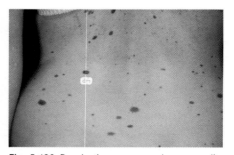

Fig. 5.130 Dysplastic naevus syndrome, predisposing to non-familial malignant melanoma. The patient shows atypical cutaneous naevi, usually exceeding 5mm in diameter, with variable pigmentation and ill defined borders.

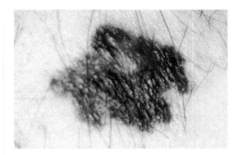

Fig. 5.131 Primary melanoma with a coastline border and multiple colours, including classic blue black pigmentation.

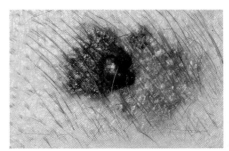

Fig. 5.132 Melanoma with an elevated nodule.

nosis. Alterations in the cyclin-dependent kinase PITSLRE have been identified in advanced melanomas [8]. The recent discovery of a role for the *BRAF* gene in melanoma illustrates the impact of large scale international collaboration [9].

Management

Treatment of primary melanoma is essentially surgical and is related specifically to the tumour thickness measurement. The primary tumour is excised with a margin of normal skin, the excision being based on the tumour thickness measurement [10]. As the primary melanoma becomes thicker (deeper), the risk for metastatic spread rises and thus survival outcomes are related specifically to the tumour thickness measurement (Fig. 5.134).

Melanoma metastasizes via the lymphatic system and also via the systemic circulation. Approximately 50% of melanomas metastasize first to the lymph nodes, thus making the management of lymph node metastases an important part of the treatment. Elective lymph node dissection (i.e. prophylactic removal of lymph nodes) is now rarely practised in the management of primary melanoma. The standard management for lymph nodes in patients with primary melanoma is an observation policy and therapeutic node dissection if lymph nodes become involved. However, selective lymphadenectomy [11] is under clinical trial at the present time. This tech-

the lesion from the granular cell layer of the epidermis to the deepest detectable melanoma cell (tumour thickness). In recent years, one additional criterion, ulceration, has been shown to be important in prognosis and is included in the AJCC/UICC classification system (Table 5.14).

While it is clear that the genetic make-up of the melanoma-prone population is very important, few melanomas can be ascribed to specific genetic defects in these populations. While 10% of melanoma patients have a first degree relative affected, less than 3% of melanomas in Australia (where the incidence of melanoma is high) can be ascribed to an inherited gene defect [3]. Familial melanoma is even more rare in lower incidence countries.

Loss-of-function mutations in the human melanocortin-1 receptor (MC1-R) have been associated with red hair, fair skin and decreased ability to tan [5], all physical characteristics which affect susceptibility to skin cancer. About 20% of melanoma-prone families possess germline mutations in the *CDKN2A* gene, which encodes p16INK4A [6]. Mutations in the gene encoding CDK4 have been identified but are extremely rare [7].

Genes identified as having a role in sporadic melanoma development include *CDKN2A* and *PTEN*, while chromosomal regions 1p, 6q, 7p and 11q may also be involved [6]. About 20% of melanomas possess mutations in the *p53* gene. Nodular melanomas display amplification of the *MYC* oncogene. Inactivation of p16INK4A is associated with a poorer prog-

Classification		Surgical excision margins
Tis	*in situ* melanoma/no invasion of the dermis	5 mm
T1	≤ 1 mm (in thickness)	10 mm
T2	1.1 mm – 2.0 mm	10 mm
T3	2.1 mm – 4.0 mm	Minimum 10 mm, maximum 20 mm
T4	> 4 mm	Minimum 20 mm, maximum 30 mm
Each T level is classified: A – if ulceration is present B – if no ulceration is present		There is no evidence that a margin greater than 1 cm improves survival but it may decrease local recurrence.

Table 5.14 Classification of melanoma (American Joint Committee on Cancer/International Union Against Cancer) and corresponding recommended excision margins.

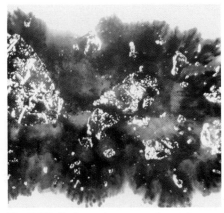

Fig. 5.133 Surface microscopy of a melanoma, showing pseudopods, blue-grey veil and multiple colours.

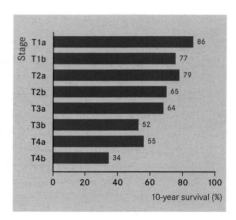

Fig. 5.134 Ten-year relative survival for melanoma, according to stage.

nique enables mapping of the lymphatics in the skin by lymphoscintigraphy: radioactive tracer is injected at the site of the primary and its flow through the skin to the first lymph node that takes up the tracer (the sentinel node) is identified. This lymph node is then removed for histopathological examination; only patients with positive lymph nodes are subjected to full lymph node dissection. However, pending completion of an international trial, the survival benefit of this technique is unknown.

Metastatic melanoma

The greater the number of nodes involved, the higher the risk of systemic metastases and poor prognosis. As the thickness of the melanoma increases and as the number of lymph nodes involved rises, the risk of systemic metastases becomes greater. Melanoma metastasizes widely, with the lungs, liver and brain being the most common sites. Vitiligo (a skin condition characterized by failure to form melanin) is a favourable prognostic sign in metastatic melanoma. At the present time, only a small proportion of people (<5%) live more than two years once systemic metastases become evident [12]. The mainstay for the treatment of systemic metastases is chemotherapy. However, no highly effective single agent or combination has yet been developed and metastatic melanoma is characterized by drug resistance [13]. Spontaneous regression of melanoma, as a result of natural and induced immune rejection, is seen in about 0.4% of cases and this has lead to increasing interest in immunotherapy [14] (*Medical oncology*, p281). At the present time this modality remains experimental, although response rates of 15-20% to cytokines, such as interferon-α and interleukin-2, have been reported, and clinical trials of vaccines containing whole cells, lysates, dendritic cells or melanoma-associated antigens, such as MAGE, TRP and MART, are underway [15].

REFERENCES

1. Ferlay J, Bray F, Parkin DM, Pisani P (2001) *Globocan 2000: Cancer Incidence and Mortality Worldwide (IARC Cancer Bases No. 5)*, Lyon, IARCPress.

2. IARC (1992) *Solar and Ultraviolet Radiation (IARC Monographs on the Evaluation of Carcinogenic Risks to Humans, Vol. 55)*, Lyon, IARCPress.

3. Aitken JF, Duffy DL, Green A, Youl P, MacLennan R, Martin NG (1994) Heterogeneity of melanoma risk in families of melanoma patients. *Am J Epidemiol*, 140: 961-973.

4. Steiner A, Pehamberger H, Wolff K (1987) In vivo epiluminescence microscopy of pigmented skin lesions. II. Diagnosis of small pigmented skin lesions and early detection of malignant melanoma. *J Am Acad Dermatol*, 17: 584-591.

5. Schaffer JV, Bolognia JL (2001) The melanocortin-1 receptor: red hair and beyond. *Arch Dermatol*, 137: 1477-1485.

6. Pollock PM, Trent JM (2000) The genetics of cutaneous melanoma. *Clin Lab Med*, 20: 667-690.

7. Goldstein AM, Chidambaram A, Halpern A, Holly EA, Guerry ID, Sagebiel R, Elder DE, Tucker MA (2002) Rarity of CDK4 germline mutations in familial melanoma. *Melanoma Res*, 12: 51-55.

8. Halachmi S, Gilchrest BA (2001) Update on genetic events in the pathogenesis of melanoma. *Curr Opin Oncol*, 13: 129-136.

9. Davies H, Bignell GR, Cox C, Stephens P, Edkins S et al. (2002) Mutations of the *BRAF* gene in human cancer. *Nature*, 417: 949-954.

10. National Health and Medical Research Council, ed. (1999) *Clinical Practice Guidelines. The Management of Cutaneous Melanoma*.

11. Morton DL (2001) Lymphatic mapping and sentinel lymphadenectomy for melanoma: past, present and future. *Ann Surg Oncol*, 8: 22S-28S.

12. Coates AS (1992) Systemic chemotherapy for malignant melanoma. *World J Surg*, 16: 277-281.

13. Helmbach H, Rossmann E, Kern MA, Schadendorf D (2001) Drug-resistance in human melanoma. *Int J Cancer*, 93: 617-622.

14. Weber JS, Aparicio A (2001) Novel immunologic approaches to the management of malignant melanoma. *Curr Opin Oncol*, 13: 124-128.

15. Hersey P (2002) Advances in the non-surgical treatment of melanoma. *Expert Opin Investig Drugs*, 11: 75-85.

WEBSITE

The Melanoma Foundation, Australia:
http://www.med.usyd.edu.au/medicine/melanoma/

THYROID CANCER

SUMMARY

> Cancer of the thyroid gland is relatively rare, but incidence is increasing in most developed countries. About 120,000 cases occur annually.

> Apart from ionizing radiation, environmental causes have not been well characterized. In Eastern Europe (Belarus, Ukraine, Russia), several hundred children developed thyroid cancer following the Chernobyl accident.

> Prognosis is usually good (around 90% five-year survival for some tumour types), even when lymph node metastases are present.

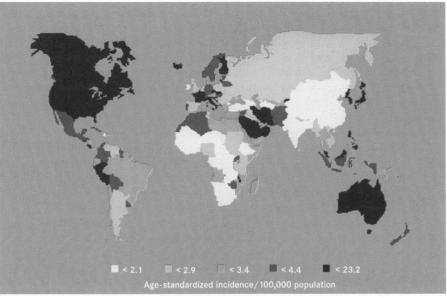

< 2.1   < 2.9   < 3.4   < 4.4   < 23.2

Age-standardized incidence/100,000 population

Fig. 5.135 Global differences in the incidence of thyroid cancer in women.

Definition
Most thyroid cancers are well-differentiated malignancies, which are predominantly papillary (80-85%), and to a lesser extent, follicular (10-15%) and Hürthle cell carcinomas (3-5%). Anaplastic carcinoma and medullary carcinoma are rare.

Epidemiology
Carcinoma of the thyroid gland is an uncommon cancer although it is the most common malignancy of the endocrine system (Fig. 5.135). Generally, thyroid cancer accounts for approximately 1% of total cancer cases in developed countries. There are about 122,000 new cases per year worldwide.

Incidence of this disease is particularly high in Iceland and Hawaii, where the rate is nearly twice that in North European countries, Canada and USA. In Hawaii, the incidence rate of thyroid cancer in all ethnic groups is higher than in the same ethnic group living in their country of origin and is particularly high among Chinese males and Filipino females. Thyroid tumours are rare in children, less than one case per million per year in most developed countries; the age-specific incidence rates increase rapidly with age (Fig. 5.137). In the past three decades, incidence rates have been increasing in most developed countries, while mortality rates have been slowly decreasing. In the year 2000, the annual mortality rate per 100,000 people was 0.3 for men and 0.6 for women [1]. Thyroid cancer causes some 26,000 deaths every year.

Etiology
An association between thyroid cancer and exposure to ionizing radiation was already suggested in 1950 [2]. Many studies have documented the increased risk of papillary or follicular thyroid carcinoma in individuals exposed to X- and γ-rays [3]. The risk of radiation-induced cancer is considerably greater in those exposed as young children than as adults. Before the Chernobyl accident, epidemiological studies appeared to indicate that radioactive iodines were much less carcinogenic than external X- or γ- irradiation. This is not confirmed by the study of persons exposed as children to fall-out from the Chernobyl accident in the most contaminated territories in Belarus, Ukraine and Russia, where a dramatic increase in thyroid cancer incidence attributable to radioactive iodines has been observed. Iodine deficiency is thought to be involved in the development of thyroid cancer because thyroid cancer incidence rates

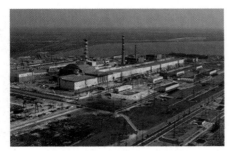

Fig. 5.136 The Chernobyl nuclear power plant following the 1986 accident. A marked increase in the incidence of thyroid cancer in children has been observed in areas exposed to radioactive iodine.

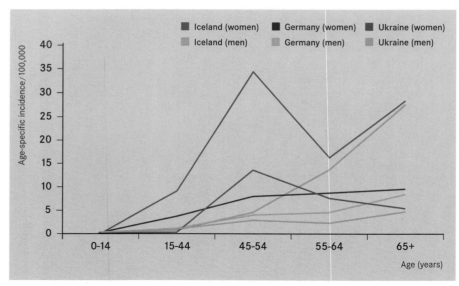

Fig. 5.137 Age-specific incidence of thyroid cancer in men and in women in the Ukraine, Iceland and Germany. Incidence is higher in women and shows a marked peak.

are high in mountainous areas, such as the Alps, Andes, and Himalayas, where severe iodine deficiency was or still is common [4]. However, several high-risk populations live on islands (such as Hawaii and Iceland), where iodine intake is generally high. The relationship between iodine intake and risk of thyroid cancer appears to be complex, since both deficiency and excess may inhibit the synthesis of thyroid hormones and cause goitre [5]. The two main types of thyroid carcinoma (papillary and follicular) may be linked to iodine-rich and iodine-deficient diets, respectively [6]. Other dietary factors, including cruciferous and goitrogenic vegetables [7], may play a role in thyroid carcinogenesis.

Thyroid cancer occurs approximately three times more frequently in women than in men, reaching a maximum at about age 45. Hormonal factors may play a role in etiology. Results from epidemiological studies, however, have been inconsistent: some have found an association between parity and risk of thyroid cancer while others did not. The most current data suggest that menstrual and reproductive factors are weakly related to thyroid cancer risk [8]. Apart from irradiation in childhood, goitre and benign nodules

are the strongest risk factors with a relative risk of approximately 3 and 30, respectively [9]. The role of hypothyroidism and hyperthyroidism is less clear.

Detection

Thyroid cancer commonly causes no obvious symptoms in its early stages. The vast majority of cancers become clinically evident as thyroid nodules. However, only a minority of all thyroid nodules is malignant. Many nodules are found in asymptomatic patients on physical examination of the neck. Some cases have a history of rapid increase in size and/or pain in the region of the nodule. Hoarseness, dyspnoea and dysphagia reflect local invasion of the recurrent laryngeal nerve, trachea and oesophagus, respectively. A small subset of patients presents with palpable cervical lymphadenopathy without an identifiable thyroid primary. High-resolution ultrasonography is useful for size assessment of nodules and for detection of unpalpable nodules. Differences in echogenicity, vascularity or tests of thyroid function cannot distinguish benign from malignant nodules. The single most important diagnostic procedure is the fine needle aspiration biopsy, performed under ultrasound guidance.

Pathology and genetics

Thyroid follicular cells give rise to both well-differentiated cancers and also anaplastic cancers. Parafollicular or C-cells are the cells of origin for medullary thyroid cancer. Stromal and immune cells of the thyroid are responsible for sarcoma and lymphoma, respectively. Approximately 90% of malignant thyroid nodules are well-differentiated cancers. They are further classified into papillary and follicular carcinomas, Hürthle cell carcinomas and others. Papillary and follicular cancers have the lowest degree of clinical malignancy. Papillary carcinoma has a propensity to invade lymphatic spaces and leads to microscopic multifocal lesions in the gland and a high incidence of regional lymph node metastases. Follicular carcinoma is unifocal and thickly encapsulated. It has a propensity to invade veins and not lymphatics.

Hürthle cell carcinoma, insular carcinoma and medullary thyroid carcinoma are considered to be of intermediate differentiation and consequently to exhibit an intermediate degree of clinical malignancy.

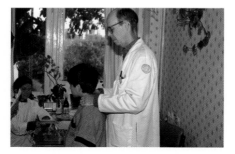

Fig. 5.138 Clinical examination of the thyroid gland of a child at risk following radioactive exposure as a result of the Chernobyl accident.

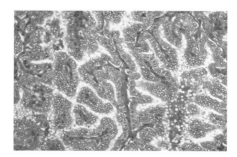

Fig. 5.139 Histopathological features of a papillary thyroid carcinoma.

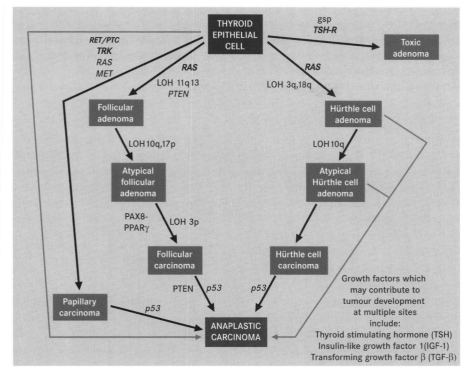

Fig. 5.140 Proposed genetic model of thyroid tumour formation. Genes in bold type have a well-established role. Adapted from D.L. Learoyd et al. (2000) *World J Surg*, 24, 923-933.

Insular carcinoma invades both lymphatics and veins, and nodal and distant metastases are common. Approximately 33% of Hürthle cell carcinomas show histological evidence of malignancy or invasive growth. The remainder behave as adenomas and may be treated conservatively.

There is evidence of familial risk in a small percentage of papillary and follicular thyroid carcinomas. The associations of Gardner syndrome (familial adenomatous polyposis) and Cowden disease (familial goitre and skin hamartomas) with differentiated thyroid carcinoma provide well-defined examples. About 25 to 35% of all medullary thyroid carcinomas are identified as a component of one of the clinical syndromes. These syndromes include: multiple endocrine neoplasia type 2A (MEN2A) which is associated with medullary thyroid carcinoma, pheochromocytoma and hyperparathyroidism; multiple endocrine neoplasia type 2B (MEN2B) which is associated with medul-

lary thyroid carcinoma, pheochromocytoma, mucosal neuromas, and marfanoid-like features; and familial medullary thyroid carcinoma.

The genes implicated in the pathogenesis of thyroid carcinoma generally form a subset of important cell growth and differentiation regulatory factors that can be separated into membrane and nuclear factors. Two different mechanisms are involved in the genesis of papillary thyroid and medullary thyroid carcinomas. As a result of intrachromosomal rearrangements, the *RET* proto-oncogene becomes attached to the promoter of one of three genes expressed constitutively in the follicular cell, which results in the so-called "papillary thyroid carcinoma oncogene" (*RET/PTC1*, *2*, and *3*). Germline point mutations of the *RET* proto-oncogene, which is normally expressed in the thyroid parafollicular cell, are found in more than 95% of individuals with hereditary medullary thyroid carcinoma (codons 609, 611, 618, 620, or

634). Mutation of codon 634 is the most commonly observed and is found in about 80% of all patients with hereditary medullary thyroid carcinoma. A germline point mutation in the tyrosine kinase portion of the *RET* receptor (codon 918) has been identified in 95% of individuals with MEN2B [10].

Management

Patients with malignant lesions diagnosed on the basis of fine needle aspiration, as well as patients with a suspicious aspiration, combined with other risk factors (such as prior radiation exposure or local symptoms) should have surgical resection. It has been recommended that total thyroidectomy should be performed at around the age of six years in children who are MEN2A gene carriers and shortly after birth in children with the MEN2B mutation [11]. Benign nodules can be monitored by ultrasound examination. Acceptable surgical procedures include lobectomy, subtotal thyroidectomy, near-total thyroidectomy and total thyroidectomy. Modified radical neck dissection is indicated in case of lymph node metastases. All patients who have undergone a total or near-total thyroidectomy for a papillary or follicular carcinoma of greater than 1.5 cm should be considered candidates for radioiodine ablation [12].

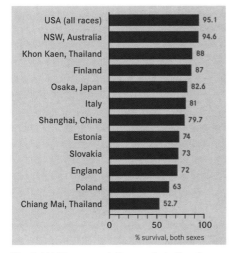

Fig. 5.141 Five-year relative survival after diagnosis of thyroid cancer.

In contrast to other solid neoplasms, the presence of regional lymph node metastases with a well-differentiated thyroid cancer has no strong correlation with overall survival. Independent predictors of prognosis include patient's age, gender, tumour size, histological grade and type, local invasion, multicentricity and the presence of systemic metastatic disease. Five-year relative survival rates for this type of malignancy vary greatly according to histological type, ranging from 98% for papillary carcinoma and 92% for follicular carcinoma, to 11% for anaplastic carcinoma [13]. Overall five-year survival rates vary significantly geographically (Fig. 5.141).

REFERENCES

1. Ferlay J, Bray F, Parkin DM, Pisani P, eds (2001) *Globocan 2000: Cancer Incidence and Mortality Worldwide (IARC Cancer Bases No. 5)*, Lyon, IARCPress.

2. Duffy BJ, Fitzgerald PJ (1950) Thyroid cancer in childhood and adolescence. Report of twenty-eight cases. *J Clin Endocrinol Metab*, 10: 1296-1308.

3. Shore RE (1992) Issues and epidemiological evidence regarding radiation-induced thyroid cancer. *Radiat Res*, 131: 98-111.

4. Franceschi S, Boyle P, Maisonneuve P, La Vecchia C, Burt AD, Kerr DJ, MacFarlane GJ (1993) The epidemiology of thyroid carcinoma. *Crit Rev Oncog*, 4: 25-52.

5. Braverman LE (1990) Iodine induced thyroid disease. *Acta Med Austriaca*, 17 Suppl 1: 29-33.

6. Williams ED, Doniach I, Bjarnason O, Michie W (1977) Thyroid cancer in an iodide rich area: a histopathological study. *Cancer*, 39: 215-222.

7. Franceschi S, Talamini R, Fassina A, Bidoli E (1990) Diet and epithelial cancer of the thyroid gland. *Tumori*, 76: 331-338.

8. Negri E, Dal Maso L, Ron E, La Vecchia C, Mark SD, Preston-Martin S, McTiernan A, Kolonel L, Yoshimoto Y, Jin F, Wingren G, Rosaria GM, Hardell L, Glattre E, Lund E, Levi F, Linos D, Braga C, Franceschi S (1999) A pooled analysis of case-control studies of thyroid cancer. II. Menstrual and reproductive factors. *Cancer Causes Control*, 10: 143-155.

9. Franceschi S, Preston-Martin S, Dal Maso L, Negri E, La Vecchia C, Mack WJ, McTiernan A, Kolonel L, Mark SD, Mabuchi K, Jin F, Wingren G, Galanti R, Hallquist A, Glattre E, Lund E, Levi F, Linos D, Ron E (1999) A pooled analysis of case-control studies of thyroid cancer. IV. Benign thyroid diseases. *Cancer Causes Control*, 10: 583-595.

10. Hofstra RM, Landsvater RM, Ceccherini I, Stulp RP, Stelwagen T, Luo Y, Pasini B, Hoppener JW, van Amstel HK, Romeo G (1994) A mutation in the RET proto-oncogene associated with multiple endocrine neoplasia type 2B and sporadic medullary thyroid carcinoma. *Nature*, 367: 375-376.

11. Gagel RF, Goepfert H, Callender DL (1996) Changing concepts in the pathogenesis and management of thyroid carcinoma. *CA Cancer J Clin*, 46: 261-283.

12. Fraker DL, Skarulis M, Livolsi V (1997) Thyroid tumors. In: DeVita VTJ, Hellman S, Rosenberg SA eds, *Cancer Principles and Practice of Oncology*, Philadelphia, Lippincott-Raven Publishers, 1629-1652.

13. Gilliland FD, Hunt WC, Morris DM, Key CR (1997) Prognostic factors for thyroid carcinoma. A population-based study of 15,698 cases from the Surveillance, Epidemiology and End Results (SEER) program 1973-1991. *Cancer*, 79: 564-573.

WEBSITES

The British Thyroid Association:
http://www.british-thyroid-association.org/

The European Thyroid Association:
http://www.eurothyroid.com/

KIDNEY CANCER

SUMMARY

> Cancer of the kidney is the 15th most common cancer in the world and most prevalent in developed countries. Close to 190,000 cases are diagnosed each year worldwide and men are generally affected more frequently than women.

> Tobacco smoking is an established cause. Excess body weight (obesity) has also been identified as a risk factor, particularly in women.

> Patients with late stage diagnosis face a poor prognosis. Recent advances in imaging allow the early detection of asymptomatic tumours. The five-year survival rate is approximately 50%.

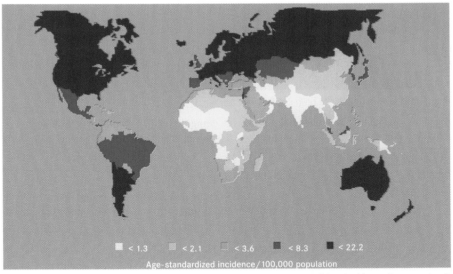

Fig. 5.142 Global burden of kidney cancer in men, showing a generally higher incidence in more developed countries.

Definition

In adults, 85-90% of cases of kidney cancer are renal cell carcinomas, a very heterogeneous group of tumours (mainly adenocarcinomas) which arise from cells of the proximal convoluted renal tubule. Transitional cell carcinoma is a less common tumour type that arises from the transitional cell epithelium in the renal pelvis, ureter and urethra. Wilms tumour (nephroblastoma) is an embryonal malignancy that afflicts 1 in 10,000 children.

Epidemiology

The incidence of kidney cancer is considerably higher in developed countries than in less developed countries (Fig. 5.142) and appears to be increasing over the past decade [1,2]. More than 189,000 new cases are diagnosed worldwide each year. In Western Europe, for example, kidney cancer is the sixth most frequently occurring cancer, incidence being particularly high in the Bas-Rhin region of France [3]. Incidence is also exceptionally high in the Czech Republic

and among Scandinavian populations. Kidney cancer is relatively less common among Asian and African peoples, although renal cell carcinoma appears to be increasing in black American men [4]. Men are affected by kidney cancer more than women, the sex ratio being 1.6-2.0:1 [5]. Most cases occur between ages 50-70, but kidney cancer may be diagnosed over a broad age range including young adults [1]. Wilms tumour is responsible for 5-15% of childhood cancers, affecting females slightly more than males. This tumour occurs with highest frequency in the black population of USA and Africa, and with lowest in Eastern Asia [1]. Kidney cancer causes the deaths of more than 91,000 people each year.

Etiology

Kidney cancer has consistently been found to be more common in cigarette smokers than in non-smokers. The association was first established as causative for transitional cell carcinoma of the bladder

and has now been extended to renal cell carcinomas, the risk increasing two-fold for heavy smokers [6]. An increased risk of renal cell carcinoma has been linked to obesity, particularly in women, as has diuretic therapy, again especially in women [7]. Leather tanners, shoe workers and dry cleaning employees have an increased risk as reported in some studies, as do workers exposed to asbestos and trichloroethylene. The influence of beverages, in particular coffee and alcohol, has not been clearly determined despite many studies. Phenacetin is carcinogenic: patients with kidney damage secondary to phenacetin-containing analgesic abuse have an increased risk of transitional cell carcinoma (*Medicinal drugs*, p48). Patients with multicystic kidney disease consequent on long-term dialysis, adult polycystic kidney disease and tuberous sclerosis also have an increased propensity to develop renal cell carcinoma and von Hippel-Lindau disease, an autosomal dominant condition, is a predisposing factor.

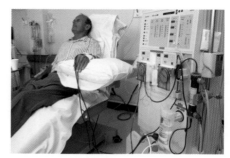

Fig. 5.144 A patient receiving kidney haemodialysis: long-term dialysis predisposes to acquired cystic disease of the kidney which may increase the risk of subsequent cancer.

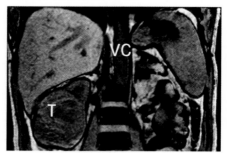

Fig. 5.145 Magnetic resonance image of a renal cell carcinoma (T), with a tumour thrombus in the inferior vena cava (VC).

Detection

Kidney cancer commonly causes no obvious symptoms in its early stages. Subsequently, symptoms include haematuria, loin pain and a palpable kidney mass [8] and these usually indicate patients with advanced disease. As a consequence of increasing use of renal imaging techniques, increasing numbers of asymptomatic, incidental tumours are being detected [5]. Diagnosis of renal cell carcinoma may be preceded by paraneoplastic syndromes, the systemic and humoral manifestations of the disease, which result from the overproduction of normal kidney proteins or hormones (e.g. renin, erythropoietin, prostaglandins) or inappropriate expression of non-kidney factors (e.g. parathyroid hormone). Symptoms may include hypertension, fever, anaemia, erythrocytosis (elevated number of red blood cells), abnormal liver function and hypercalcaemia (abnormally high calcium levels) [2, 8].

The presence of a tumour may be initially defined by intravenous urogram. Computed tomography (CT) is the imaging procedure of choice for diagnosis and staging [1]; scanning of the abdomen and pelvis confirms tumour extent, lymph node status and contralateral kidney functionality. Selective renal arteriography via percutaneous femoral artery catheterization may be used for diagnosis and staging [1]. Less invasive than arteriography is magnetic resonance imaging (MRI), which can also be used to assess thrombus of renal vein or vena cava involvement (Fig. 5.145). Chest radiographs (commonly with CT) and technetium-99m radiopharmaceutical bone scans are employed to determine whether lung or skeletal metastases are present.

Pathology and genetics

Renal cell carcinoma (Figs. 5.146, 5.147) is commonly represented by adenomas, although there is some controversy over the difference between renal cortical adenoma and renal cell adenocarcinoma [1]. In terms of renal cell carcinoma histology, grade I cells have a lipid-rich cytoplasm and a small peripheral nucleus. As grade advances from I to IV, the nuclear pleomorphism increases and the lipid-rich cytoplasm reduces. The tumour is initially capsulated (in 50-60% of diagnosed cases), tends to spread to lymph nodes (10% of cases diagnosed) or may metastasize to the lungs, bone, brain and liver (20-30% of cases). There is a tendency for the tumour to spread within the renal vein and into the inferior vena cava, extending in extreme cases into the right atrium [8]. Transitional cell carcinoma accounts for 5-8% of kidney tumours [8] and is derived from the renal pelvis transitional cell epithelium, which is identical to that of the bladder and ureter; 50% of patients with renal transitional cell carcinoma also develop the same tumour type of the bladder.

Cytogenetics and molecular biology have allowed significant advances to be made in the differentiation and staging of kidney cancer tumours, which may be histologically complex and heterogeneous [9].

Cytogenetics have shown, for example, that the two main types of renal cell carcinomas, clear cell (non-papillary) carcinoma and papillary carcinoma, are genetically distinct (Table 5.15), although there can often be difficulties in distinguishing them histologically. Corresponding changes in transitional cell carcinoma have been less well-defined. The papillary form has a better prognosis than the non-papillary [9]. Mitochondrial DNA changes have been observed in early-stage oncocytic and chromophobe tumours [10], but are not yet used clinically.

Von Hippel-Lindau disease is characterized by the development of multiple tumours, including bilateral renal cell carcinoma, pheochromocytomas, hemangioblastomas of the central nervous system, retinal angiomas and pancreatic cysts [1,11]. Von Hippel-Lindau patients have a >70% lifetime risk for renal cell carcinoma and it is the cause of death in 15-50% of cases. Such patients thus require regular screening; currently some 30-50% of patients with von Hippel-Lindau disease who are identified with renal cell carcinoma as a result of symptoms have metastases on presentation, and hence respond poorly to treatment. Most families with von Hippel-Lindau disease (80%) have mutations in the *VHL* gene, a probable tumour suppressor gene. Sporadic forms of renal cell carcinoma, as well as familial forms, are asso-

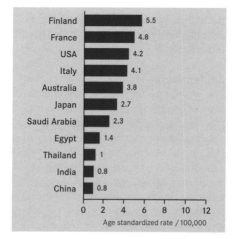

Fig. 5.143 Mortality from kidney cancer in various countries.

Stage	Clear cell carcinoma	Papillary carcinoma
Adenoma	Loss of 3p Partial trisomy of 5q Loss of Y chromosome	Loss of Y chromosome Trisomy of 7, 17 Gain of 3p Gain of 7, 12, 16, 17, 20
Carcinoma	*p53* mutations Loss of 8, 9, 13, 14, 6q, 10q, 18q, 11, 17/17p Gain of 12, 20 Loss of *VHL* function	Loss of 6q, 9, 11, 14q, 17/17p, 21 Gain of 8, 20 Loss of *MET* function
Metastatic tumours		Excess of minichromosomes, comprising 7q31 containing the *MET* oncogene

Table 5.15 Genetic alterations in renal cell carcinoma.

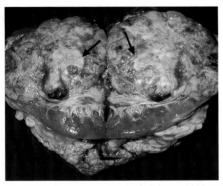

Fig. 5.146 Surgical specimen of a bisected kidney showing a large renal cell carcinoma. Much of the kidney has been replaced by tumour tissue.

ciated with structural alterations of the short arm of chromosome 3 and with *VHL* gene mutations [1,11].

Wilms tumour of the kidney occurs in both sporadic and familial forms. It has a specific syndrome associated with abnormalities including aniridia (absence of the iris), hemihypertrophy (overgrowth of one half of the body or a body part), and cryptorchidism (failure of the testes to descend into the scrotum). A number of loci involved in the development of Wilms tumour have been characterized, key amongst these being *WT1*, a tumour suppressor gene located on chromosome 11p [12].

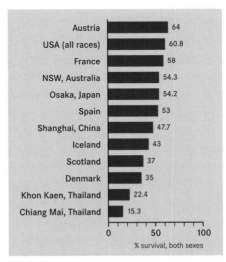

Austria 64
USA (all races) 60.8
France 58
NSW, Australia 54.3
Osaka, Japan 54.2
Spain 53
Shanghai, China 47.7
Iceland 43
Scotland 37
Denmark 35
Khon Kaen, Thailand 22.4
Chiang Mai, Thailand 15.3

0   50   100
% survival, both sexes

Fig. 5.148 Five-year relative survival after diagnosis of kidney cancer.

Management

Radical nephrectomy (removal of the kidney, perinephric fat, adjacent lymph nodes and often the adrenal gland) is currently the main therapy for renal cell carcinoma. This procedure has been shown to produce better survival rates than simple nephrectomy (kidney removal only), since involvement of regional lymphatics and periaortic lymph nodes has been noted in almost 25% of patients [1]. Treatment for transitional cell carcinoma is radical nephrou-reterectomy, although more conservative therapy may be appropriate for smaller low-grade tumours. In patients possessing a single kidney, or in the case of bilateral simultaneous tumour, either partial nephrectomy or radical nephrectomy with dialysis and possible later transplantation is indicated [1]. However, immunosuppression associated with transplantation raises the risk of potential tumour recurrence (*Immunosuppression*, p68).

Accurate staging depends on histological evaluation of the resected tumour. Up to 30% of patients present with metastases at diagnosis or relapse following surgery. Metastatic kidney cancer is extremely resistant to systemic therapy [13]. A potential reason for this is the high level of expression of the multi-drug resistance gene *MDR1* which encodes P-glycoprotein (Box: *Resistance to cancer chemotherapy*, p285) in both normal proximal tubules and in tumour

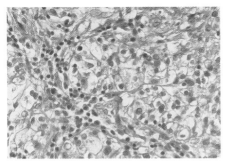

Fig. 5.147 Clear cell carcinoma of the kidney showing a monomorphic proliferation of distinctive tumour cells, with an abundant clear, lipid-containing cytoplasm, arranged in a trabecular pattern.

tissue [14]. Most chemotherapeutic and hormonal agents appear to show little efficacy, although there is some controversy over the efficacy of vinblastine and 5-fluorouracil as single agents or in combination therapy [13,8]. In contrast, in the treatment of transitional cell carcinoma, cisplatin combination therapy seems to be effective.

For the systemic treatment of metastatic kidney cancer, interferon-α and interleukin-2 have been shown to elicit a modest response rate of 10-15% [8], allowing complete response in some patients and an increased survival benefit in others. Although overall survival rates are poor (Fig. 5.148), the five-year survival for patients with early stage tumours is greater than 80% [8]. The indication of renal vein/inferior vena cava involvement reduces five-year survival rates to 25-50%, whilst regional lymph node involvement or extracapsular extension also indicates a much reduced rate of 15-50%. The presence of distant metastases or stage IV cancer carries a very poor prognosis (5% five-year survival rate) [1].

REFERENCES

1. Richie JP, Kantoff PW, Shapiro CL (1997) Renal cell carcinoma. In: Holland JF, Bast RC, Morton DL, Frei E, Kufe DW, Weichselbaum RR eds, *Cancer Medicine*, Williams and Wilkins.

2. Godley PA, Ataga KI (2000) Renal cell carcinoma. *Curr Opin Oncol*, 12: 260-264.

3. Ferlay J, Bray F, Parkin DM, Pisani P, eds (2001) *Globocan 2000: Cancer Incidence and Mortality Worldwide (IARC Cancer Bases No. 5)*, Lyon, IARCPress.

4. McLaughlin JK, Blot WJ, Devesa SS, Fraumeni FJ (1996) Renal cancer. In: Schottenfeld D, Fraumeni, JFJ eds, *Cancer Epidemiology and Prevention*, New York, Oxford University Press, 1142-1155.

5. Chow WH, Devesa SS, Warren JL, Fraumeni JF, Jr. (1999) Rising incidence of renal cell cancer in the United States. *JAMA*, 281: 1628-1631.

6. Doll R (1996) Cancers weakly related to smoking. *Br Med Bull*, 52: 35-49.

7. Schmieder RE, Delles C, Messerli FH (2000) Diuretic therapy and the risk for renal cell carcinoma. *J Nephrol*, 13: 343-346.

8. Watkin N, Christmas TJ (1998) Renal Tumours. In: Morris D, Kearsley J, Williams C eds, *Cancer: a comprehensive clinical guide*, Harwood Academic Publishers.

9. Bernheim A, Vagner-Capodano A, Couturier J, et le Groupe Francais de Cytogenetique Oncologique (2000) De la cytogénétique à la cytogénomie oncologique. *Medecine/Sciences*, 16: 528-539.

10. van den Berg, Dijkhuizen T (1999) Classification of renal cell cancer based on (cyto)genetic analysis. *Contrib Nephrol*, 128: 51-61.

11. Couch V, Lindor NM, Karnes PS, Michels VV (2000) von Hippel-Lindau disease. *Mayo Clin Proc*, 75: 265-272.

12. Hata J (1999) Wilms tumor and the WT1 gene. *Contrib Nephrol*, 128: 62-74.

13. Motzer RJ, Russo P (2000) Systemic therapy for renal cell carcinoma. *J Urol*, 163: 408-417.

14. Vogelzang NJ, Stadler WM (1998) Kidney cancer. *Lancet*, 352: 1691-1696.

WEBSITES

NCI Kidney Cancer Homepage:
http://www.cancer.gov/cancer_information/cancer_type/kidney/

The Kidney Cancer Association (USA):
http://www.nkca.org/

TUMOURS OF THE NERVOUS SYSTEM

SUMMARY

> Tumours of the nervous system account for less than 2% of all malignancies (about 175,000 cases per year worldwide); the incidence does not vary markedly between regions or populations.

> Etiology is largely unknown; the only unequivocal cause is therapeutic irradiation, but occurrence in these circumstances is very rare.

> The nervous system is frequently involved in inherited tumour syndromes, including neurofibromatosis (*NF1/NF2* germline mutations), von Hippel-Lindau disease (*VHL*), tuberous sclerosis (*TSC1/TSC2*) and Li-Fraumeni syndrome (*p53*).

> Glioblastomas are the most common brain tumours and mainly affect adults. These tumours are surgically incurable and largely resistant to radiation and chemotherapy; only 3% of patients survive more than 3 years.

> Embryonal tumours, including cerebellar medulloblastomas, retinoblastomas and peripheral neuroblastoma, predominantly afflict children, ranking second after leukaemia as the most common types of paediatric cancer.

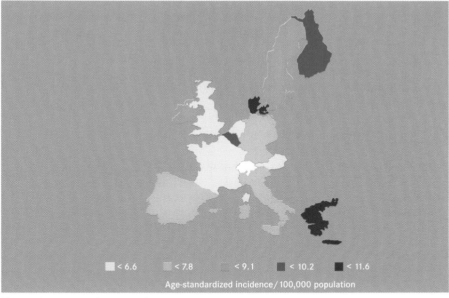

< 6.6   < 7.8   < 9.1   < 10.2   < 11.6

Age-standardized incidence/100,000 population

Fig 5.149 Incidence of cancers of the brain and nervous system in men, in Europe.

Definition

The majority of tumours of the central nervous system (CNS) are derived from glial cells (gliomas), the most malignant and frequent being glioblastoma. Malignant embryonal tumours typically manifest in children and occur in the central nervous system (medulloblastomas) and the sympathetic nervous system and adrenal gland (neuroblastomas). Tumours originating from the brain coverings (meningiomas) are usually benign.

Epidemiology

The age distribution of brain tumours is bimodal, with a peak incidence in children and a second larger peak in adults aged 45-70 [1]. In most developed countries, brain tumours are the 12th most frequent cause of cancer-related mortality in men [2]. Geographical variation in incidence is less than for most other human neoplasms [2] (Fig. 5.149). However, incidence tends to be higher in more developed countries. In most North American and European countries, incidence rates for malignant tumours of the nervous system are 6-8 new cases per 100,000 population per year. Highest rates are observed in Sweden, Greece, Iceland and Croatia. In multiracial communities, both adults and children of African or Asian descent tend to be less frequently affected than whites. It has been reported that white Americans have a 3.5 times greater risk of glioblastoma and germ cell tumours than African Americans [1]. However, the lower incidence recorded for Singapore and Japan may be due to inadequate registration.

Generally, incidence rates are higher for men; in particular, malignant brain tumours occur more frequently in males while the benign meningiomas occur predominantly in females. During the past decade, the incidence of glioblastomas in the elderly has increased by 1-2% per year but to some extent this may be due to the introduction of high-resolution neuroimaging. The brain is also a frequent site of metastases, with carcinomas of the breast and lung as most frequent primary tumours.

Etiology

With the exception of brain tumours associated with inherited cancer syndromes and the very rare cases caused by therapeutic irradiation, no causative environmental or lifestyle factors have been unequivocally identified. Radiation-induced meningiomas may follow low-dose irradiation for tinea capitis (a fungal infection of the scalp) and high-dose irradiation for primary brain tumours [3]. Children who received prophylactic CNS irradiation for acute lymphoblastic leukaemia seem to have an increased risk of developing malignant gliomas.

Tumour (WHO Grade)	Typical location	Age at clinical manifestation (% of cases)			Five-year survival (% of patients)	Genetic alterations
		0-20 yrs	20-45 yrs	>45 yrs		
Pilocytic astrocytoma (Grade I)	Cerebellum, optic nerve	74	20	6	>85	*NF1* (neurofibro-matosis cases)
Low grade diffuse astrocytoma (Grade II)	Cerebral hemispheres	10	61	29	>50	*p53* mutation
Glioblastoma (Grade IV)	Cerebral hemispheres	3	25	72	<3	*EGFR* amplification, *PTEN* mutation, p16 deletion, LOH chromosome 10
Oliogodendroglioma (Grade II/III)	Cerebral hemispheres	8	46	46	>50	LOH 1p, 19q
Ependymoma (Grade II)	Ventricles, spinal cord	37	38	25	<30	*NF1* (spinal tumours)
Medulloblastoma (Grade IV)	Cerebellum	74	23	3	>50	Isochromosome 17, mutations of *p53*, *PTCH*, ß-catenin
Neuroblastoma (Grade IV)	Abdomen	>95			>90 (<1 yr old) 20-50 (>1 yr)	LOH 1p, 11q, *MYCN* amplification, trisomy 17q

Table 5.16 Summary of epidemiological data on intracranial tumours.

Some studies have suggested an increased incidence of CNS neoplasms associated with certain occupations, including farming, fire-fighting, metal-working and the rubber and petrochemical industries, and with those who work as anatomists, pathologists and embalmers, but most of these reports have not been confirmed and causative agents have not been identified. Suggestions that radio-frequency radiation generated by mobile phones and microwave telecommunications may play a role in the etiology of malignant gliomas remain to be substantiated. Similarly, the role of diet in brain tumour etiology, and specifically involvement of *N*-nitroso compounds (which are potent neuro-carcinogens in rodents) formed in nitrite-preserved food, is unclear.

The nervous system is frequently affected in inherited tumour syndromes, often in association with extraneural tumours and skin lesions (Table 5.17).

Detection

Signs and symptoms largely depend on the location of the neoplasm and include paresis (slight/incomplete paralysis), speech disturbances and personality changes. Patients with oligodendroglioma often have a long history of epileptic seizures. Eventually, malignant brain tumours cause life-threatening intracranial pressure that may result in visual disturbance and ultimately lead to unconsciousness and respiratory arrest. Since the brain does not contain pain receptors, headache is only present if the tumour infiltrates the meninges. The presence of symptoms usually leads to a detailed neurological examination, using techniques such as computed tomography (CT) and magnetic resonance imaging (MRI).

Pathology and genetics

The WHO classification of tumours of the nervous system contains more than 50 clinico-pathological entities with a great variation in biological behaviour, response to therapy and clinical outcome [4]. The most frequent ones are listed in Table 5.16. Of all intracranial tumours, approximately 60% are of neuroepithelial origin (gliomas), 28% are derived from the brain coverings (meningiomas) and 7.5% are located in cranial and spinal nerves. Lymphomas and germ cell tumours account for 4% and 1% respectively.

Astrocytic tumours

Tumours of astrocytic origin constitute the largest proportion of gliomas. They vary greatly in morphology, genetic profile and clinical behaviour.

Pilocytic astrocytoma (WHO Grade I) is the most frequent CNS neoplasm in children, and is predominantly located in the cerebellum and midline structures, includ-

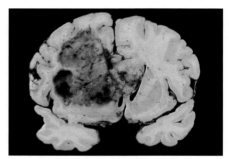

Fig 5.150 A large glioblastoma multiforme in the left frontal lobe, extending into the corpus callosum and the contralateral white matter.

ing the optic tract, brain stem and spinal cord. It infiltrates adjacent brain structures but grows slowly and usually has a favourable prognosis with five-year survival rates of more than 85% (WHO Grade I). Some pilocytic astrocytomas occur in the setting of neurofibromatosis type 1 (NF1), particularly those of the optic nerve (optic glioma). Other astrocytomas usually develop in the cerebral hemispheres of adults and diffusely infiltrate adjacent brain structures.

Low grade diffuse astrocytomas (WHO grade II) occur in young adults and grow slowly. However, they diffusely infiltrate the brain and cannot, therefore, be completely surgically resected. Morphologically, tumour cells resemble differentiated astrocytes. Mutations in *p53* are found in two-thirds of cases and are considered an early event. The five-year survival rate is more than 60%.

Anaplastic astrocytomas (WHO grade III) often develop from low-grade astrocytomas, grow relatively fast and typically progress to glioblastoma within two to three years, accompanied by genetic alterations, including loss of heterozygosity (LOH) on chromosome 19.

Glioblastomas (WHO grade IV)

This is the most frequent and most malignant nervous system tumour. Secondary glioblastomas develop by malignant progression from low-grade and anaplastic astrocytoma and are characterized by *p53* mutations and LOH on chromosome 10q. Primary glioblastomas are more frequent (>80% of cases) and develop rapidly in the elderly (mean age, 55 years), with a short clinical history of less than three months. Their genetic profile includes amplification and overexpression of the *EGF* receptor gene, *PTEN* mutations, p16^{INK4A} deletions and loss of chromosome 10. Both glioblastoma types diffusely infiltrate the brain, including the opposite hemisphere and show high cellularity and large areas of necrosis despite excessive vascular proliferation.

Oligodendrogliomas

These neoplasms develop from myelin-producing oligodendroglial cells or their precursors and are typically found in the cerebral hemispheres of adults, often including the basal ganglia. Histologically, they are isomorphic, with a typical honeycomb pattern and delicate tumour vessels ("chicken wire" pattern). Anaplastic oligodendrogliomas (WHO Grade III) show features of anaplasia and high mitotic activity and carry a less favourable prognosis. Genetic hallmarks of oligodendrogliomas are LOH on chromosomes 1p and 19q. Oligodendrogliomas that carry these genetic alterations show a remarkable sensitivity to chemotherapy.

Ependymomas

These gliomas develop from the ependymal lining of the cerebral ventricles and

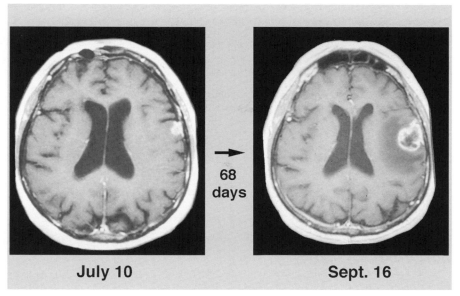

July 10 → **68 days** → **Sept. 16**

Fig. 5.151 An MRI scan of a primary glioblastoma in a 79 year-old patient. A small cortical lesion rapidly developed into a full-blown glioblastoma with perifocal oedema and central necrosis.

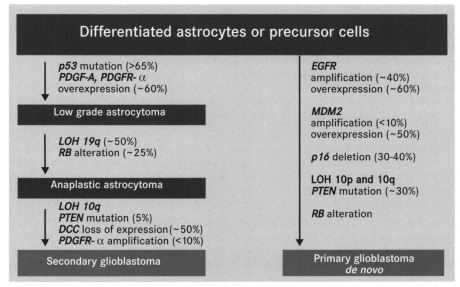

Differentiated astrocytes or precursor cells

p53 mutation (>65%)
*PDGF-A, PDGFR-*α overexpression (~60%)
↓
Low grade astrocytoma

LOH 19q (~50%)
RB alteration (~25%)
↓
Anaplastic astrocytoma

LOH 10q
PTEN mutation (5%)
DCC loss of expression (~50%)
*PDGFR-*α amplification (<10%)
↓
Secondary glioblastoma

EGFR amplification (~40%) overexpression (~60%)

MDM2 amplification (<10%) overexpression (~50%)

p16 deletion (30-40%)

LOH 10p and 10q
PTEN mutation (~30%)

RB alteration
↓
Primary glioblastoma *de novo*

Fig 5.152 Genetic pathways in the evolution of primary and secondary glioblastoma.

Syndrome	Gene	Chromosome	Nervous system	Skin	Other tissues
Neurofibromatosis 1	NF1	17q11	Neurofibromas, MPNST, optic nerve gliomas, astrocytomas	Café-au-lait spots, axillary freckling	Iris hamartomas, osseous lesions, phaeochromocytoma, leukaemia
Neurofibromatosis 2	NF2	22q12	Bilateral vestibular schwannomas, peripheral schwannomas, meningiomas, meningioangiomatosis, spinal ependymomas, astrocytomas, micro-hamartomas, cerebral calcifications	-	Posterior lens opacities, retinal hamartoma
von Hippel-Lindau	VHL	3p25	Haemangioblastomas	-	Retinal haemangioblastomas renal cell carcinoma,
Tuberous sclerosis	TSC1 TSC2	9q34 16p13	Subependymal giant cell astrocytoma, cortical tubers	Cutaneous angiofibroma ("adenoma sebaceum") peau de chagrin, subungual fibromas	Cardiac rhabdomyomas, adenomatous polyps of the duodenum and the small intestine, cysts of the lung and kidney, lymphangioleiomyomatosis, renal, angiomyolipoma
Li-Fraumeni	p53	17p13	Astrocytomas, glioblastomas, medulloblastomas	-	Breast carcinoma, bone and soft tissue sarcomas, adrenocortical carcinoma, leukaemia
Cowden	PTEN (MMAC1)	10q23	Dysplastic gangliocytoma of the cerebellum (Lhermitte-Duclos), megalencephaly	Multiple trichilemmomas, fibromas	Hamartomatous polyps of the colon, thyroid neoplasms, breast carcinoma
Turcot	APC	5q21	Medulloblastoma	-	Colorectal cancer
	hMLH1 hPSM2	3p21 7p22	Glioblastoma	Café-au-lait spots	Colorectal cancer
Naevoid basal cell carcinoma syndrome (Gorlin)	PTCH	9q31	Medulloblastoma	Multiple basal palmar and plantar pits	Jaw cysts, ovarian fibromas, skeletal abnormalities

Table 5.17 Major familial tumour syndromes involving the nervous system.

the central canal of the spinal cord. They manifest preferentially in children and young adults and usually have an intraventricular or spinal location. Histologically, they are cellular, with typical perivascular rosettes. Spinal ependymomas show a high frequency of mutations in the neurofibromatosis gene NF2.

Glioneuronal tumours
This group of brain tumours is less frequent and generally carries a favourable prognosis. Some manifest preferentially in children (desmoplastic infantile astrocytoma/ganglioglioma, dysembryoplastic neuroepithelial tumour), others preferentially in adolescents and adults (gangliocytoma, ganglioglioma, central neuro-

cytoma). They often cause a long-term history of epileptic seizures.

Embryonal tumours
These neoplasms are derived from embryonal or fetal precursor cells, typically manifest in children, and are highly malignant but often respond to radio- or chemotherapy. In the central nervous system, cerebellar medulloblastomas are most common. The peak age at manifestation is 3-6 years; only 20% develop in adults. Occasionally, they occur in the setting of inherited cancer syndromes, including Turcot syndrome (in association with familial polyposis colon cancer) and naevoid basal cell carcinoma syndrome (associated with PTCH germline muta-

tions). Neuroblastomas originate from migrating neuroectodermal cells targeted for the adrenal medulla and sympathetic nervous system, which are the principal

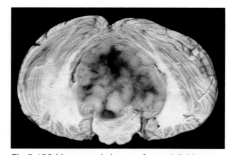

Fig 5.153 Macroscopic image of a medulloblastoma of the cerebellar vermis, compressing the brainstem.

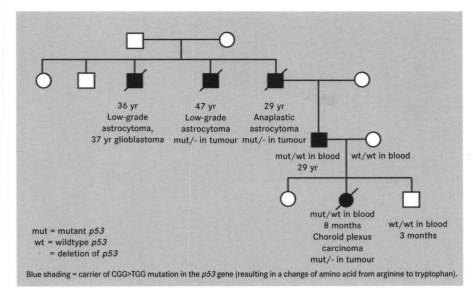

mut = mutant *p53*
wt = wildtype *p53*
- = deletion of *p53*

Blue shading = carrier of CGG>TGG mutation in the *p53* gene (resulting in a change of amino acid from arginine to tryptophan).

Fig. 5.154 Pedigree of a family with by Li-Fraumeni syndrome, caused by a germline mutation in codon 248 of the *p53* tumour suppressor gene. Blood samples of affected family members have a mutation in one allele. In tumours, the second allele is usually deleted. This family shows a remarkable clustering of brain tumours.

tumour sites. They manifest as an abdominal mass almost exclusively in children less than 10 years old, with a peak incidence of 1-4 years. Tumours in very young children and tumours outside the adrenal medulla have a better prognosis, and some lesions regress spontaneously. Amplification of the *N-MYC* gene indicates a poor prognosis.

Tumours of peripheral nerves
Most of these tumours develop from myelin-producing Schwann cells and are termed neurinomas or schwannomas. Bilateral acoustic schwannomas are diagnostic of the inherited neurofibromatosis type 2. They are benign (WHO Grade I) and rarely recur after surgical resection. Neurofibromas and malignant peripheral

nerve sheath tumours represent typical manifestations of the neurofibromatosis type 1 syndrome.

Meningiomas
These slowly growing, usually benign, neoplasms develop from arachnoidal cells in the meninges. They preferentially affect women, particularly those located in the spine. Meningiomas do not infiltrate the brain but may cause symptoms of intracranial pressure due to compression of adjacent brain structures (WHO Grade I). Preferential sites are the cerebral hemispheres. Meningiomas can often be cured by surgical resection. Malignant meningiomas are much less frequent; they may infiltrate the brain and often recur locally.

Outlook
Although not very frequent, brain tumours contribute significantly to morbidity, often affect children and overall have a poor prognosis. Due to marked resistance to radiation and chemotherapy, the prognosis for patients with glioblastomas is very poor. The majority of patients die within 9-12 months and less than 3% survive more than 3 years. Many genetic alterations involved in the development of nervous tissue tumours have been identified and may lead to novel therapeutic approaches, including gene therapy.

REFERENCES

1. Lantos PL, Louis DN, Rosenblum MK, Kleihues P (2002) Tumours of the nervous system. In: Graham DI, Lantos PL eds, *Greenfield's Neuropathology, Seventh Edition*, London, Arnold.

2. Ferlay J, Bray F, Parkin DM, Pisani P (2001) *Globocan*

2000. Cancer Incidence and Mortality Worldwide (IARC Cancer Bases No. 5), Lyon, IARCPress.

3. Preston-Martin S, Mack WJ (1996) Neoplasms of the nervous system. In: Schottenfeld D, Fraumeni, JF eds, *Cancer Epidemiology and Prevention*, pp. 1231-1281. New

York, Oxford University Press.

4. Kleihues P and Cavenee WK (2000) *World Health Organization Classification of Tumours. Pathology and Genetics of Tumours of the Nervous System*. Lyon, IARCPress.

Cancer management

Once cancer is diagnosed, the patient may require medical treatment and specialized care for months, and often years. The principal modes of therapy – surgery, radiotherapy and chemotherapy – may be given alone or in combination. Strong emphasis is now placed on the development of specialized cancer centres in which evidence-based multimodality therapy is applied, subject to evaluation by appropriately designed trials. After successful treatment, specific rehabilitation may be needed.

When cancer treatment is not curative, maintaining the highest possible quality of life is paramount. For many patients, supportive and palliative care are essential and this often involves a range of professional services that extends beyond the discipline of oncology.

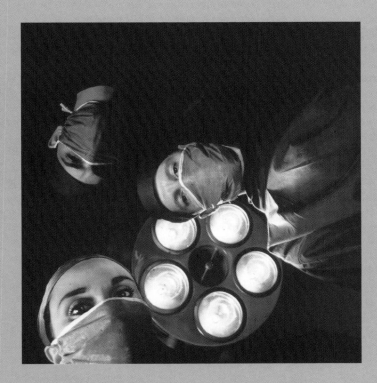

SURGICAL ONCOLOGY

SUMMARY

> Surgical oncology is emerging as a specialist discipline; recent advances include more precise identification of the tumour margin, leading to reduced local recurrence.

> New technology has facilitated minimal invasive surgery, laparoscopy and fibreoptic endoscopy.

> The greatly elevated cancer risk in individuals with familial cancer syndromes increasingly raises the prospect of preventive surgery, e.g. mastectomy in carriers of *BRCA1/2* mutations and colectomy in patients with familial adenomatosis coli.

> Surgical management is underpinned by recognition of the whole patient, and not merely focused on tumour excision.

Although surgery for cancer was available for many years prior to the advent of other therapies, the discipline of surgical oncology is not yet recognized in all countries as a speciality. Rather, surgical oncology is a concept which has developed recently, evolving with the emergence of radiotherapy and chemotherapy as separate modalities (*Radiotherapy*, p277 and *Medical oncology*, p281). The surgeon, who in the past was performing solo in the treatment of patients with cancer, has now become part of a team of players working together in a complex programme of multimodal anticancer therapies.

Since a surgical oncologist cannot hope to master the whole field of solid cancers, especially in view of the high technical demands of such surgery, subspecialization in organ-based groupings, such as upper gastrointestinal and colorectal subspecialities, has become necessary. Hyperspecialization into hepato-pancreato-biliary, endocrine and vascular surgery has also developed. Tentative attempts to develop proce-dure-based subgroupings, with new specializations for surgeons devoted to one type of procedure, such as organ transplantation or video laparoscopy, have generally failed. There is now a tendency to recruit surgeons who focus on one, or a few, organ sites. These specialists bring with them not only basic knowledge of the biology of cancer but the ability to participate in multidisciplinary research and to collaborate with colleagues from other disciplines.

However, with the growing evidence that cancer is rarely an organ-limited disease, both a disease-orientated approach and an organ-orientated approach are necessary to ensure optimal care for the cancer patient. Surgical oncologists have promoted the standardization of surgical practice aiming at the increase of life expectancy. Their participation in multi-centre clinical trials has provided the opportunity to compare clinical results of surgery and outcomes in the treatment of cancer [1,2].

Ethical and organizational aspects

Treatment of patients with cancer, of all ages, requires a specific ethical and psychological approach. Most patients move through a state of denial and later acceptance as the diagnosis and treatment of the disease progresses. A decision to perform surgery may be made when the disease has already adversely affected the quality of the patient's life. Cancer is often considered as a mutilating, self-destructive process and surgery is viewed frequently as either a last chance salvage procedure or an additional insult to a ravaged body. Thus, from the patient's perspective, the prospect of surgery is seen as a new burden, but also a chance of cure. Surgeons involved in the care of cancer must help patients to regain their autonomy in decision-making and self-determination. This insight has value as a prelude to obtaining informed consent for surgery and particularly before proposing to a patient that he or she should enter a clinical trial. In practice, patients often have greater confi-

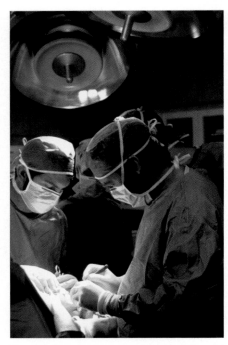

Fig. 6.1 Surgery can cure patients with solid tumours when the tumour is confined to the anatomic site of origin.

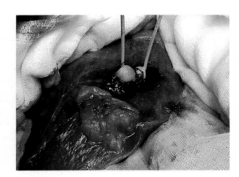

Fig. 6.2 A patient undergoing electrolysis treatment for an unresectable liver tumour. Two platinum electrode catheters deliver a low dose electric current causing local tumour ablation.

dence in a well-structured and coordinated multidisciplinary team than in a single physician.

The changing relationship between patients and surgeons due to the dissemination of knowledge and to public awareness of cancer has given rise to new attitudes towards operative risk. Many surgeons involved in the care of cancer patients have had to change their "surgeon-centric" focus to a position of a surgical oncologist committed to an integrated approach to treatment of cancer which merges organ-orientated and disease-orientated specializations. Such surgeons are therefore better placed to face new challenges.

There is a general trend towards centralizing the care of cancer patients in hospitals where it is possible to muster multidisciplinary teams. Radiation therapy and cytotoxic chemotherapy are often centralized to oncology clinics with oncological surgeons having the opportunity to focus on the surgical part of the treatment. However, since it is unrealistic and undesirable to deprive general surgery of its role in the treatment of cancer patients, it remains essential to improve the knowledge and expertise of general surgeons in oncological practice.

Context

Surgery for prevention of cancer

Surgical resection of tumours with severe dysplasia is a strategy for the prevention of cancer (Table 6.1). One striking example is total coloproctectomy in young asymptomatic patients with familial adenomatous polyposis (Fig. 6.4). Another example is total pancreatectomy in a patient with intraductal multifocal papillary mucinous tumour of the pancreas with areas of moderate to severe dysplasia (Fig. 6.5). Liver transplantation for advanced liver cirrhosis, from which small, undetectable hepatocellular carcinomas may developed [3], may be considered a means to prevent liver cancer.

Surgery for cancer cure

Local control of the tumour, which means the total eradication of the primary tumour and disease involving regional lymphatics, is indispensable for obtaining a cure. Surgery is often the most appropriate procedure for obtaining this goal and, from this point of view, remains the cornerstone in treatment [4]. Curative surgery is no longer synonymous, however,

Underlying condition	Associated cancer	Prophylactic treatment
Cryptorchidism	Testicular	Orchidopexy
Familial colon cancer FAP, familial adenomatous polyposis, or HNPCC, hereditary nonpolyposis colorectal cancer	Colon	Colectomy
Ulcerative colitis	Colon	Colectomy
Multiple endocrine neoplasia MEN 1, MEN2	Medullary cancer of the thyroid	Thyroidectomy
Familial breast cancer BRCA1, BRCA 2	Breast	Mastectomy
Familial ovarian cancer BRCAI	Ovary	Oophorectomy

Table 6.1 Surgery as a means of cancer prevention. V.T. DeVita et al., (1997) *Cancer: Principles and practice of oncology* © Lippincott, Williams & Wilkins.

with mutilating surgery. The general philosophy of cancer surgery has become more conservative than in the past, as long as such conservation remains compatible with an adequate resection of the tumour. The preoperative assessment, however, is of the utmost importance before subjecting a patient to a potentially hazardous operative procedure.

Conservative surgery in breast cancer is a conspicuous example of how the need for adequate treatment has been reconciled with preservation of the female breast and improved quality of life. Radical mastectomy, although effective, was accompanied by the psychological trauma of breast amputation. This promoted evaluation of

more conservative procedures (Table 6.2) and it became apparent that partial mastectomy alone was followed by significant local recurrence rates. Results in the 1980s and 1990s demonstrate that overall and disease-free survival from breast cancer are equivalent for mastectomy and breast-conserving surgery with postoperative radiotherapy for women with early breast cancer [5]. Breast conservation therapy as an alternative to mastectomy is especially important since, as a consequence of mammographic screening, the average size of invasive tumours has decreased while the incidence of noninvasive breast carcinoma has increased. In the case of stomach cancer, surgery is

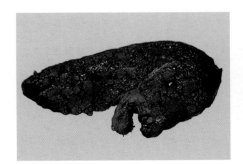

Fig. 6.3 The liver of a cirrhotic patient demonstrating multifocal hepatocellular carcinoma.

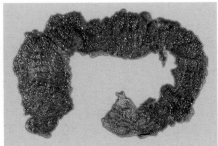

Fig. 6.4 Operative specimen of total coloproctectomy for familial adenomatous polyposis in a 14 year old boy; numerous polyps are evident.

Year	Radical mastectomy (%)	Modified radical mastectomy (%)
1972	47.9	27.7
1976	25.5	51.9
1977	20.9	55.4
1981	3.4	72.3

In a radical mastectomy, all the breast tissue is removed together with the pectoralis minor and major muscles and the axillary contents; the pectoralis major is preserved in the modified procedure. American College of Surgeons, Commission on Cancer, Chicago, 1982.

Table 6.2 Halsted radical mastectomy and modified radical mastectomy in the treatment of breast cancer; use of the less drastic modified procedure has steadily increased.

the only possible curative treatment and results of gastrectomy have improved since 1970 (Table 6.3) [4]. Comparison of five-year survival shows dramatic differences between Japanese and American results (100% for Japan and 50% for the USA for stage I cancer), which may in part due be to differences in classification of stage or in surgical technique. In Japan, extended lymph node dissection is standard procedure and total gastrectomy and dissection of adjacent organs are more commonly performed.

Palliative cancer surgery
Indications for palliative surgery have decreased during the last decades with the increasing emergence of interventional techniques. Endoscopic and radiological technology has enabled significant palliation of disabling symptoms, particularly in the context of lumen-occluding compression by the tumour.

Technological advances
Surgical instrumentation has evolved steadily over the past two decades. Fibre-optic endoscopy, along with other new technologies, has had a significant impact on the development of modern surgery. Laparoscopy (endoscopic examination of the interior of the abdomen) has become a mainstay in the diagnosis of intraperitoneal non-Hodgkin lymphoma and peritoneal carcinomatosis (widespread carcinoma in the abdominal cavity). Combined with ultrasonography, it plays an increasingly important role in the staging of many cancers, such as hepatic and pancreatic tumours [6]. Moreover, new procedures are still being explored in the treatment of cancer. Early results of laparoscopic resection of colonic carcinoma seem to be promising, although the sporadic reports of port site recurrences need further investigation. Peripheral lung metastases can be resected through thoracoscopy by

wedge resection. However, more specific data are required to justify adoption of laparoscopic and thoracoscopic procedures as standard operations in the field of cancer. Oncological principles should not be compromised solely to accommodate the technically complex tasks associated with video-endoscopic techniques.
Over recent years, non-operative ablative techniques have also emerged. These are designed to facilitate local destruction of tumours either by chemical or physical agents, such as arterial chemoembolization, alcohol injection, cryotherapy, radiofrequency ablation, electrolysis (Fig. 6.2) and chemo-hyperthermia [7]. These procedures can be used not only for palliation but also with a curative intent, as an alternative to, or in combination with, surgical resection, according to the stage of the tumour and the general condition of the patient.
Liver transplantation is now considered the best modality of treatment in carefully selected cirrhotic patients with small hepatocellular carcinoma confined to the liver (Fig. 6.3). Although still controversial, this new strategy, which treats both tumour and cirrhosis, is now meeting with increasing success and is becoming more accepted in developed countries. Nevertheless, its application on a large scale remains limited by the persistent shortage of donors and thus of organs available for transplantation. Liver transplantation with living, related donors has become a valuable alternative to reduce the pressure on the significant shortage of cadaveric liver grafts and has been applied to carefully selected patients with a limited range of malignant liver tumours. In Asian countries (particularly Japan and Hong Kong) where transplantation from cadaveric donors is nearly non-existent, this new strategy is progressively being developed by specialized centres.

Role of surgical oncology in multi-modality therapy
Surgery remains the primary option for the cure of many cancers. However, on occasions, curative resection is impossible or the prognosis following resection remains unsatisfactory. To combat such

Period	Resectability (%)	Mortality (%)	5-yr survival (%)
Before 1970	37	15	38
Before 1980	53	13	52
Before 1990	48	5	55

Table 6.3 Survival and mortality following stomach cancer surgery have improved significantly.
A.J.A. Bremers et al. (1999) *Cancer Treatment Reviews*, 25: 333-353.

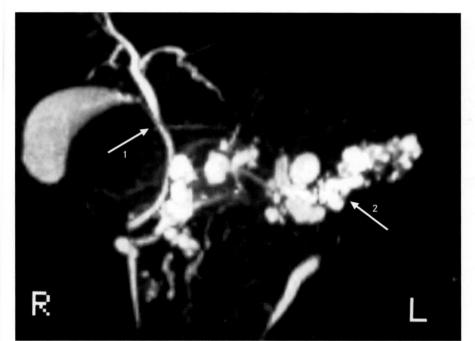

Fig. 6.5 Contrast-enhanced magnetic resonance imaging (MRI) of an intraductal papillary mucinous tumour of the pancreas in an adult patient who was subsequently treated by total pancreatectomy. 1 = common bile duct; 2 = pancreatic duct with multiple dilations caused by the presence of tumour tissue; R = right, L = left.

The future

Typically within more developed countries, there is now a range of fully equipped and staffed specialist cancer hospitals or major centres with specialized cancer units. Despite this infrastructure, in many countries, surgical oncology still remains apart on both a local and national level. Adoption of new technologies in cancer surgery should be guided by scientific evidence of benefit for the patient and cost-effectiveness in relation to current practice. During the evaluation phase, access to the technology should be restricted to multi-centre controlled clinical trials within a critical academic oncology climate. Such a programme of action will safeguard continuing progress in outcomes of cancer care, while at the same time keeping the economic burden within reasonable and sustainable limits [2].

expectation of poor outcome, adjuvant therapies combining chemotherapy and radiotherapy have been developed and, when added to surgery, may be regarded as an integral part of modern surgical oncology.

Neoadjuvant use of radiotherapy has been developed to help downstage tumours such as rectal carcinoma. Some irresectable tumours may become resectable following such treatment. Similar results can be obtained by chemotherapy in the management of large, awkwardly placed hepatic colorectal metastatic disease, and this can transform certain tumours from irresectable to resectable lesions. Neo-adjuvant therapy may also decrease the rate of regional recurrence after curative resection of aggressive carcinomas, exemplified by pancreatic exocrine adenocarcinoma [8].

The goal of cytoreductive surgery is to remove as much as possible of the tumour mass. Such elimination of large portions of known malignant deposits is referred to as "debulking". Cytoreductive surgery is widely employed as the primary treatment of ovarian cancer, with both five-year survival and median survival better for patients with small residual masses. Some of these findings may, however, be a reflection of patients selected for surgery rather than a treatment-related change in the natural history of disease. Cytoreductive surgery is usually combined with subsequent chemotherapy and radiotherapy. There is increasing use of cytoreductive surgery and intraperitoneal chemotherapy for peritoneal carcinomatosis from ovarian cancer. Recent advances in intraoperative radiotherapy have the potential to offer additional strategies in the management of inaccessible or poorly resected cancers, typified by tumours of the biliary tract. Biliary cholangiocarcinomas can be managed by the placement of intraoperative radiotherapeutic sources as adjuvant treatment following either resection or failed resection.

TELEMEDICINE

The prospects for telemedicine in cancer treatment primarily involve information distribution for quality assurance and sharing of medical technology resources. The Internet provides a powerful platform for information and knowledge distribution worldwide. Routine use of telemedicine is currently limited to developed countries. The impact of telemedicine in developing countries remains limited since Internet access is often restricted. In developed countries, sharing of medical technology resources among health care institutions is likely to increase markedly with the development of advanced Internet-based services. These may include remote diagnosis, telemedical services such as remote image processing (including 3D or virtual reality for diagnosis or training), remote therapy planning (e.g. in radiation therapy) and expert system counterchecks (e.g. to monitor treatment courses) which may improve treatment outcome at affordable costs.

Today, with modern network capacities no longer limiting electronic medical data transfer, the management of huge quantities of information and quality assurance are the major challenges in advanced medical informatics. Although much effort has been directed towards the development of electronic patient records, no truly authoritative standard has thus far evolved (European Committee for Standar- dization, Technical Committee for Health Informatics, http://www.centc251.org/).

In developed countries, most hospitals rely on electronic data processing as the means of delivering services. Individual medical departments often employ their own digital information systems. In most instances, these applications will have been implemented over many years without reference to sharing, and communication, even within the hospital information system, may not be practicable due to proprietary communication standards. In effect, within a single health care institution, relevant patient information is distributed in numerous information systems without proper exchange capabilities. Attempts have been made to utilize Web technology to create integration platforms, with HL 7 as the communication standard (Health Level 7, http:// www.HL7.org). However, disadvantages apply with respect to data handling, security and speed of performance. An alternative, as integration middleware, may be CORBA (Object Management Group, http://www.omg.org/) but commercial applications still have to prove their value in clinical routine.

Only broad distribution of electronic infrastructures in health care will allow the integration of beneficial telemedical services into medical practice. In developed countries, the evolution of electronic patient records promises extensive advantages in terms of quality assurance and cost-effectiveness of patient treatment. In developing countries, ubiquitous access to Internet information sources will help tremendously in the distribution of medical standards and knowledge (Ricke J and Bartelink H, *Eur J Cancer* 36, 827-834, 2000; Wootton R ed., *European telemedicine* 1998/99. Kensington publications, London 1999).

REFERENCES

1. Vetto J, ed. (1999) *Current Practice and Therapy in Surgical Oncology*, Hagerstown, MD, Lippincott Williams & Wilkins Publishers.

2. Feig BW, Berger DH, Fuhrman GM, eds (1998) *The M.D. Anderson Surgical Oncology Handbook*, Hagerstown, MD, Lippincott Williams & Wilkins Publishers.

3. Mion F, Grozel L, Boillot O, Paliard P, Berger F (1996) Adult cirrhotic liver explants: precancerous lesions and undetected small hepatocellular carcinomas. *Gastroenterology*, 111: 1587-1592.

4. Bremers AJ, Rutgers EJ, van de Velde CJ (1999) Cancer surgery: the last 25 years. *Cancer Treat Rev*, 25: 333-353.

5. Fisher B (1999) From Halsted to prevention and beyond: advances in the management of breast cancer during the twentieth century. *Eur J Cancer*, 35: 1963-1973.

6. Berry DP, Maddern GJ (2000) Other in situ ablative techniques for unresectable liver tumours. *Asian J Surg*, 23: 22-31.

7. Luck AJ, Maddern GJ (1999) Intraoperative abdominal ultrasonography. *Br J Surg*, 86: 5-16.

8. Partensky C, Maddern GJ (1999) Pancreatectomy after neoadjuvant chemoradiation for potentially resectable exocrine adenocarcinoma of the pancreas. In: Mornex F, Mazeron, JJ, Droz, JP, Marty, M eds, *Concomitant Chemoradiation: Current Status and Future*, Paris, Elsevier.

WEBSITES

Society of Surgical Oncology (USA):
http://www.surgonc.org

European Society for Surgical Oncology:
http://www.esso-surgeonline.be/

World Federation of Surgical Oncology Society:
http://www.wfsos.com/index.htm

On-line Medical Dictionary (CancerWeb):
http://cancerweb.ncl.ac.uk/omd/

RADIOTHERAPY

SUMMARY

> Radiotherapy is fundamental to the optimal management of cancer patients; its efficacy is affected by technical (the nature and delivery of the beam) and biological factors (tumour susceptibility modulated by hypoxia and drugs).

> Provision of radiotherapy services is central to national cancer control strategies, requiring long-term planning and appropriate assessment of health care resources.

> Without recourse to sophisticated technology, effective radiotherapy for many cancers can be comprehensively provided at moderate cost.

It is estimated that 50% of all patients who are diagnosed with cancer in the world would currently benefit at some stage of their illness from radiotherapy. This could be either as part of radical therapy with curative intent or as palliation for pain or other symptoms. The delivery of radiotherapy requires long-term planning in the construction of facilities as well as specialized doctors, physicists and technicians [1]. In many parts of the world facilities are very poor, even though upgrading is well within many health service budgets. The increasing reliability of modern equipment together with the reducing costs of the associated sophisticated computer planning facilities should result in considerable global improvement over the next decade.

Radiobiology

Radiotherapy is defined as the use of ionizing radiation for the treatment of malignant disease. Modern high energy X-ray machines deliver radiation which is up to one hundred times more penetrating than the X-rays used for diagnosis and can be delivered using tight beams to well defined areas in the body. This allows for the treatment of deep-seated tumours with minimal radiation being delivered to surrounding normal tissue. Although the majority of treatments given in this way use X- or gamma rays, ionizing radiation can also be given by electron beam accelerators or particle accelerators.

The biological basis for the therapeutic effect of radiation has been examined extensively in both cell culture and animal tumours. Although there are correlations from the laboratory, most clinical radiotherapy regimens are based on experience rather than biological modelling. There is considerable heterogeneity between tumours which defies rigid prediction.

Cell survival curves after the administration of different doses of radiation have been used to explore the best way to enhance selectivity between normal and malignant cells. Radiation causes profound DNA damage which is then repaired in most cells (*Carcinogen activation and DNA repair*, p89). The amount of damage depends on the type of radiation used and is increased in the presence of oxygen. Many tumours are hypoxic, simply because they have outgrown their blood supply (*Invasion and metastasis*, p119) and this renders such tumours more resistant to radiation damage. Different techniques to overcome this problem, such as the use of hyperbaric oxygen, hypoxic cell sensitizers and neutron radiation, have had only limited success. It is

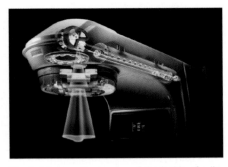

Fig. 6.6 Schematic drawing of the inside of a linear accelerator, indicating the wave-guide in which electrons are accelerated before hitting a target. ©Varian Medical Systems.

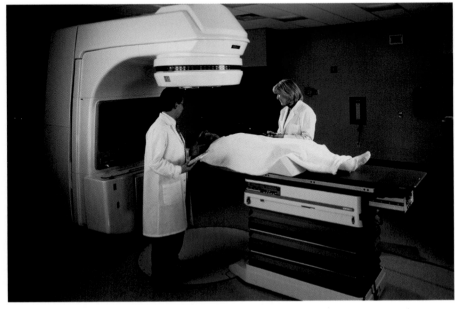

Fig. 6.7 A patient being prepared for treatment on a modern linear accelerator. © Varian Medical Systems.

Equipment	Energy	50% depth dose (depth at which electron beam ionization is 50%)	Approximate machine cost (million US$)
Orthovoltage	50-250 KeV	4 cm	0.2
Cobalt	1.25 MeV	9 cm	0.6
Linear accelerator	4-20 MeV	15 cm	1.0
Particle accelerator	4-20 MeV	5-20 cm	20 - 50

Table 6.4 Characteristics of radiotherapy equipment.

likely that as more is understood about the molecular genetics of cancer, the effects of radiation will be more accurately predictable. This will allow for more tailored and appropriate radiation schedules and doses, with better efficacy and less toxicity.

Equipment

Radiotherapy equipment is complex and varied [2]. The penetrating power of a radiotherapy beam is defined in terms of its energy and is measured in electron volts (eV). The simplest type of equipment is a low energy orthovoltage machine that basically represents an enhanced diagnostic X-ray machine. It can produce a beam of up to 250KeV. The problem in using a standard X-ray tube to produce a beam of higher energy is the heat gener-

ated at the target site (the site at which X-rays are generated by electron bombardment). Even with elaborate water cooling systems, target degradation occurs rapidly at higher voltages. Although the penetration of such low voltage beams is only 1-4 cm, they are effective at treating superficial cancers of the skin and for palliating bone metastases. The application of multiple orthovoltage fields was used to treat deep tumours in the past, but severe skin reactions and the large volume of normal tissue irradiated posed severe problems.

Isotope-based radiotherapy using gamma ray-emitting sources produces beams with a higher energy. Initially radium was the source used, but this was superseded by cobalt. Cobalt machines produce an energy of 1.25 MeV and are very reliable.

The cobalt source is housed in a lead box with a shutter, which is opened electrically. The only mechanical failure to be addressed involves malfunction of the shutter mechanism. However there are problems with radiological protection as the sources need to be changed every five years because of radioactive decay. There have also been several bizarre incidents in developing countries where stolen cobalt heads have been sold for scrap metal resulting in highly radioactive home and office furniture.

Linear accelerators (Fig. 6.7) are now the "gold standard" for radiotherapy provision. Electrons are accelerated down a linear wave-guide of about a metre in length and then hit a target where their kinetic energy is transferred into X-rays. Such machines can reliably produce beams of up to 20MeV energy. These beams pass directly through the skin surface causing little or no skin reaction. In order to deliver maximal quantities of radiation to deep tumours while keeping normal tissue dose low it is necessary to use more than one beam. The amount of energy given up by each beam diminishes as it penetrates. With modern equipment and computer planning facilities, excellent dose distribution can usually be achieved in most parts of the body using three fields. The characteristics of the radiation produced and the approximate equipment costs are shown in Table 6.4.

The process by which the volume to be irradiated is identified by the radiotherapist is called "planning". Information is taken from clinical examination, plain X-rays, computed tomography (CT) and magnetic resonance imaging (MRI) scans and used to identify the target high dose volume. A simulator (a diagnostic apparatus with the same characteristics as a treatment machine) is used to check the anatomical relationships. In many situations, computed tomography planning systems allow direct marking of the volume on a computed tomography scan.

For small volume, very accurate fields, such as those used for laryngeal or pituitary tumours, some form of patient immobilization shell is required. This is a thin perspex mask made to fit each patient

Tumour	Total Dose (Gy)	Duration of treatment (weeks)	No. of fractions (dose (Gy) per fraction)
Prostate cancer	64	6	32 (2)
Glioblastoma	60	6	30 (2)
Oesophageal cancer	60	6	30 (2)
Laryngeal cancer	60	6	30 (2)
Pituitary tumour	50	5	25 (2)
Lung cancer	50	4	20 (2.5)
Hodgkin disease	40	4	20 (2)
Bone metastases	8	1	1 (8)

Table 6.5 Radiotherapy treatment appropriate to particular cancers.

individually and onto which marks for the entry and exit points have been made. In this way, the set-up is reproduced identically each day with no inaccuracy caused by slight shifts in the patient's position or changes in skin shape or contour due to weight loss that may occur during treatment. Radical radiotherapy is usually fractionated into small daily doses given five days a week. This allows a lethal dose to be given to the tumour, whilst the normal tissues have time to recover and repair the DNA damage caused by radiation.

The relative merit of cobalt machines as compared to linear accelerators is often debated. In the past there have been concerns regarding capital cost, reliability and clinical need for linear accelerator technology in the developing world [3]. Recent technical advances in beam collimation, conformal therapy, modular design and the ability to construct national and indeed international computer networks now favour linear accelerators as the workhorse for radiotherapy provision in developed countries. Although there are some who still consider cobalt effective [4], most organizations, including the UK's Royal College of Radiologists, consider linear accelerators to be the way forward [5].

Dosimetry

Radiation can be measured in several ways. In the early days, techniques such as film blackening, skin erythema and measuring changes in chemicals contained in pastilles placed on the skin, gave an approximate indication of dose. In 1937 the "Roentgen" was defined, reflecting the energy of the beam measured in an ionization chamber. This did not, however, reflect absorbed dose in a target volume in a patient. The "Rad" was the first unit of absorbed dose, with 1 rad representing the absorption of 100 ergs of energy per gram of tissue. The current unit using the S.I. system (International System of Units) is the Gray (Gy) which is the equivalent of 100 rads. Most fractionation schemes are expressed in centi-Gray (cGy), which is the same as 1 rad.

Different types of radiation – X-rays of different energy, neutrons and particles – have different biological effects on tissue even though the same dose may be given. This has to be taken into account in radiation safety calculations. For radiological protection the "Sievert" is used. This is calculated from the absorbed dose in cGy multiplied by a quality factor Q, which is 1.0 for most X-rays, 10 for neutrons and 20 for alpha particles.

In prescribing radiation, the timing, fractionation and volume to be treated are all interdependent. Many radical radiotherapy plans use a dose of approximately 60 Gy given in 30 daily fractions of 2Gy each day, Monday to Friday, over six weeks. Palliative treatments may be given with much larger fractions over a short period of time, using a lower total dose. For control of bone pain, a single large fraction of 8 Gy may be used. When the size of each fraction is increased the amount of normal tissue damage also rises because of the reduced time for the normal repair processes to work. Therefore the biological effects of giving the same total dose over a short period of time are much greater than giving it over a longer period of time. Various complex formulae have been developed to relate time dose and fraction size. The radiotherapist chooses a dose based on the type of tumour, whether treatment is radical or palliative and the volume and type of normal tissue included (Table 6.5).

The total amount of radiation tolerated by different parts of the body varies enormously. There are several tissues in the body that have a poor capacity to repair following exposure to radiation. The most sensitive are the lens of the eye, the spinal cord, lung, kidney and small intestine. Depending on the patient's general condition and expectation of cure, it is often necessary to construct elaborate plans to avoid these structures. More recently, conformal plans which correspond precisely to the shape of the tumour have become widely available (Fig. 6.8). Such plans reduce normal tissue toxicity and allow the actual tumour dose to be escalated, increas-

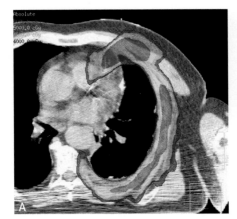
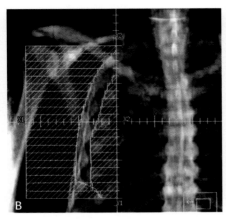
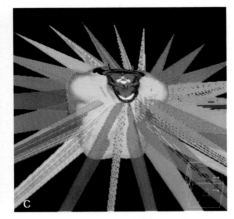

Fig. 6.8 Conformal radiotherapy to a pleural mesothelioma. **A** The calculated dose distribution in the axial or transverse view. **B** An example of one Beam's Eye View (BEV). The BEV at this particular gantry angle has a crescent shape that conforms to the target volume. **C** Different Beam's Eye Views (BEVs) that are delivered in one conformal X-ray arc field. ©Varian Medical Systems

CANCER EDUCATION IN MEDICAL COURSES

The Edinburgh Declaration of 1988 (World Conference on Medical Education, *Lancet* 2:464, 1988) aimed to change the character of medical education so that "it truly reflects the defined needs of the society in which it is situated". The total burden of cancer on the global community and the health care professions is increasing. These realities are prompting increased efforts in cancer control, and medical student cancer education must be an integral part of this effort. The International Union Against Cancer (UICC) monograph (Robinson E et al., *Cancer Education for undergraduate medical students : curricula from around the world*, UICC, Geneva 1994) describes global concerns about the status of medical student education about cancer, and provides a series of model curricula.

The continued orientation of most medical student curricula around traditional department-discipline areas rather than community or patient needs inhibits the development of clinical service-based integrated teaching. It also inhibits the incorporation of new knowledge about cancer biology and epidemiology and improved cancer treatments into medical student education. Medical educators stress the importance of medical students' experience as a major determinant of lifetime approaches to cancer. Initial perspectives may not be greatly affected by postgraduate training. For many doctors, their only formal cancer education is that gained as a medical student, partly because cancer management and control does not fall squarely on any of the individual postgraduate educational bodies. It is clearly important that medical students should be appropriately educated about cancer. The joint UICC/WHO statement (Undergraduate education in cancer, UICC/WHO Workshop, Geneva, 1981), to the effect that "in most countries there is a significant gap between the actual cure rates of various cancers and the maximum cure rates obtaining through utilizing current available knowledge", is sobering. An important first step in the reform of medical student cancer education is the appointment of a cancer education committee or co-ordinator in all medical schools. A reorganization of the existing syllabus with the introduction of problem-based learning relating to cancer biology, cancer prevention, diagnosis, treatment and symptom control, would rectify many of the deficiencies identified in surveys of medical student cancer education.

---

ing the chance of tumour eradication, provided no metastases are present.

Brachytherapy

This literally means "short distance treatment" and is used to describe techniques where radioactive sources are placed directly through or in contact with a tumour. Such systems for the treatment of cervical cancer are very effective. This cancer is common in many parts of the developing world and, if better education could result in earlier presentation, more women would be curable by this relatively low-tech procedure. Basically rods of caesium or other isotope are placed directly into the uterus with further radioactive material inserted into the vaginal vault. In this way a pear-shaped deposition of high intensity radiation is delivered over a two- to three-day period. More sophisticated after-loading systems are available in which the isotope, in the form of cobalt or iridium beads, is inserted into guides by a hydraulic system. This reduces unwanted exposure of staff and relatives to radiation.

Iridium 191 wires are flexible and can be inserted directly into tumours of the tongue, buccal mucosa, anus and breast. This gives a very high dose of radiation precisely to the tumour. The wires remain in position for three to five days and the results are often as good as found with more expensive external radiotherapy systems.

Side effects of radiotherapy

Most patients tolerate radiotherapy relatively well. Problems arise from the intrinsic sensitivity of normal tissue inevitably included in the treatment volume. Mucous membranes became oedematous and painful, skin reaction leads in extreme cases to ulceration and scarring. Abdominal radiation causes enteritis and diarrhoea. The general acute effects of radiation include radiation sickness and general debility. Good nursing care with drugs to control sickness, headaches, diarrhoea and oedema can effectively control most problems. The delivery of high quality radiotherapy requires teamwork between a range of professionals to maximize its benefits and reduce the severity of its side effects.

REFERENCES

1. Porter A, Aref A, Chodounsky Z, Elzawawy A, Manatrakul N, Ngoma T, Orton C, Van't Hooft E, Sikora K (1999) A global strategy for radiotherapy: a WHO consultation. *Clin Oncol (R Coll Radiol)*, 11: 368-370.

2. Price P, Sikora K, eds (2000) *Treatment of Cancer*, 4th Edition, London, Chapman and Hall.

3. Borras C, Stovall J, eds (1993) *Design Requirements for Megavoltage Radiotherapy X-Ray Machines for Cancer Treatment in Developing Countries*, New Mexico: Los Alamos Laboratories.

4. Van Dyk F, Battista J (1996) Cobalt 60: an old modality, a renewed challenge. *Curr Oncol* 3: 23-34.

5. Royal College of Radiologists (1998) *Equipment, Workload and Staffing for Radiotherapy in the UK*, London

WEBSITES

International Society of Radiology:
http://209.67.209.116/

The Royal College of Radiologists (UK):
http://www5.red.net/enquiries/college/page0001.html

European Association and Congress of Radiology:
http://www.ecr.org/

Cancer BACUP (UK): Understanding Radiotherapy:
http://www.cancerbacup.org.uk/info/radiotherapy.htm

MEDICAL ONCOLOGY

SUMMARY

> The efficacy of chemotherapy varies markedly depending upon the malignancy. Some, such as testicular seminoma, leukaemias and malignant lymphomas are highly responsive, while minimal response tumours include those of the brain (glioblastoma), lung and pancreas.

> WHO has identified a list of essential anticancer drugs.

> Drugs are typically used in combination, based on and progressively improved by randomized trials.

> Inherent or induced drug resistance limits efficacy.

> Most currently-used drugs inhibit DNA synthesis and/or cell division, inducing apoptosis. Drugs that target tumour-specific signalling pathways, including the tryrosine kinase inhibitor Gleevec for stromal tumours and acute myeloid leukaemia, are being developed.

> New approaches include gene therapy and novel strategies for immunotherapy, but clinical results thus far are largely disappointing.

CHEMOTHERAPY

The use of chemotherapy to treat cancer began in 1943 following the observation of leukopenia (reduction in number of leukocytes) in military personnel exposed to mustard gas after an explosion of a battleship in Bari harbour. This alkylating agent was adapted for intravenous use and produced dramatic but short-lived responses in patients with lymphoma and leukaemia. Other agents, such as the folic acid and pyrimidine inhibitors, followed and the armamentarium rapidly grew. It was recognized that drug resistance developed when single agents were used, so combi-

nation chemotherapy became standard. During the 1950s and 1960s, major strides were made in the treatment of leukaemias, lymphomas and choriocarcinomas with many patients being completely cured. New drugs were discovered following extensive screening programmes – the vinca alkaloids from the periwinkle, the anthracyclines from fungi and platinum drugs from experiments on the effects of electric currents on bacterial growth. The 1970s and 1980s brought effective drug combinations for testicular cancer and many childhood malignancies. Thus chemotherapy is now given in the setting of paediatric malignancy, germ cell tumours (Cancers of the male reproductive tract, p208) and some types of lymphoma (Lymphoma, p237) with curative intent. Chemotherapy may be administered prior to surgery (neoadjuvant) to facilitate resection and prevent metastasis or after surgical debulking (adjuvant) to reduce the risk of distant relapse. Adjuvant chemotherapy for breast and colon cancer was proven to be beneficial in large-scale randomized trials followed by sophisticated meta-analyses [1]. The value of chemotherapy in improving the quality of life of patients, by palliating symptoms and pain, even in the absence of survival advantage, is evident.

New drugs have been launched and new combinations put together. However, many challenges remain (Table 6.6). Despite many new agents becoming available, often at great cost, the gains in terms of cure rates have been small. Fashions for high dose chemotherapy with

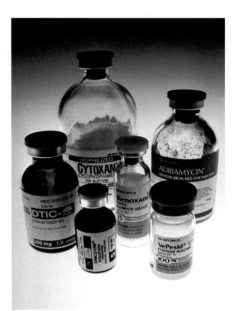

Fig. 6.9 Chemotherapeutic drugs for injection may be available as ampoules (as shown) or ready-prepared in a syringe.

High complete response	High complete response	Low complete response
High cure	Low cure	Low cure
Hodgkin disease	Acute myeloid leukaemia	Non small cell lung cancer
Acute lymphoblastic leukaemia	Breast cancer	Colon cancer
Testicular cancer	Ovarian cancer	Stomach cancer
Choriocarcinoma	Small cell lung cancer	Prostate cancer
Childhood cancer	Sarcoma	Pancreatic cancer
Burkitt lymphoma	Myeloma	Glioblastoma

Table 6.6 Chemotherapy for advanced cancer: the current situation.

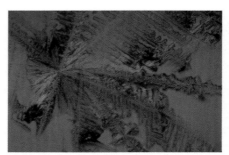

Fig. 6.10 Crystals of cisplatin: more than 90% of patients with advanced germ cell tumours are curable since the introduction of cisplatin-based chemotherapy.

bone marrow transplantation, the use of marrow support factors, biological therapies such as monoclonal antibodies or cytokines, have resulted in little overall gain but considerable expense. The driving force for medical oncology comes from the USA, which spends 60% of the world's cancer drug budget but has only 4% of its population (Fig. 6.11). Huge cultural differences exist in the use of chemotherapy, with USA-trained physicians following aggressive regimens for patients who in other countries would simply be offered palliative care. This has created a tremendous dilemma for those responsible for health care budgets. For example, the use of paclitaxel in patients with metastatic breast cancer will prolong survival by six months at a cost of US$12,000. In many countries this would far exceed the total health care consumption throughout a cancer patient's life. Yet the pressure to use expensive patented drugs is enormous. Conferences, travel and educational events sponsored by the drug industry rarely give a real perspective on the effective prioritization of cancer care for poorer countries.

The biological basis

In respect of their molecular structure, drugs currently used in cancer chemotherapy represent an enormous range of structural diversity. Anticancer drugs may be characterized as being toxic to, and hence able to cause the death of, dividing cells. Many agents for which a mechanism or mechanisms of action is relatively clear interfere with biological processes necessary for cell division, specifically including the synthesis of DNA or RNA (Fig. 6.12). Antimetabolites limit synthesis of nucleic acid precursors. In this way methotrexate inhibits dihydrofolate reductase, thereby limiting synthesis of reduced folate, which is necessary for production of purines and pyrimidines. Similar agents include 5-fluorouracil and cytarabine. After synthesis, the macromolecular processing of DNA is dependent upon topoisomerases and these enzymes are specifically inhibited by a number of classes of drugs, including anthracyclines (doxorubicin, daunorubicin and epirubicin), epipodophyllotoxins (etoposide and teniposide) and the camptothecins (irinotecan and topotecan). Some drugs cause structural damage to mature DNA, as exemplified by alkylating agents (cyclophosphamide, chloroambucil and procarbazine) and platinum derivatives (cisplatin and carboplatin). Functioning of the mitotic spindle is variously affected by vinca alkaloids (vincristine and vinblastine) and the taxanes (paclitaxel and related compounds). Hormonal agents such as tamoxifen affect proliferation of hormonally responsive cells and are thus effective in breast cancer. Otherwise, pharmacological mechanisms such as those summarized above often fail to account for the marked differences in responsiveness of particular tumour types to the various agents, and for

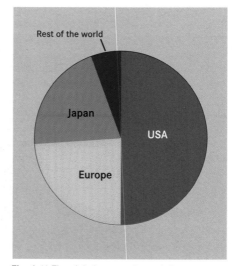

Fig. 6.11 The global cancer drug market.

which no mechanistic insight may be available.

Cytotoxic drugs evoke drug resistance. Tumours (relative to normal tissue) may be inherently resistant or acquire resistance as a consequence of treatment. Such resistance may be anticipated to include drugs of similar structure, but often extends to multiple classes of structurally unrelated agents (Box: *Resistance to cancer chemotherapy*, p285). The phenomenon has been extensively studied experimentally, by selection of cell populations able to proliferate in the presence of a high drug concentration. While relevant processes have been revealed, including production of the multidrug resistant protein 1 (which mediates drug transport out of cells), the extent to which these processes limit patient responses is still being determined.

Delivery

Increasingly, chemotherapy can be given entirely in a day care or outpatient setting. This reduces costs and is preferred by most patients and their families. Prior to initiation, the goal of therapy must be realistically defined. Prognostic factors such as the stage of the disease, the sites of metastases, the general medical condition of the patient, the willingness to accept any likely toxicity and the availability of the necessary facilities to treat complications must all be considered. It is essential to carefully document the degree of involvement at key sites so that the response to drugs can be measured. Although a particular tumour may be curable in some circumstances, not all patients with that tumour type will be cured. The risk-benefit concept needs to be discussed beforehand. Increasingly, cancer patients are being given more information about their disease and the options available. An honest appraisal of cost-effectiveness is vital in countries where the full cost of drugs is paid for by the patient. Cancer chemotherapy requires access to laboratory facilities to monitor at least blood counts, liver and renal function and tumour markers. Nurse-led chemotherapy suites are very effective and liked by patients. Clear protocols must be in place and adapted to local circumstances.

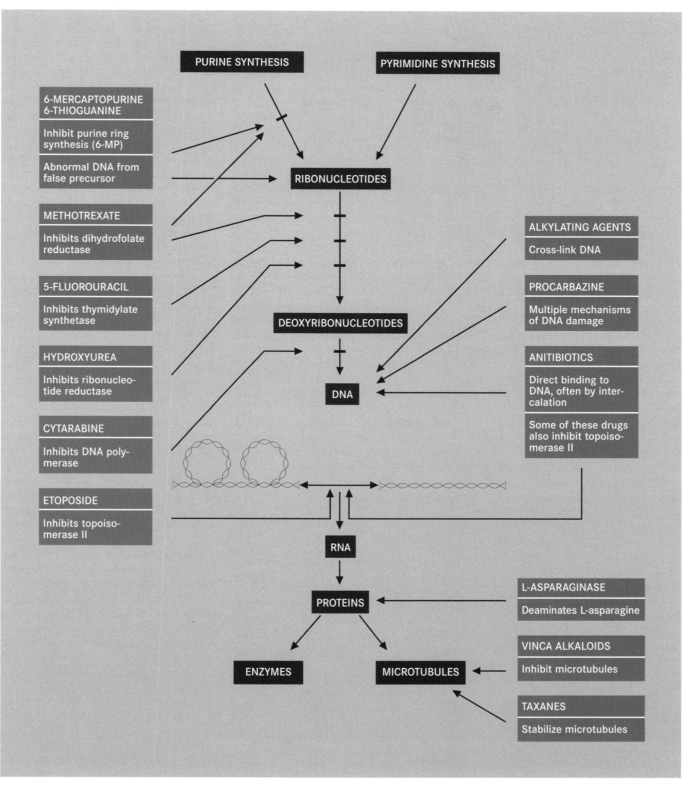

Fig. 6.12 Summary of the mechanisms and sites of action of selected cancer chemotherapeutic drugs.

Responsiveness (in decreasing order of efficacy)	Cancer
Category 1	Germ cell, leukaemias, lymphomas, choriocarcinoma
Category 2	Breast, colorectal, ovarian, osteosarcoma, Ewing's sarcomas, Wilms tumour
Category 3	Lung, bladder, prostate, stomach, cervical
Category 4	Head and neck
Category 5	Liver, melanoma, pancreatic, brain, renal, thyroid

Table 6.7 Categorization of cancer by effectiveness of chemotherapy.

For many curable cancers, the initial therapy is the most important. Any dose reduction, delay or drug substitution can adversely affect response rate. Managers and patients must understand that reducing the drug dosage or number of cycles to save money is unacceptable. Adjuvant chemotherapy is now of proven value in breast and colon cancer. Again, rigid adherence to protocols is essential to maximize results.

Recently several high cost drugs have been marketed for common cancers. Although capable of a significant response rate in patients with metastatic disease, such responses may be of short duration and may only prolong survival by weeks. To what extent some of these new agents should replace older and cheaper generic agents has not yet been determined in well designed trials with relevant endpoints, which include cost benefit analysis [2]. Inevitably this will have a subjective element and will vary with the overall allocation of cancer treatment resources in a country.

Categories of effectiveness

Protocols for drug use, and the determination of which agents should be used in the treatment of which cancers, has fre-quently been determined empirically. Clinical trials are developed for this purpose, and recognized standards, extending from informed patient consent through to adequate statistical analysis, have been established for such trials. Often, cytotoxic drugs are employed (usually in combination) at the maximum possible dose. Dosage is limited by toxicity: the consequence of the agent reaching, and hence affecting, normal tissue. Certain toxicity, such as hair loss, may be of limited significance but death of proliferating cells in the gut, bone marrow or other sites may provoke nausea, myelosuppression or other adverse effects.

There are more than 200 types of cancer and these respond variably to chemotherapy. Tumours can be split into five categories with regard to the relative usefulness of chemotherapy (Table 6.7). This provides a basis for examining the overall health gain of defined interventions. This will of course change as new drugs with greater efficacy are introduced.

Category 1: Tumours for which there is evidence that the use of a single or a combination of drugs used alone or with other therapeutic modalities will result in cure as defined by a normal life span in some and prolongation of survival in most patients.

Category 2: Tumours where the average survival is prolonged when chemotherapy is used as an adjuvant to local surgery or radiotherapy in the early stages of disease.

Category 3: Tumours where there is evidence that a single drug or a combination will produce clinically useful responses in more than 20% of patients. Prolongation of survival occurs in most responding patients but may be of short duration.

Category 4: Tumours where local control may be improved by using chemotherapy before, during or after surgery and radiotherapy.

Category 5: Tumours for which there are currently no effective drugs. Objective responses occur in less than 20% of patients and there is no evidence of survival benefit in randomized controlled trials when compared to best supportive care.

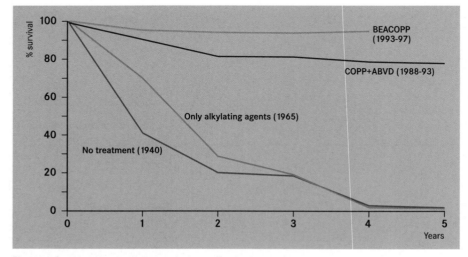

Fig. 6.13 Combination chemotherapy is more effective than a single agent for treatment of Hodgkin disease. (ABVD = adriamycin [doxorubicin], bleomycin, vinblastine and dacarbazine; BEACOPP = bleomycin, etoposide, adriamycin [doxorubicin], cyclophosphamide, oncovin [vincristine], procarbazine and prednisone; COPP = cyclophosphamide, oncovin [vincristine], procarbazine and prednisone).

RESISTANCE TO CANCER CHEMOTHERAPY

While many anticancer drugs, either alone or in combination, dramatically affect the course of malignant disease, success is far from universal. Certain tumour types are relatively refractory to anticancer drugs. In other instances, a marked response to treatment occurs but, over time, the disease process recurs and drugs, both those originally used and agents not previously employed, are ineffective. This phenomenon is referred to as "drug resistance", sub-categorized as either inherent or acquired, as appropriate.

To understand, and ultimately circumvent, drug resistance, massive resources have been directed toward elucidating mechanisms. The primary focus has been malignant tumour cell cultures which are resistant to particular drugs, or cell populations which acquire resistance as a result of being cultured in the presence of progressively increasing drug concentrations. Such cultures partially reflect the clinical behaviour of tumours, particularly to the extent that cultures "selected" using one drug also exhibit resistance to some, but not all, other drugs.

Mechanisms of drug resistance in cultured cells have been elucidated. Typically, resistance is attributable to mutation or altered expression of genes whose products mediate the transport of a drug(s) into or out of the cell, the metabolism and hence the intracellular concentration of the drug, and the structural or enzymatic protein to which the drug binds to cause cytotoxicity, sometimes called the target. Thus the multidrug resistance gene MDR1 encodes P-glycoprotein which mediates the transport of a family of "natural product drugs" (including vinca alkaloids and epipodophyllotoxins, but excluding, for example, cisplatin) out of the cell thereby reducing their intracellular concentration and hence cytotoxicity (Tan B et al., Curr Opin Oncol, 12: 450-458, 2000). Agents tending to inhibit P-glycoprotein, and hence restore drug sensitivity, have been identified (Szabó D et al., Anticancer Res, 20: 4261-4274, 2000; Persidis A, Nat Biotechnology, 17: 94-5, 1999). Depending upon drug concentrations employed in the selection process, overexpression of P-glycoprotein may be achieved through increased concentration of messenger RNA with or without amplification of the MDR1 gene. Altered expression of genes affecting apoptosis may also account for resistance (e.g. Helmbach H et al., Int J Cancer, 93: 617-22, 2001). Gene amplification and related effects are restricted to malignant cells, and are considered to reflect the genomic instability that is characteristic of cancer biology.

Exploitation of drug resistance mechanisms to improve clinical outcome for patients with relevant cancers has been limited. Surveys have been undertaken to establish overexpression of "resistance" genes in particular tumour types, and such studies may be applied to individual tumours as a basis for designing therapy.

Drug resistance mechanisms operating in clinical cancer are demonstrable. However, the findings overall are complex: few specific generalizations can be made and effective therapy is often restricted to individual cases. Likewise, the results of clinical trials of MDR1 inhibitors, or novel drugs specifically developed to circumvent particular resistance processes, have not become the dominant features of cancer chemotherapy. However, accumulated knowledge tends to confirm the efficacy of drug combinations rather than single agents as offering the best basis for cancer chemotherapy. Indeed, the vulnerability of single agents to resistance mechanisms has been demonstrated in relation to the drug STI-571 ("Gleevec") which was developed to specifically inhibit the gene product which has a critical role in the etiology of chronic myeloid leukaemia (McCormick F, Nature, 412, 281-282, 2001).

Class of compound	Resistance mechanism(s)
Antimetabolites Methotrexate	Defect in active transportation Polyglutamation defect Increased DHFR
5-Fluorouracil (5-FU)	Alterations in activating enzymes Increased thymidylate synthase Increased dUMP
Alkylating agents Mustard derivatives	Decreased cellular uptake Increased cellular gluathione Enhanced DNA repair
Nitrosoureas	Enhanced DNA repair via guanine-O^6-alkyl transferase Decreased cellular uptake
Platinum derivatives	Increased cellular gluathione Enhanced DNA repair
Anthracyclines and like agents	P-glycoprotein Altered topoisomerase-II activity Increased cellular gluathione
Natural alkaloids Taxanes	Alterations in tubulin P-glycoprotein

Table 6.10 Some causes of cytotoxic drug resistance.

Most of the world's most common cancers fall into category 3 (Table 6.7).

Prioritizing cancer care

Chemotherapy is only one of many approaches to cancer control (*Cancer control*, p303). In all environments, skilled prioritization is necessary to maximize the overall benefit of medical intervention. This must include the prevention, education, early diagnosis, and the other treatment modalities outlined elsewhere. Recently, the WHO has published its recommendations for prioritizing anticancer drugs with the creation of an essential drugs list [3]. The drugs were banded by their utility in treating category 1, 2 and 3 tumours and related to the global incidence of the responding tumours. Thirteen drugs were identified which provide beneficial outcomes against certain cancers, with a further four drugs necessary to treat leukaemia. Thus 17 drugs can be considered as the first priority (Table 6.8). All are generic and relatively cheap and should be made widely available before the more recent, heavily promoted high cost drugs are purchased.

A second group of drugs is listed as priority 2. These have well documented benefits in certain clinical situations but are not truly essential, as either drugs from priority 1 can be used as substitutes or their effects are only palliative. Cheaper and simpler forms of palliation with radiotherapy or analgesics may be more appropriate in low resource environments. Few of these drugs are available as generics.

The practical problems in assessing the role of a particular drug are exemplified by the case of the taxanes – paclitaxel and docetaxel. A randomized controlled trial in the USA demonstrated a 13-month survival advantage for women given paclitaxel and cisplatinum as first-line treatment for ovarian cancer when compared to cyclophosphamide and cisplatinum, the previously most widely used treatment [4]. The additional cost of paclitaxel per quality-adjusted life year may be as much as US$ 20,000 per patient. Whether to recommend the routine use of paclitaxel in this situation must relate to the total health care economy of a country [5]. Of course the wealthy will simply buy the drug or go abroad for it, but state health care systems will increasingly have to take rationing decisions - something politicians try to avoid. The suggestion is often made that the pharmaceutical industry should make more effort to create a pricing structure that reflects local economies. Unfortunately parallel importing – the purchasing of a drug in a low-priced country and exporting it to one in which the price is high and selling it for profit – is a flourishing trade. This makes imaginative pricing schemes unpopular with major manufacturers who would see price erosion in their most profitable markets.

The drugs in the priority 3 group are recent, expensive and some are of low efficacy. About 50% of patients with metastatic breast cancer respond to docetaxel but the duration of benefit is usually only about six months. A similar order of benefit is seen with gemcitabine for non-small cell lung cancer, irinotecan for colorectal cancer and luteinizing hormone-releasing hormone (LHRH) agonists for prostate cancer. Manufacturers disseminate positive information through press releases and by using public relations agencies which support patient advocacy groups, as well as the more conventional advertising in medical journals. This fuels demand and disturbs the financing of public sector drug supply. Education of political decision-makers as well as the public is essential to correct this imbalance. A good example is the common desire to invest in stem cell rescue systems in the developing world. Although there is compelling evidence for a strong relationship between dose intensity of chemotherapy and tumour response rate, there is no good randomized data to show that dose escalation with bone marrow support pro-

The WHO essential cancer drug list	
Bleomycin	Procarbazine
Chlorambucil	Tamoxifen
Cyclophosphamide	Vincristine
Doxorubicin	Vinblastine
Etoposide	Cytarabine
5-Fluorouracil	Dactinomycin
Methotrexate	Daunorubicin
Prednisolone	6-Mercaptopurine
Cisplatinum	Plus two anti-emetics

Table 6.8

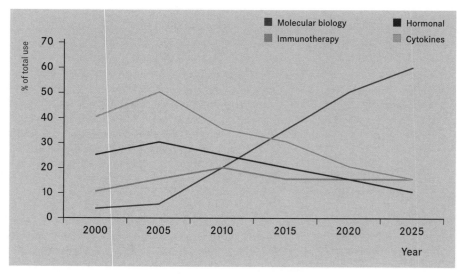

Fig. 6.14 Prediction for likely changes in approaches to chemotherapy, 2000 – 2025.

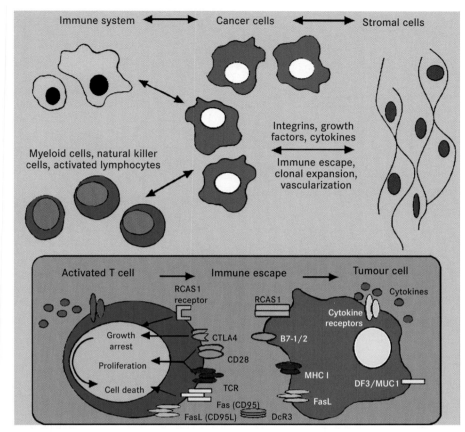

Fig. 6.15 Tumour cells are under selective pressure to escape the body's growth-restricting mechanisms. Upper panel: complex three-way interactions occur between tumour cells, their microenvironment and the immune system. Neighbouring stromal cells transfer nutrients and growth-stimulatory signals to cancer cells and stimulate vascularization. Cells of the innate and adaptive immune systems may attack cancer cells. Lower panel: different mechanisms may lead to evasion or counter-attack of cancer cells towards the immune system, including impaired antigen presentation, limited activation of cytotoxic T-cells, expression of Fas ligand which kills tumour-infiltrating cytoxic T-cells, natural killer cells, granulocytes or macrophages and production of mucins which block T-cell proliferation.

duces more cures in common cancers. The cost is enormous, often exceeding US$ 50,000 per patient.

Drugs for supportive care
Most effective cancer chemotherapy has significant side-effects. Effective antiemetics are available and should be routinely administered in advance with most chemotherapy combinations. Steroids (prednisolone or dexamethasone), a dopamine receptor antagonist (domperidone, metoclopramide) and a 5-hydroxytryptamine (5-HT3) receptor antagonist (ondansetron, granisetron) are essential. Local pricing should be used to determine choice within each category.

Neutropenia (subnormal levels of circulating neutrophils) and the risk of infection is one of the most common dose-limiting side-effects of cancer chemotherapy, leading to reduced dosages, delayed cycles and reduced effectiveness. Recombinant colony stimulating factors are available which mobilize marrow stem cells. There is little evidence that their routine use enhances the overall effectiveness of standard chemotherapy and yet two are billion dollar blockbusters.

A wide range of relatively cheap drugs is available for the relief of the many symptoms experienced by cancer patients. Especially important are the opioid analgesics, which are often strictly controlled and unavailable in many countries. The education of politicians, legislators and health care professionals is necessary to reduce the immense amount of needless suffering caused globally by inadequate analgesic use (*Palliative care*, p297).

Future developments
Several pieces of technology are coming together to drive forward chemotherapy in the next decade [6]. Molecular biology has provided some remarkable new targets for drug design. The Human Genome Project will yield huge volumes of information to categorize cancer risk and to define likely responses to treatment (Box: *Impact of the Human Genome Project,* p324). Understanding and measuring gene expression patterns will lead to novel agents to interfere with signal transduction, gene transcription, apoptosis and angiogenesis. Gene therapy (*Box: Gene therapy for cancer,* 289) holds promise to correct the basic defects that lead to cancer. It is likely that use of new therapeutic approaches centring on molecular biology will increase rapidly in the near future (Fig. 6.14) but advances will be expensive to implement. There is no doubt that the treatment of cancer is set to improve dramatically over the next decade. The greatest challenge facing all of us is how to fund the implementation of an equitable system of cancer care in an increasingly material world.

IMMUNOTHERAPY

Treatment of cancer with vaccines to stimulate the host's own immune system to reject the cancer has been a goal of tumour immunologists for much of the 20th century. Apart from vaccines and the administration of other agents such as bacterial products, which constitute "active" immunotherapy, exogenous immunity may be provided by the giving of antibodies or lymphoreticular cells in "passive" immunotherapy. Progress has been substantial but there is still a long way to go before immunotherapy is accepted as an important modality in the treatment of cancer. The problems largely stem from the fact that most cancer antigens (proteins displayed on the tumour cell surface which elicit a response from the host immune system) are also expressed in normal tissue, albeit at different levels or developmental stages (e.g. reappearance of fetal antigens such as alpha-fetoprotein and carcinoembryonic antigen). This lack of "foreignness" has meant that immunization against tumours has proved difficult. It is also clear that the method by which the antigen is presented to the immune system is critical in that T-cells can be "tolerized" to the tumour antigen, rather than activated. Immune responses can be qualitatively different and vary in their ability to reject tumours. The determinants of these different responses by the immune system are becoming better understood and are becoming incorporated into the design and administration of vaccines. On the other hand, the plasticity of the genome of tumour cells allows for the rapid generation of antigen-loss variants, which in some cases exceeds the adaptive processes of the immune system. Products of the tumour cell may have direct suppressive effects on immune responses. Certain tumour cells also appear resistant to programmed cell death induced by the immune cells.

Problems to be overcome in immunotherapy

There are inherent problems which limit the effectiveness of immune therapy (Fig. 6.15). Cancer cells can receive nutrients and growth-stimulatory signals from neighbouring stromal cells and stimulate neovascularization. Cells of both the innate (or non-specific, e.g. myeloid cells such as macrophages and neutrophils) and adaptive (or acquired, requiring the production of antibodies, e.g. lymphoid cells such as T-, B- and natural killer cells) immune systems may attack cancer cells. Myeloid cells can attack tumour cells in an antigen- and major histocompatibility complex (MHC)-independent way, for example, natural killer (NK) cells are triggered by cells lacking MHC class I molecules. In contrast, cytotoxic T lymphocytes

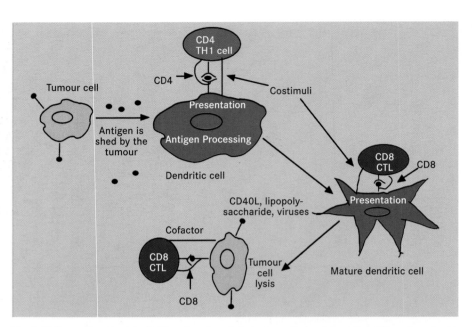

Fig. 6.16 Generation of cytotoxic T lymphocyte activity is dependent on interaction with mature dendritic cells (a distinct set of antigen-producing cells). CTL = cytotoxic T cell, THL = T-helper cell.

must be activated by antigen-derived peptides presented by MHC molecules. The lack of "foreignness" of a tumour is reflected in the number of precursor T-cells that are available in the host to reject the tumour. The higher the number of T-cells that recognize the tumour, the more likely it is that tumour rejection will occur. An extreme example of this is the rejection of allotransplants (grafts between two genetically different individuals) due to the host's possession of a high frequency (approximately 1 in 300) of precursors against alloantigens. Although it is unlikely that immunization against a single tumour cell antigen will achieve this frequency of T-cells, it is quite possible that immunization against several antigens will summate to these levels.

It has long been suspected that T-cells in cancer patients were tolerant to tumour antigens. Impaired antigen presentation results in limited cytotoxic T lymphocyte activation. This may follow from the expression of decoy receptor DcR3 on cancer cells and the neutralization of Fas ligand (CD95L) produced by cytotoxic T lymphocytes and natural killer cells (Fig. 6.15, lower panel). Expression of Fas ligand may kill tumour-infiltrating cytotoxic T

lymphocytes, natural killer cells, granulocytes or macrophages. Mucins, such as DF3/MUC1, or the new ligand RCAS1 (a growth inhibitory molecule expressed in many ovarian and uterine carcinomas), may block T-cell proliferation, adding to the arsenal of weapons that tumours may use to evade control by the immune system.

Measurement of tolerance has been facilitated by the introduction of tetramer technology. Tetramers are formed by linking biotinylated human leukocyte antigen (HLA) class I molecules to avidin and then adding peptides to the complex that are recognized by T-cells. Studies in transgenic mouse models and in melanoma patients have shown that tolerance of T-cells appears to correlate with low avidity of the T-cell receptor for the corresponding antigen [7].

In addition to the requirement for a high frequency of high avidity T-cells targeted against the antigen, it is also important that the responding T-cells produce cytokines, such as IFN-γ and IL-2, that recruit type 1 helper T-cell (TH1)-mediated responses, rather than IL-4- and IL-10-recruited type 2 helper T-cell (TH2) responses, which induce antibody pro-

GENE THERAPY FOR CANCER

Technology developed for manipulation of genetic material in an experimental context gave rise to the notion of altering gene structure or expression in the context of clinical treatment. Adenosine deaminase deficiency was the first inherited disease for which clinical gene therapy was performed (Blaese RM et al., *Science*, 270: 475-80, 1995). Infusion of T-cells in which the adenosine deaminase gene had been retrovirally transferred led to sustained detection of transduced and functional T-cells at least in two cases. Advancing knowledge about the genetic lesions present in cancer cells has allowed the emergence of gene therapy as a new method of intervention against cancer, which is targeted at the level of gene expression. Gene therapy has the potential to achieve a much higher level of specificity of action than conventional drug therapeutics owing to pinpoint targeting of control and regulatory mechanisms of gene expression (Gomez-Navarro J et al., *Eur J Cancer*, 35: 2039-2057, 1999).

A number of strategies for cancer gene therapy have been developed to the point of phase I or II trials:

Mutation compensation – includes replacement of a deficient function, e.g. of a tumour suppressor gene (e.g. retinoblastoma) by administering the wild-type gene, or ablating the function of a dominant oncogene (e.g. E1A). However, tumours are typically heterogeneous in their patterns of oncogene/tumour suppressor gene expression and possess more than one abnormality. Development of such therapy may require the "permanent" expression of the modified gene.

Molecular chemotherapy – includes delivery of a gene which is toxic to a cancer cell (e.g. thymidine kinase), or increases its sensitivity to conventional therapies (e.g. the *P450* gene sensitizes breast cancer to cyclophosphamide), or protects bone marrow from myelosuppression induced by chemotherapy. Problems to be overcome include a low transfection rate when the vector is injected loco-regionally, dose-limiting toxicity and the appearance of drug-resistant subpopulations.

Genetic immunopotentiation – attempts to enhance the anti-tumour activity of cells of the immune system (e.g. tumour-infiltrating lymphocytes) or to increase the immunogenicity of the tumour cell itself (e.g. transfer of granulocyte-macrophage colony stimulating factor (GM-CSF), the B7 family of co-stimulatory molecules, or major histocompatibility complex (MHC)). Obstacles to success include low transfer rate, tolerance of tumour antigens, and inhibition of immune response.

The promise of gene therapy has been realized in limited contexts. Primary immunodeficiencies have long been considered as a possible experimental field for gene therapy. As noted, adenosine deaminase deficiency was the first inherited disease for which clinical gene therapy was performed. The low number of cells transduced with the required gene, however, was not sufficient to provide sustained clinical benefit.

Nevertheless, Severe Combined Immunodeficiencies (SCID) represent unique conditions in which currently available vectors can still be considered for a therapeutic approach. This assumption is based on the expected selective advantage conferred to transduced cells in this setting. X-linked SCID is characterized by an absence of mature T and natural killer (NK) lymphocytes due to gamma c chain cytokine receptor deficiency. The ability of gamma c chain-transduced CD34+ cells from SCID-X1 patients to mature into T-cells (Hacein-Bey S et al., *Blood*, 92: 4090-7, 1998), as well as NK cells (Cavazzana-Calvo M et al., *Blood*, 88: 3901-9, 1996), sets the basis for a clinical trial of *ex-vivo* gene transfer into CD34+ cells from SCID-X1 patients.

The clinical trial was approved in January 1999 and initiated in March of the same year. Five patients were enrolled. *Ex-vivo* gene transfer led to an infection rate of CD34+ cells of 40% and 14 - 26.5 x 10^6/kg CD34+ cells were infused back to the

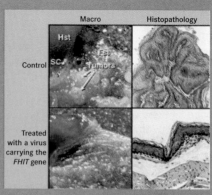

Fig. 6.17 Tumours are evident in the forestomach (Fst) and at the squamocolumnar junction (SCJ) with the hindstomach (Hst) in mice who possess only one normal copy of the *FHIT* tumour suppressor gene. Oral administration of a virus carrying a wildtype *FHIT* gene results in a substantial reduction in numbers and size of these tumours, and near normal stomach epithelia. K.R. Dumon et al. (2001) *Proc Natl Acad Sci USA* 98:3346-51.

patients without prior chemoablation. In all patients but one, T lymphocyte counts were detected from day 30 and rose progressively to reach values ≥ 3500/µl for the first two patients (Cavazzana-Calvo M et al., *Science*, 288: 669-72, 2000) and about 4800/µl for the fourth patient. These results are promising, although preliminary, and may open the door to treatment of other immunodeficiencies, and possibly cancer, by *ex-vivo* gene transfer.

Website:
Clinical trials in human gene transfer, Office of Biotechnology Activities, NIH:
http://www4.od.nih.gov/oba/clinicaltrial.htm

duction. It is clear that tumour cells are not passive targets for destruction by the immune system but become selected partly on the basis of products which inhibit host responses (Table 6.9).

Principles of immunotherapy

The considerations above and the experience gained from past studies on immunotherapy suggest it is possible to formulate principles that might apply irrespective of the cancer under study.

Immunization at sites removed from the tumour reduces the influence of the tumour on the antigen-presenting cell. Administration of a vaccine can be optimized in terms of dose, frequency and duration. Adjuvants (substances mixed with an antigen to enhance the immune response to this antigen) may increase numbers of antigen-presenting cells and processing thereby.

Induction of high affinity T-cell responses is becoming an important objective and underlies much of the interest in the use of dendritic cell vaccines. This is because studies in several animal models have shown it is possible to break tolerance by immunization with the antigen displayed on dendritic cells that have been activated by suitable agents, such as CD40 ligand, TNF-α and others [8-10]. Figure 6.16 illustrates recent concepts of how helper T-cells may act to cause maturation of dendritic cells to a stage where they can induce cytotoxic T-cell activity. Dendritic cells are induced to mature by interaction with helper T-cells which express the CD40 ligand. Dendritic cells can also be matured by lipopolysaccharide, TNF-α and viruses. Activated cytotoxic T lymphocytes can kill tumour cells expressing the relevant antigens. Tumour cells may inhibit dendritic cell maturation by release of factors such as interleukin IL-10 and vascular endothelial growth factor.

Immunization with low doses of antigen, such as with plasmid DNA, also appears to favour the induction of high affinity T-cells. The optimal antigens to be used in vaccines will differ between different types of cancer but in general the aim is to include antigens that are expressed at relatively high concentrations on the tumour cell

Mechanism	Factors involved
Inhibition of antigen presentation	Vascular endothelial growth factor (VEGF), interleukin-10 (IL-10)
Inhibition of cytokine production	IL-10, transforming growth factor-β (TGF-β) α- melanocyte-stimulating hormone
Tolerance of T cells	Tumour antigen, hydrogen peroxide, lack of co-stimulation
Inhibition of migration of leukocytes from blood vessels	Prostaglandin E2, VEGF
Tumour-mediated destruction of T cells	Fas Ligand, Tumour necrosis factor-related apoptosis-inducing ligand (TRAIL)
Resistance of tumour cells to killing	IL-10, immunoselection of human leukocyte antigen (HLA) and antigen loss variants

Table 6.9 Mechanisms involved in inhibition of host immune responses to tumours.

and against which there are relatively high numbers of precursor cells [11-13]. Increasing the relative numbers of T-cells targeted against a particular antigen has not proven an easy task and approaches to this include depletion of overall T-cell numbers prior to immunization. The most effective antigens in animal models have been individual-specific antigens. The same may apply in humans but use of autologous tumours cells or tumour extracts (derived from the host's own tumour) has practical difficulties in most patients. The general aim, however, is to use antigens in the vaccine which will increase the number of T-cells above the required threshold for rejection of the tumour.

Cancer vaccine trials

Melanoma remains the most studied human cancer, in terms of potential for treatment by immunotherapy. A number of phase III (comparison of the relative value of the new drug with the current standard treatment) and phase I/II trials (initial evaluation of a drug's safety and pharmacokinetics, generally in patients with advanced disease/focus on the activity of the new product as a single agent in a noncomparative, open study) have been conducted. Multiple centres have reported phase III trials based on use of whole cells or lysates of whole cells [14]. Most recently, the emphasis in vaccine development has shifted to the use of well-defined antigens in vaccines, such as peptide epitopes recognized by T-cells or whole proteins [7]. Immunotherapy with dendritic cells is also being tested in a number of centres. The objective of inducing apoptosis by the TNF family of ligands has received very little attention as a therapeutic strategy in immunotherapy but may hold the key to whether the immunotherapy is successful or not. Interferon-α2 (IFN-α2) is able to induce TRAIL (TNF-related apoptosis-inducing ligand) (Apoptosis, p113) on a variety of different lymphocytes such CD4 T-cells, natural killer cells and monocytes [15].

Broad perspectives

Insights into the complexity of tumour cells and the host immune system are gradually evolving. The lack of foreignness of most tumour antigens, tolerance of the immune system to the antigens and release of immunosuppressive factors by tumour cells provides a formidable problem to development of effective vaccine therapy. Most of the existing phase III trials are based on use of whole cell or lysates of whole cells and were initiated before some of the more recent concepts in tumour immunology were known. The results of three randomized trials in patients with melanoma have shown no substantial benefit from vaccine therapy but several major studies have yet to be completed. The advent of many "start-up" biotechnology companies and new information about cancer antigens has generated many new approaches in cancer vaccine therapy, particularly in the use of dendritic cell vaccines. The next few years promise therefore to be an exciting period in the evolution of immunotherapy.

HORMONAL THERAPY

Adjuvant endocrine therapy is a standard component in the management of tumours of the breast and prostate gland. In breast cancer, anti-estrogenic treatment is recommended for all post-menopausal women with newly-diagnosed metastatic disease if the tumour biopsy shows evidence of estrogen receptor (ER) or progesterone receptor (PR) expression. Similarly, this treatment is given if the receptor status is unknown, whereas ER/PR-negative carcinomas are not treated since they cannot be expected to respond. For many years, tamoxifen has been the drug of choice as many clinical trials have shown that it significantly increases progression-free survival; it may also prevent or delay the development of breast cancer in high-risk women [16]. As second-line treatment, the selective aromatase inhibitor anastrozole has been shown to be similarly effective. About one-quarter of breast carcinomas overexpress the HER2/neu protein (the *ERBB2* gene product) and these may respond to therapy with a monoclonal antibody (Herceptin) that binds to the receptor.

Prostate cancer was the first human neoplasm to be successfully treated with hormonal therapy, which has been used in the treatment of advanced disease for more than six decades. Androgen suppression may be achieved by luteinizing hormone-releasing hormone (LHRH) agonists or surgical orchidectomy. The majority of patients with metastatic prostate cancer show an initial response, often with significant relief of symptoms, but treatment is rarely curative and in most cases tumours become resistant to anti-androgen therapy.

Hormonal therapy, commonly with progestational agents, is also indicated and useful in the treatment of metastatic cancer of the endometrium, being associated with significant improvements in survival.

REFERENCES

1. Early Breast Cancer Trialists' Collaborative Group (1992) Systemic treatment of early breast cancer by hormonal, cytotoxic, or immune therapy. 133 randomised trials involving 31,000 recurrences and 24,000 deaths among 75,000 women. *Lancet*, 339: 71-85.

2. NCI/ASCO (1998) Integrating economic analysis into cancer clinical trials: the National Cancer Institute-American Society of Clinical Oncology Economics Workbook. *J Natl Cancer Inst Monogr*, 1-28.

3. Sikora K, Advani S, Koroltchouk V, Magrath I, Levy L, Pinedo H, Schwartsmann G, Tattersall M, Yan S (1999) Essential drugs for cancer therapy: a World Health Organization consultation. *Ann Oncol*, 10: 385-390.

4. McGuire W, Neugut AI, Arikian S, Doyle J, Dezii CM (1997) Analysis of the cost-effectiveness of paclitaxel as alternative combination therapy for advanced ovarian cancer. *J Clin Oncol*, 15: 640-645.

5. Sikora K (1999) Developing a global strategy for cancer. *Eur J Cancer*, 35: 24-31.

6. Sikora K (1998) Cancer. In: Marinker M, Peckham,M eds, *Clinical futures*, London, BMJ Books, 74-95.

7. Hersey P (2003) Principles in immunotherapy of melanoma. In: Thompson JF, Morton DL, Kroon, BBR eds, *Textbook of Melanoma: Pathology, Diagnosis and Management*, Martin Dunitz.

8. Lanzavecchia A (1998) Immunology. Licence to kill. *Nature*, 393: 413-414.

9. Sotomayor EM, Borrello I, Tubb E, Rattis FM, Bien H, Lu Z, Fein S, Schoenberger S, Levitsky HI (1999) Conversion of tumor-specific CD4+ T-cell tolerance to T-cell priming through *in vivo* ligation of CD40. *Nat Med*, 5: 780-787.

10. Diehl L, den Boer AT, Schoenberger SP, van der Voort EI, Schumacher TN, Melief CJ, Offringa R, Toes RE (1999) CD40 activation *in vivo* overcomes peptide-induced peripheral cytotoxic T-lymphocyte tolerance and augments antitumor vaccine efficacy. *Nat Med*, 5: 774-779.

11. Boon T, van der Bruggen P (1996) Human tumor antigens recognized by T lymphocytes. *J Exp Med*, 183: 725-729.

12. Rosenberg SA (1999) A new era for cancer immunotherapy based on the genes that encode cancer antigens. *Immunity*, 10: 281-287.

13. Gilboa E (1999) The makings of a tumor rejection antigen. *Immunity*, 11: 263-270.

14. Hersey P (2002) Advances in non-surgical treatment of melanoma. *Expert Opin Investig Drugs*, 11:75-85.

15. Nguyen T, Thomas WD, Zhang XD, Sanders J, Hersey P (2000) Immunologically mediated tumor cell apoptosis. The role of TRAIL in T cell and cytokine mediated responses to melanoma. *Forum (Genova)*, 10: 243-252.

16. O'Regan RM, Jordan VC (2002) The evolution of tamoxifen therapy in breast cancer: selective oestrogen-receptor modulators and downregulators. *Lancet Oncol*, 3: 207-214.

WEBSITES

Drug Information: a guide to prescription and over-the-counter medications (USA):
http://www.nlm.nih.gov/medlineplus/druginformation.html

US Food and Drug Administration Oncology Tools website:
http://www.fda.gov/cder/cancer/

American Society of Clinical Oncology:
http://www.asco.org

REHABILITATION

SUMMARY

> Rehabilitation involves restoring cancer patients to their highest achievable level of physical and psycho-intellectual capacity despite the impact of disease, thus improving quality of life.

> Medical, physical, cultural, financial and emotional needs of individuals must be considered.

> A comprehensive interdisciplinary team provides the optimal means.

Definition

Contemporary medicine places an emphasis on comprehensive patient care. In the cancer patient, this encompasses not only the patient's immediate condition and treatment, but also longer-term effects, physical disabilities, vocational issues and social reintegration.

Rehabilitation is the process of returning a person to their highest level of function following illness, injury or other debilitating events, the physical, psychological, social and vocational effects of which can lead to impairment, disability or handicap [1].

Impairment results from a loss or abnormality of physiological or anatomical structure or function [2]. These can be the clinical features or manifestations of a disease, such as weakness or confusion from a brain tumour [3].

A disability is a restriction or lack of ability to perform a task or activity within the normal range. This is the functional consequence of the impairment. An example may be the inability to walk due to weakness caused by a brain tumour.

A handicap results from the interaction of a person with their environment leading to a disadvantage in performing a role otherwise normal for an individual. An example would be the inability to continue work as a mail carrier due to the inability to walk from weakness caused by a brain tumour.

Cancer rehabilitation is the process by which those with cancer maximize their function and minimize their disability from the impairments of cancer, while attempting to maintain their quality of life (Table 6.11). Quality of life can be defined as a sense of well-being from current life experiences "in the context of the value systems in which they live, and in relation to their goals and concerns." [5].

Overall perspective

Due to earlier diagnosis and improvements in treatment, people are living longer following the diagnosis of cancer. The average five-year survival rate for cancer patients is 50% in developed countries, 30% in developing countries. However, cancer patients are frequently left with deficits in mobility, cognition and self-care. Cancer rehabilitation helps people live better with cancer. There is thus an increasing need for rehabilitation professionals to care for cancer patients and survivors [4].

Cancer rehabilitation can improve quality of life by eliminating or decreasing the

Objectives of cancer rehabilitation
Maximize functional abilities.
Minimize disability from cancer-related impairments.
Maintain quality of life.
Provide treatments for symptom control.

Table 6.11

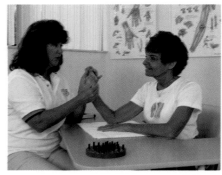

Fig. 6.18 Occupational therapy focuses on the restoration of bodily functions, mechanical movements and increasing patients' quality of life.
Von Kantor and Associates, Fort Lauderdale, USA.

Year	Physiatrists certified	
	No. certified in that year	Total certified
1975	65	1,163
1978	114	1,469
1980	101	1,709
1985	166	2,378
1990	287	3,454
1995	298	4,940
1998	317	5,886
1999	334	6,220

Table 6.12 The number of physiatrists (physical medicine and rehabilitation specialists) certified by the American Board of Physical Medicine and Rehabilitation has increased six-fold since 1975.

"burden of care" needed for cancer patients. Quality of life is subjectively defined by each individual but usually includes a sense of dignity. Dignity may simply be using a commode rather than a bedpan, being able to dress oneself, or being able to get from bed to chair with little assistance. Cancer rehabilitation strives to enable patients to keep their respect and dignity.

Due to the aggressive nature of many cancers, treatment has rightly been the focus of most clinicians. However, there can also be tremendous disability associated with cancer and its treatments, and thus rehabilitation is appropriate for patients throughout their disease. It is important that the primary care physician, medical oncologist, surgeon, radiation oncologist and palliative care physician are aware of the benefits of rehabilitation, minimizing disability as early as possible in the course of the disease. However, unlike diseases and injuries traditionally seen in rehabilitation medicine, cancer can be progressive in nature, and medical interventions may be ongoing.

Cancer rehabilitation must balance the benefits of continued rehabilitation therapies with the physiological effects of tumour progression and advanced cancer treatments. With advanced cancer, further therapies may not be able to make appreciable differences in function and actually prevent patients from doing things they want to do by expending their limited time and energy resources. Therefore, as with many other treatments for cancer patients, it is very important to recognize when "enough is enough". In patients with advanced cancer, rehabilitation can often provide an objective view of the patient through their functional abilities and activity, thus providing important information for palliative care-type decisions (*Palliative care*, p297).

It is important to know of further planned cancer treatments as these can impact upon the patient's condition and abilities. Aggressive chemotherapy can result in fatigue, decreased nutritional intake and immunosuppression, which can affect function as well as participation in a rehabilitation programme. Surgery to debulk

or remove tumour can lead to neurological and musculoskeletal deficits, not to mention other complications associated with major surgery in a high-risk population. If major surgery is planned for the near future, therapy to address current functional deficits may be wasted as other deficits may be acquired after surgery. It may therefore often be advantageous to delay intensive rehabilitation until these treatments are completed.

Responsibility for rehabilitation
Due to complex medical, physical, social, financial and emotional issues, cancer rehabilitation is best facilitated by a comprehensive interdisciplinary team. Effective communication and teamwork is essential in formulating and carrying out plans to achieve successful rehabilitation outcomes. Team members may include a physiatrist (i.e. a physical medicine and rehabilitation specialist), the primary care physician, a medical oncologist, surgeon, radiation oncologist, physical therapist, occupational therapist, speech therapist, case manager, social worker, nutritionist, rehabilitation nurse and chaplain (Table 6.13).

The physiatrist can diagnose and treat deficits in neuromuscular function, prescribe physical, occupational and speech therapies, prescribe therapeutic modalities such as tens (a method of producing electroanalgesia through electrodes applied to the skin) and ultrasound, perform joint and soft tissue injections for symptom control, perform electrodiagnostic studies, and coordinate the comprehensive rehabilitation programme created by the interdisciplinary team to meet the needs of the patient (Table 6.14).

The physical therapist can evaluate patient strength, range of motion and functional mobility, and follow this by appropriate treatments.

The occupational therapist can evaluate deficits in activities of daily living such as feeding, grooming, bathing, dressing and toileting, and again follow this with appropriate treatments.

The speech therapist can evaluate deficits in communication, cognition and swallowing. Proposed treatments may

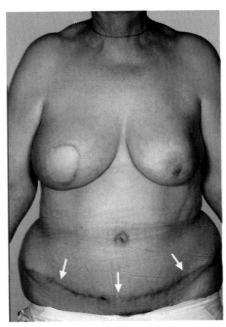

Fig. 6.19 In the TRAM flap procedure, the trans rectus abdominus muscle, which lies in the lower abdomen, is used to reconstruct the breast after mastectomy. Arrows indicate the resulting abdominal scar.

include oral strengthening exercises, use of laryngeal or oesophageal speech techniques, alternative communication devices, aphasia education and swallowing strategies.

A nutritionist or dietician can evaluate the current nutritional status of the patient and make recommendations on dietary needs based on maintaining current activity level and also, if possible, increasing strength and endurance. Dietary recommendations may include supplements or additional tube feeding if the nutritional needs of the patient are not being met.

Rehabilitation nursing provides the necessary medical and surgical nursing care for complicated rehabilitation inpatients. They must also reinforce mobility and self-care techniques taught by the other therapists and provide family education in skin care, bowel and bladder management, medication administration, feeding tube use, wound care and many other patient care issues.

The social worker assists with issues of patient and family adjustment to the cancer and its associated disability. Frequently, community resources, family and friends need to be mobilized for a safe discharge of the patient from hospital. The social worker is familiar with agencies and charities that can provide financial assistance as well as equipment and services, if needed.

The case manager can assist patients with home health and equipment referrals, obtain insurance approvals for inpatient rehabilitation hospitalization, and address questions regarding insurance coverage.

The chaplain can provide supportive spiritual services to patients and their families who are having a difficult time coping with the uncertainty of their disease.

It is feasible for knowledgeable primary care physicians, oncologists, or surgeons to coordinate appropriate rehabilitation care. However the time and resources necessary to put together the appropriate rehabilitation team are often not available.

The context of cancer rehabilitation

As previously stated, cancer rehabilitation should occur throughout the course of the disease to lessen and prevent disability. A rehabilitation programme can be prescribed prior to surgery or treatment to improve conditioning or toleration of the treatment. Specific therapies may be prescribed to maintain strength or range of motion in an area that may be adversely affected by proposed treatments. A rehabilitation programme is often initiated dur-

Interdisciplinary rehabilitation team
Physiatrist (rehabilitation physician)
Primary care physician, medical oncologist, surgeon, radiation oncologist
Rehabilitation nurse
Physical therapist
Occupational therapist
Speech therapist
Nutritionist
Case manager
Social worker
Chaplain

Table 6.13

ing active ongoing treatment to limit the adverse physical affects of the treatment and also provide the patient with an active role that he/she can play in the recovery process. Rehabilitation frequently occurs after surgery or chemotherapy when the effects of disease and treatment have led to deconditioning or specific functional deficits. Rehabilitation for advanced cancer patients with significant tumour burden may focus on therapies designed to improve basic mobility and self-care.

Finally, rehabilitation for terminal cancer patients may focus on family training for basic care-giving, bowel and bladder issues, skin care, pain control, and palliative care measures.

Cancer rehabilitation can be performed in various settings depending on the extent of the cancer and the extent of the disability. For ambulatory patients with focal weaknesses, physical and occupational therapists can improve mobility and self-care issues. For patients requiring hospitalization, a comprehensive interdisciplinary team may be used to coordinate mobility, self-care, cognitive, nutritional and patient care issues prior to discharge and return home. For advanced cancer patients, the same interdisciplinary team can help teach family members and carers how to move and care for the patient, enabling the patient to spend quality time in familiar surroundings.

Outpatient therapies can be obtained in the office, clinic or therapy gym. Inpatient rehabilitation can occur in a rehabilitation unit that is part of a general hospital or can occur in a free standing rehabilitation hospital with cancer patient experience. Due to extensive medical issues in advanced cancer patients, it is beneficial to have ready access to surgical and medical consultants as well as medical oncologists for urgent assistance. End-stage cancer rehabilitation can be given in the rehabilitation unit, palliative care unit or hospice. At any stage of disease, quality of life is the goal of cancer rehabilitation, which can also be arranged at home as long as it is safe for the patient and family.

Rehabilitation interventions
Physical therapy for strengthening, range of motion exercises, gait training.
Occupational therapy for training in activities of daily living such as bathing, grooming, dressing, toileting.
Speech therapy for cognitive assessment and training, swallowing evaluation and treatment.
Orthotic devices for functional assistance and pain control.
Pharmacological treatments for pain, spasticity, bowel and bladder control.
Joint injections, trigger point injections, botulism toxin injections for symptom control.

Table 6.14

CASE EXAMPLES

A 90-year-old patient with lower leg malignant fibrohistiocytoma is one month post-resection, with resulting difficulties in balance and gait. After appropriate tests and studies are performed to rule out post-operative infection, deep venous thrombosis or cancer recurrence, a review of the patient's history reveals that he is tripping over the toes of his affected leg. Physical examination reveals weakness in the ankle and toe dorsiflexors of the affected leg. An orthotist (specialist in orthopaedic appliances) may be contacted to fabricate an ankle foot orthosis, providing dorsiflexion assistance. Physical therapy can then provide gait training with the orthosis and a device such as a cane or walker. Stretching exercises of the ankle plantar flexors will also be important to prevent a plantar flexion contracture. These measures can reduce the fall risk in this elderly patient. Finally, occupational therapy can evaluate the patient and make sure he can dress his lower extremities, providing an adaptive reacher or other equipment as necessary.

A 42-year-old woman with breast cancer treated with modified radical mastectomy followed by transrectus abdominus muscle flap reconstruction is now suffering right shoulder stiffness and right arm swelling, 8 weeks after surgery. Assuming appropriate tests and studies have been performed to rule out recurrence of disease, post-operative wound infection or venous thrombosis, a likely diagnosis would be lymphoedema, secondary to surgical lymph node dissection. Examination of the right upper extremity would include assessment of strength, sensation, and range of motion. A quantitative measurement of oedema may be accomplished by circumferential measurements of the arm at measured distances from the elbow and wrist. Deficits in range of motion can be addressed with a physical or occupational therapy exercise programme. Lymphoedema can be treated with compression wrapping, a compres-

sion garment and/or manual lymph drainage exercises. Medications to treat neuropathic pain may be prescribed. Finally, patient education in lymphoedema management and prevention with recommendations on activity modification can be reinforced.

A 60-year-old male patient with metastatic renal cell cancer to the spine with resulting spinal cord compression and paraplegia (paralysis of the legs and lower part of the body) is hospitalized for palliative radiation treatments to the spine. The patient's deficits resulting from his paraplegia may include impaired mobility and self care, impaired sensation to his lower trunk, and neurogenic bowel and bladder (dysfunction of the bowel and bladder due to a malfunction of the relevant nerves). Although his prognosis is poor, a brief concentrated inpatient rehabilitation programme can greatly improve his quality of life by teaching him how to do more for himself, and teaching loved ones how to care for him when he becomes unable to do so. Physical therapy can instruct the patient on bed mobility, on transfer techniques from the bed to wheelchair, on wheelchair use, and also provide a range of motion exercises for spasticity management. Occupational therapy can instruct the patient in upper extremity techniques to facilitate bathing, grooming, toileting and dressing as a paraplegic. Rehabilitation nursing can teach the patient and family a skin maintenance programme, urinary catheterization for bladder management, as well as techniques and medications to manage neurogenic bowel. Patient and family education would also be beneficial in the areas of deep venous thrombosis prevention, autonomic dysreflexia prevention and management, and energy conservation. An in-patient rehabilitation programme with concomitant radiation therapy may be completed within 1-2 weeks, resulting in a paraplegic patient who is able to perform wheelchair mobility and self care without physical assistance.

A 33-year-old patient with left frontal glioblastoma multiforme has been treated

with craniotomy (operation on the skull) for tumour resection with resulting right hemiplegia and aphasia (speech dysfunction). The patient may have deficits in mobility, self-care and communication. He may be depressed. He may also have dysphagia and be at risk from aspiration (breathing foreign material into the lungs). A speech therapist can assess his speech and cognition, providing assisted communication as appropriate. A swallow evaluation with radiographic contrast can provide evidence of aspiration, and diet modifications, swallowing strategies, or a feeding tube may be recommended. Physical therapy can address mobility issues such as transfers from bed to chair and ambulation as appropriate. A cane, walker or wheelchair may be necessary depending on the degree of weakness. Occupational therapy can address self-care abilities associated with the hemiparesis such as feeding, grooming, bathing, and toileting. Both physical therapy and occupational therapy can provide a stretching and strengthening programme for the affected side. Rehabilitation nursing can assist in assessment of bowel and bladder function and assessment of skin integrity. It will be necessary to teach the patient and family how to maintain these areas in the home setting. When the patient has reached a level of functioning with mobility and self-care that is safe for home discharge, it may be beneficial to continue some therapies as an outpatient. These can reinforce concepts and techniques learned in the hospital and also provide an opportunity to problem-solve difficulties encountered in the home setting. With the nature of this tumour, it is likely that further neurologic deterioration in the future will lead to further functional deficits. It is important to plan for this decline, providing the patient and family with necessary education and equipment. It is also possible that this patient will have brain irradiation, repeat surgery or chemotherapy, all of which require further rehabilitation assistance.

REFERENCES

1. Garden FH, Gillis TA (1996) Principles of Cancer Rehabilitation. In: Braddom RL, Buschbacher R.M. eds, *Physical Medicine and Rehabilitation*, Philadelphia, Saunders, 1199-1214.

2. World Health Organization (1980) *International Classification of Impairments, Disabilities, and Handicaps*, Geneva, WHO.

3. Levin V, Gillis TA, Yadav R, Guo Y (2002) Rehabilitation of Patients with Neurological Tumours and Tumour-related Disabilities. In: Levin V ed., *Cancer in the Nervous System*. *2nd Edition*, Oxford University Press.

4. Conference Report (2001) Cancer Rehabilitation in the New Millenium (Supplement). *Cancer*, 92: 970-1048.

5. WHO QOL Group (1998) The World Health Organization Quality of Life Assessment (WHO QOL): development and general psychometric properties. *Soc Sci Med*, 46: 1569-1585.

WEBSITE

American Academy of Physical Medicine and Rehabilitation:
http://www.aapmr.org/

PALLIATIVE CARE

SUMMARY

> Central to palliative care are symptom relief and support for the patients and their families, including regard for emotional, cultural and other needs.

> A role for palliative care is best considered early in the course of disease, possibly at diagnosis.

> Optimal palliative care depends on adequate infrastructure (personnel, facilities, drugs) and methodology (modes of delivery, dose adjustment by the patient); its outcome should be evaluated.

> Adequate pain control is an essential component of cancer care. Supportive treatment is not limited to immediate medical needs but should also take account of individual and community traditions.

Death from cancer, which is usually preceded by significant morbidity, may occur:
- at the time of diagnosis (especially when diagnosed at an advanced stage as is the norm in less industrialized countries);
- during treatment with some major symptoms the direct result of anticancer treatment (surgery, radiotherapy, chemotherapy);
- when disease is progressive with less or no effectiveness for anticancer treatment (even if available).
In all stages, the patient needs comprehensive care and a patient with an eventually fatal disease requires good palliative care from the time of diagnosis. Comprehensive care should proceed concurrently with anticancer treatment, whether with curative or palliative intent. This approach to palliative care – as relevant to the entire care of a patient with probably eventually fatal disease – is in sharp contrast to other models of cancer care, specifically including those in which palliative care is squeezed into a small section of the overall management.

Principles of palliative care

Goals for patients with probably incurable disease should relate to optimum quality of life as well as achievable prolongation of life, but not to immortality. Hope is not fostered by unrealistic goals; rather, these foreshadow emotional despair.

Decisions should concern the overall care of the patient, including anticancer therapies, where evidence indicates that personal benefit should ensue (tumour response closely but not wholly parallels patient benefit) and truly informed consent is given by the patient under normal circumstances, or by a duly qualified representative if the patient is incompetent [1-4].

Advances in palliative medicine and palliative nursing in the last two decades have markedly increased the options for therapy that may be provided to patients with complications of advanced disease, such as gastrointestinal obstruction. Apart from these broad considerations, the following specific issues must be addressed in the context of palliative care for a particular patient:
- relief of major symptoms in all stages of disease, especially cancer pain relief;
- comprehensive care for patients actually close to death;
- support for family during the illness and after the death of the patient.

The adequacy of palliative care

Evaluation of palliative care may be related to structural issues (e.g. personnel, facilities, drugs), processes (modes of delivery of care) or outcomes [5]. In practice, evaluation properly involves a combination of all three categories which may be assessed at the local, national and international level [6].

Evaluation should include consideration of:
- availability of essential drugs, notably oral morphine;
- availability of educated professionals who can serve as a resource for existing health services and families, and education/training systems [7];
- evidence of sound decision-making with due regard for the patient's wishes;
- measurement of major symptoms and their relief (especially pain), in the course of anticancer treatment as well as on cessation.

The USA has undertaken significant research in "End of Life Care", which has highlighted deficiencies. An authoritative Committee on Care at the End of Life prepared a comprehensive report for the Institute of Medicine, Washington, DC, entitled *Approaching Death* [8]. This report offers a blueprint for change relevant at a global level. Especially significant is the model of care proposed ("mixed management") with palliative care in its core dimensions present from time of diagnosis of eventually fatal illness, and not tied to prognosis (involving failure of all available anticancer treatment). This constitutes a radically new approach, with far reaching implications for clinical practice, education, research, quality assurance and administrators (and funding agencies), and for specialist palliative care practitioners.

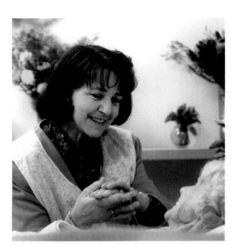

Fig. 6.20 At all stages of disease, the cancer patient needs comprehensive care. Mary Potter Hospice, North Adelaide, South Australia.

Cancer pain relief varies and in some instances is largely deficient, even in countries with adequate resources and specialist palliative care services. The barriers to cancer pain relief have been codified and include physician attitudes, availability of crucial drugs, and community barriers, particularly in relation to the use of morphine. Fear of patients becoming addicted often remains a barrier at the physician level, and also at the community level, despite the fact that such addiction is virtually unknown if opioid drugs are used correctly for cancer pain relief. The renowned Wisconsin Cancer Pain Initiative involved drug regulators as well as health professionals in its initial stages and has shown to the satisfaction of all that increased availability of morphine for cancer pain relief did not increase drug diversion in the community.

In less developed countries, the public health approach to pain relief may be the only basis for palliative care, the benefit being not merely islands of excellence, but general population coverage. This approach has proved valuable in countries such as Spain, where the service set up in Catalonia is a model of excellence relying on mobilization of the community and its resources within mainstream health care [9].

Nations should be encouraged to develop national guidelines indicating the importance of cancer pain relief; such guidelines exist in many countries today. WHO guidelines have stressed the importance of:

- a national policy to make drugs available for cancer pain relief;
- actual availability of drugs at the community level as well as in hospitals;
- an education programme.

These may be regarded as three sides of a triangle and must all be present if cancer pain relief is to be achieved. Drugs such as oral morphine should be available readily, with ease of prescription and no geographic or time restrictions. Use of morphine as part of the treatment of cancer pain relief should be dictated by the nature and severity of the pain and not by the prognosis.

The International Narcotics Control Board has strongly supported the liberalization of the availability of morphine for cancer pain relief and has taken the "ensuring of an adequate supply of controlled drugs for medical purposes" as "a principal objective of the international drug control treaties" [10]. Unfortunately, the dramatic increases in morphine use in the last ten years are frequently not correlated with the incidence of advanced cancer: pain relief is almost certainly seriously inadequate, but data are scarce.

Some procedural changes have been found to improve the likelihood of cancer pain relief:

- the listing of pain as a vital sign to be measured in hospital charts;
- public education to increase the expectations of pain relief;
- some system of cancer pain monitoring at a community and national level;
- projecting cancer care as a social justice issue: WHO has recognized cancer pain relief as a right.

There is now the need for a coherent initiative to consolidate the earlier gains achieved by WHO and to prevent unnecessary suffering for many more people worldwide, particularly where strategies for cancer pain relief at low cost exist.

The organization of palliative care

Good palliative care is not necessarily dependent upon the existence of specialist palliative care services, but implies the mobilization of services and recognition of priorities within whatever the mainstream health care system is. In some developed countries, specialist palliative care services are a prominent feature of health care delivery and serve as catalysts and resources for patients and families with problems more difficult than average.

Reference has already been made to the public health approach with mobilization of the whole health care system to care for those patients with eventually fatal disease at all locations. This implies allocation of adequate resources to patients in this category.

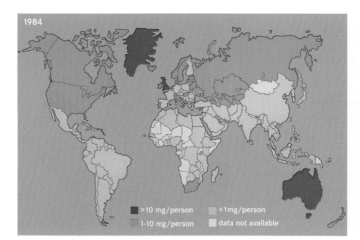
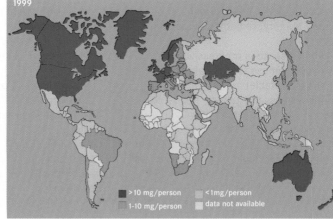

Fig. 6.21 Worldwide morphine consumption nearly tripled between 1984 and 1999, largely as a result of increasing emphasis by WHO on the need to use morphine in the treatment of cancer-related pain.

WHO has recommended that in developed countries one half of the available resources for cancer care should be devoted to palliative care, i.e. that the resources available for palliative care should equal the combined resources available for all anticancer treatment – surgery, radiotherapy and chemotherapy. WHO recommended that in less developed countries at least 80% of resources should be available for palliative care, noting that there is no other measure which can improve the quality of life of the population as much as widely available palliative care.

Palliative care and cancer pain worldwide

Global improvements in palliative care do not depend so much upon the creation of specialized palliative care services separate from mainstream health care, but upon the permeation of the whole health care system by the principles of palliative care. This in turn is dependent upon a major planning exercise with administrative, education and research implications. Specialized demonstration programmes are justified to assist in this undertaking. There is now a vast store of information concerning developments in palliative care internationally, whether involving specialized palliative care services or mainstream health care systems and guidelines have been developed by relevant authorities, including the International Association of Hospice and Palliative Care.

There are problems in all contexts, but improvements have begun to be recognized. Less developed countries vary with regard to palliative care services. In developed countries the problem is that of patchy application of the vast body of

COMPLEMENTARY AND ALTERNATIVE MEDICINE

A majority of cancer patients in most developed countries probably use complementary therapies as adjuncts to mainstream care for symptom management and quality of life. A smaller proportion use "alternative" remedies, unproved methods that typically are invasive, biologically active, and often promoted as literal alternatives to evidence-based oncology treatment. These methods tend to involve considerable travel and expense. Many are associated with significant risks of adverse events or substantial delays in receipt of needed care. Many alternatives, such as high-dose vitamin C supplements, special diets, shark cartilage, Iscador, and laetrile, have been studied and found ineffective.

Conversely, the benefits of some complementary therapies are well documented. Randomized trials support the value of hypnosis and acupuncture for pain and nausea, of relaxation therapies, music therapy and massage for anxiety, pain and depression, of yoga, tai chi and meditation for improved strength and stability. These and other complementary therapies increasingly are provided in mainstream cancer programmes. Some complementary therapies, such as psychological support, humour therapy and spiritual assistance, have been available for decades as "supportive" care in oncology

medicine. In this sense, complementary medicine may be seen as an extension and expansion of earlier efforts to focus on patients' broader needs (Cassileth BR, *The Alternative Medicine Handbook: The Complete Reference Guide to Alternative and Complementary Therapies*, WW Norton & Company, 1998).

Botanicals hold largely untapped promise, requiring serious research to document their value against cancer or capacity to enhance well-being (Duke JA, *The Green Pharmacy*, New York, Rodale Press, 1997; Tyler VE, *Herbs of Choice: The Therapeutic Use of Phytomedicinals*, 1993 and Tyler VE, *The Honest Herbal: A Sensible Guide To The Use of Herbs and Related Remedies*, 1994, both by Pharmaceutical Press).

However, many herbal remedies are toxic or contaminated, or interact negatively with pharmaceuticals. St. John's Wort, for example, a useful herb for mild and moderate depression, is now known to decrease blood levels of protease inhibitors, cyclosporine and other immunosuppressive drugs, birth control pills, cholesterol medications, Coumadin, and chemotherapeutic agents. Such problems require that oncologists remain vigilant to potential interactions many, if not most, of which, remain undocumented. It is probably safest for patients to stop herbs and other nonprescription products during receipt of cancer treatments.

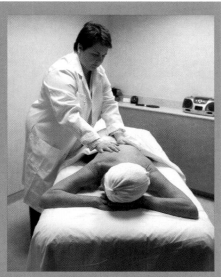

Fig. 6.23 Massage as a form of relaxation therapy

Both the helpful and the problematic components of complementary and alternative medicine are likely to persist in cancer medicine. The challenge for the physician and for the patient is to promote and utilize beneficial complementary therapies and discard disproved alternatives. In recent years, increasingly greater integration of complementary and conventional medicine has occurred, creating integrative medicine. This synthesis of the best of complementary therapies and mainstream care lights the way to the more comprehensive, humane, and needed cancer care that hopefully will characterize the future of oncology.

EMERGING ISSUES IN PALLIATIVE CARE

1. Adequacy of resources for care (especially and at least pain relief) from time of diagnosis of probably incurable cancer, in comparison with resources for anticancer treatment (surgery radiotherapy, chemotherapy and the related diagnostic and monitoring processes).
This is an issue throughout the world but precise information is needed. It is worth the attention of health economists with an understanding of WHO principles.

2. Being allowed to die – and allowing oneself to die: an issue in high technology environments.
Attention should be given to the circumstances in which futile treatment should neither be initiated nor maintained.

3. Education of professionals, especially doctors, with respect to the clinical science, attitudes and skills essential for contemporary palliative care.
The courage and excellence of the USA national programme for doctors throughout the country may have global significance.

4. Increasing incidence of cancer (especially the less curable types), notably in less industrialized countries, associated with the ageing of the population and continuing high levels of cigarette smoking and industrial pollution.
In such circumstances the balance between attempts to cure and care becomes more crucial, and delivery of care must be efficient, effective and sustainable at the level of the whole population in need: a massive challenge.

5. Assessment of adequacy of palliative care at total community level.

6. Ethical issues relating to the disparity of care available in different circumstances throughout the world (differences between countries and within countries): can we continue to tolerate such disparities in this millennium?
Daniel Callaghan, the founder of the revered Hastings Institute for Ethics has recently written: "The greatest importance of palliative care medicine is not simply the benefit it can bring at the end of life, but its recasting of the goals of medicine, trying to better balance care and cure, and in all of life not just at its end... Most needed is what I call a 'sustainable medicine'... that accepts death as part of the human condition, that is not obsessed with the struggle against disease, that understands progress as learning better how to live with, and die with, mortality as a fundamental mark of the human condition" (Callaghan D, *J Palliat Care*, 8: 3-4, 2000; Callaghan D, *The troubled dream of life*, New York, 1993).

existing clinical science. Whether or not appropriate patients are referred to specialist palliative care services, as should be the case in difficult situations, depends on referral patterns and this fact may impede the delivery of optimum palliative care.

The obstacles to the achievement of a "good" level of cancer pain relief community-wide in all countries, but especially developing countries, include not only the diffusion of knowledge regarding cancer pain relief, policy change concerning drug availability, and education of health professionals and the public, but also more subtle and sensitive issues. There are countless examples of delays in implementation which are only explicable in terms of cultural factors which must be respected and understood.

Some of these profound issues are spiritual and philosophical, and are felt especially keenly in developing countries. Questions such as the following may be unspoken, or rarely articulated:

- Does the adoption of a recognized strategy for cancer pain relief run the risk of damaging the spiritual fabric of our society, of destroying our way of thinking about the meaning of life, of suffering, of death?
- When we are so short of resources, why should we spend so much time, money and trouble on pain treatment in those who can no longer work, instead of trying to cure more people?
- Why is cancer pain relief still so poor in the West, even in prestigious cancer centres?

These matters need discussion in situations of trust, and in an atmosphere of partnership.

It is essential that those seeking to introduce the WHO approach to pain relief are deeply aware of the personal, cultural and spiritual context into which this new mode of thinking and acting is to be introduced. The beneficial outcomes to the patients and their families are so significant that these outcomes themselves may be the key tool for change: such change must come from within the community. However, wise leadership from senior administrators and clinicians can have dramatic consequences.

The challenge now in achieving better levels of global cancer pain relief is a more appropriate understanding of the psychological matrix within which the means to relieve that pain must operate. Awareness of the total ecological matrix – with its historical, social, economic, psychological and spiritual components – is essential if cancer pain relief is to be achieved. In some respects, psychological and spiritual development in some so-called developing countries is far in advance of the rest of the globe – and there is a need for all to recognize exchange-in-partnership as the most promising means of advance for the third millennium.

Those working in the policy area of health care and with patients should

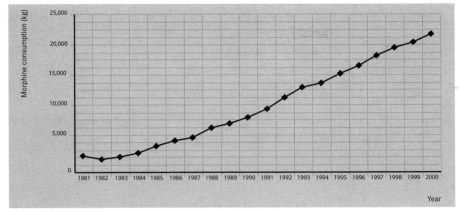

Fig. 6.22 The worldwide medical consumption of morphine is increasing.

understand not only the technical aspects but also the cultural and spiritual significance of new approaches to the patient experiencing pain, the need for recognition (not hiding) of the pain, and the obligation to relieve relievable distress, without denying (and indeed confirming) the precious values forming the fabric of society. Cancer pain relief, and palliative care in general, give expression to the compassion which is one of the most basic values within all human societies.

REFERENCES

1. Doyle D, Hanks GW, MacDonald N, eds (1997) *Oxford Textbook of Palliative Medicine, 2nd Edition*, Oxford, Oxford University Press.

2. World Health Organization (1986). *Cancer Pain Relief and Palliative Care*, Geneva, WHO.

3. World Health Organization (1996). *Cancer Pain Relief and Palliative Care*, Geneva, WHO.

4. World Health Organization (1998). *Symptom Relief in Terminal Illness*, Geneva, WHO.

5. Higginson I, ed. (1993) *Clinical Audit in Palliative Care*, Oxford, Radcliffe Medical Press.

6. World Health Organization (2002). *National Cancer Control Programmes: Policies and Management Guidelines, 2nd Edition*, Geneva, WHO.

7. American Medical Association Institute of Ethics (1999) *EPEC Project. Education for Physicians on End of Life Care*, Chicago.

8. Field MJ, Cassel CK, eds (1997) *Approaching Death: Improving Care at the End of Life (Committee on Care at the End of Life, Division of Health Care Services, Institute of Medicine)*, Washington, D.C., National Academy Press.

9. Gomez-Batiste X, Fontanals MD, Roca J, Borras JM, Viladiu P, Stjernsward J, Ruis E (1996) Catalonia WHO demonstration project on palliative care implementation 1990-1995: Results in 1995. *J Pain Symptom Management*, 12: 73-78.

10. International Narcotics Control Board (1999) *Report of the International Narcotics Control Board for 1999*, Vienna, United Nations Publications.

WEBSITES

The Macmillan Cancer Relief charity, UK:
http://www.macmillan.org.uk/framed.html

National Hospice and Palliative Care Organization, USA:
http://www.nhpco.org/

International Association of Hospice and Palliative Care, USA:
http://www.hospicecare.com

American Pain Foundation:
http://www.painfoundation.org/

Education for Physicians on the End of Life Care (EPEC):
http://www.epec@ama-assn.org

The WHO Collaborating Center for Policy and Communications:
http://www.medsch.wisc.edu/painpolicy

Cancer Pain Release (publication of the WHO global communications programme to improve cancer pain control and palliative and supportive care):
http://www.whocancerpain.wisc.edu/

Cancer control

The negative impact of cancer on individuals and communities can be greatly reduced through cancer control programmes. The scope of cancer control extends from prevention and screening to management of disease, rehabilitation and palliative care. Implementation of cancer control measures requires political will, resource mobilization, and a shared strategy involving governmental and nongovernmental organizations, in particular health services and community and patient groups. This challenge has been addressed by WHO through recommendations for the establishment of National Cancer Control Programmes. They focus particularly on the needs of developing countries and include global perspectives for a successful fight against cancer.

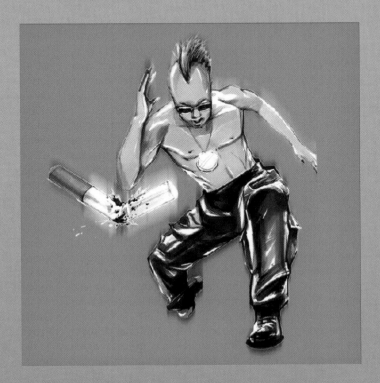

CANCER CONTROL: A GLOBAL OUTLOOK

SUMMARY

> The aim of cancer control is a reduction in the incidence of the disease and of the associated morbidity and mortality, as well as improved quality of life for cancer patients and their families.

> Prevention, screening and early diagnosis, treatment and palliative care are the principal approaches to cancer control.

> Progress in cancer control requires not only sound knowledge of the disease process, but also an understanding of the psychological, social, economic and organizational factors which govern how that knowledge can be put to effective use.

The world cancer burden is expected to increase from the current level of about 10 million new cancer cases diagnosed annually to about 15 million in 2020, largely because of demographic changes and the effects of tobacco, as well as other risk factors. It will take time for cancer control measures, even if efficiently applied and based on well-planned strategies, to have a major impact on these figures. However, prevention could reduce the load by about 2 million by 2020, and 6.5 million by 2040. In contrast, the impact of both screening and treatment is likely to be small; even by 2040, half the potential reduction in cancer deaths from 16 to 8 million would be due to prevention, and much less from more effective screening and treatment. It is clear therefore that, although on a short-term basis we cannot ignore applying effective therapies, for maximum impact on the cancer problem we must change the priority to prevention. The prevention of cancer should be set within the context of prevention of all noncommunicable diseases caused by shared risk factors, while the links between specific infectious agents and certain cancers will also permit some of the principles of control of communicable diseases to be adopted.

WHO approach to cancer control

The increasing magnitude of noncommunicable diseases, including cancer, represents one of the major health challenges to global development in the new century. To respond to this growing challenge, WHO has given cancer control a high priority in its programme of work and in technical collaboration with countries. WHO has also developed, in close collaboration with its Member States and other partners, a global strategy for the prevention and control of noncommunicable diseases in which cancer control is one of four major priorities. The strategy places emphasis on the rising impact of cancer on developing countries and the disproportionate suffering it causes in poor and disadvantaged populations. The global strategy was endorsed by the 53rd World Health Assembly (May 2000), and in its resolution WHA53.17 the Assembly urges Member States to establish effective national programmes, and requests WHO to provide the necessary technical support and to coordinate global partnerships and alliances for advocacy, capacity building and collaborative research. WHO is committed to the promotion of National Cancer Control Programmes as the most effective national-level strategy for reducing the morbidity and mortality from cancer and improving quality of life of cancer patients and their families [1]. Medical knowledge is now sufficiently advanced to permit the prevention of at least one-third of all cancers, the cure of a further one-third, given early diagnosis and the administration of effective therapy, and the adequate control of pain and other symptoms, with palliative care for the remainder.

The development of National Cancer Control Programmes is a process which involves the review of the current disease

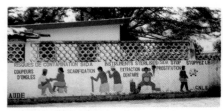

Fig. 7.1 AIDS information for the general public at a health centre in Côte d'Ivoire. Effective linkages with control programmes for HIV/AIDS and other diseases could facilitate the establishment of effective National Cancer Control Programmes.

and health care situation, evaluation of the potential impact of various disease control strategies (prevention, early diagnosis/screening, treatment and palliative care), the setting of goals and priorities and the allocation of resources. As cancer has increased in incidence in many countries, several have recognized the need to initiate National Cancer Control Programmes. However, others have not yet done so. Because of the increasing importance of noncommunicable diseases, including cancer, in all countries WHO is committed to securing recognition of the importance of cancer among all Member States. This in turn creates further needs, towards which WHO can make important contributions by:
- Updating and disseminating information on effective strategies for cancer prevention and control;
- Developing background documentation on planning National Cancer Control Programmes;
- Working with interested countries in the development and evaluation of their National Cancer Control Programmes;
- Encouraging countries to share experience and learn from successes and failures and promote networking at subregional, regional and global levels.

Goals of National Cancer Control Programmes

To reduce the burden of cancer, a country must be prepared to allocate a certain priority to cancer control activities, and possess a basic public health and health care infrastructure. Prevention of cancer has to be set within the context of prevention of other noncommunicable diseases, as there are a number of risk factors in common. Furthermore, cancer detection and screening and the management of detected cancers (without which screening will fail) have to be set within the existing health infrastructure. No country can afford a cancer care system that is independent of other health care facilities. Such a cancer care system must be capable of covering the total population.

Personnel involved in formulating and implementing the overall strategy should be health professionals with experience in disease control and large-scale health programmes, together with cancer experts and other health service workers. This will involve collaboration between the relevant Ministry of Health, those in charge of existing cancer programmes, and representatives of appropriate nongovernmental organizations. Ultimately, the Programme should involve the general public, whose knowledge and awareness of the problem can and should become a major force in combating cancer.

Political commitment to the adoption and implementation of these policies is essential. It should be the responsibility of health leaders to convince political leaders, health practitioners and the public of the magnitude of the current and (especially) the future national cancer problem, and to outline what can be done to overcome it. Different objectives and priorities will be set in different countries, according to the national cancer burden and the resources available. However, the processes to be undertaken in all countries are similar, whether a National Cancer Control Programme is to be introduced for the first time or an existing programme is to be revised to make it more effective.

Components of National Cancer Control Programmes

Matters essential to National Cancer Control Programmes are the subject of chapters in earlier sections of this Report, particularly chapters outlining prevention and management (4 and 6). Such activities are discussed here in relation to difference in impact and priority according to the needs and situations of different communities and countries.

REORGANIZATION OF THE CERVICAL CANCER SCREENING PROGRAMME IN CHILE

In 1985, with the assistance of WHO, a National Cancer Control Programme was established by the Ministry of Health, Chile, with cervical cancer as one of the main priorities. During the previous two decades, opportunistic annual screening for cervical cancer had not achieved the expected benefit. Therefore, in 1987 a public health-oriented cervical screening programme was launched, based on screening women aged 26 to 64 by Pap smear every three years. Health service managers at that time were reluctant to apply the ministry's approach. Consequently the decision was made to focus effort and resources in a demonstration area, the Metropolitan Area of Santiago, which include one-third of the population of the country.

The approach adopted in the Metropolitan Area involved a series of training workshops for health professionals concerned with the programme at every level of care. Each workshop was assisted by a physician expert in education and health communications and aimed at a gradual implementation of the strategies. The participants received motivational input, updated information on the programme and were trained how to assess the current situation, compare it to the desired situation and develop specific strategies to bridge the existing gaps. In a follow-up workshop some months later, evaluation of progress and constraints encountered were discussed and subsequent tasks were planned accordingly. The first strategy implemented was to motivate the female health care providers within the health care system to be screened. The second strategy was to monitor the follow-up of women with abnormal Pap smears in the various levels of care, as they were a key group to track programme deficiencies. Additional strategies involved offering screening to women in the target group from easily accessible and progressively larger female populations.

Seven years later in a consensus meeting, the programme was expanded to cover the whole country. According to biannual national surveys, coverage of the target group by Pap smear had risen from 40% in 1990 to 66% in 1997. The age adjusted mortality rate decreased from 13.3 in 1970 to

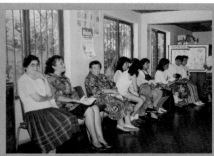

Fig. 7.3 Education of women about cervical cancer screening in a primary health care clinic in Chile as part of the regular activities of the centre.

7.7 per 100,000 women in 1999, with an apparently higher rate of reduction in the last five years. The programme emphasized network organization, timeliness of diagnosis and treatment, reliability of Pap smear, and low cost screening promotion strategies at the community level. During the initial years, financial support for the programme was minimal. Additional funding from the government was provided only after six years and this was mainly for upgrading equipment at the secondary level and for supporting community-based, low cost promotion activities.

UICC: A UNIQUE ROLE IN GLOBAL CANCER CONTROL

Founded in 1933, the International Union Against Cancer (Union International Contre le Cancer) plays a critical role in inaugurating and supporting effective cancer control strategies at local, regional, national and international levels. Its objectives are to advance scientific and medical knowledge in research, diagnosis, treatment and prevention of cancer, and to promote all other aspects of the campaign against cancer throughout the world. One of the Union's strengths is the wide spectrum of its membership, being composed of nearly 300 cancer organizations, institutes, societies, associations and Ministries of Health in 85 developed and developing countries.

Core activities

As the only global nongovernmental organization dedicated to cancer control, UICC is uniquely qualified to stimulate and strengthen coordination and collaboration with other concerned organizations and groups, creating a global sense of responsibility. The UICC World Conferences for Voluntary Cancer Organizations, initiated by the UICC Cancer Organizations, Public Education, and Patient Services (COPES) Programme, are one example of such collaboration. COPES is devoted to establishing a worldwide network of voluntary cancer organizations and to providing support to strengthen their services. Another core activity of UICC is the Committee on International Collaborative Activities, which works in collaboration with WHO, IARC and other relevant bodies to stimulate cancer leagues to take an interest in supporting cancer registration and to assist in establishing national cancer control plans and comprehensive cancer centres. In so doing, UICC promotes standardized data collection, better and cheaper services as well as increased survival rates through a comprehensive national health care programme that ranges from patient information to palliative care for the entire population.

Emphasis on prevention and reduction of disparities

The strategies recently set up by UICC for the new century call for a greater emphasis on public health, prevention, risk reduction, information awareness campaigns and carefully selected screening programmes. As lung cancer is the world's leading preventable cause of death, UICC's focus is to curb tobacco use by promoting comprehensive tobacco control programmes and providing technical assistance and advocacy training for cancer leagues and institutions in developing countries seeking to fight the use of tobacco products. Building the capacity of nongovernmental organizations and cancer leagues and catalysing the optimal use of current knowledge are other goals of UICC, in order to reduce existing disparities in cancer prevention and care. In many parts of the world, cancer patients are diagnosed at an advanced stage and do not have access to early detection or screening for early-stage cancer. UICC facilitates the education of health professionals with a focus on common cancers that have an easily applicable medical intervention (cervical, breast, colorectal cancers etc.). The Union has the means, through its membership, to become a clearing house and conduit for lifesaving cancer interventions, by promulgating the transfer of clinical and programme techniques from places that already have them to places that do not.

Sharing knowledge

UICC Fellowships and world standard publications such as the *International Journal of Cancer*, the *TNM Classification of Malignant Tumours* (Sobin L and Wittekind C, 5th edition, John Wiley & Sons, New York, 1997) and the *Manual of Clinical Oncology* (R. Pollock et al., 7th edition, John Wiley & Sons, New York, 1999) all make UICC a reference point and a resource in the dissemination of knowledge about cancer and its application to patient care.

Through its Information Network (http://www.uicc.org), and by supporting and strengthening local access to the Internet, the Union contributes to making information uniformly applicable and available across the world. An example of a free Internet-based service is the UICC Telepathology Consultation Centre, which helps pathologists around the world to get a second opinion in difficult tumour cases. Information dissemination is also effected via meetings, workshops and symposia. The UICC Quadrennial Cancer Congress is instrumental in improving uniform standards in cancer care by providing a digest of state-of-the-art in all cancer disciplines while attracting attention to challenges in developing countries.

Voluntarism

An integral part of UICC, voluntarism constitutes a way for organizations to achieve maximum effectiveness when they want to reach deep into the community. An objective of UICC is to teach institutions and leagues how to recruit, train, motivate and manage volunteers, and to be a proponent worldwide for voluntarism by creating a global awareness campaign through its members.

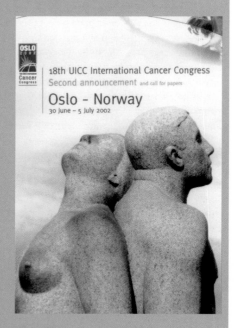

Fig. 7.4 Poster advertising the UICC International Cancer Congress, 2002.

Prevention of cancer

Every country should give high priority to tobacco control in its fight against cancer. Unchecked, smoking will cause more than 10 million deaths from cancer (predominantly lung cancer) in the next decade [2]. Given the multi-faceted impact of diet on cancer, in many countries the aim must be to encourage consumption of locally produced vegetables, fruit and agricultural products, and avoid the adoption of Western style dietary habits. Dietary and alcohol policies and measures to increase physical exercise and reduce obesity should be developed in a local context [3].

Since other common noncommunicable diseases share the same lifestyle-related risk factors, action to prevent cancer should focus on controlling these risk factors in an integrated manner. This requires close coordination with programmes for the prevention of other related noncommunicable diseases, mainly cardiovascular diseases, chronic obstructive pulmonary diseases and diabetes. The structure and mechanisms necessary to ensure such collaboration will vary from one country to another according to the epidemiological situation, disease control priorities, available resources and existing initiatives. In some countries, a national structure within the Ministry of Health charged with health promotion and disease prevention is given the responsibility of planning, implementing and evaluating primary prevention initiatives in close coordination with - and active contribution by - the National Cancer Control Programme as well as other noncommunicable disease prevention programmes. Continuing surveillance of levels and patterns of risk factors is of fundamental importance to planning and evaluating primary prevention activities.

There is a great need for effective and carefully evaluated school education programmes for tobacco abstinence and healthy dietary habits. Very few countries have such education programmes that are effective [2]. National Cancer Control Programmes can help to ensure that governments take the necessary actions to guarantee that the public has the motivation to adopt healthy personal habits.

In some countries, steps may be needed to avoid exposure to known carcinogens in industries transferred from developed countries. Prevention of infectious disease is relevant. Hepatitis B vaccination should be included to prevent future cancers of the liver in many countries. Strengthening *Schistosomiasis* control programmes is the most feasible approach to reduce the incidence of bladder cancer in certain countries.

Early detection of cancer – early diagnosis and population screening

The strategy of early diagnosis is a public and health professional awareness activity. A public health education campaign teaches people to recognize early signs of the disease and urges them to seek prompt medical attention. Health professionals, especially primary health workers, are trained to identify cases that are suspicious and refer them for rapid diagnosis.

Because of the considerable resources involved, population screening programmes should be undertaken as a component of early detection only where their effectiveness has been demonstrated, where resources (personnel, equipment, etc.) are sufficient to cover at least 70% of the target group, where facilities exist for confirming diagnoses and for treatment and follow-up of those with abnormal results, and where prevalence of the disease is high enough to justify the effort and costs of screening. At present, population screening can only be advocated widely for cancer of the cervix by Pap smear; such screening should be done in all developed countries and in those developing countries where it is feasible. Population screening for breast cancer by mammography should only be considered in countries with high rates of breast cancer and that can afford the high technology cost, and which have the skilled professionals required, due to the much lower effectiveness of breast screening [4]. In such programmes, efforts should concentrate on women at greatest risk of developing invasive cancer, i.e. those aged 30 and over for cervical cancer and those aged 50-69 for breast cancer.

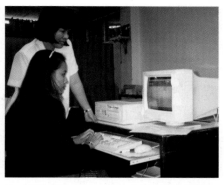

Fig. 7.2 Training of a cancer registry clerk in Khon Khaen, Thailand. Population-based cancer registries or vital statistics systems are necessary to assess changes in incidence and mortality.

Treatment of cancer

A National Cancer Control Programme should establish guidelines for integrating treatment resources with programmes for screening and early diagnosis, and provide therapeutic standards for the most important cancers in the country.

The efficacy of treatment varies depending on cancer type, and this should influence priorities. Some treatments require sophisticated technology that is available only in locations with substantial resources. Since the cost of establishing and maintaining such facilities is high, it is desirable that they should remain concentrated in relatively few places in a country to avoid draining resources that could be devoted to other aspects of the National Cancer Control Programme.

WHO has established an essential drug list for oncology, based on generically available drugs that enable those cancers with a high priority for therapy to be treated in most countries [5]. WHO supports the introduction of radiotherapy based largely on cobalt units in appropriate centres. In all countries, measures must be taken to ensure access to therapy for those patients with treatable cancers, and ensure that adequate standards of care are followed.

WHO TOBACCO FREE INITIATIVE

The Tobacco Free Initiative is a WHO cabinet project created to focus international attention, resources and action on the global tobacco pandemic that kills more than four million people every year. It is estimated that tobacco will kill 10 million people a year by 2030 and that over 70% of these deaths will occur in the developing world.

Globalization of marketing and trade in tobacco products means that all countries need to take strong action individually and together if their populations are to become free of the burden of tobacco-related disease and death. WHO has initiated work on the Framework Convention on Tobacco Control - the world's first set of multilaterally negotiated rules focusing on global tobacco control. Currently being negotiated by 191 countries, the treaty will be ready for ratification no later than 2003. This new legal instrument will address issues as diverse as tobacco advertising and promotion, agricultural diversification, tobacco product regulation, smuggling, excise tax levels, treatment of tobacco dependence, second-hand smoke and tobacco free areas.

The challenge comes in seeking global and national solutions in tandem for a problem that cuts across national boundaries, cultures, societies and socioeconomic strata. The Framework Convention on Tobacco Control process seeks to activate all those areas of governance that have a direct impact on public health.

Science and economics will mesh with legislation and litigation. Health ministers will work with their counterparts in finance, trade, labour, agriculture and social affairs ministries to give public health the place it deserves.

The Framework Convention on Tobacco Control process also involves building up the national capacities of countries to undertake tobacco control activities. This includes technical assistance on legislation but extends to many other areas. In collaboration with the World Bank, the Tobacco Free Initiative has been looking into the issue of the economics of tobacco control. The work demonstrates that the economic fears that have deterred policymakers from taking action are largely unfounded. Policies that reduce the demand for tobacco, such as a decision to increase tobacco taxes, would not cause long-term job losses in the vast majority of countries. Nor would higher tobacco taxes reduce tax revenues; rather, revenues would climb in the medium term. Such policies could, in sum, bring unprecedented health benefits without harming economies.

Some of the projects that the Tobacco Free Initiative is involved in extend to surveillance. In collaboration with the USA Centers for Disease Control and Prevention, the Global Youth Tobacco Survey has been implemented in over 50 countries. The Global Health Professionals Tobacco Survey monitors tobacco use, assesses behaviours in providing cessation support to patients and assesses knowledge of health effects of tobacco. Advocacy for policy change is the cornerstone of the Tobacco

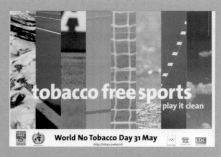

Fig. 7.5 Poster for Tobacco Free Sports, World No Tobacco Day 2002.

Free Initiative's communications and information work. "Tobacco Kills - Don't be Duped", a two-year United Nations Foundation-sponsored project on media and nongovernmental organization advocacy for policy change, was launched in 1999 and is being piloted in over 25 countries. World No Tobacco Day, May 31st, focuses on different themes every year. The theme for 2002 was Tobacco Free Sports. The United States Centers for Disease Control and Prevention, the International Olympic Committee, the Federation Internationale de Football Association (FIFA), Olympic Aid and other regional and local sports organizations joined WHO in this campaign. Tobacco free events organized all over the world included the 2002 Salt Lake City Winter Olympic Games in the USA and the 2002 FIFA World Cup in the Republic of Korea and Japan.

These and other areas of work all have a single purpose - to cut back on tobacco consumption and to save lives.

Palliative care

Since palliative care services can be provided relatively simply and inexpensively, they should be available in every country. Palliative care should be given high priority, especially in countries where the majority of patients are diagnosed with cancer at an advanced stage and cure for most of them is likely to remain impossible for

years to come. Health care providers should be trained to deliver palliative care, both within health care facilities and in patients' homes. Guidelines for the relief of cancer pain have been drawn up by and are available from WHO; the widespread availability of morphine for oral administration is critical to pain relief, and should be ensured by appropriate legislation [6,9].

Managing the development of a National Cancer Control Programme

Although countries differ in their preparedness to initiate national cancer control programmes, all, even the most technologically advanced, have to set priorities and decide how best to allocate the available resources. This requires several carefully-managed steps, which include:

- Assessing the magnitude of the cancer problem, i.e. performing a situation analysis
- Determining priorities and setting measurable cancer control objectives
- Evaluating possible strategies for cancer control
- Appointing a National Cancer Control Programmes coordinator
- Performing a policy review to ensure that appropriate decisions are made
- Formulating an action plan with measurable monitoring and evaluation indicators
- Mobilizing (and reallocating) necessary resources.

The initial situation analysis is essential for understanding the magnitude of the cancer problem and for setting priorities and reallocating resources. This is based on:
- demographic (population) data
- data on cancer morbidity, incidence and mortality
- data on other diseases
- information on health care facilities and human resources.

Role of cancer registries in National Cancer Control Programmes

Cancer registries can contribute to surveillance by:
- Assessing the current magnitude of the cancer burden and its likely future evolution
- Providing a basis for research on cancer causes and prevention
- Providing information on prevalence and trends in risk factors
- Monitoring the effects of early detection/screening, treatment, and palliative care.

Cancer registries can also provide a focus of epidemiological expertise with the responsibility of providing data on a continuing basis on incidence, prevalence, mortality, methods of diagnosis, stage distribution, treatment patterns and survival. In planning a Programme, a critical step is to obtain political commitment from the government. Perhaps equally important is to ensure the availability of leadership by a nationally respected and knowledge-able individual with good management skills. The cancer policy provides the framework for a balanced cancer control programme, defining broad aims, principles, objectives, their relative priority and indicating the resources and programmes required to carry out the policy. Priorities for the Programme are determined by the local situation, epidemiological trends and the existence of cost-effective interventions. Among locally prevalent cancers, those that are preventable and those that are amenable to early detection and treatment should be identified. Resources must be allocated accordingly and should be provided by the government and supplemented by nongovernmental organizations and, if necessary, by special fund-raising. A key issue is the reallocation of resources from unproductive areas to areas with greater potential for success. A classic example is high frequency of cervical cytology screening of young, and therefore low-risk, women versus low intensity screening of older,

THE CANCER CONTROL PROGRAMME OF KERALA, INDIA

The National Cancer Control Programme of India was formulated in 1984, focusing on (a) primary prevention of tobacco-related cancers, as 50% of all cancer in India was due to tobacco use, (b) early detection of cancers at accessible sites, as the three major forms of cancer were accessible (cancer of the cervix, breast and oral cavity) (c) augmentation of treatment facilities, and (d) establishment of equitable pain control and a palliative care network throughout the country, as more than 80% of cancer patients presented at a very late stage. Kerala, a state in south-western India with a population of 31 million, was the first state in the Indian union to formulate a state-wide cancer control programme, and did so in 1988 as a 10-year action plan. The state programme was prepared with the same goals as the National Cancer Control Programme of India and was developed with advice from WHO. The programme consisted of creation of awareness of risk factors and early warning signals. This empowers the population to seek healthy lifestyles and examinations supported by medical procedures to detect and diagnose the disease in early stages and receive treatment in institutions designed for this purpose.

Tobacco control included two state-wide programmes targeted at teenagers via the school system. A programme carried out in 1993-4 "One Lakh Tobacco Free Homes" resulted in 126,000 homes being declared tobacco-free. During the past two years, a similar programme has been implemented in over 6,000 schools. With respect to early detection, as high technology, expensive methods were beyond the means of this state, the programme stressed education followed by diagnosis. Awareness via opportunistic early detection clinics was organized with the support of the government and voluntary organizations. Self-examination methods were emphasized, particularly for cancers of the oral cavity and breast. Over 12,600 village level cancer control volunteers were trained to promote awareness of cancer and detect early signs of disease, to advocate and motivate people to undergo diagnostic screening tests and therapy, and to extend financial support. This activity covered 85 villages in the state. Early Cancer Detection Centres were developed to serve as focal points for coordination and implementation of early detection programmes in the state. Emphasis was given to the improvement of therapy hand-in-hand with the improvement of early cancer detection. In addition, two nodal centres for pain control and palliative care have been set up in the State and 16 peripheral centres are networked under the guidance of these main centres. Morphine tablets have been available since 1991 and the local manufacture of morphine tablets has begun.

Upon evaluation, this programme has achieved a reduction in tobacco consumption, downstaging of advanced tumours, augmentation of comprehensive therapy programmes and networking of palliative care centres.

CANCER CONTROL IN THE USA: CENTERS FOR DISEASE, CONTROL AND PREVENTION

One of the focuses of the Centers for Disease Control and Prevention (CDC) is developing, implementing, supporting and evaluating cancer prevention and control efforts in the USA.

CDC's many activities related to cancer include the following: cancer registries, cancer risk and behavioural surveillance systems, tobacco control, comprehensive cancer control and occupational, environmental and infectious disease-related cancers. CDC's educational initiatives and interventions include those for breast, cervical, colorectal, prostate, skin, and ovarian cancers, for infectious-disease related cancers (e.g. hepatitis C-related liver cancer and *Helicobacter pylori*-related stomach cancer) and tobacco-related cancers (e.g. lung and oral cancers). Recognizing the importance of physical activity and nutrition in preventing disease, including cancer, CDC also has programmes in physical activity and nutrition.

Developing and strengthening cancer surveillance systems

Cancer registry data are used to identify and monitor cancer trends, gaps, disparities, barriers and successes, to develop and guide state-wide, comprehensive cancer prevention and control plans, to prioritize allocation of resources, to serve as the basis for research, and to evaluate prevention and control efforts. Such data are, therefore, the foundation upon which all cancer prevention and control efforts should be based.

Many countries, including the USA, need to establish, support or strengthen an integrated, nationwide cancer surveillance system and use the system's data as a basis for decision making. In a step towards development of such a system in the USA, CDC launched the National Program of Cancer Registries Cancer Surveillance System (NPCR-CSS) in January 2001. The system will receive, assess, enhance, aggregate and share data from the National Program of Cancer Registries-funded programmes. Established in 1992, the National Program of Cancer Registries supports registries in 45 states, 3 territories, and the District of Columbia. The goal of the NPCR-CSS is to maximize the benefits of state- and territory-based cancer registries by providing feedback for improving data quality and usefulness and to provide public-use data for regional and national studies.

Once cancer registries are established, decision- and policymakers should support and strengthen them in the following ways:
- Provide adequate funding and staffing to ensure that registries are fully equipped and that their personnel are adequately trained so as to provide complete, timely, accurate data, obtain certification of data and conduct research.
- If needed, develop, enact, and implement legislation and regulations that strengthen and support registries.
- Ensure that the data are certified as meeting standards for completeness, timeliness, and quality.
- Encourage integration of cancer registry data with those of other relevant data systems, such as geographic information or behaviour and risk factor surveillance systems. Linked data may provide more clues to risk factors for cancer, how to prevent cancer and how to increase survival and improve the health care delivery system.
- Use registry data to develop and review policies and programmes, develop and update comprehensive cancer control plans, allocate scarce resources and evaluate the effectiveness of actions taken.

Preventing tobacco use

Use of tobacco products is the single most preventable cause of disease (including cancer) and death, yet tobacco use remains a problem worldwide. In 1999, CDC launched the National Tobacco Control Program. The programme provides funds to all 50 states, the District of Columbia, and USA territories to conduct tobacco control activities. It has the following goals:
- Eliminate exposure to environmental tobacco smoke.
- Prevent initiation of tobacco use among young people.
- Promote quitting of tobacco use among adults and young people.
- Eliminate disparities in tobacco use among various populations.

The programme's goals are being achieved through four components: community interventions, anti-tobacco marketing in the media, policy and regulation, and surveillance and evaluation.

For tobacco control programmes to succeed, decision-makers and policymakers need to provide leadership, support research evaluating tobacco control efforts, and support training of health care professionals. CDC has developed and disseminates *Best Practices for Comprehensive Tobacco Control Programs* (http://www.cdc.gov/tobacco/bestprac.htm).

A new approach: comprehensive cancer control.

Globally, cancer control activities are fragmented, uncoordinated and often categorized and funded by cancer type. In the USA, CDC has been supporting development of an integrated approach called comprehensive cancer control. This includes surveillance, policy, research, education and intervention programmes, services, and evaluation. By integrating these activities and services, health agencies, policymakers and others can better prioritize, maximize use of limited resources, reduce duplication of or unnecessary efforts, evaluate and improve the effectiveness of all actions. The approach also aims to increase cooperation and collaboration among risk-factor and cancer-specific programmes and activities (including surveillance systems).

CDC and its partners have developed a comprehensive cancer control framework (http://www.cdc.gov/cancer/ncccp/cccpdf/09Abed67-78.pdf) that will help states and other entities address major cancers, establish priorities and apply limited resources. CDC currently is providing USA states, territories and tribes with guidance and, in some cases, funding to develop and implement comprehensive cancer control programmes.

high-risk women. Further details on planning are provided in the National Cancer Control Programmes handbook [1].

Achievements of effective National Cancer Control Programmes

National Cancer Control Programmes permit a better use of available funds, ensure a sound scientific basis to programme components, and promote social justice by ensuring equitable coverage of the population. Development of a Programme following an internationally accepted framework results in an understanding of the broader issues by both health care professionals and the general public. Of particular importance in many countries are avoiding the misuse of available resources, both public and personal, and an ethical obligation to relieve suffering at reasonable costs.

Barriers to effective National Cancer Control Programmes

There are a number of potential barriers to an effective Programme. These may include competing interests that could prevent the resources intended for cancer control being allocated to this purpose. In addition, the future patient is unknown and under-represented, so the importance of prevention may be downgraded as there is a lack of knowledge on the potential for prevention, both among health professionals and the public. Further, in both early detection and therapy, there tends to be excess reliance on high technology, with a failure to recognize the potential for contribution from low technology approaches. In the palliative care area, although the principles have been carefully set out by WHO, there may be a failure to ensure the availability of oral morphine, and also a failure to ensure that morphine is prescribed correctly, both in hospital and in home care. Other major barriers include:

- Lack of essential drugs and minimum standards of health care in low-income countries and disadvantaged populations
- Lack of appropriate human resources
- Lack of effective linkages with control programmes of other diseases (other noncommunicable diseases, HIV/AIDS, reproductive health etc.)
- Lack of effective intersectional approaches necessary for primary prevention
- Insufficient involvement of the community and nongovernmental organizations.

Monitoring impact of cancer control

As part of Programme planning, mechanisms must be set up to monitor the impact of cancer control activities. In general, this is best centred on a population-based cancer registry and an established vital statistics system. However, it is possible to set up ad hoc mechanisms, especially if the programme is initially concentrating on a few cancer sites. The basic measures are:

- Trends in cancer incidence - to assess the impact of prevention (and screening for those cancers detected in the precursor stage, especially cervical)
- Trends in cancer mortality - to assess the impact of screening and treatment
- Change in tumour stage - to assess the impact of early detection
- Change in cancer survival - to assess the impact of treatment.

These should be supplemented by process measures, such as reduction in the prevalence of smoking in adults, and take-up of smoking in children and adolescents, measurement of the proportion of the target population receiving screening, and the proportion of patients with curable cancers receiving therapy, and the proportion of those with non-curable cancers receiving oral morphine. Process measures can be applied in all countries. In countries without population-based cancer registries or vital statistics systems, it will be impossible to assess changes in incidence and mortality.

REFERENCES

1. World Health Organization (2002) *National Cancer Control Programmes: Policies and Management Guidelines, 2nd Edition.* Geneva, WHO.

2. World Health Organization (1998) *Guidelines for Controlling and Monitoring the Tobacco Epidemic,* Geneva, WHO.

3. WHO/FAO (2003) *Expert Consultation on Diet, Nutrition, and the Prevention of Chronic Diseases.* Geneva, WHO. *In preparation.*

4. IARC (2002) *Breast Cancer Screening (IARC Handbooks of Cancer Prevention, Vol. 7),* Lyon, IARCPress.

5. Sikora K, Advani S, Koroltchouk V, Magrath I, Levy L, Pinedo H, Schwartsmann G, Tattersall M, Yan S (1999) Essential drugs for cancer therapy: a World Health Organization consultation. *Ann Oncol,* 10: 385-390.

6. World Health Organization (1996) *Cancer Pain Relief,* Geneva, WHO.

7. World Health Organization (1998) *Symptom Relief in Terminal Illness,* Geneva, WHO.

8. World Health Organization (1998) *Cancer Pain Relief and Palliative Care in Children,* Geneva, WHO.

9. World Health Organization (2000) *Achieving balance in national opioids control policy – guidelines for assessment.* Geneva, WHO.

WEBSITE

The WHO Programme on Cancer Control: http://www.who.int/cancer/

CANCER CONTROL IN DEVELOPING COUNTRIES

SUMMARY

> More than 50% of the world's cancer burden, in terms of number of cases and deaths, occurs in developing countries.

> Some developing countries, particularly in Asia and South America (e.g. China, India, Thailand, Brazil, Peru, Costa Rica), have established effective diagnosis and treatment facilities, but such progress has been severely limited in many regions of Africa.

> Primary prevention measures targeting the most common cancers prevalent in the region, should be a mandatory component of National Cancer Control Programmes.

> Since a large proportion of cancer in developing countries is only detected late in the course of disease, efforts to achieve earlier diagnosis through improved awareness and diagnosis are warranted. Delivery of adequate palliative care and pain relief are equally important.

More than half of the global cancer burden is experienced in developing countries, although incidence rates in such countries are low compared to those in developed countries [1-3]. This burden of disease necessitates rational planning and appropriate investment in prevention and early detection. There is an equal requirement for the evolution of basic health services in a phased manner, taking due account of available technical and financial resources, which are often limited in developing countries.

A review of the current status of cancer control across the world reveals a widely varying level of progress in respect of primary prevention activities, early detection initiatives, and cancer-related health care including infrastructure and human resources. While the developed countries of Europe, North America, Australia and Japan have organized, sophisticated health care systems for cancer control, very little has been achieved in this domain in many sub-Saharan African countries, where even basic requirements for delivering minimal cancer care are lacking. On the other hand, certain countries in Asia (e.g. China, India, Israel, Iran, Jordan, Oman, Philippines, Viet Nam, Thailand, Singapore) and South America (e.g. Argentina, Brazil, Bolivia, Peru, Costa Rica, Cuba) have been successful in establishing and furthering basic facilities for diagnosis and treatment of cancer in at least some regions within these respective countries. This certainly provides a foundation for further expansion of cancer control activities.

Cancer information systems

Information systems providing data on cancer incidence (population-based cancer registries) and survival, as well as mortality (death registration) are useful for a reliable situation analysis and formulation of cancer control strategies. Incidence and mortality data are valuable for monitoring and evaluating the effectiveness of cancer control measures. Such data, while not totally lacking, are far from comprehensive (Table 7.1). The establishment of population-based cancer registries in developing countries has been a very haphazard process. Some countries have an official policy to support cancer registries, but in most developing countries with cancer registries, this outcome has followed a localized initiative of research-oriented clinicians and pathologists.

As indicated by the International Association of Cancer Registries listing, (http://www.iacr. com.fr/iacrweb.htm), 131 population cancer registries exist in 65 developing countries in Africa, Latin America and Asia. Some of them cover national populations (e.g. Israel, Oman, Costa Rica), while most are confined to certain regions or capital cities. The reliability and completeness of data reported from these registries are variable. Incidence data pertaining to 34 populations in 21 developing countries were reported in volume VII of *Cancer Incidence in Five*

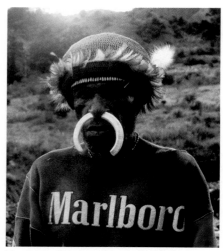

Fig. 7.6 A tribesman from a rural area of West Java, Indonesia, wearing a sweatshirt sponsored by a tobacco company. Smoking prevalence in men in this area has been reported to be 84%.
M. Imperi (2000) *Brit. Med J,* 321, cover photo, with permission from the BMJ Publishing Group.

Continents [4] while volume VIII will be reporting on 57 populations in 22 countries. Population-based cancer survival data, which reflect the average prognosis for a given cancer, and hence are indicative of the efficiency of cancer health services in a particular region, are available for only 11 populations in 6 developing countries [5,6].

In contrast, cancer mortality data from only 10 Asian countries, 8 countries in South America and the Caribbean and a single country in the African continent were reported to the WHO Cancer Mortality Data Bank in or around 1995. In certain instances, these data covered the countries only partially. It is quite likely that many of these existing mortality registration systems are incomplete to varying degrees in terms of their ability to capture all deaths and relevant information on cause of death. Limited relative frequency information (which may provide a restricted and biased insight on cancer patterns in a given region) obtained from hospital cancer registries or medical records departments is available from some developing countries lacking reliable incidence data. However, medical records departments are either rudimentary or do not exist in many sub-Saharan African countries and are poorly developed in many countries in Asia.

The importance of establishing and maintaining information systems, particularly population-based cancer registries, to support and evaluate cancer control programmes is clear. The organization of population-based cancer registries covering selected regions with particular cancer health services seems to be the most feasible approach in the short term. Much more sustained and coordinated efforts are required to develop a reliable mortality registration system for the entire country. The evolution of a network of cancer registries under the National Cancer Registry Programme of India provides a good example.

Primary prevention efforts

There are no dedicated and sustained primary prevention programmes for cancer in many developing countries. However, there is wide recognition that efforts should be made to create awareness at the community level. Thus individuals may be encouraged to adopt healthy lifestyles, based on informed choice, as a means to control common cancers. There has been very little focus in developing countries on educational initiatives concerned with cancer prevention, such as tobacco control, guidelines on diet and alcohol consumption, avoidance of exposure to certain infections, promotion of physical activity and so on. Thus far, health education

for cancer has been largely the outcome of periodic, sporadic activities by cancer societies or cancer treatment establishments.

The implementation of fiscal measures, such as taxation, impacting upon tobacco and alcohol control, is the responsibility of Finance Ministries in many countries. Such decisions may be influenced by revenue considerations, commercial and agricultural pressures, and least of all, by public health concerns and advocacy. Pricing policies for tobacco and alcohol are important factors influencing consumption, and are relevant to cancer prevention. To a large extent, pricing may have contributed to preventing large increases in the consumption of processed tobacco products such as cigarettes in many sub-Saharan African countries and in the Indian subcontinent. Long-term policies to provide alternative agricultural and commercial employment for those previously involved in tobacco production, marketing and sales have so far received very little attention in those countries where the tobacco industry is a major contributor to the economy.

Legislative measures may impinge on advertising, health warnings, sales and consumption of tobacco products and alcohol, as well as reducing occupational exposure to hazardous substances. Often, there is no lack of enactment of such legislation by governments. However, very little attention has been paid to the means of implementing these measures by the various agencies concerned with their enforcement. In fact, exist-

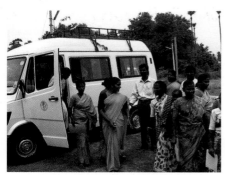

Fig. 7.7 Women participating in WHO cervical cancer screening in Ambillikai, South India (supported by the Bill and Melinda Gates Foundation).

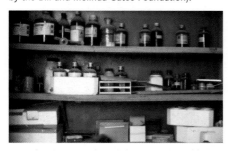

Fig. 7.8 The medicine cupboard in a health care centre in Burkina Faso. Resources are scarce and essential medicines are often in short supply.

ing legislative measures often remain to be implemented or enforced in many countries, sometimes for want of better awareness, willingness and coordination among different agencies.

Though some 31 high and intermediate-risk developing countries have implemented hep-

Regions	Number of countries with data available for the 1990s		
	Incidence data published[1]	Population-based cancer survival[2]	Mortality data[3]
Africa (56 countries)	8	None	1
Central and South America (21 countries)	6	None	5
Caribbean (8 countries)	3	1	2
Asia (44 countries)	13	5	7

[1] Based on *Cancer Incidence in Five Continents*, Volume VIII, peer-reviewed papers and registry reports.
[2] References [5, 6]
[3] WHO Cancer Mortality Database (as available on http://www-depdb.iarc.fr/who/menu.htm)

Table 7.1 Availability of cancer incidence, survival and mortality data from South America, Africa and Asia.

Regions	Number of countries providing cancer control services[1]		
	Pathology services	Screening programmes	Radiotherapy
Africa (56 countries)	49	None	20
Central and South America (21 countries)	21	5	16
Caribbean (8 countries)	8	1	5
Asia (44 countries)	43	1	32

[1] R. Sankaranarayanan, communication based on personal observation.

Table 7.2 Diagnostic and radiotherapy facilities in developing countries.

atitis B vaccination as part of an immunization programme, coverage needs to be further improved. In sub-Saharan Africa, where there is a high risk of HBV infection, only four countries have so far implemented HBV vaccination. Lack of adequate financial resources is a major impediment to the adoption of HBV vaccination in many high-risk developing countries.

Referral, detection, treatment and care facilities

A cancer control programme cannot be developed and be functional in a country without a network of laboratories and hospitals providing basic diagnostic and treatment facilities for cancer patients. Nor can a cancer control programme work without a framework for appropriate referral practices across the three levels of care, namely primary, secondary and tertiary. In developing countries where such basic facilities exist (e.g. Algeria, Argentina, Brazil, China, Costa Rica, Cuba, Egypt, India, Jordan, Kenya, South Korea, Philippines, Singapore, South Africa, Thailand, Tunisia, Viet Nam, Zimbabwe, etc.), diagnostic and treatment services have been mostly established in the tertiary care sector.

Diagnosis and early detection

The minimum diagnostic facilities required for cancer detection include histopathology, basic imaging services (here restricted to conventional diagnostic radiology and ultrasonography), and basic endoscopy. These will contribute to diagnosis and to assessing the clinical extent of disease, as well as indicating therapeutic options and prognosis. The basic clinical resources include surgical services for radical excision of tumours, radiotherapy and chemotherapy to the extent of providing selected essential drugs for adjuvant or mainstay treatment.

Early detection may be achieved through screening, case-finding and health education [7]. Many developing countries do not have sustained and focused activity directed towards early detection in their health services. Screening requires a committed infrastructure and is cost-intensive. It is not feasible to introduce screening programmes in many developing countries due to technical and financial constraints. A few South American countries, such as Brazil, Chile, Cuba, Costa Rica, Mexico and Colombia, and Singapore in Asia, have introduced cervical cancer screening with cytology, variously covering either national or selected urban populations [8]. However, most of these programmes have not been associated with reductions in incidence and mortality. Cuba has introduced an oral cancer screening programme, which again is yet to be associated with a reduction in incidence or mortality from oral cancer [9]. Singapore and Cuba have limited breast cancer early detection facilities in their health services.

Review of the availability of diagnostic and treatment services in developing countries (Table 7.2) indicates that the level of such services is particularly poor in sub-Saharan Africa, where there are extremely limited facilities for histopathology. Most countries in the region have a single pathology laboratory with one or two pathologists. Only in six countries are there more than two histopathology services and more than four pathologists in the entire country. In most countries, the laboratories are equipped with old, malfunctioning equipment and staffed by two or less locally trained technicians, with no quality control procedures of any sort. There are no continuing education/re-orientation opportunities available for these personnel.

In many sub-Saharan African countries, other facilities like conventional diagnostic radiology (let alone computerized imaging systems), ultrasonography and endoscopy are available only to a very limited extent in the public health services. If these are available at all, they are not within the reach of most people as they are located in the capitals and require out-of-pocket payments.

Surgery

Surgery plays an important role in the diagnosis and treatment of cancer generally. Removal of the tumour mass is curative for many localized solid cancers. Facilities for simple diagnostic and therapeutic surgery are available in the district hospitals of many countries in Asia and Latin America and facilities for more radical surgical procedures are offered in university hospitals and other tertiary care centres in these countries. A large number of trained surgeons are also available.

THE INTERNATIONAL AGENCY FOR RESEARCH ON CANCER: CANCER RESEARCH FOR CANCER CONTROL

The International Agency for Research on Cancer (IARC, http://www.iarc.fr) is part of the World Health Organization. IARC's mission is to coordinate and conduct research on the causes of human cancer and the mechanisms of carcinogenesis, and to develop scientific strategies for cancer control. The Agency is involved in both epidemiological and laboratory research and disseminates scientific information through publications, meetings, courses and fellowships. The Agency's work has four main objectives.

Monitoring global cancer occurrence
IARC is studying cancer incidence, mortality and survival in numerous countries and is thus playing a leading role in cancer registration worldwide. IARC supports and coordinates cancer registries throughout the world, being involved in initial advice and planning, the provision of training and the production of training manuals, guides and computer software, as well as in the collection and analysis of data. The Agency provides the secretariat for the International Association of Cancer Registries (which links registries in over 100 countries) and for the European Network of Cancer Registries. Collaboration is most active with developing countries, often including field studies to identify the causes of cancer that are important locally. Data from cancer registries throughout the world are published regularly in the *Cancer Incidence in Five Continents Series* and the *GLOBOCAN* and *EUCAN* databases which are also produced in electronic format (http://www .dep.iarc.fr).

Identifying the causes of cancer
Since the Agency's creation, a strong emphasis has been put on cancer etiology.

In laboratory investigations, epidemiological studies and working group meetings, more than 800 agents and exposures have been examined with the aim of unambiguously identifying those which cause cancer in humans. IARC's prestigious series of *Monographs on the Evaluation of Carcinogenic Risks to Humans* (http://monographs.iarc.fr/) are authoritative reports on risks posed by these agents and exposures. Recent Monographs have included *Man-made Vitreous Fibres, Non-ionizing Radiation Part 1, Some Thyrotropic Agents* and *Some Industrial Chemicals*.

Elucidation of the mechanisms of carcinogenesis
IARC laboratory research concentrates on the interaction of carcinogens with DNA, with the aim of elucidating mechanisms of carcinogenesis. Particular emphasis is placed on identifying carcinogen-induced, endogenous and inherited mutations in transforming tumour suppressor genes. For example, IARC maintains the p53 Mutation Database, which contains over 16,000 published mutations in the *p53* tumour suppressor gene (http://www.iarc.fr/p53/). This knowledge not only gives insights into the biology of cancer, but also helps to identify stages where it may be possible to intervene to prevent progression to clinical disease. IARC has research collaborations with scientists and with research and public health institutions in over 60 countries.

Developing scientific strategies for cancer control
IARC's programmes are aimed at finding approaches to preventing cancer. This includes both primary prevention and early detection of cancers. The role of IARC among cancer research institutes is characterized by its focus on cancer prevention, by its emphasis on studies that combine epidemiological and laboratory approaches, and by the special

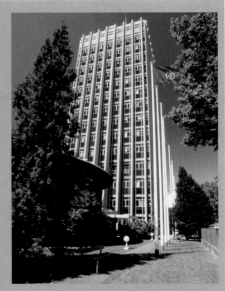

Fig. 7.10 The International Agency for Research on Cancer in Lyon, France.

forum and support it provides for international collaborations. In 1996, IARC established a programme to evaluate cancer prevention strategies, the results of which are published as the IARC *Handbooks of Cancer Prevention*. The first volumes in this series deal primarily with chemoprevention of cancer, e.g. *Retinoids, Sunscreens*, whilst subsequent titles include *Weight Control and Physical Activity* and *Breast Cancer Screening*. Although the implementation of measures to control cancer is not a central part of its mission, the Agency takes part in interventions with the aim of testing their effectiveness in preventing cancers or in the early diagnosis of tumours. For example, the Gambia Hepatitis Intervention Study, conducted in The Gambia, is designed to assess the effectiveness of vaccination of newborn infants against hepatitis B virus in preventing cancer and other diseases of the liver. The Agency is not as a rule involved with research into cancer treatments.

Treatment facilities are not widely available in most of sub-Saharan Africa. Surgical services are very limited, with only a few departments (e.g. general surgery, gynaecology, orthopaedics, urology etc.) attached to university hospitals providing limited services as part of their overall services for a variety of diseases, and then for paying patients only. The surgical services available are often limited to abdominal and pelvic surgical procedures, mastectomy, excision of superficially located tumours and biopsy procedures. Committed surgical oncology services catering for the needs of cancer patients are available only

CANCER CONTROL IN A RURAL DISTRICT IN WESTERN INDIA

The Tata Memorial Centre, Mumbai, India, is the apex body for cancer control in Western India and one of the major Comprehensive Cancer Centres in India. It has encouraged the initiative of a voluntary body called Ashwini Rural Cancer Research and Relief Society in cancer control in an industrially and educationally backward rural region of western India. The Society wished to organize a rural Comprehensive Cancer Centre in Barshi town in Solapur District, Maharashtra, to provide multidisciplinary services encompassing cancer prevention, early detection, treatment, pain relief and continuing care to the rural poor as well as to conduct community-oriented cancer control research. Thus the Nargis Dutt Memorial Cancer Hospital was set up in 1982. The Tata Memorial Centre, under the aegis of its rural cancer extension project, provided continuing technical assistance to organize and develop the clinical and community extension services of this hospital.

A basic cancer surgical facility with an outpatient clinic and an operating theatre was first organized while the Tata Memorial Centre trained two surgeons in the principles and practice of surgical oncology, as well as other medical and paramedical personnel. A health education programme was initiated in the rural districts surrounding the hospital to create cancer awareness. Soon a histopathology and a cytology laboratory were established followed by endoscopy and radiological facilities. Ultrasound equipment was added in 1987. Thus basic diagnostic and surgical facilities were organized initially along with community awareness programmes.

A population-based cancer registry to monitor cancer incidence in part of the rural district (Barshi, Paranda, Bhum Tehsils) served by the hospital was established in 1987 with assistance from the Indian Council of Medical Research. This started providing reliable cancer incidence data from rural India for the first time. The results from the registry revealed that cervical cancer was responsible for half of the cancer burden in women. Meanwhile the cancer awareness efforts culminated in an increasing proportion of women with cervical cancers diagnosed in earlier clinical stages as years passed.

A radiotherapy facility with a Theratron Phoenix telecobalt unit, brachytherapy equipment, a treatment planning system and a radiation physics laboratory was initiated in 1992 with assistance from Ratan Tata Trust in Mumbai. A committed medical oncology service was inaugurated in 1995. A CT scanner was added in 1999. The technical staff for these facilities were trained by the Tata Memorial Centre.

The Nargis Dutt Hospital initiated a non-randomized controlled intervention study in 1995 to evaluate the outcome of focused health education on the early detection of uterine cervical cancer, in collaboration with IARC. This initiative, now in its sixth year, has resulted in early detection and increased survival, followed by a non-significant reduction in death from cervical cancer in the district receiving health education as compared to the control district.

The Hospital has now grown into a Comprehensive Cancer Centre with 80 in-patient beds and a patient dormitory, catering for the cancer care needs of approximately 8 million people living in the surrounding districts of Solapur, Osmanabad, Latur, Ahmed Nagar, Beed and Aurangabad in Maharashtra state, Western India. The institution is headed by a chairman and is staffed by two surgical oncologists, a radiation oncologist, a physician, two anaesthetists, a pathologist, three resident medical officers, an epidemiologist, two pathology/cytology technicians, three laboratory technicians, a physicist, three radiographers, twelve oncology nurses and some health workers. Around 1,400 new cancer patients are registered annually, and around 6,000 follow-up visits are carried out. The

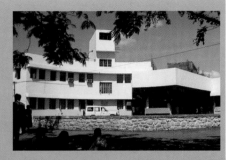

Fig. 7.11 The Nargis Dutt Memorial Cancer Hospital, Barshi.

laboratories process around 1,700 specimens for histology, and around 4,000 radiological imaging procedures are carried out annually. Around 400 major and 550 minor cancer surgical procedures and around 400 endoscopic procedures are carried out annually. Around 700 patients receive radiotherapy and 500 receive some form of chemotherapy.

In 1999, the Nargis Dutt Hospital initiated a randomized intervention trial involving 160,000 women to evaluate the comparative efficacy and cost-effectiveness of cervical screening approaches such as visual inspection with acetic acid, low intensity cervical cytology, and HPV testing in cervical cancer prevention in collaboration with the Tata Memorial Centre and IARC.

The Nargis Dutt Hospital has grown into a major community cancer centre providing comprehensive cancer control services, encompassing detection, treatment and prevention services, to a large rural population in Central India. The programmes are financially sustained by the revenue generated by the Hospital, non-recurring government grants, research grants and voluntary donations. Services are provided free of charge or subsidized for approximately half of the registered patients. The rural cancer control model developed by the Tata Memorial Centre and the Nargis Dutt Hospital is ideal for replication in many low resource settings.

in the capitals/urban areas of four sub-Saharan African countries.

Radiotherapy

Radiotherapy services are capital-intensive requiring considerable outlay for equipment, buildings and other infrastructure, as well as for trained personnel. Proper maintenance and calibration of equipment are essential to ensure sustained delivery of good quality, safe treatment. It has been shown that the acquisition of these services is related to the per capita gross national income of countries, with some regional variations. The cost of initiating (average cost of a cobalt unit is US$ 500,000 and a linear accelerator costs US$ 1.2 million) and sustaining radiotherapy services, the lack of trained personnel (radiotherapists, radiation physicists and technicians) and the necessity of having allied oncology services (diagnosis, pathology and surgery), in a sound hospital environment have been major factors limiting the provision of adequate radiotherapy services in most developing countries, particularly in sub-Saharan Africa.

In spite of significant expansion of radiotherapy services in the last decade, there is a major discrepancy in the availability of radiotherapy equipment between developing and developed countries [10,11]. For instance, Italy has more machines (200) than the whole of Africa (155). Currently, a total of 2,233 mega-voltage machines (671 linear accelerators and 1,562 cobalt machines) are available in developing countries, to serve a population of 5.5 billion people [12]. In contrast, 4,472 machines (3,902 linear accelerators and 670 cobalt machines) are available in developed countries, to serve a population of 1.5 billion people.

As with other areas of cancer control, Africa is the least developed region in terms of available radiotherapy services [10]. A total of 155 radiotherapy machines are available in Africa, accounting for 7% of machines in the developing world. These are located in 23 of the 56 African countries, and Egypt, South Africa, Algeria, Tunisia, Morocco and Libya account for 80% of these (125 machines). At any given time, a proportion of the radiotherapy facilities in the 16 sub-Saharan countries, other than South Africa, may not be functioning due to equipment breakdown or lack of radi-

ation source or lack of trained personnel. Many countries have inadequate or non-existent radiotherapy services. The rapid acquisition of comprehensive radiotherapy services is an unrealistic goal if there are limited technical and financial resources. It may be more prudent for some countries, particularly sub-Saharan countries, to form consortia to organize good quality, sustainable radiotherapy services in selected locations, which can thus be shared and subsidized by neighbouring countries.

Indigenous production of cheap and robust radiotherapeutic equipment and radioactive sources is important in the context of setting up radiotherapy services in developing countries. Countries like Brazil, China and India have established some capabilities in this domain.

Chemotherapy

A WHO consultation has proposed a list of 24 essential cancer chemotherapeutic drugs: ideally 17 drugs should be available for the treatment of the 10 most common cancers and 8 others should be available only where the resources and facilities exist for the treatment of paediatric cancers and leukaemias [13]. These drugs are not widely available in most sub-Saharan African countries and in some Asian and South American countries. Where available, these drugs are not subsidized, and hence not within the reach of many needy cancer patients. Expensive drugs subject to import duties, together with the limited efficacy of these agents in the context of most disseminated cancers, are major impediments to the gradual development of cancer chemotherapy in health services. It is impossible and unrealistic to subsidize cancer chemotherapeutic drugs in view of the extremely limited total health care resources available for cancer control in developing countries. Indigenous production of these drugs will go a long way in decreasing the costs of cancer chemotherapy. Currently, only a few developing countries, such as Brazil, China, Cuba, India, South Korea and South Africa, produce a sufficiently wide range of cancer chemotherapeutic drugs to have a great impact on costs. Basic facilities for diagnosis and chemotherapy are available in the tertiary care centres in most other developing

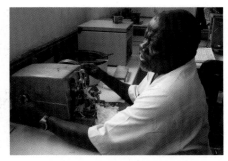

Fig. 7.9 A technician at a microtome, preparing histological slides in Luanda, Angola. Pathology laboratories are limited in many regions of sub-Saharan Africa.

countries in Asia and South America. However, these are often restricted to urban centres, causing accessibility problems for rural populations.

Comprehensive care

Comprehensive Cancer Centres, providing preventive, diagnostic, therapeutic, supportive and follow-up cancer care under one roof, are an important and effective organizational level in the delivery of cancer care, and are usually tertiary care centres. In most developed countries, cancer care is predominantly delivered through such centres established in different regions to cater for a defined population catchment area. Establishment and maintenance of Comprehensive Cancer Centres require considerable financial and technical resources. These Centres serve as apex bodies for cancer control in large regions, if sufficient attention is paid to incorporating extension services such as preventive oncology, community participation, palliative care (particularly in the home), and continuing follow-up care. In fact, some of the best models of cancer control activities in developing countries have been built around regional Comprehensive Cancer Centres, which have developed and directly implemented regional cancer control programmes (e.g. India, Thailand, Viet Nam, Peru). Such Centres are being increasingly developed in health services in Asia and Latin America, whereas there are few in Africa. More than 70% of the patients diagnosed

CANCER CONTROL IN GUINEA, WEST AFRICA

Guinea is situated on the Atlantic coast of West Africa and has an area of 246,000 km². The estimated population was around 7.5 million in 1999, with an annual growth rate of 3%. The crude death rate is around 14 per 1,000 and the infant mortality rate around 134 per 1,000. Guinea has a fairly well developed primary health care system, but all health services levy charges.

A population-based cancer registry was organized in 1990 to register incident cancer cases among the residents of Conakry, the capital. The registry reported an overall average annual rate of 83.3 per 100,000 males and 110.5 per 100,000 females, during 1992-1994. The common cancers in males were liver (age-standardized rate per 100,000 population 32.6), prostate (8.1 per 100,000 population) and stomach (6.2 per 100,000 population); the predominant cancers in females were cervix (46.0 per 100,000 population), liver (12.5 per 100,000 population) and breast (10.9 per 100,000 population). Only a quarter of the registered cancers were microscopically verified.

The department of pathology at the University Hospital of Donka, Conakry, is the only histopathology service in the entire country. This is staffed by a Guinean pathologist trained in France and a locally trained laboratory technician. This laboratory processes around 800 pathology specimens annually. Basic materials such as alcohol, formalin, stains and paraffin are always in short supply. The laboratory is equipped with an old but functioning microtome, a binocular microscope, a histiokinette and other materials, which are mostly donated from abroad.

The University Hospital of Donka and the Central Hospital of Ignace Deen in Conakry, the capital of Guinea, provide most of the cancer diagnostic and treatment services in Guinea, though some limited surgery is possible in a few provincial hospitals. Conventional radiology, ultrasonography and endoscopy services are available in these hospitals. Clinically inoperable cases are not usually subjected to biopsy. Cancer treatment is mostly limited to surgery for early cervix, breast, ovarian and stomach cancers and other operable superficial cancers. There are no thoracic or neurosurgical facilities. A medical oncology/haematology oncology service has been recently organized in the University Hospital of Donka, staffed by a physician. A restricted spectrum of cancer chemotherapeutic drugs is available from this service on payment. There is no radiotherapy service available in Guinea. If patients can afford it, they are referred to Senegal or France for such treatment. In practical terms, very little can be offered for inoperable tumours. Charges are levied for all services in the public health care services in Guinea. There is some coordination and collaboration between the histopathology, surgery, gynaecology and medical oncology services in these two hospitals.

A state-of-the-art private hospital with advanced medical, surgical and imaging

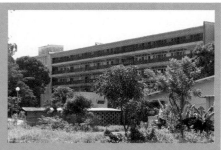

Fig. 7.12 The University Hospital of Donka, Conakry.

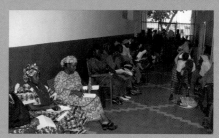

Fig. 7.13 Women awaiting screening for cervical cancer at the University Hospital of Donka, Conakry.

facilities mostly serves expatriates and affluent Guineans who can afford the services.

There is no officially proclaimed national cancer control programme in Guinea. HBV vaccination is not part of the immunization protocol in Guinea. A limited experimental intervention to reduce exposure to aflatoxins has been organized in a small region near Kindia. There are no early detection programmes for cervical cancer. A formal evaluation of visual inspection with acetic acid for early detection of cervical dysplasia and their treatment with cryotherapy is ongoing in collaboration with IARC.

with cancer in sub-Saharan Africa do not receive or complete the prescribed treatment. In regions of Asia and Latin America, the proportion of newly diagnosed cancer patients not receiving, or not completing, prescribed treatment ranges from 20% to 40%. Comparative studies of cancer survival in 11 developing country populations indicate that the average five-year survival associated with cancers such as colon and rectum, larynx, breast, cervix, ovary, urinary bladder, kidney, testis, lymphoma and leukaemia are 10-25 years behind those in the USA, Western Europe and Japan [5,6].

Consensus policies on approaches to diagnosis, treatment and palliative care of cancer on a site by site basis for major cancers, taking into account the resources available, are important in developing cancer control programmes and may prove extremely useful in optimizing use of resources. Such policies are generally lacking in most developing countries.

Palliative care

A large proportion of cancers in developing countries are diagnosed at advanced stage and thus palliative care merits a major place in the overall cancer strategy. WHO has catalyzed a major awareness and orientation of palliative care and this initiative has resulted in substantial improvements in the delivery of care [14-16]. Homecare concepts have gained currency. The "three-step analgesic ladder" approach and the availability of oral morphine for pain relief have significantly advanced palliative care. However, progress has not been uniform throughout the world, particularly in comparison to more developed countries. Thus even now, cancer pain remains unrelieved in a significantly large proportion of cancer patients, particularly in sub-Saharan Africa, mostly due to inadequacy or non-availability of opioid analgesics, particularly oral morphine.

Human resource development

The existing human resources for cancer control (oncologists, pathologists, epidemiologists, oncology nurses, technicians, administrative personnel) are limited in many developing countries, particularly in sub-Saharan Africa, certain countries of the Middle East and in some developing countries in Asia and Latin America. For instance, in the whole of francophone sub-Saharan Africa, there are not more than sixteen pathologists, four trained radiation oncologists and six medical oncologists. Similarly, there are only a small number of technicians trained in laboratory technology, radiology technology etc. There are only nine countries sub-Saharan Africa where regular training programmes exist for personnel concerned with aspects of cancer control. Generally, inadequacy of training of personnel is an impediment in developing countries.

Conclusion

A strict appraisal of the current situation in each developing country would allow a realistic review of resources available and their allocation for cancer control. The theory and practice of cancer control should be addressed in relation to specific needs: primary prevention, early detection, therapy, pain and symptom relief, psycho-social rehabilitation and health services development [17]. In the context of several competing health care priorities in low resource settings, the goal of having a National Cancer Control Programme, as advocated by WHO, to establish priorities, must be evaluated pragmatically. A National Cancer Control Programme provides a framework for rational and integrated implementation of cancer control activities taking into account the facilities already existing, and focusing on vertical investment to augment the necessary health care services. Introducing basic diagnostic services, basic cancer surgical facilities and palliative care should be the initial goals for implementing cancer programmes where current development is poor. Once achieved, this should form the nucleus for future expansion into other areas including prevention, diagnosis, treatment and continuing care, as well as information services. Investment in more capital-intensive areas should follow the establishment of basic services.

REFERENCES

1. Ferlay J, Bray F, Parkin DM, Pisani P, eds (2001) *Globocan 2000: Cancer Incidence and Mortality Worldwide (IARC Cancer Bases No. 5)*, Lyon, IARCPress.

2. Parkin DM, Bray FI, Devessa SS (2001) Cancer burden in the year 2000. The global picture. *Eur J Cancer*, S4-S66.

3. Pisani P, Bray F, Parkin DM (2002) Estimates of the worldwide prevalence of cancer for 25 sites in the adult population. *Int J Cancer*, 97: 72-81.

4. Parkin DM, Whelan SL, Ferlay J, Raymond L, Young J, eds (1997) *Cancer Incidence in Five Continents, Vol. VII (IARC Scientific Publications No. 143 and IARC Cancerbase No. 2)*, Lyon, IARCPress.

5. Sankaranarayanan R, Black RJ, Parkin DM, eds (1998) *Cancer Survival in Developing Countries (IARC Scientific Publication, No. 145)*, Lyon, IARCPress.

6. Chia KS, Du WB, Sankaranarayanan R, Sankila R, Seow A, Lee HP (2001) Population-based cancer survival in Singapore, 1968 to 1992: an overview. *Int J Cancer*, 93: 142-147.

7. Sankaranarayanan R (2000) Integration of cost-effective early detection programs into the health services of developing countries. *Cancer*, 89: 475-481.

8. Sankaranarayanan R, Budukh AM, Rajkumar R (2001) Effective screening programmes for cervical cancer in low-and middle-income developing countries. *Bull World Health Organ*, 79:954-962.

9. Fernandez-Garrote L, Sankaranarayanan R, Lence Anta JJ, Rodriguez-Salva A, Parkin DM (1995) An evaluation of the oral cancer control programme in Cuba. *Epidemiology*, 6: 428-431.

10. Levin CV, El Gueddari B, Meghzifene A (1999) Radiation therapy in Africa: distribution and equipment. *Radiother Oncol*, 52: 79-84.

11. Tatsuzaki H, Levin CV (2001) Quantitative status of resources for radiation therapy in Asia and Pacific region. *Radiother Oncol*, 60: 81-89.

12. International Atomic Energy Agency (2002) *Directory of Radiotherapy Centres*, Vienna, IAEA.

13. Sikora K, Advani S, Koroltchouk V, Magrath I, Levy L, Pinedo H, Schwartsmann G, Tattersall M, Yan S (1999) Essential drugs for cancer therapy: a World Health Organization consultation. *Ann Oncol*, 10: 385-390.

14. World Health Organization (1986) *Cancer Pain Relief*, Geneva, WHO.

15. World Health Organization (1990) *Cancer Pain Relief and Palliative Care*, Geneva, WHO.

16. World Health Organization (1998) *Manual on the Prevention and Control of Common Cancers*, Geneva, WHO.

17. World Health Organization (2002) *National Cancer Control Programmes: Policies and Managerial Guidelines*, 2nd edition, Geneva, WHO.

WEBSITES

CANCER*Mondial*:
http://www-dep.iarc.fr/

International Association of Cancer Registries:
http://www.iacr.com.fr/

Directory of ongoing research in cancer prevention:
http://www-dep.iarc.fr/prevent.htm

ENCR (European Network of Cancer Registries):
http://www-dep.iarc.fr/encr.htm

PERSPECTIVES AND PRIORITIES

SUMMARY

> Current smoking levels and the adoption of unhealthy lifestyles, together with a steadily increasing proportion of elderly people in the world, will result in a doubling of new cancer cases, from 10 million worldwide in 2000 to 20 million in 2020, with an annual death toll then reaching 12 million.

> Strategies exist to reduce the predictable burden of cancer through research, education, prevention, early detection, treatment and palliative care. Political will and international collaboration are now required for effective cancer control.

> Application of existing knowledge, technology and control strategies could prevent at least a quarter of all cancer cases, and cure at least a third of all cancercases in the next 20 years.

Thanks to social and economic advances that the world has witnessed during the late 20th century, humanity is facing rapid change and many challenges. During the last five decades, food supply has more than doubled and increased much faster than population growth; per capita gross domestic product in real terms has risen by at least two and a half times, and adult literacy by more than 50% since 1970. Dramatic increases have been observed in the number and proportion of children at school and the proportion of chronically undernourished children has declined considerably. These changes are having a major impact on global disease patterns and on the health and quality of life of human beings. Without question, the face of humanity is being rapidly reshaped due to political, economic and sociocultural interaction; the world of 2050 will be radically different from today's and will be almost unrecognizable from that of 1950.

Population health is no exception to this dynamic evolution, with global changes influencing and conditioning the way individuals and communities live, work and age.

Increasing life expectancy and population ageing

Globally, life expectancy at birth has increased from 45 years in 1950 to 66 years in 2000 and is expected to reach about 77 years in 2050 [1,2]. By 2025, the majority of countries, covering about 96% of total world population, will have a life expectancy at birth of greater than 60 years; for no country will it be less than 50 years (Fig. 7.14). The global population is expected to increase by 60% during the next 50 years, from 6 billion people in 2000 to 9.4 billion people in 2050; the number of people aged 60 years and above will more than triple, from 610 million to 1.9 billion, during this period.

With a slow and steady decline in fertility rates, the population of the world is thus ageing rapidly. The median age of the global population will have risen from 23.5 years in 1950 to 36.5 years in 2050. The global proportion of the population aged 60 years and over will increase from 10% in 2000 to more than 20% in 2050. The most rapid increase is, however, expected among the number of "oldest-old" - those aged 80 years and over. This population will increase by a factor of five between 2000 and 2050. The number of centenarians is increasing at an accelerating rate. In France, for example, the estimated number of centenarians was about 200 in 1950, and 8,500 in 2000, and will reach 150,000 by 2050. The life span of many individuals extends beyond the age of 115 in some countries.

In the early 1950s, the great majority of the global population died before the age of 50; today, the great majority is dying after the age of 50. It has been estimated that among 100 persons aged 20 years in 1955, at least 60 will be able to celebrate their 65th birthday and that among 100 persons aged 20 years in 1995, at least 80 persons will have that privilege. This represents an increase of more than 30% in survival chances between the two generations and has been achieved through advances in medicine and public health, in science and technology and above all in the adaptation and application of medico-scientific know- ledge for the improvement of health for all. These advances offer real hope for a longer, and hopefully a healthier future for humankind [3].

While extending life expectancy is desirable in itself, it is equally important that increased expectancy is accompanied by freedom from any prospect of years of suffering as a consequence of chronic diseases, pain or disability. Individuals are becoming conscious about their health expectancy, defined as life expectancy in good health. Unfortunately, while much is known about the determinants of population health in terms of life expectancy, very little is known about human longevity - the maximum duration of an individual's life and its determinants.

Cancer trends and prognosis

WHO reported that in 2000 [4] there were more than 6 million deaths caused by cancer, i.e. about 12% of a total of more than 55 million deaths from all causes worldwide. Infectious and parasitic diseases accounted for about 26% and diseases of the circulation for about 30% of total deaths. During the period 1985-1997, the number of deaths from cancer is estimated to have increased by 35%, from 4.5 million deaths in 1985 to 6.1 million deaths in 1997 [5] (Fig. 7.17). Deaths from circulatory diseases increased by about 30%, from 11.5 million to 15.1 million. These increases were not, however, geographically uniform. From 1985 to 1997, in more developed countries, there was a slight decline in the number of deaths due to circulatory diseases, but an increase of about 9% in the number of deaths due to cancer. During the same period, in developing countries the number of deaths increased

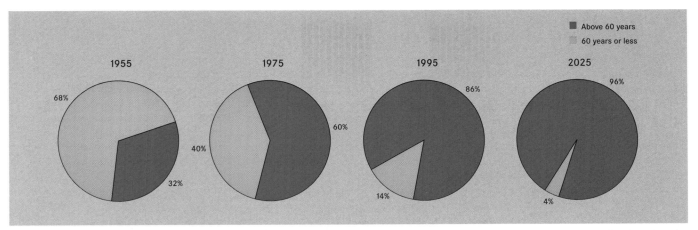

Fig. 7.14 Worldwide life expectancy at birth is steadily increasing. It is estimated that by 2025, approximately 90% of the total population of all WHO Member States (representing >90% of the global population) will live for 60 years or more. *WHO World Health Report, 1998.*

by at least 62% both for circulatory diseases and for cancers.

In 2000, there were 6.2 million cancer deaths, 10.1 million new cases of cancer and 22.4 million persons living with cancer worldwide [6]. This represents a global increase of about 22% in cancer deaths and in cancer incidence during the period 1990-2000. By 2020, the number of new cancer cases is expected to reach at least 15 million a year and cancer deaths 10 million a year. WHO in 1998 [5] reported that in 1960 cancer was one of the five leading health problems in three of the six WHO regions (The Americas, Europe and Western Pacific). Moreover, it will be one of the top five leading health problems by 2025 in all the WHO regions, except for the Africa region. Cancer is emerging as a major problem globally, both in more developed and in less developed countries.

Priority areas for action

Opportunities are clear at national and international levels for initiatives to control and reduce incidence, mortality and avoidable suffering and pain due to cancer. With a better understanding of the causes, mechanisms and progression of cancer, vigorous implementation of proven interventions, systematic experimentation and evidence-based choice of efficient delivery procedures, it is possible to reduce the burden of cancer.
WHO (1998) [5] concludes that by taking

effective action now, cancer incidence can be reduced substantially. Even modest efforts to adapt and apply available treatments, early detection methods and healthy lifestyle approaches will have far-reaching effects on the cancer burden worldwide. Achieving these goals is predicated on a commitment to coordinate global and national priorities for research, development and implementation of cancer control strategies. It requires a broad focus. In addition to providing evidence-based, cost-effective clinical interventions targeting selected cancer sites in individual patients, the task is to deliver essential yet comprehensive evidence-based, cost-effective medical and health interventions covering prevention, diagnosis and treatment. To achieve cancer control, a cost-efficient approach is required in order to deliver programmes as a part of the existing health systems infrastructure (see: *Cancer control package and its delivery,* p323). In some instances, different measures may be appropriate for the developed and the developing world, but many aspects of prevention and treatment are relevant to almost all communities.

Prevention

From a global perspective, cancer prevention can be justifiably focused on three cancer-causing factors: tobacco, diet and infection. These factors are responsible for at least 4.6 million cancer deaths (73%)

and 7.5 million new cancer cases (75%) annually, and for at least 15.8 million persons living with cancer (72%) in 2000 [8]. Effective promotion of a healthy diet, smoking avoidance/cessation and safe sex may be complemented with improved access to prophylactic and preventive vaccination and appropriate screening for high-risk populations.

Infection is responsible for about 17% of cancer incidence worldwide (varying from about 7% in developed countries to about 25% in developing countries) [9].

Present knowledge offers means by which transmission of infectious agents, such as hepatitis B virus (HBV) and *Heliobacter pylori*, can be reduced. Preventive HBV vaccination is already available worldwide and prophylactic vaccination against hepatitis C virus (HCV) and human papillomaviruses (HPV) may be introduced in the near future. The infrastructure for existing immunization services at national and international levels could be utilized in this context.

Early detection

Early detection can lead to a rapid and complete return to health. Established methods of screening, whether technology-based or undertaken by direct inspection, have reduced the mortality of cervical cancer. HPV testing, when combined with a conventional cervical smear test, improves the identification of cancerous

ETHICS AND CANCER

Major ethical issues are inherent in almost all aspects of cancer control: primary prevention, screening and early diagnosis, treatment and terminal care. The design and management of research involving human subjects, including clinical trials, also generate important ethical questions.

Ethical problems arise in a clinical, public health or research context when choosing between alternative decisions and may entail a conflict between different values, each regarded as intrinsically "good". The first, indispensable step in ethical decision analysis is to recognize the existence of a potential ethical conflict beyond what may appear as a mere technical choice. For example, the physician's assessment of the positive and negative consequences of a cancer treatment (physical, psychological and social) may differ from that of the patient and this divergence must be fully taken into account. A current approach for the recognition and analysis of ethical problems is to view decisions in the light of three moral principles: autonomy, beneficence and justice. Autonomy dictates that personal choices by competent persons should not be constrained. Beneficence (and, prior to this, non-maleficence, *"first, do no harm"*), dictates that the decision should benefit the recipients. Justice implies that every subject should be treated equally. Ethical problems arise because these principles very often conflict when applied to specific situations. Thus, offering a patient the widest scope of therapeutic resources, consistent with beneficence, may deprive others of resources, contrary to the principle of justice. A working scheme for ethical decision analysis involves examining choices in the light of the three principles as relevant to each of the parties affected, e.g. the patient, the physician, the relatives and the scientific community. Although some moral philosophers regard this procedure as inadequate, given the complex and unique nature of ethical conflict situations, the scheme has become a popular tool within biomedical ethics committees.

Ethical problems arise in *primary prevention* influencing personal behaviour, granted the impact of tobacco smoking, alcohol drinking, diet and sexual habits upon cancer. Individual behaviour should result from personal informed choices rather than being the product of psychological pressure, however well intentioned. However, respect for autonomy as well as beneficence converge in justifying vigorous anti-tobacco initiatives.

In *secondary prevention*, the central ethical issues revolve around the level of benefit which warrants offering a screening procedure to healthy, asymptomatic individuals. Positive evidence of some benefit should be available, ideally in terms of reduced death rates. Those participating should be informed of relevant risks in a clear, balanced way. Screening for genetic predisposition to cancer in the general population is not yet feasible but genetic testing for some cancers in high-risk families is established. Multiple ethical questions remain unanswered. For instance, should a young woman at risk of familial breast cancer consent to a test to determine whether she possesses a *BRCA1* mutation, and if so, at what age? What could be the effects of a positive test on her life, marriage and child-bearing? Will recognition that she is at risk materially improve her situation? Moreover, the investigator may be involved, if testing results in awareness of the genetic status of family members who have not provided any consent.

Ethical problems in *cancer treatment* centre upon the need for more effective, safe therapies. Controlled randomized trials are necessary to ensure unbiased comparison of treatments. However, assigning patients on a random basis to the new or the old (best standard) treatment continues to raise legitimate concerns. The implicit hope when propounding a new treatment is that it is more effective than the standard one: it may be regarded as unethical not to offer such a hope to every patient. Such limitations can only be overcome by extensive discussion with the proposed participants, explaining the rationale of the investigation and the degree of hope and, at the same time, uncertainty that surrounds the alternative treatments and justifies randomization. Without this process, consent signed by a patient is not informed and is ethically unsatisfactory. Appropriate dialogue, information and communication can reduce the likelihood of patients and families relying to their detriment on untested but highly publicized treatments, and perhaps abandoning effective, if uncomfortable, therapy.

Prevailing ethical attitudes, and consequent legal dispositions, vary worldwide with respect to active interventions to terminate life for compassionate reasons. Such options are not legally available in most countries. An exception is Holland where, provided strict rules are followed to ascertain the patient's wishes, these interventions are not regarded as legally punishable, the ultimate evaluation being left to the judicial authority. There is scant evidence that cancer patients faced with a poor prognosis, when given adequate support and care, seek life-ending interventions. Hence appropriate palliative care, guaranteeing the highest possible quality of life to the patient and to those close to him or her, is currently regarded from an ethical perspective as the most acceptable course of action.

To conclude, first, there cannot be an ethically justifiable decision without informed participation of all individuals affected by the decision, however demanding this may be. Second, ethics committees, composed of representatives of all parties involved in decision-making, are essential for the protection of the individual. The terms of reference, guiding principles and operational procedures of these committees should be accessible to the community at large. Third, a continuous and critical self-scrutiny is required from all involved in order to focus on the substance of the ethical issues and quash the notion that ethical responsibility is discharged by the filling-in of a multiplicity of forms.

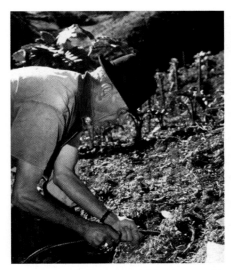

Fig. 7.15 A grandfather at work in his vegetable garden, Columbia, an example of an active, healthy lifestyle at advanced age.

abnormalities [10] but it is not yet known if this results in improved outcomes. The process of technical innovation continues to produce increasingly sophisticated, but easily adaptable, early detection techniques. A major cost in instituting any cancer screening programme is that associated with informing the community and sustaining logistics to cope adequately with initial positive findings. Education plays a critical role in motivating and increasing access to cancer screening.

Treatment
Based on the growing knowledge of the mechanisms underlying cancer, new drugs are being developed and the efficacy of new drug combinations is being assessed. Novel drugs will not necessarily eradicate tumours but, when used in combination with other agents, may turn many cases of rapidly fatal cancer into "manageable" chronic illness [11]. The potential worldwide health gain from defined interventions in cancer treatment using chemotherapy (including hormone therapy) has been assessed [8]. Seventeen drugs target those cancers which collectively account for 13.3 million (60%) persons living with cancer worldwide and 3.9 million (around 62%) annual cancer deaths. All these drugs

are also widely available as generic preparations at relatively low cost. It is also operationally feasible to give these drugs in an outpatient setting rather than in a hospital ward.

Many hospitals dealing with cancer patients are now establishing nurse-led day chemotherapy suites, as it is increasingly acknowledged that chemotherapy can be given in a day-care setting if the outcome of therapy is realistically defined and laboratory facilities are available to monitor basic markers (such as blood count, and liver and renal functions). Also required are implementation of clear protocols adapted to local circumstances which nevertheless meet scientifically demonstrable criteria, and rigid adherence to these protocols. A curable-cancer programme based on an essential drug list with a delivery system that meets the above attributes of good patient care and with a mechanism to monitor availability and performance of its components should improve efficiency and quality of cancer care worldwide.

Palliation
Individuals suffering from cancer form a burden that goes beyond the statistics of mortality and incidence, a burden that is borne by patients, their entire family and the community. In developed countries, roughly 50% of cancer patients die of the disease; in the developing world, around 80% of cancer patients have late-stage incurable disease when they are diagnosed. Clearly, the health profession has an ethical duty to prevent avoidable suffering at least through palliative care for pain relief. When cure is not possible, suitable measures to alleviate pain in terminal illness through effective palliative care are essential. Recent studies in the USA, Canada and Latin America concluded that the primary barrier to patient access to palliative care is lack of education for patients, as well as for health professionals. The situation is amenable to intervention through education and involvement of patients and their families in the provision of palliative care. Well-integrated community-based programmes that enable patients to die with dignity in a situation of their choice are achievable as a part of cancer control strategy.

The cancer control package and its delivery

In order to achieve an overall decline in cancer burden at national and international levels by reducing cancer incidence, improving cancer survival outcomes and ensuring pain control, WHO has formulated strategies that focus on education, prevention, early detection, treatment and palliative care. At the core of this cancer control strategy, there will be an essential package of cost-effective interventions for at least the following components: tobacco control, infection control, healthy eating, a curable cancer programme and palliative care. Once modalities for cancer prevention, screening and diagnosis, and treatment are chosen, it is necessary to integrate them into a comprehensive "cancer control package" that can be applied in countries at various levels of development. Provision must be made for its delivery as an integral part of the health services infrastructure. This package should include a technical protocol and operational guidelines for a cost-efficient approach to providing appropriate services to patients and the general population. Thus, a comprehensive approach may start with relevant anticancer medical interventions targeting specific types of cancers, but should evolve into a cancer control package that incorporates prevention, diagnosis, treatment and care, and takes account of genetic diversity between individuals as well as environmental and lifestyle information [7].

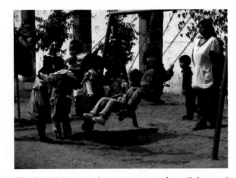

Fig. 7.16 Advances in many areas of medicine and public health will ensure a longer and healthier life span for today's children.

IMPACT OF THE HUMAN GENOME PROJECT

The Human Genome Project was initiated in 1990 in the United States by the National Human Genome Research Institute at the National Institutes of Health and the US Department of Energy. The Project is an international research effort defined by a series of specific goals (Collins FS et al., *Science*, 282:682-689, 1998) of which the major ones are: (1) to build genetic maps constructed by classical Mendelian studies of families or populations; (2) to build physical maps, constructed by analysis of the anatomic location of genes along the chromosomes; and ultimately (3) to determine the DNA sequence of the approximately 3 x 10⁹ base pairs that constitute the human genome. Centres around the USA and Europe, as well as Japan and China, are involved in this effort. The expected completion date of the finished product, without any gaps or ambiguities, is 2003, although an initial sequence and analysis has already been published (*Nature*, http://www.nature.com/genomics/human/; *Science*, http://www.sciencemag.org/feature/data/genomes/landmark.shl; http://www.hugo-international.org/hugo/). Progress can be monitored at the website http://www.ncbi.nlm.nih.gov/genome/seq, where genetic information is available in the public database GenBank.

Sequencing data obtained highlight the extreme similarity of human beings at the DNA level (99.9%). Cataloguing the 0.1% of human genetic variation is a key goal, as the data will provide information about increased susceptibility or resistance to disease. Identifying single nucleotide polymorphisms (SNPs), which are DNA sequence variations, should permit the performance of association studies that compare affected and non-affected individuals, and the specification of the genetic component of complex diseases such as cancer (Collins FS, Mansoura MK, *Cancer*, 91: 221-225, 2001). A specific programme has been started to identify SNPs in 450

samples from fully informed consenting individuals from Africa, Asia, Europe, and the Americas before colonization. These case–control studies will focus on correlation or associations between specific SNPs and diseases, and in most cases, data generated will be relevant to many populations. For example, African-American men are 32% more likely to develop prostate cancer than Caucasian men. Initially conducted on Caucasian populations, previous studies on the genetic contribution to prostate cancer have identified regions of chromosome 1 and chromosome X that are likely to harbour variations in genes that lead to increased susceptibility (Gronberg H et al., *Cancer Res*, 57: 4707-4709, 1997; Xu J et al., *Nat Genet*, 20: 175-179, 1998). A project involving the National Human Genome Research Institute, Howard University and the National Institutes of Health has recently been set up and preliminary data suggest that regions of the genome other than those previously identified might be involved in susceptibility to the disease in African-American men.

The sequencing data produced by the Human Genome Project may provide a mine of information about new genes having a role in different cancers. Revealing the complexity of cancer at the genomic level will require comparison between "normal" cell and cancer cell genomes. Moreover, new technology will be required to address the diverse kinds of genetic changes that are present in cancer cells (Futreal PA et al., *Nature*, 409, 850-852, 2001). One example is the development of gene expression profiling using cDNA microarrays (e.g. Khan J et al., *Nat Med*, 7: 673-679, 2001). Identifying associations between specific SNPs, as well as other genetic changes, and cancer will help to predict increased risk, to provide early detection, and to promote more effective treatment strategies. However, with the potential for this research to dramatically improve human health, a number of complex ethical, legal, and social issues arise. They are addressed in a specific programme established as an integral part of the Human Genome Project. Its major priorities

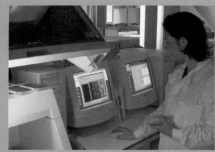

Fig. 7.18 Automatic DNA sequencing at the Sanger Centre, Cambridge, UK.

are to guarantee health insurance and employability for individuals known to be at genetic risk, and privacy of health data records.

WHO has recently published a guide which covers biological, social and ethical aspects of the recent advances in genome research and their potential benefits for human health (*Genomics and World Health*, World Health Organization, Geneva, 2002).

Websites:

The Cancer Genome Project, UK:
http://www.wellcome.ac.uk/en/1/biovencan.html

Cancer Genome Anatomy Project, USA:
http://cgap.nci.nih.gov/

The National Human Genome Research Institute, USA:
http://www.nhgri.nih.gov/

Functional genomics: the Human Genome (*Science*):
http://www.sciencemag.org/feature/plus/sfg/human/timeline.shtml

Genome Web–lists of genome sites:
http://www.hgmp.mrc.ac.uk/GenomeWeb/

The Human Genome: a guide to information resources online (NCBI):
http://www.ncbi.nlm.nih.gov/genome/guide/human/

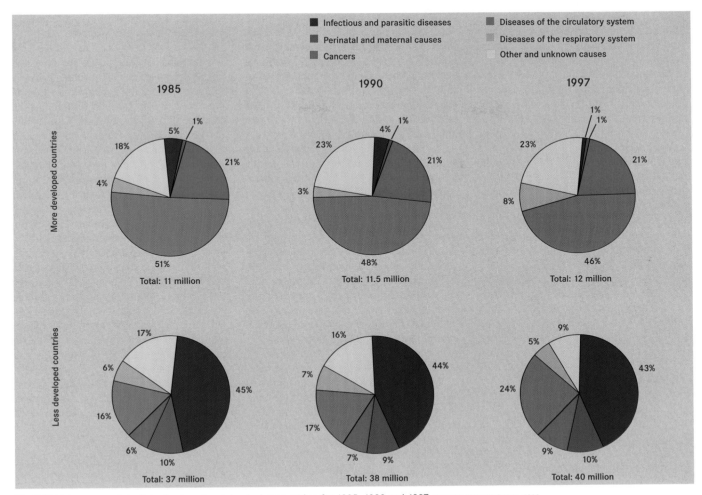

1985

More developed countries

5% 1%
21%
18%
4%
51%

Total: 11 million

1990

23% 4% 1%
21%
3%
48%

Total: 11.5 million

1997

1% 1%
23%
21%
8%
46%

Total: 12 million

Less developed countries

17%
6%
16%
6%
10%
45%

Total: 37 million

16%
7%
17%
7% 9%
44%

Total: 38 million

9%
5%
24%
9% 10%
43%

Total: 40 million

Fig. 7.17 Main causes of death in developed and developing countries, for 1985, 1990 and 1997. *WHO World Health Report, 1998.*

Equitable and effective access to care

To ensure equitable access to and provision of quality care, a cancer care delivery system has to be organized with due reference to cultural differences, individual attitudes and other determinants of access to health care. It should then be incorporated into the existing health care infrastructure in order to achieve efficiency, coordination and effective management. Ultimately, when relevant interventions are incorporated into standard medical practice, the benefits of state-of-the-art knowledge and practice will be available to all people, enhancing their health and well-being.

Effective mechanisms and procedures for improving access to health care, while maintaining and raising the quality of provision and outcome of care, pose a challenge in all countries. The elimination or rapid decline in incidence of many infectious diseases shows that sufficient experience already exists to recognize and respond to the need for change in health care delivery and management. A "primary health care" approach could be used. Experience in health care delivery is a valuable asset that can be fruitfully applied in formulating and implementing meaningful public health policies for the control of cancer and other chronic diseases.

There is enough knowledge available to analyse the cancer burden and to apply resources where they will have the greatest impact. Regardless of economic circumstances, a critical assessment of needs, appropriate planning and prioritization can curtail the toll of cancer worldwide. Additionally, an aspect of managing the development and implementation of cancer control strategies is to ensure that all members of the population benefit from such progress and that disparities are reduced. Attention must be given to ways of reducing the cost of cancer treatments and of translating laboratory research into clinical practice. Also required are improved methods of formulating and implementating public health policies and strategies that address tobacco control, infection control and healthy eating. Innovative approaches to cancer treatment, including palliative care, are required. Above all, options must be determined for integrating a cancer control strategy into each country's national health service and for establishing the best way of collaboration to convey new developments in cancer research from the laboratory into health care delivery [7].

An agenda for action

The *World Health Report 1997* [12], the *WHO Developing a Global Strategy for Cancer* and *Our Vision for Cancer* from the Imperial Cancer Research Fund [13] illustrate some approaches for dealing with this problem. Priority action proposed here takes into account information contained in these reports.

After an assessment of the global cancer situation, and based on advances in scientific knowledge and in diagnostic and treatment technologies, as well as on experience gained in adapting and applying cost-effective interventions in clinical and public health practice, the following priorities are evident:

1. To promote and sustain the commitment of political decision-makers and the support of funding agencies, health care providers, educational institutions and the media to reduce the emerging burden of suffering and deaths due to cancer.

2. To support the development and implementation of a Global Strategy for Cancer Reduction, and associated national cancer control strategies, to deliver a package of essential medical and health interventions that are cost-effective and evidence-based for tobacco control, infection control, healthy diet, screening, treatment and care.

3. To develop, test and make available guidelines and protocols for the implementation of strategies based on systematic experimentation and evidence-based choice of efficient procedures for delivery of drugs and vaccines, and the promotion of effective approaches for informing and involving health professionals and the community in cancer control.

4. To mobilize adequate financial resources to strengthen the health infrastructure so that the package can be delivered as an integral part of health services. This would ensure increased access to these services.

5. To stimulate relevant research for fuller application of existing knowledge and cost-effective methods of detection and cure, and to accelerate research into new areas.

6. To establish a global network of professional societies and an information sharing mechanism, and to ensure that current knowledge is shared, research gaps are identified and promising areas for reducing cancer burden are explored.

As "population ageing" will continue and possibly accelerate in the coming years, and as favourable economic prospects may lead to undesirable and unhealthy changes in lifestyle and behaviour, a cancer control strategy should be produced that can serve as a catalyst for change in health care delivery itself. It can be expected that the national strategies for cancer reduction that take into account cancer epidemiology, proven interventions, educational standards, existing resources and the economic status of the health system will contribute to a significant reduction in the global burden of cancer. The goal is a judicious mix of existing knowledge, technologies and available resources in order to develop cancer control programmes that can prevent at least a quarter of all cancers and cure at least a third of cancer cases. As a result of acting now, by the year 2020 countries can achieve significant reductions in cancer incidence and in mortality due to cancer. Opportunities exist - can they be exploited for the benefit of humankind?

REFERENCES

1. United Nations (1998) *World Population Projections to 2150*, New York, United Nations.

2. United Nations (1998) *World Population Prospects: the 1998 Revision*, New York, United Nations.

3. Greenfield S (2000) Boldly into a bright new era. Science, the Future, a Financial Times Guide. *Financial Times*.

4. WHO (2001) *The World Health Report 2001. Mental health: New understanding, new hope*, Geneva, World Health Organization.

5. WHO (1998) *The World Health Report 1998: Life in the 21st century. A vision for all*. Geneva, World Health Organization.

6. Ferlay J, Bray F, Parkin DM, Pisani P, eds (2001) Globocan 2000: *Cancer Incidence and Mortality Worldwide (IARC Cancer Bases No. 5)*, Lyon, IARCPress.

7. WHO (2002) *National Cancer Control Programmes. Policies and managerial guidelines, 2nd edition*. Geneva, World Health Organization.

8. Sikora K (1999) Developing a global strategy for cancer. *Eur J Cancer*, 35: 24-31.

9. Parkin DM, Pisani P, Munoz N, Ferlay J (1998) The global health burden of infection. In: Weiss RA, Beral,V, Newton, R eds, *Infections and human cancer (Vol. 33, Cancer Surveys)*, Cold Spring Harbour, Cold Spring Harbour Laboratory Press.

10. Cuzick J, Beverley E, Ho L, Terry G, Sapper H, Mielzynska I, Lorincz A, Chan WK, Krausz T, Soutter P (1999) HPV testing in primary screening of older women. *Br J Cancer*, 81: 554-558.

11. Stipp D (2000) A new way to attack cancer. *Fortune*, 141: 164-6, 168, 172.

12. WHO (1997) *The World Health Report 1997, Conquering suffering, enriching humanity*, Geneva, World Health Organization.

13. ICRF (1999) *Our Vision for Cancer: Finding Cures, Saving Lives 1995-2000*, London, Imperial Cancer Research Fund.

Contributors and Reviewers
Sources of figures and tables
Subject index

CONTRIBUTORS

Dr Alex A. Adjei
Mayo Clinic
200 First Street SW
Rochester, MN 55905
USA
Tel: +1 507 538 0548
Fax: +1 507 284 1803
adjei.alex@mayo.edu
[*Drugs targeting signal transduction pathways*]

Dr Frank Alvaro
John Hunter Children's Hospital
Locked Bag No. 1
Hunter Region Mail Centre
NSW 2310
Australia
Tel: +61 2 4921 3080
Fax: +61 2 4921 4080
falvaro@doh.health.nsw.gov.au
[*Childhood cancer*]

Dr Ala Alwan
Management of Noncommunicable Diseases
World Health Organization
Geneva
Switzerland
Tel: +41 22 791 4619
Fax: +41 22 791 4259
alwana@who.ch
[*Cancer control: a global perspective*]

Dr Alain Barbin
Unit of Endogenous Cancer Risk Factors
International Agency for Research on Cancer
150, cours Albert Thomas
69372 Lyon
France
Tel: +33 4 7273 8538
Fax: +33 4 7273 8088
barbin@iarc.fr
[*Carcinogen activation and DNA repair*]

Dr Daniele Bernardi
Centro di Riferimento Oncologico
Divisione di Oncologia Medica A
Via Pedemontana Occ. le 12
33081 Aviano (PN)
Italy
Tel: +39 434 659 284
Fax: +39 434 659 531
dbernardi@cro.it
[*Tumours associated with HIV/AIDS*]

Dr Sheila A. Bingham
MRC Dunn Human Nutrition Unit
Hills Road
Cambridge CB2 2XY
UK
Tel: +44 1223 252 760
Fax: +44 1223 252 765
sab@mrc-dunn.cam.ac.uk
[*Phyto-estrogens and cancer*]

Dr Paolo Boffetta
Unit of Environmental Cancer Epidemiology
International Agency for Research on Cancer
150, cours Albert Thomas
69372 Lyon
France
Tel: +33 4 7273 8441
Fax: +33 4 7273 8320
boffetta@iarc.fr
[*Tobacco, Tobacco control,
Occupational cancer,
Alcohol drinking,
Environmental pollution,
Lung cancer, Oesophageal cancer,
Bladder cancer*]

Dr Sandra Boivin-Angele
DNA Repair Group
International Agency for Research on Cancer
150, cours Albert Thomas
69372 Lyon
France
Tel: +33 4 7273 8317
Fax: +33 4 7273 8322
angele@iarc.fr
[*ATM and breast cancer*]

Freddie I. Bray
Unit of Descriptive Epidemiology
International Agency for Research on Cancer
150, cours Albert Thomas
69372 Lyon
France
Tel: +33 4 7273 8375
Fax: +33 4 7273 8650
bray@iarc.fr
[*Globocan 2000,
Global burden of cancer*]

Dr Eduardo Bruera
Symptom Control and Palliative Center
The University of Texas M.D. Anderson
Cancer Center, 1515 Holcombe Boulevard,
Box 0008 Houston, TX 77030
USA
Tel: +1 713 792 6084
ebruera@mail.mdanderson.org
[*Rehabilitation*]

Dr Elisabeth Cardis
Unit of Radiation and Cancer
International Agency for Research on Cancer
150, cours Albert Thomas
69372 Lyon
France
Tel: +33 4 7273 8508
Fax: +33 4 7272 8054
cardis@iarc.fr
[*Radiation*]

Dr Barrie R. Cassileth
Integrative Medicine Service
Memorial Sloan-Kettering Cancer Center
1275 York Avenue
New York, NY 10021
USA
Tel: +1 212 639 8629
Fax: +1 212 794 5851
Cassileth@mskcc.org
[*Complementary and alternative medicine*]

Dr Maria Cavazzana-Calvo
Laboratoire de Thérapie Cellulaire et
Génétique, INSERM U429
Hôpital Necker EM
149 Rue de Sèvres
75015 Paris
France
Tel: +33 1 4449 5068
Fax: +33 1 4273 0640
cavazzan@necker.fr
[*Gene therapy*]

Dr Pascale A. Cohen
Faculté de Pharmacie
15 Avenue Charles Flahault
34093 Montpellier
France
Tel: +33 4 67548613
Fax: +33 4 67548610
pascale.cohen@ibph.pharma.univ-montpl.fr
[*Implications for cancer of the
Human Genome Project*]

Dr Catherine Cohet
Unit of Environmental Cancer Epidemiology
International Agency for Research on Cancer
150, cours Albert Thomas
69372 Lyon
France
Tel: +33 4 7273 8657
Fax: +33 4 7273 8320
cohet@iarc.fr
[*Geographic variation in mutation patterns*]

Dr Vera Luiz da Costa e Silva
Tobacco Free Initiative
World Health Organization
Geneva
Switzerland
Tel: +41 22 791 2442
costaesilvav@who.int
[Tobacco Free Initiative]

Dr Louis J. Denis
Oncology Centre Antwerp
Lange Gasthuisstraat 35-37
2000 Antwerp
Belgium
Tel: +32 3223 5350
Fax: +32 3223 5352
Louis.denis@skynet.be
[Prostate cancer, Screening for prostate cancer]

Dr Suzanne Eccles
Tumour Biology and Metastasis
McElwain Laboratories
Cancer Research UK Centre for Cancer
Therapeutics
Institute of Cancer Research
Cotswold Road
Belmont, Sutton SM2 5NG
UK
Tel: +44 20 8722 4210
Fax: +44 20 8643 0223
suzan@icr.ac.uk
[Invasion and metastasis]

Dr Hashem B. El-Serag
Gastroenterology and Health Services
Research
Baylor College of Medicine and the Houston
VA Medical Center 2002 Holcombe Boulevard
(152) Houston, TX 77030
USA
Tel: +1 713 794 8640
Fax: +1 713 748 7359
hasheme@bcm.tmc.edu
[Stomach cancer prevention and screening]

Jacques Ferlay
Unit of Descriptive Epidemiology
International Agency for Research on Cancer
150, cours Albert Thomas
69372 Lyon
France
Tel: +33 4 7273 8490
Fax: +33 4 7273 8650
ferlay@iarc.fr
[Globocan 2000, Global burden of cancer]

Dr Alain Fischer
Laboratoire de Thérapie Cellulaire et
Génétique
INSERM U 429
Hôpital Necker EM
149 Rue de Sèvres
75015 Paris
France
Tel: +33 1 4449 4822
Fax: +33 1 4273 5070
fischer@necker.fr
[Gene therapy]

Dr Silvia Franceschi
Unit of Field and Intervention Studies
International Agency for Research on Cancer
150, cours Albert Thomas
F-69372 Lyon
France
Tel: +33 4 7273 8402
Fax: +33 4 7273 8345
franceschi@iarc.fr
[Infectious agents, HPV vaccination]

Dr Emil J. Freireich
Adult Leukemia Research Program
The University of Texas MD Anderson
Cancer Center
1515 Holcombe Boulevard, Box 0055
Houston, TX 77030
USA
Tel: +1 713 792 2660
Fax: +1 713 794 1812
efreirei@mdanderson.org
[Leukaemia]

Dr David Goldgar
Unit of Genetic Epidemiology
International Agency for Research on Cancer
150, cours Albert Thomas
69372 Lyon
France
Tel: +33 4 7273 8318
Fax: +33 4 7273 8342
goldgar@iarc.fr
[Genetic susceptibility]

Dr David Y. Graham
Department of Medicine
Veterans Affairs Medical Center (111D)
2002 Holcombe Boulevard.
Houston, TX 77030,
USA
Tel: +1 713 795 0232
Fax: +1 713 790 1040
dgraham@bcm.tmc.edu
[Stomach cancer prevention and screening]

Dr Keith Griffiths
Tenovus Cancer Research Centre
University of Wales College of Medicine
Heath Park, Cardiff CF4 4XX
UK
Tel: +44 1 633 680 765
Fax: +44 1 633 681 359
ProfKGriffiths@aol.com
[Prostate cancer, Prostate cancer screening]

Dr Salima Hacein-Bey
Laboratoire de Thérapie Cellulaire et
Génétique, INSERM U 429
Hôpital Necker EM
149 Rue de Sèvres
75743 Paris
France
Tel: +33 1 4449 5068
Fax: +33 1 4273 0640
[Gene therapy]

Dr Pierre Hainaut
Unit of Molecular Carcinogenesis
International Agency for Research on Cancer
150, cours Albert Thomas
69372 Lyon
France
Tel: +33 4 7273 8532
Fax: +33 4 7273 8322
hainaut@iarc.fr
[Oncogenes and tumour suppressor genes,
Cell cycle, Liver cancer, Food contaminants,
Oesophageal cancer, Geographic variation in
mutation patterns]

Dr Janet Hall
DNA Repair Group
International Agency for Research on Cancer
150, cours Albert Thomas
69372 Lyon
France
Tel: +33 4 7273 8596
Fax: +33 4 7273 8322
hall@iarc.fr
[Carcinogen activation and DNA repair, ATM
and breast cancer]

Dr Peter Hersey
Immunology and Oncology Unit
Room 443, David Maddison Building
King and Watt Streets
Newcastle, NSW 2300
Australia
Tel: +61 2 4923 6828
Fax: +61 2 4923 6184
Peter.Hersey@newcastle.edu.au
[Immunotherapy]

Dr Rudolf Kaaks
Hormones and Cancer Group
International Agency for Research on Cancer
150, cours Albert Thomas
69372 Lyon
France
Tel: +33 4 7273 8553
Fax: +33 4 7273 8361
kaaks@iarc.fr
[Reproductive factors and hormones]

Dr Keiichi Kawai
Kyoto Prefectural University of Medicine
and Yukawa Gastroenterological Hospital
2-10-2 Dogashiba-cho
Tennnoji-ku, Osaka
Japan
Fax: +81 6 6628 4707
[Stomach cancer prevention
and screening]

Dr Ausrele Kesminiene
Unit of Radiation and Cancer
International Agency for Research on Cancer
150, cours Albert Thomas
69372 Lyon
France
Tel: +33 4 7273 8662
Fax: +33 4 7272 8054
kesminiene@iarc.fr
[Thyroid cancer]

Dr Greg Kirk
Viral Epidemiology Branch
Division of Cancer Epidemiology
and Genetics
National Cancer Institute
6120 Executive Boulevard
EPS - 8003, MSC 7248
Rockville, MD 20852
USA
Tel: +1 301 496 8115
Fax: +1 301 402 0817
kirkg@mail.nih.gov
[HBV vaccination and liver cancer]

Dr Paul Kleihues
Director
International Agency for Research on Cancer
150, cours Albert Thomas
69372 Lyon
France
Tel: +33 4 7273 8577
Fax: +33 4 7273 8564
kleihues@iarc.fr
[Tumours of the nervous system]

Dr Stener Kvinnsland
International Union Against Cancer
(UICC)
3, rue du Conseil-Général
CH-1205 Geneva
Switzerland
Tel: +47 5597 6300
Fax: +47 5597 2046
skvi@haukeland.no
[UICC]

Dr René Lambert
International Agency for Research on Cancer
150, cours Albert Thomas
69372 Lyon
France
Tel: +33 4 7273 8499
Fax: + 33 4 7273 8650
lambert@iarc.fr
[Colorectal cancer,
Colorectal cancer screening]

Dr Françoise Le Deist
Laboratoire de Thérapie Cellulaire et
Génétique, INSERM U 429
Hôpital Necker EM
149 Rue de Sèvres
75015 Paris
France
Tel: +33 1 4449 5088
Fax: +33 1 4273 0640
ledeist@necker.fr
[Gene therapy]

Dr J. Norelle Lickiss
Sydney Institute of Palliative Medicine
Royal Prince Alfred Hospital
Missenden Road
Camperdown, NSW 2050
Australia
Tel: +61 2 9515 6111
Fax: +61 2 9515 7464
norelle@pal.cs.nsw.gov.au
[Palliative care]

Dr Julian Little
Epidemiology Group
Department of Medicine
and Therapeutics
University of Aberdeen
Foresterhill House Annexe
Foresterhill, Aberdeen AB25 2ZD
UK
Tel: +44 1224 554 485
Fax: +44 1224 849 153
j.little@abdn.ac.uk
[Cervical cancer screening]

Dr Guy Maddern
University of Adelaide
Department of Surgery
The Queen Elizabeth Hospital
Woodville Road,
Woodville, SA 5011
Australia
Tel: +61 8 8222 6756
Fax: +61 8 8222 6563
guy.maddern@.adelaide.edu.au
[Surgical oncology]

Dr Norio Matsukura
First Department of Surgery
Nippon Medical School
1-1-5 Sendagi, Bunkyo-ku
Tokyo 113-8603
Japan
Tel: +81 3 3822 2131 (Ext 6767)
Fax: +81 3 5685 0989
matsun@nms.ac.jp
[Stomach cancer]

Dr Heidi K. Mattock
International Agency for Research on Cancer
150, cours Albert Thomas
69372 Lyon
France
Tel: +33 4 7273 8429
Fax: +33 4 7273 8022
heidimattock@yahoo.com

Dr William H. McCarthy
Sydney Melanoma Unit
Level 3, Gloucester House
Royal Prince Alfred Hospital,
Missenden Road
Camperdown, NSW 2050
Australia
Tel: + 61 2 9515 6060
Fax: + 61 2 9515 6060
bill@mel.rpa.cs.nsw.gov.au
[Melanoma]

Dr Anthony B. Miller
Division of Clinical Epidemiology
German Cancer Research Centre
Im Neuenheimer Feld 280
D-69120 Heidelberg
Germany
Tel: +49 6221 42 2202
Fax: +49 6221 42 2203
a.miller@dkfz-heidelberg.de
[Cancer control: a global perspective]

Georgia Moore
Centers for Disease Control and Prevention
National Center for Environmental Health
1600 Clifton Road, NE, MS E19
Atlanta, GA 30341 USA
Tel: +1 404 498 1812
Fax: +1 404 498 1313
gbm7@cdc.gov
[*CDC*]

Dr Nubia Muñoz
International Agency for Research on Cancer
150, cours Albert Thomas
F-69372 Lyon
France
nubia@iarc.fr
[*Infectious agents, HPV vaccination*]

Dr M. Krishnan Nair
Director
Regional Cancer Institute
Medical College Campus
Thiruvanthapuram 695 011
Kerala India
Tel: +91 471 442541
Fax: +91 471 447454
[*Cancer control: a global perspective*]

Dr Craig R. Nichols
Division of Hematology/Medical Oncology
Oregon Health and Sciences University
3181 S.W. Sam Jackson Park Road
Portland, OR 97201-3098 USA
Tel: +1 503 494 6346
Fax: +1 503 494 4285
nicholsc@ohsu.eud
[*Cancer of the testis*]

Dr Murray Norris
Children's Cancer Institute Australia
PO Box 81
Randwick, NSW 2031
Australia
Tel: +61 2 9382 1813
Fax: +61 2 9382 1850
m.norris@unsw.edu.au
[*The molecular determination of minimal residual disease*]

Dr Hiroko Ohgaki
Unit of Molecular Pathology
International Agency for Research on Cancer
150, cours Albert Thomas
69372 Lyon
France
Tel: +33 4 7273 8534
Fax: +33 4 7273 8564
ohgaki@iarc.fr
[*Stomach cancer*]

Dr Kola Okuyemi
Departments of Family Medicine and
Preventive Medicine
University of Kansas Medical Center
3901 Rainbow Boulevard
Kansas City, KA 66160-7370
USA
Tel: +1 913 588 1938
Fax: +1 913 588 1910
kokuyemi@kumc.edu
[*Pharmacological approaches to smoking cessation*]

Dr Christian Partensky
Fédération des Spécialités Digestives
Hôpital Edouard Herriot, Lyon
France
Tel: +33 4 7211 6261
Fax: +33 4 7211 6259
christian.partensky@chu-lyon.fr
[*Surgical oncology*]

Dr Frederica Perera
Columbia Center for Children's Environmental Health
Columbia University School of Public Health
60 Haven Avenue, B-109
New York City, NY 10032
USA
Tel: +1 212 304 7280
Fax: +1 212 544 1943
fpp1@columbia.edu
[*Molecular epidemiology*]

Dr Roger R. Reddel
Children's Medical Research Institute
214 Hawkesbury Road
Westmead
Sydney, NSW 2145
Australia
Tel: +61 2 9687 280
Fax: +61 2 9687 2120
rreddel@cmri.usyd.edu.au
[*Telomerase*]

Dr Elio Riboli
Unit of Nutrition and Cancer
International Agency for Research on Cancer
150 cours Albert Thomas
69372 Lyon
France
Tel: +33 4 7273 8411
Fax: +33 4 7273 8419
riboli@iarc.fr
[*Diet and nutrition*]

Dr Jerry Rice
International Agency for Research on Cancer
150 cours Albert Thomas
69372 Lyon
France
rice@iarc.fr
[*Medicinal drugs, Immunosuppression*]

Dr Jens Ricke
Strahlenklinik
Charite Campus Virchow-Klinikum
Humboldt University
Augustenburger Platz 1
D-13353 Berlin
Germany
Tel: +49 30 4505 7001
Fax: +49 30 4505 7901
jens@charite.de
[*Telemedicine*]

Dr Rengaswamy Sankaranarayanan
Unit of Descriptive Epidemiology
International Agency for Research on Cancer
150, cours Albert Thomas
69372 Lyon
France
Tel: +33 7273 8599
Fax: +33 4 7273 8650
sankar@iarc.fr
[*Head and neck cancer, Oral cancer screening, Cancer control in developing countries*]

Dr Annie J. Sasco
Unit of Epidemiology for Cancer Prevention
International Agency for Research on Cancer
150, cours Albert Thomas
69372 Lyon
France
Tel: +33 4 7273 8412
Fax: +33 4 7273 8342
sasco@iarc.fr
[*Breast cancer, Tobacco control*]

Dr Cecilia Sepúlveda
Programme on Cancer Control
World Health Organization
Geneva
Switzerland
Tel: +41 22 791 3706
Fax: +41 22 791 4297
sepulvedac@who.ch
[*Cancer control: a global perspective*]

Dr Ki Shin
Section of Physical Medicine and Rehabilitation
Department of Palliative Care and
Rehabilitation Medicine
The University of Texas MD Anderson
Cancer Center
1515 Holcombe Boulevard, Box 0008
Houston, TX 7703 USA
Tel: +1 713 745 2327
Fax: +1 713 792 6092
kshin@mdanderson.org
[Rehabilitation]

Dr Karol Sikora
Department of Cancer Medicine
Imperial College School of Medicine
Hammersmith Hospital, Du Cane Road
London W12 OHS UK
Tel: +44 20 8383 3060
Fax: +44 20 8383 1708
karol.sikora@astrazeneca.com
[Radiotherapy, Medical oncology]

Dr Leslie H. Sobin
Division of Gastrointestinal Pathology
Armed Forces Institute of Pathology
Washington, DC 20306 USA
Tel: +1 202 782 2880
Fax: +1 202 782 9020
sobin@aifp.osd.mil
[TNM]

Dr Michele Spina
Division of Medical Oncology A
National Cancer Institute
via Pedemontana occ.le 12
33081 Aviano (PN) Italy
Tel: +39 434 659 284
Fax: +39 434 659 531
oma@ets.it
[Tumours associated with HIV/AIDS]

Dr Kenneth Stanley
Programme on Cancer Control
World Health Organization
Geneva
Switzerland
[Cancer control: a global perspective]

Dr Bernard W. Stewart
SEH Cancer Control Program
Locked Bag 88
Randwick, NSW 2031
Australia
Tel: +61 2 9382 8249
Fax: +61 2 9382 8334
StewartB@sesahs.nsw.GOV.AU
[Reduction of UV, Apoptosis,
Multistage carcinogenesis]

Dr Muthu Subramanian
Former Director, WHO
601 Regency Drive
Franklin Park, NJ 08823 USA
Tel: +1 732 821 8859
Fax: +1 732 821 9557
muthusub@att.net
[Perspectives and priorities]

Dr Martin H.N. Tattersall
Blackburn Building, D06
University of Sydney
Sydney, NSW 2006
Australia
Tel: +61 2 9351 3675
Fax: + 61 2 9351 4317
mtatt@med.usyd.edu.au
[Cancer education in medical courses]

Dr Umberto Tirelli
Division of Medical Oncology A
National Cancer Institute
via Pedemontana occ.le 12
33081 Aviano (PN)
Italy
Tel: +39 434 659 284
Fax: +39 434 659 531
utirelli@ets.it
[Tumours associated with HIV/AIDS]

Dr Harri Vainio
Unit of Chemoprevention
International Agency for Research on Cancer
150, cours Albert Thomas
69372 Lyon
France
Tel: +33 4 7273 8418
Fax: +33 4 7273 8319
vainio@iarc.fr
[Chemoprevention, Precursor lesions]

Dr Stacey Vandor
National Cancer Institute
6130 Executive Boulevard
Rockville, MD 20852 USA
Tel: +1 301 594 6786
vandors@od.nci.nih.gov
[NCI]

Dr Andrew C. von Eschenbach
Director
National Cancer Institute
6116 Executive Boulevard
Bethesda, MD 20892-8322
USA
Tel: 1 301 496 5615
Fax: 1 301 402 0338
[Prostate cancer,
Screening for prostate cancer]

Dr Yoshiyuki Watanabe
Department of Social Medicine
and Cultural Sciences
Research Institute for Neurological
Diseases and Geriatrics
Kyoto Prefectural
University of Medicine
Kawaramachi-Hirokoji
Kamigyo-ku, Kyoto 602-8566
Japan
Tel: +81 75 251 5770
Fax: +81 75 251 5799
watanabe@basic.kpu-m.ac.jp
[Stomach cancer prevention and screening]

Dr Naohito Yamaguchi
Cancer Information and Epidemiology Division
National Cancer Center Research Institute
5-1-1 Tsukiji, Chuo-ku
Tokyo 104-0045
Japan
Tel: +81 3 3547 5245
Fax: +81 3 3546 0630
nyamaguc@info.ncc.go.jp
[Cancer control in Japan]

Dr Hiroshi Yamasaki
School of Science and Technology
Kwansei Gakuin University
1, 2-chome Gakuon, Sanda
Hyogo 69-13972
Japan
Tel: +81 795 65 8734
Fax: +81 795 65 8734
yhyamasaki@ksc.kwansei.ac.jp
[Multistage carcinogenesis,
Cell-cell communication]

Dr Graham A.R. Young
Kanematsu Laboratories
Royal Prince Alfred Hospital
Camperdown, Sydney
NSW 2050
Australia
Tel: +61 2 9515 8863
Fax: +61 2 9515 6255
graham@kan.rpa.cs.nsw.gov.au
[Lymphoma]

REVIEWERS

Dr Sandra E. Brooks
405 W. Redwood Street, 3rd Floor
Division of Gynecologic Oncology
University of Maryland School of Medicine
Baltimore, MD 21201
USA
Tel: +1 410 328 2076
Fax: +1 410 328 8389
sbrooks@umm.edu
[Cancers of the female reproductive tract]

Dr Richard P. Gallagher
Cancer Control Research Program
British Columbia Cancer Agency
600, West 10th Avenue,
Vancouver BC, V5Z 4E6
Canada
Tel: +1 604 877 6098 ext 3056
Fax: +1 604 877 1868
rickg@bccancer.bc.ca
[Reduction of exposure to UV radiation]

Dr Phillip C. Hoffman
University of Chicago Medical Center
Department of Medicine
Section of Hematology Oncology
5841 S Maryland Avenue, MC 2115
Chicago, IL 60637-1470
USA
Tel: +1 773 702 6149
Fax: +1 773 702 0963
phoffman@medicine.bsd.uchicago.edu
[Lung cancer]

Dr Clement W. Imrie
Upper Gastrointestinal Unit
Lister Department of Surgery
Royal Infirmary
16, Alexandra Parade
Glasgow
Lanarkshire G31 2ER
UK
Tel: +44 141 211 4293
Fax: +44 141 211 4991
clemimrie@hotmail.com
[Pancreatic cancer]

Dr Anthony B. Miller
Division of Clinical Epidemiology
German Cancer Research Centre/Deutsches
Krebsforschungszentrum
Im Neuenheimer Feld 280
D 69120 Heidelberg
Germany
Tel: +49 6221 42 2202
Fax: +49 6221 42 2203
a.miller@dkfz-heidelberg.de
[Chapters 1, 2, 4, 5, 7]

Dr Indraneel Mittra
Tata Memorial Hospital
Tata Memorial Centre
Dr Ernest Borges Road
Parel, Bombay 400 012
India
Tel: +91 22 414 6750
Fax: +91 22 414 6937
imittra@bom7.vsnl.net.in
[Surgical oncology]

Dr Marshall Posner
Head and Neck Oncology Program
Dana-Farber Cancer Institute
SW430H, 44 Binney Street
Boston, MA 02115
USA
Tel: +1 617 632 3090
Fax: +1 617 632 4448
marshall_posner@dfci.harvard.edu
[Head and neck cancer]

Dr Roger Stupp
University Hospital CHUV
Multidisciplinary Center for Oncology
Rue du Bugnon 46
1011 Lausanne
Switzerland
Tel: +41 21 314 0156
Fax: +41 21 314 0737
Roger.Stupp@chuv.hospvd.ch
[Chapter 6]

Dr Peter Swann
Department of Biochemistry
and Molecular Biology
University College London
Gower Street
London WC1E6BT
UK
Tel: +44 207 679 7117 ext2329
Fax: +44 207 679 7193
p.swann@biochem.ucl.ac.uk
[Chapter 3]

Dr Alistair M. Thompson
Department of Surgery
and Molecular Oncology
Ninewells Hospital and Medical School
University of Dundee
Dundee DD1 9SY, Scotland UK
Tel: +44 1382 660 111
Fax: +44 1382 496 361
a.m.thompson@dundee.ac.uk
[Breast cancer, Oesophageal cancer,
Stomach cancer]

Dr Nicholas J. Vogelzang
University of Chicago Cancer Research Center
5841 S. Maryland Avenue, MC 1140
Chicago, IL 60637-1470
USA
Tel: +1 773 702 6180
Fax: +1 773 702 0595
nvogelza@medicine.bsd.uchicago.edu
[Kidney cancer]

SOURCES OF FIGURES AND TABLES

Figures

1.1 & 1.2 GLOBOCAN 2000*

1.3 WHO/TDR Image Library/Crump

1.4 GLOBOCAN 2000*

1.5 CDC Public Health Image Library, Atlanta, USA/Dr. Edwin P. Ewing, Jr.

1.6 Anna White, Coordinator, Global Partnerships for Tobacco Control, PO Box 19405, Washington, DC 20036, USA

1.7 & 1.8 GLOBOCAN 2000*

1.9 & 1.10 IARCPress

2.1 IARCPress

2.2 B.W. Stewart, Australia

2.3 SPL/Cosmo

2.4 WHO Digital Photo Library/H. Anenden

2.5 Reprinted from *Eur J Cancer*, Vol. 35, F. Levi, F. Lucchini, E. Negri, P. Boyle, C. La Vecchia C, Cancer mortality in Europe, 1990-94, and an overview of trends from 1955 to 1994, 1477-1516, copyright 1999, with permission from Elsevier Science

2.6 P. Boffetta, IARC/American Cancer Society, E.C. Hammond (1966) *Natl Cancer Inst Monogr*, 19:127-204; T. Hirayama (1985) A cohort study of cancer in Japan. In Blot WJ, Hirayama T, Hoel DG eds. *Statistical Methods in Cancer Epidemiology*. Hiroshima, Radiation Effects Research Foundation, 73-91

2.7 Reprinted from *Eur J Cancer Prev*, Vol. 8, M. Pandey, A. Mathew, M.K. Nair, Global perspective of tobacco habits and lung cancer: a lesson for third world countries, 271-279, Copyright 1999, with permission from Elsevier Science

2.8 Adapted from C.J.L. Murray et al., Tobacco, in C.J.L. Murray and A.D. Lopez (1996)*Quantifying Global Health Risks: the Burden of Disease Attributable to Selected Risk Factors*. Cambridge, Harvard University Press

2.9 A.D. Lopez N.E. Collishaw, T. Piha (1994) A descriptive model of the cigarette epidemic in developed countries. *Tobacco Control*, 3:242-247, with permission from the *BMJ* Publishing Group

2.10 P. Boffetta, IARC

2.11 A.M. Thompson, UK

2.12 P. Boffetta, IARC/*IARC Monographs* Programme

2.13 D. Jernigan, Marin Institute, California, USA

2.14 Adapted from A.J. Tuyns, J. Estève, L. Raymond, F. Berrino, E. Benhamou et al. (1988) Cancer of the larynx/hypopharynx, tobacco and alcohol: IARC international case-control study in Turin and Varese (Italy), Zaragoza and Navarra (Spain), Geneva (Switzerland) and Calvados (France), *Int J Cancer*, 41(4):483-491

2.15 D. Jernigan, Marin Institute, California, USA

2.16 Graphics and Audiovisual section, NCI Office of Cancer Communications, USA

2.17 - 2.19 IARCPress

2.20 Groupe Charbonnages de France; HBL Audiovisuel/ Synchro

2.21 & 2.22 IARCPress

2.23 Pan Photographics, Via Le Pietre 15, Vico Equense, NA 80069, Italy

2.24 WHO Digital Image Library/PAHO/Armando Waak

2.25 Pascale Dia, IARC

2.26 WHO Digital Image Library/H. Anenden

2.27 - 2.31 R. Montesano, IARC

2.32 IARCPress/T.W. Kensler, Department of Environmental Health Sciences, Johns Hopkins School of Hygiene and Public Health, Baltimore, MD 21205, USA

2.33 H. Ohgaki, IARC

2.34 Wellcome Trust Medical Photographic Library, UK

2.35 IARCPress

2.36 "Chernobilinterinform" 1996, 255620 Chernobilinterin -form, 1996 (25560, Chernobil, Kiev region, B. Chmelnitcky street, 1a)

2.37 Pan Photographics, Via Le Pietre 15, Vico Equense, NA 80069, Italy

2.38 NRPB (2001) *ELF Electromagnetic fields and he risk of cancer*, Vol. 12. No. 1, National Radiogical Protection Board, Chilton Didcot, Oxon OX11 OPQ, UK

2.39 H. N. Ananthaswamy, Department of Immunology, The University of Texas M.D. Anderson Cancer Center, 1515 Holcombe Blvd., Houston, Texas 77030, USA

2.40 USA Environmental Protection Agency

2.41 Public Health Image Library CDC, USA/Dr Erskine Palmer

2.42 Wellcome Trust Medical Photographic Library, UK

2.43 By permission of Oxford University Press, H. zur Hausen (2000) Papillomaviruses causing cancer, *J Natl Cancer Inst*, 92(9): 695

2.44 & 2.45 IARCPress

2.46 Public Health Image Library, CDC, USA/Dr Edwin P. Ewing, Jr.

2.47 & 2.48 S. Franceschi, IARC

2.49 Copyright of the American Society for Investigative Pathology. F. Chisari (2000), Viruses, Immunity and Cancer: Lessons from Hepatitis B, *Am J Pathol*, 156, 1118-1131

2.50 IARCPress

2.51 Public Health Image Library, CDC, USA/Dr Edwin P. Ewing, Jr.

2.52 Istituto Nazionale dei Tumori, Milan, Italy; Deutsches Krebsforschungszentrum, Heidelberg, Germany; National Institute of Public Health and Environmental Protection (RIVM), Bilthoven, Netherlands

2.53 T. Norat and E. Riboli, IARC

2.54 D. Graham, USA/Adapted from Fig. 2, S. Tsugane, M. Akabane, T. Inami, S. Matsushima, T. Ishibashi et al. (1991) Urinary salt excretion and stomach cancer mortality among four Japanese populations. *Cancer Causes Control*, 2:165-8, with kind permission of Kluwer Academic Publishers

2.55 IARCPress

2.56 B.W. Stewart, Australia

2.57 EPIC study/Dr Riboli, IARC

2.58A Map derived from FAO food consumption statistics/ T. Norat, E. Riboli, IARC.

2.58B GLOBOCAN 2000*

2.59 Public Health Image Library, CDC, USA/James Gathany

2.60 Courtesy of the Multi-Organ Transplant Programme, UK

2.61 & 2.62 N.L. Harris, Department of Pathology, Warren 2, Massachusetts General Hospital, Fruit Street, Boston, MA 02114, USA

2.63 R.D. Brunning, Department of Laboratory Medicine and Pathology, University of Minnesota Hospital, 420 Delaware Street SE, Box 609, Minneapolis, MN 55455-0385, USA

2.64 C. A. Clarke (2001) Changing incidence of KS and NHL among young men in San Francisco, *AIDS*, 15(14): 1913-1914, copyright Lippincott Williams & Wilkins

2.65 E.J. Stanbridge and W. K. Cavanee, Tumor Suppressor Genes, in, R. Weinberg, ed (1989) *Oncogenes and the Molecular Origins of Cancer*, Cold Spring Harbor Laboratory Press

2.66 & 2.67 Wellcome Trust Medical Photographic Library, UK.

2.68 C. Bonnardel, IARC

2.69 IARCPress

2.70 Wellcome Trust Medical Photographic Library, UK

2.71 Reprinted with permission from Elsevier Science. Collaborative Group on Hormonal Factors in Breast Cancer (1996) Breast cancer and hormonal contraceptives: collaborative reanalysis of individual data on 53 297 women with breast cancer and 100 239 women without breast cancer from 54 epidemiological studies, *Lancet*, 347, 1713-27

2.72 WHO/TDR Image Library/Crump

3.1 C. Harris, National Cancer Institute, NIH, Bethesda, MD 20892-4255, USA

3.2 E.R. Fearon and B. Vogelstein (1990) A genetic model for colorectal tumorigenesis, *Cell*, 61: 759-767

3.3 Reprinted from *Eur J Cancer*, Vol. 35(3), M. Ilyas, J. Straub, IP Tomlinson, W.F. Bodmer, Genetic pathways in colorectal and other cancers, 335-35, Copyright (1999), with permission from Elsevier Science

3.4 Y. Nakanuma, Second Department of Pathology, Kanazawa University School of Medicine, Takaramachi 13-1 920-8640

3.5 L.H. Sobin, USA

3.6 N.J. Carr, Department of Cellular Pathology, Southampton General Hospital, Tremona Road, Southampton SO16 6YD, UK

3.7 A. Barbin, IARC

3.8 B.W. Stewart, Australia

3.9 - 3.11 Reprinted with permission from *Nature*. J.H. Hoeijmakers (2001) Genome maintenance mechanisms for preventing cancer. *Nature* 411, 366-374, Copyright (2001) Macmillan Magazines Ltd.

3.12 J.R. Jass, Pathology Department, Grad. Med. School, University of Queensland, Herston Road, 4006 Brisbane, Queensland, Australia

3.13 Adapted from C.R. Boland, F.A. Sinicrope, D.E. Brenner, J.M. Carethers (2000) Colorectal cancer prevention and treatment. *Gastroenterology*, 118(2 Suppl 1): S115-28

3.14 J. Hall, IARC

3.15 P. Hainaut, IARC

3.16 B. W. Stewart, Australia.

3.17 Courtesy of J. Couturier, Unité de Cytogénétique, Institut Curie, 26, rue d'Ulm, 5248 Paris, France

3.18 Adapted from P.H. Rabbitts, Tumour suppressor genes, in J. Kendrew and E. Lawrence, eds (1994) *The Encyclopaedia of Molecular Biology*, Blackwell Science

3.19 P. Hainaut, IARC

3.20 Loréal Recherche, Centre Charles Zviak, 92583 Clichy, France

3.21 P. Hainaut, IARC

3.22 P. Hainaut, IARC/RasMol software, version 2.6; coordinate file for p53:DNA crystal data 1TUP in the Protein Brookhaven Database. Data from Y. Cho, S. Gorina, P.D. Jeffrey, N.P. Pavletich. Crystal structure of a p53 tumor suppressor-DNA complex: understanding tumorigenic mutations (1994) Science, 265(5170): 346-355

3.23 P. Hainaut, IARC

3.24 P. Hainaut, IARC/IARC TP53 gene mutation database, R6, 2002

3.25 C.A. Rubio, Gastrointestinal and Liver Pathology, Department of Pathology, Karolinska Institute, 171 76 Stockholm, Sweden

3.26 S. Zeitlin and K. Sullivan, Department of Cell Biology, The Scripps Research Institute 10550 N. Torrey Pines Road, La Jolla, CA 92037, USA

3.27 & 3.28 P Hainaut, IARC

3.29 J.W. Shay, W.E.Wright, University of Texas Southwestern Medical Center, Department of Cell Biology Room K2-206 5323 Harry Hines Boulevard, Dallas, TX 75390-9039, USA. The centromere and telomere probes were provided by S. Gryaznov at the Geron Corporation, Menlo Park, CA, and the digital image was taken by Y. Zou

3.30 & 3.31 H. Yamasaki, Japan

3.32 M. Mesnil and H. Yamasaki (2000) Bystander effect in herpes simplex virus-thymidine kinase/ganciclovir cancer gene therapy: role of gap junctional intercellular communication. *Cancer Res*, 60: 3989-3999

3.33 J. F.R. Kerr and B.V. Harmon (1991) Definition and incidence of apoptosis, in *Apoptosis: the Molecular Basis of Cell Death*, eds L.D. Tomei and F.O. Cope. Cold Spring Harbour Laboratory Press, 5-29

3.34 Reprinted with permission from *Nature*. B.B. Zhou, S.J. Elledge (2000) The DNA damage response: putting checkpoints in perspective. *Nature*, 408: 433-439, Copyright (2000) Macmillan Magazines Ltd.

3.35 IARCPress

3.36 N.J. Carr, Department of Cellular Pathology, Southampton General Hospital, Tremona Road. Southampton SO16 6YD, UK

3.37 Reprinted with permission from *Nature*, M.O. Hengartner (2000) The biochemistry of apoptosis, *Nature*, 407, 770-6. Copyright (2000) Macmillan Magazines Ltd.

3.38 J.C. Bourdon, Department of Surgery and Molecular Oncology, Ninewells Hospital, University of Dundee, Scotland, UK

3.39 Adapted from A.A. Adjei, USA

3.40 Reprinted from *Eur J Cancer*, Vol. 36, Beavon I, The E-cadherin complex in tumour metastasis: structure , function, regulation, 1607-1620. Copyright (2000), with permission from Elsevier Science

3.41 Reprinted from *Eur J Cancer*, Vol. 36, J.A. Wyke, Overview-burgeoning promise in metastasis research, 1589-1594. Copyright 2000, with permission from Elsevier Science

3.42 C. Fenoglio-Preiser, Department of Pathology, University of Cincinnati, School of Medicine, 231 Bethesda Avenue, POB 670529, Cincinnati, OH 45267-0529, USA

3.43 R.C. Janzer, Division of Neuropathology, University Institute of Pathology, 27 rue du Bugnon, CH 1011 Lausanne, Switzerland

3.44 R.D. Rubens, Clinical Oncology Unit, Guys Hospital, London SE1 9RT, UK

3.45 S. Eccles, UK

4.1 Reprinted from R. Doll, R. Peto, K. Wheatley, R. Gray, I. Sutherland (1994) Mortality in relation to smoking: 40 years' observations on male British doctors. *BMJ*, 309(6959): 901-911, with permission from the *BMJ* Publishing Group

4.2 Adapted from F. Faggiano, T. Partanen, M. Kogevinas, P. Boffetta (1997) *Socioeconomic differences in cancer incidence and mortality (IARC Scientific Publication 138)*, 65-176.

4.3 R. Peto, S. Darby, H. Deo, P. Silcocks, E. Whitley et al. (2000) Smoking, smoking cessation, and lung cancer in the UK since 1950: combination of national statistics with two case-control studies. *BMJ*, 321(7257): 323-329.with permission from the *BMJ* Publishing Group

4.4 T. Lancaster, L. Stead, C. Silagy, A. Sowden (2000) Effectiveness of interventions to help people stop smoking: findings from the Cochrane Library. *BMJ*, 321(7257): 355-358, with permission from the *BMJ* Publishing Group. Original data from Silagy et al. (2000) *Nicotine replacement therapy for smoking cessation*, Cochrane Library, Issue 3, Oxford: Update Software

4.5 R. Peto, Z.M. Chen, J. Boreham (1999) Tobacco the growing epidemic. *Nat Med 5* (1);15-17 and B.Q. Liu, R. Peto, Z.M. Chen, J. Boreham, Y.P. Wu et al. (1998) Emerging tobacco hazards in China: 1. Retrospective proportional mortality study of one million deaths. *BMJ*, 317(7170):1411-22

4.6 "La verité si j'fume" courtesy of la Fédération Nationale des Centres de Lutte Contre le Cancer and Aventis Pharma SA; "Il suffit de dire NON", courtesy of the Association Tunisienne de Lutte Contre le Cancer; "Quanto ti costa fumare?", Istituto Nazionale per la Ricerca sul Cancro, Genoa, Italy; "Merci de ne pas fumer" & "Animals Smoking", copyright of Comité National Contre le Tabagisme, 31, avenue Michel Bizot, 75012 Paris, France, www.cnct.org; "NO smoking", courtesy of the Japan Public Health Association

4.7 Centers for Disease Control and Prevention (2000) *Mortality and Morbidity Weekly Report*, 49:1066-1069, http://www.cdc.gov/mmwr

4.8 Graphics and Audiovisual section, NCI Office of Cancer Communications, USA

4.9 P. Boffetta, IARC/Adapted from K. Magnus, A. Andersen, A.C. Hogetveit (1982) Cancer of respiratory organs among workers at a nickel refinery in Norway. *Int J Cancer*, 30(6): 681-685

4.10 Reprinted with permission from Elsevier Science, J. Peto, J.T. Hodgson, F.E. Matthews, J.R. Jones (1995) Continuing increase in mesothelioma mortality in Britain. *Lancet*, 345(8949): 535-539

4.11 Anti-Cancer Council of Victoria, Australia/IARCPress

4.12 Graphics and Audiovisual section, NCI Office of Cancer Communications, USA

4.13 The Cancer Council New South Wales and the NSW Health Department, Australia

4.14 GLOBOCAN 2000*

4.15 & 4.16 WHO (2000) Vaccines, Immunization and Biologicals, 1997 data http://www.who.int/vaccinessurveillance/graphics/htmls/hepbprev.htm and http://www.who.int/vaccinessurveillance/graphics/htmls/hepb.htm

4.17 J.Y. Scoazec, France

4.18 G. Kirk, USA/Adapted from P. Pisani, D.M. Parkin, N. Muñoz, J. Ferlay (1997) Cancer and infection: estimates of the attributable fraction in 1990. *Cancer Epidemiol Biomarkers Prev*, 6(6): 387-400

4.19 G.Kirk, USA.

4.20 IARCPress

4.21 W.J. Edmunds, G.F. Medley, D.J. Nokes, A.J. Hall and H.C. Whittle (1993) The influence of age on the development of the hepatitis B carrier state. *Proc R Soc Lond B*, 253, 197-201. With permission from The Royal Society.

4.22 - 4.24 IARCPress

4.25 Graphics and Audiovisual section, NCI Office of Cancer Communications, USA

4.26 C.R. Boland, F.A. Sinicrope, D.E. Brenner, J.M. Carethers (2000) Colorectal cancer prevention and treatment.

Gastroenterology, 118(2 Suppl 1): S115-28, with the permission of W.B. Saunders Company

4.27 IARCPress

4.28 B. Marincek, Institut für Diagnostische Radiologie, UniversitätsSpital, Ramistrasse 100, CH-8091 Zürich, Switzerland

4.29 R. Sankaranarayanan, IARC

4.30 Copyright GE Medical Systems

4.31 P. Pisani, IARC

4.32 D.M. Parkin et al. (2001) Eur J Cancer, 37, suppl.8: S4-66

4.33 A. M. Thompson, UK

4.34 Wellcome Trust Medical Photographic Library, UK

4.35 Graphics and Audiovisual section, NCI Office of Cancer Communications, USA

4.36 Reprinted from *Radiol Clin North Am, 38,* L. Tabar, B. Vitak, H.H. Chen, S.W. Duffy, M.F. Yen et al., The Swedish Two-County Trial twenty years later. Updated mortality results and new insights from long-term follow-up, 625-651, copyright (2000), with permission from Elsevier Science

4.37 Wellcome Trust Medical Photographic Library, UK

4.38 D.M. Parkin et al. (2001) Eur J Cancer, 37, suppl.8: S4-66

4.39 R. LiPuma, Prostate Cancer Education Council, 300 South Jackson Street, Suite 540 Denver, CO 80209, USA.

4.40 C.A. Rubio, Gastrointestinal and Liver Pathology, Department of Pathology, Karolinska Institute, 171 76 Stockholm, Sweden

4.41 D.M. Parkin et al. (2001) Eur J Cancer, 37, suppl.8: S4-66

4.42 Prévention et Biologie, SA, 29-33 Rue de Metz, 94170 Le Perreux, France

4.43 D.M. Parkin et al. (2001) Eur J Cancer, 37, suppl.8: S4-66

4.44 IARCPress

4.45 D.M. Parkin et al. (2001) Eur J Cancer, 37, suppl.8: S4-66

4.46 Adapted from M.R. Law, J.K. Morris, N.J. Wald (1999) The importance of age in screening for cancer. *J Med Screen*, 6(1): 16-20, with permission from the *BMJ* Publishing Group

4.47 R. Sankaranarayanan, IARC

4.48 IARCPress

4.49 - 4.52 R. Sankaranarayanan, IARC

4.53 A & B H. Ohgaki, IARC

4.53C R. Lambert, IARC

4.54 D.M. Parkin et al. (2001) Eur J Cancer, 37, suppl.8: S4-66

4.55 Adapted from Table 2, Y. Tsubono and S. Hisamichi (2000) Screening for gastric cancer in Japan. *Gastric cancer*, 3: 9-18. Copyright Springer-Verlag

5.1 GLOBOCAN 2000*

5.2 Graphics and Audiovisual section, NCI Office of Cancer Communications, USA

5.3 B.W. Stewart, Australia

5.4 D.M. Parkin et al. (2001) Eur J Cancer, 37, suppl.8: S4-66

5.5 J.A. Baron and T.E. Rohan, Tobacco, in D. Schottenfeld and J.F. Fraumeni Jr. eds (1996) *Cancer Epidemiology and Prevention, 2nd edition*, Oxford University Press, UK

5.6 P. Boffetta, IARC/Adapted from J.H. Lubin, W.J. Blot (1984) Assessment of lung cancer risk factors by histo-logic category. *J Natl Cancer Inst*, 73: 383-389

5.7 B. Marincek, Institut für Diagnostische Radiologie, UniversitätsSpital, Ramistrasse 100, CH-8091 Zurich, Switzerland

5.8 F. Berger and J.Y. Scoazec, Laboratoire d'Anatomo-Pathologie, Hôpital Edouard Herriot, Place d'Arsonval, 69437 Lyon France

5.9 P. Boffetta, IARC

5.10 IARC/SEER/Osaka Cancer Registry†

5.11 IARCPress/Department of Pathology, University of Zurich, Switzerland

5.12 GLOBOCAN 2000*

5.13 Wellcome Trust Medical Photographic Library, UK

5.14 Von Kantor & Associates Inc., Ft. Lauderdale FL, USA/www.lectureslides.com

5.15 A. M. Thompson, UK

5.16 & 5.17 F. Berger and J.Y. Scoazec, Laboratoire d'Anatomo-Pathologie, Hôpital Edouard Herriot, Place d'Arsonval, 69437 Lyon France

5.18 P. Kleihues, IARC

5.19 D.M. Parkin et al. (2001) Eur J Cancer, 37, suppl.8: S4-66

5.20 Von Kantor & Associates Inc., Ft. Lauderdale FL, USA/www.lectureslides.com

5.21 IARC/SEER/Osaka Cancer Registry†

5.22 IARCPress

5.23 GLOBOCAN 2000*

5.24 D.M. Parkin et al. (2001) Eur J Cancer, 37, suppl.8: S4-66

5.25 N. Matsukura, Japan

5.26 H. Ohgaki, IARC

5.27 F. Berger and J.Y. Scoazec, Laboratoire d'Anatomo-Pathologie, Hôpital Edouard Herriot, Place d'Arsonval, 69437 Lyon France

5.28 IARC/SEER/Osaka Cancer Registry†

5.29 GLOBOCAN 2000*

5.30 IARCPress

5.31 Reprinted from European Journal of Cancer, Vol 35, No 3, Ilyas M, Straub J, Tomlinson IPM, Bodmer W, Genetic pathways in colorectal and other cancers, 335-351, copyright (1999), with permission from Elsevier Science

5.32 - 5.34 F. Berger and J.Y. Scoazec, Laboratoire d'Anatomo-Pathologie, Hôpital Edouard Herriot, Place d'Arsonval, 69437 Lyon France

5. 35 C. Fenoglio-Preiser, Department of Pathology, University of Cincinnati, School of Medicine, 231 Bethesda Avenue, POB 670529, Cincinnati, OH 45267-0529, USA

5.36 IARC/SEER/Osaka Cancer Registry†

5.37 & 5.38 GLOBOCAN 2000*

5.39 IARCPress

5.40 B. Marincek, Institut für Diagnostische Radiologie, UniversitätsSpital, Ramistrasse 100, CH-8091 Zurich, Switzerland

5.41 - 5.43 F. Berger and J.Y. Scoazec, Laboratoire d'Anatomo-Pathologie, Hôpital Herriot, place d'arsonval, 69437 Lyon

5.44 IARC/SEER/Osaka Cancer Registry†

5.45 GLOBOCAN 2000*

5.46 D.M. Parkin et al. (2001) Eur J Cancer, 37, suppl.8: S4-66

5.47 L. Denis, Belgium, and K. Griffiths, UK

5.48 & 5.49 F. Berger and J.Y. Scoazec, Laboratoire d'Anatomo-Pathologie, Hôpital Edouard Herriot, place d'Arsonval, 69437 Lyon France

5.50 Adapted from Figure 4C. Abate-Shen, M.M. Shen (2000) Molecular genetics of prostate cancer. *Genes Dev*, 14(19): 2410-2434

5. 51 GLOBOCAN 2000*

5.52 P. Kleihues, IARC

5.53 M.K. Rosenblum, Department of Pathology, Memorial Sloan Kettering Cancer Center, 1275 York Avenue, New York NY 10021, USA

5.54 F. Berger and J.Y. Scoazec, Laboratoire d'Anatomo-Pathologie, Hôpital Edouard Herriot, place d'Arsonval, 69437 Lyon France

5.55 Adapted from Figure 6, R.S. Chaganti, J. Houldsworth (2000) Genetics and biology of adult human male germ cell tumors. *Cancer Res*, 60(6): 1475-1482

5.56 IARC/SEER/Osaka Cancer Registry†

5.57 GLOBOCAN 2000*

5.58 WHO/TDR Image Library/Crump

5.59 & 5.60 R. Sankaranarayanan, IARC

5.61 F. Berger and J.Y. Scoazec, Laboratoire d'Anatomo-Pathologie, Hôpital Edouard Herriot, Place d'Arsonval, 69437 Lyon France

5.62 IARC/SEER/Osaka Cancer Registry†

5.63 GLOBOCAN 2000*

5.64 F. Berger and J.Y. Scoazec, Laboratoire d'Anatomo-Pathologie, Hôpital Edouard Herriot, Place d'Arsonval, 69437 Lyon France

5.65 IARC/SEER/Osaka Cancer Registry

5.66 M. Esteller, J. Xercavins, J. Reventos (1999) Advances in the molecular genetics of endometrial cancer. *Oncology Reports* 6 (6): 1377-1382

5.67 GLOBOCAN 2000*

5.68 B. Marincek, Institut für Diagnostische Radiologie, UniversitätsSpital, Ramistrasse 100, CH-8091 Zurich, Switzerland

5.69 Wellcome Trust Medical Photographic Library, UK

5.70 F. Berger and J.Y. Scoazec, Laboratoire d'Anatomo-Pathologie, Hôpital Edouard Herriot, Place d'Arsonval, 69437 Lyon France

5.71 IARC/SEER/Osaka Cancer Registry†

5.72 GLOBOCAN 2000*

5.73 & 5.74 IARC Press

5.75 D.M. Parkin et al. (2001) Eur J Cancer, 37, suppl.8: S4-66

5.76 A.M. Thompson, UK

5.77 F. Berger and J.Y. Scoazec, Laboratoire d'Anatomo-Pathologie, Hôpital Edouard Herriot, Place d'Arsonval, 69437 Lyon France

5.78 C. Fenoglio-Preiser, Department of Pathology, University of Cincinnati, School of Medicine, 231 Bethesda Avenue, POB 670529, Cincinnati, OH 45267-0529, USA

5.79 M. Werner, Institute of Pathology, Technische Universität München, Ismaninger Strasse 22, D-81675 Munich, Germany

5.80 IARC/SEER/Osaka Cancer Registry†

5.81 GLOBOCAN 2000*

5.82 P. Brennan, IARC/ Adapted from P. Brennan, O. Bogillot, S. Cordier et al. (2000) Cigarette smoking and bladder cancer in men: a pooled analysis of 11 case-control studies. *Int J Cancer*, 86(2): 289-294

5.83 WHO/ TDR Image Library/ Manderson

5.84 & 5.85 F. Berger and J.Y. Scoazec, Laboratoire d'Anatomo-Pathologie, Hôpital Edouard Herriot, Place d'Arsonval, 69437 Lyon France

5.86 Reprinted from *Urologic Clinics of North America*, 27(1), R. Lee and M.J. Droller, The natural history of bladder cancer, 1-13, copyright (2000), with permission from Elsevier Science

5.87 IARC/SEER/Osaka Cancer Registry†

5.88 - 5.90 GLOBOCAN 2000*

5.91 - 5.93 R. Sankaranarayanan, IARC

5.94 F. Berger and J.Y. Scoazec, Laboratoire d'Anatomo-Pathologie, Hôpital Edouard Herriot, Place d'Arsonval, 69437 Lyon France

5.95 IARC/SEER/Osaka Cancer Registry†

5.96 D. Sidransky (1997) Tumor suppressor genes, in V.T. DeVita Jr., et al., eds, *Cancer: Principles and Practice of Oncology, 5th edition*, Lippincott-Raven, p 737

5.97 GLOBOCAN 2000*

5.98 Wellcome Trust Medical Photographic Library, UK

5.99 L.A.G. Ries, M.P. Eisner, C.L. Kosary, B.F. Hankey, B.A. Miller, L. Clegg, B.K. Edwards eds (2001) *SEER Cancer Statistics Review, 1973-1998*, National Cancer Institute, Bethesda, MD

5.100 GLOBOCAN 2000*

5.101 E.S. Jaffe, Laboratory of Pathology, NIH, Building 10, Room 2N-202, 10 Center Drive MSC-1500, Bethesda, MD 20892-1500, USA

5.102 F. Berger and J.Y. Scoazec, Laboratoire d'Anatomo-Pathologie, Hôpital Edouard Herriot, Place d'Arsonval, 69437 Lyon France

5.103 H. Stein, Institut für Pathologie, Freie Universität Berlin, Universitätsklinikum Steglitz, Hindenburgdamm 30, D 12200 Berlin, Germany

5.104 E.S. Jaffe, Laboratory of Pathology, NIH, building 10, Room 2N-202, 10 Center Drive MSC-1500, Bethesda, MD 20892-1500, USA

5.105 Reprinted by permission from A.A. Alizadeh, M.B. Eisen, R.E. Davis, C. Ma, I.S. Lossos et al. (2000) Distinct types of diffuse large B-cell lymphoma identified by gene expression profiling. *Nature*, 403(6769): 503-511. Copyright 2000, Macmillan Magazines Ltd.

5.106 & 5.107 IARC/SEER/Osaka Cancer Registry†

5.108 GLOBOCAN 2000*

5.109 Los Alamos National Laboratory/SPL/Cosmos

5.110 L.A.G. Ries, M.P. Eisner, C.L. Kosary, B.F. Hankey, B.A. Miller et al., eds (2001) *SEER Cancer Statistics Review, 1973-1998*, National Cancer Institute, Bethesda MD, USA

5.111 A & B R.D. Brunning, Department of Laboratory Medicine and Pathology, University of Minnesota Hospital, 420 Delaware Street S.E., Box 609, Minneapolis, MN 55455-0385, USA

5.112 Adapted from a figure by J. Melo, Department of Haematology, ISCM, Hammersmith Hospital, Ducane Road, London W12 ONN, UK

5.113 A & B G. Flandrin, Laboratoire Central de Hématologie, Hôpital Necker, 149 rue de Sèvres, F-75743 Paris, France

5.114 R.D. Brunning, Department of Laboratory Medicine and Pathology, University of Minnesota Hospital, 420 Delaware Street S.E., Box 609, Minneapolis, MN 55455-0385, USA

5.115 With permission of J.A. Squire, from V.D. Markovic, D. Bouman, J. Bayani, J. Al-Maghrabi, S. Kamel-Reid et al. (2000) Lack of BCR/ABL reciprocal fusion in variant Philadelphia chromosome translocations: a use of double fusion signal FISH and spectral karyotyping. *Leukemia*, 14(6):1157-1160

5.116 B. Hirsch, Department of Laboratory Medicine and Pathology, University of Minnesota School of Medicine, 420 Delaware St. SE, Minneapolis, MN 55455, USA

5.117 J.W. Vardiman, Department of Pathology, University of Chicago Medical Center, 5841 South Maryland Ave., MC0008 Romm TW-055, Chicago, IL 60637-1470, USA

5.118 IARC/SEER/Osaka Cancer Registry†

5.119 & 5.120 GLOBOCAN 2000*

5.121 Graphics and Audiovisual section, NCI Office of Cancer Communications, USA

5.122 G. Zamboni, Dept of Pathology, University of Verona, Strada Le Grazie, I-37134 Verona, Italy

5.123 G. Klöppel, Institute of Pathology, University of Kiel, Michaelistrasse 11, D-24105 Kiel, Germany

5.124 P. Vogt, Department of Pathology, University Hospital USZ, Schmelzbergstrasse 12, CH-8091 Zurich, Switzerland

5.125 F. Berger and J.Y. Scoazec, Laboratoire d'Anatomo-Pathologie, Hôpital Edouard Herriot, Place d'Arsonval, 69437 Lyon France

5.126 IARC/SEER/Osaka Cancer Registry†

5.127 GLOBOCAN 2000*

5.128 Data from New South Wales Central Cancer Registry†, Australia

5.129 B.W. Stewart, Australia

5.130 - 5.134 W. McCarthy, Australia

5.135 GLOBOCAN 2000*

5.136 International Atomic Energy Agency, Vienna

5.137 GLOBOCAN 2000*

5.138 International Atomic Energy Agency, Vienna

5.139 F. Berger and J.Y. Scoazec, Laboratoire d'Anatomo-Pathologie, Hôpital Edouard Herriot, Place d'Arsonval, 69437 Lyon France

5.140 Adapted from Figure 2, D.L. Learoyd , M. Messina, J. Zedenius, B.G. Robinson (2000) Molecular genetics of thyroid tumours and surgical decision making. *World J Surg*, 24, 923-933

5.141 IARC/SEER/Osaka Cancer Registry†

5.142 & 5.143 GLOBOCAN 2000*

5.144 Wellcome Trust Medical Photographic Library, UK

5.145 B. Marincek, Institut für Diagnostische Radiologie, UniversitätsSpital, Ramistrasse 100, CH-8091 Zurich, Switzerland

5.146 Public Health Image Library, CDC, USA/Dr Edwin P. Ewing, Jr.

5.147 F. Berger and J.Y. Scoazec, Laboratoire d'Anatomo-Pathologie, Hôpital Edouard Herriot, Place d'Arsonval, 69437 Lyon France

5.148 IARC/SEER/Osaka Cancer Registry†

5.149 J. Ferlay, F.I. Bray, R. Sankila, D.M. Parkin eds (1999) *EUCAN90: Cancer Incidence Mortality and Prevalence in the European Union (IARC Cancer Bases No. 4)*, Lyon, IARCPress

5.150 P. Kleihues, IARC

5.151 P.C. Burger, Pathology Building, Room 706, The Johns Hopkins Hospital, 600 Wolfe Street, Baltimore, MD 21287, USA

5.152 H. Ohgaki, IARC

5.153 P. Kleihues, IARC

5.154 A. Vital, Laboratory of Neuropathology, Victor Segalen University, Bordeaux 2, 146, rue Leo-Saignat, 33076 Bordeaux, France

6.1 Wellcome Trust Medical Photographic Library, UK

6.2 - 6.5 G. Maddern, Australia

6.6 Varian Medical Systems, Palo Alto, USA

6.7-6.8 Varian Medical Systems UK Ltd.

6.9 & 6.10 Graphics and Audiovisual section, NCI Office of Cancer Communications, USA

6.11 K. Sikora, UK

6.12 Modified from C.M. Haskell, ed (1995) *Cancer Treatment, 4th Edition*, W.B. Saunders/Reprinted from W.E. Ross et al., *Pharmacology and Therapeutics*, copyright 1987, Vol. 32, p. 89, with permission from Elsevier Science

6.13 H. Stein, Institut für Pathologie, Freie Universität Berlin, Universitätsklinikum Steglitz, Hindenburgdamm 30, D-12200 Berlin, Germany

6.14 K. Sikora, UK

6.15 A. Villunger and A. Strasser (1999) The great escape: is immune evasion required for tumor progression? *Nat Med*, 5(8): 874-5

6.16 P. Hersey, Australia

6.17 K.R. Dumon, H. Ishii, L.Y. Fong, N. Zanesi, V. Fidanza et al., (2001) FHIT gene therapy prevents tumor development in Fhit-deficient mice. *Proc Natl Acad Sci USA* , 98: 3346-3351. Copyright (2001) National Academy of Sciences, USA

6.18 Von Kantor and Associates Inc., Fort. Lauderdale FL, USA/www.lectureslides.com

6.19 A. M. Thompson, UK

6.20 Courtesy of the Palliative Care Council of South Australia

6.21 Adapted from WHO (1996) Cancer Pain Relief, 2nd edition, Geneva, World Health Organization/data for 1999 from David E. Joranson, Pain & Policy Studies Group, WHO Collaborating Center for Policy and Communications and the International Narcotics Control Board, United Nations Demographic Yearbook, 1999.

6.22 Data from David E. Joranson, Pain & Policy Studies Group, WHO Collaborating Center for Policy and Communications

6.23 B. Cassileth, USA

7. 1 & 7.2 IARCPress

7.3 C. Sepulvéda, WHO

7.4 International Union Against Cancer (UICC), 3, rue du Conseil-Général, CH-1205 Geneva, Switzerland

7.5 Tobacco Free Initiative (TFI), World Health Organization, Avenue Appia 20 1211, Geneva 27 Switzerland

7.6 M. Imperi (2000) *BMJ*, 321, cover photo, with permission from the *BMJ* Publishing Group.

7.7 E. Lucas, IARC

7.8 WHO/TDR Image Library/Haaland

7.9 R. Sankaranarayanan, IARC

7.10 G. Mollon, IARC

7.11 - 7.13 E. Lucas, IARC

7.14 WHO (1998) *The World Health Report 1998. Life in the 21st Century: A Vision for All*. Geneva, World Health Organization, p39

7.15 & 7.16 WHO/HPR/TDR Image Library/Crump

7.17 WHO (1998) *The World Health Report 1998. Life in the 21st Century: A Vision for All*. Geneva, World Health Organization, p44

7.18 Wellcome Trust Medical Photographic Library, UK

Tables

2.1 & 2.2 Reprinted from *Eur J Cancer Prev*, Vol. 8, M. Pandey, A. Mathew, M.K. Nair. Global perspective of tobacco habits and lung cancer: a lesson for third world countries, 271-9, Copyright 1999, with permission from Elsevier Science

2.3 Adapted from N.J. Wald and A.K. Hackshaw (1996) *Br Med Bulletin*, 52 (1): 3-11 (and from the American Cancer Study (CPSII)), by permission of Oxford University Press

2.4 H. Boeing, Alcohol and risk of cancer of the upper gastrointestinal tract: first analysis of the EPIC data. In: E. Riboli and R. Lambert eds (2002) *Nutrition and Lifestyle: Opportunities for Cancer Prevention (IARC Scientific Publications No. 156)*. Lyon, IARCPress

2.5 & 2.6 P. Boffetta, IARC

2.7 - 2.10 J. Rice, IARC/*IARC Monographs* Programme

2.11 P. Boffetta, IARC

2.12 P. Boffetta, IARC/WHO European Centre for Environment and Health, 1995

2.13 - 2.15 J. Rice, IARC/*IARC Monographs* Programme

2.16 IARCPress/UNSCEAR, 1994

2.17 E. Cardis, IARC

2.18 S. Franceschi, IARC

2.19 J. Rice, IARC/*IARC Monographs* Programme

2.20 & 2.21 D. Goldgar, IARC

2.22 S. Franceschi, F. Parazzini, E. Negri, M. Booth, C. La Vecchia, V. Beral, A. Tzonou and D. Trichopoulos (1991) Pooled analysis of 3 European case-control studies of epithelial ovarian cancer III. Oral contraceptive use. Int J. Cancer, 49: 61-65

3.1 Adapted from H. Marquardt, Chemical carcinogenesis, in H. Marquardt, S.G. Schafer, R. McClellan and F. Welsch, eds (1999). *Toxicology*, Academic Press, San Diego, 151-178

3.2 & 3.3 P. Hainaut, IARC

3.4 H. Yamasaki, Y. Omori, M.L. Zaidan-Dagli, N. Mironov, M. Mesnil et al. (1999) Genetic and epigenetic changes of intercellular communication genes during multistage carcinogenesis, *Cancer Detect and Prev*, 23: 273-279

3.5 & 3.6 S. Eccles, UK

3.7 Reprinted by permission from *Nature*, L.A. Liotta, E.C. Kohn (2001) The microenvironment of the tumour-host interface, *Nature*, 411: 375-379, copyright 2001, Macmillan Magazines Ltd.

3.8 A. Sasco, IARC

4.1 & 4.2 C.J.L. Murray, A.D. Lopez, Assessing the burden of disease that can be attributed to specific risk factors. In *Ad Hoc Committee on Health Research Relating to Future Intervention Options. Investing in Health Research and Development*. World Health Organization, Geneva, 1996

4.3 A. Sasco, IARC

4.4 IARC (1999) *Re-evaluation of some Organic Chemicals, Hydrazine and Hydrogen Peroxide (IARC Monographes Vol. 71)*, Lyon, IARCPress

4.5 USA EPA (2000) *Latest Findings on National Air Quality: 1999 Status and Trends*, US Environmental Protection Agency

4.6 WHO (1999) *Air Quality Guidelines*, Geneva, WHO

4.7 S. Yamamura (2001) Drinking water guidelines and standards, in *United Nations synthesis report on arsenic in drinking water*, United Nations (draft), http://www.who.int/water_sanitation_health/Arsenic/ArsenicUNReptoc.htm

4.8 B.W. Stewart, Australia

4.9 Adapted from Table 1, Prophylactic vaccines under development, in A. Kols and J. Sherris (2000) *HPV Vaccines: Promise and Challenges*. Alliance for Cervical Cancer Prevention, PATH

4.10 & 4.11 S. Franceschi and N. Muñoz, IARC

4.12 H. Vainio, IARC

4.13 & 4.14 L. Denis, Belgium

4.15 & 4.16 R. Lambert, IARC

4.17 R. Lambert, IARC/Adapted from J.S. Mandel, J.H. Bond, T.R. Church, D.C. Snover, G.M. Bradley et al. (1993) Reducing mortality from colorectal cancer by screening for fecal occult blood. Minnesota Colon Cancer Control Study. *N Engl J Med*, 328:1365-1371

4.18 IARC Working Group on Cervical Cancer Screening (1986) Summary chapter, *Screening for Cancer of the Uterine Cervix. (IARC Scientific Publication No. 76)*, Lyon, IARCPress

4.19 R. Sankaranarayanan, IARC

5.1 P. Boffetta, IARC

5.2 A. Sasco, IARC/Data from Table 36.2-23, Cancer of the Breast, in V.T. DeVita Jr. et al., eds (1997) *Cancer: Principles and Practice of Oncology, 5th Edition*, Lippincott-Raven

5.3 H. Ohgaki, IARC

5.4 L. Raymond, J. Young M. Parkin S. Whelan and J. Ferlay , (1997) *Cancer Incidence in Five Continents, Vol. VII*, IARCPress

5.5 L.A.G. Ries, M.P. Eisner, C.L. Kosary, B.F. Hankey, B.A. Miller et al., eds (2001) *SEER Cancer Statistics Review, 1973-1998*, National Cancer Institute, Bethesda MD, USA

5.6 & 5.7 P. Hainaut, IARC

5.8 L. Denis, Belgium

5.9 T. Shimoda, Department of Clinical Laboratory, National Cancer Center Hospital, 5-1-1 Tsukiji Chuo Ku, 104-0045 Tokyo, Japan

5.10 Adapted from Anon. (1997) A clinical evaluation of the International Lymphoma Study Group classification of non-Hodgkin's lymphoma. The Non-Hodgkin's Lymphoma Classification Project. *Blood*, 89: 3909-3918

5.11 G. Young, Australia

5.12 & 5.13 G. Klöppel, Institute of Pathology, University of Kiel, Michaelistrasse 11, D-24105 Kiel, Germany

5.14 W. McCarthy, Australia

5.15 Data from E. van den Berg, T. Dijkhuizen (1999) Classification of renal cell cancer based on (cyto)genetic analysis. *Contrib Nephrol*, 128: 51-61; A. Bernheim, A. Vagner-Capodano, J.Couturier, et le Groupe Français de Cytogénétique Oncologique (2000) De la cytogénétique à la cytogénomie oncologique. *Médecine/Sciences*, 16: 528-539

5.16 & 5.17 P. Kleihues, IARC

6.1 Table 15-12, p301, S. Rosenberg, Principles of cancer management: surgical oncology, in V.T. DeVita Jr., S. Hellman, S.A. Rosenberg, eds (1997) *Cancer: Principles and Practice of Oncology, 5th edition*, copyright Lippincott, Williams & Wilkins

6.2 G.H. Sakorafas (2001) Breast cancer surgery—historical evolution, current status and future perspectives. *Acta Oncol*, 40(1): 5-18

6.3 A.J.A. Bremers, E.J.Th. Rutgers, C.J.H. van de Velde (1999) Cancer surgery: the last 25 years. Cancer Treat Rev, 25: 333-353

6.4 - 6.8 K. Sikora, UK

6.9 P. Hersey, Australia

6.10 Adapted from S.J. Clarke, Drug resistance, in J.F. Bishop, ed (1999) *Cancer Facts. A Concise Oncology Text*, Australia, Harwood Academic Publishers, 67-71

6.11 K. Shin, USA

6.12 J.A. DeLisa, *Cancer*, Vol. 92, No. 4 Suppl., 2001, pp. 970-974. Copyright (2001) American Cancer Society. Reprinted by permission of Wiley-Liss, Inc., a subsidiary of John Wiley & Sons, Inc.

6.13 & 6.14 K. Shin, USA

7.1 & 7.2 R. Sankaranarayanan, IARC

Note:
* GLOBOCAN 2000 J. Ferlay, F.I. Bray, D.M. Parkin, P. Pisani (2001) *Globocan 2000: Cancer Incidence and Mortality Worldwide (IARC Cancer Bases No. 5)*, Lyon, IARCPress.
† IARC/SEER/Osaka Cancer Registry.
R. Sankaranarayanan, R.J. Black and D.M. Parkin (1998) *Cancer survival in developing countries (IARC publication No. 145)*, Lyon, IARCPress;
F. Berrino, R. Capocaccia, J. Esteve, F. Berrino, J. Capocaccia et al. (1999) *Survival of cancer patients in Europe: the EUROCARE-2 study (IARC Publication No. 151)*, Lyon, IARCPress;
L.A.G. Ries, M.P. Eisner, C.L. Kosary, B.F. Hankey, B.A. Miller et al., eds (2001) *SEER Cancer Statistics Review, 1973-1998*, National Cancer Institute. Bethesda, MD; http://seer.cancer.gov/csr/1973_1999/
Osaka Cancer Registry, Japan: data for 1992 used. http://www.mc.pref.osaka.jp/ocr_e/ocr/

SUBJECT INDEX

p27, 105, 106
p53 germline mutation, 190
p53 mutation, 44, 85, 105, 267
p53, 22, 27, 44, 54, 59, 72, 73, 91, 94, 98-105, 107, 114, 115, 120, 164, 185, 186, 191, 196, 199, 201, 204, 206, 210, 217, 219, 225, 226, 230, 248, 250, 255, 263, 265, 268, 315
Paclitaxel, see taxanes
Palliative care, 297, 308, 323
Pancreatic cancer, 13, 22, 24, 45, 72, 73, 120, 131, 248, 250, 251, 273, 281, 284
Papanicolaou smear, 88, 167, 216
Papillary thyroid carcinoma, 258
para-Chloro-ortho-toluidine, 35
Passive smoking, see environmental tobacco smoke
Patched, 54
PAX8, 259
Peau de chagrin, 268
Penicillium, 44
Peptic ulcer, 131
Perchloroethylene, 85
Peripheral vascular disease, 131
Peritoneum, 34, 124
Pesticides, 34, 35, 42, 43, 44, 45, 137, 140, 189, 238
Petroleum, 36, 40
Peutz-Jegher syndrome, 72, 199, 251
Peutz-Jeghers polyp, 86
P-glycoprotein, see MDR1
Phaeochromocytoma, 72, 268
Pharmaceutical industry, 286
Pharyngeal cancer, 24, 29, 30, 34, 57, 62, 65, 131, 154, 232
Phenacetin, 48, 49
Philadelphia chromosome, 244, 245
Phosphoinositide-3-kinase (PI3K), 117
Photofluoroscopy, 176, 195
Phyto-estrogens, 78, 209
Pilocytic astrocytoma, 266
Piroxicam, 152
Pituitary tumour, 85, 278
Platelet derived growth factor (PDGF), 117, 267
Platelet derived growth factor receptor (PDGFR), 123, 267
Platinum derivatives, 285
Platinum drugs, 49, 91, 186, 197, 206, 208, 212, 214, 219, 221, 222, 263, 282, 286
Pleura, 34, 37
PMS1, 73
PMS2, 73
Poly(ADP-ribose)polymerase (PARP), 93
Polychlorinated biphenyls, 35, 42, 45, 140, 228, 248
Polycyclic aromatic hydrocarbons, 25, 27, 33, 38, 45, 46, 63, 91, 138, 139, 228, 230
Polycystic kidney disease, 262
Polymerase chain reaction, 246
Polymorphisms, 31, 66, 80, 90, 111, 185, 209, 235, 324
Polynucleotide kinase (PNK), 93
Population ageing, 320
pRb, 105, 107
Prednisolone, 286, 287
Prednisone, 286

Premalignant lesions, 73, 84, 163, 170, 172, 175, 185, 199, 216, 224
Primary (de novo) glioblastoma, 267
Procarbazine, 48, 50, 241, 282, 283, 286
Progesterone receptors, 291
Progesterone, 85, 191
Prognostic factors, 123, 124, 282
Programmed cell death, see apoptosis 84
Promoter hypermethylation, 101, 105, 186, 250
Promutagenic DNA adducts, 89
Prophylactic vaccination, 144, 148
Prostaglandins, 151, 290
Prostate cancer screening, 160
Prostate cancer, 12, 35, 62, 73, 77, 85, 105, 111, 120, 121, 154, 160, 208, 221, 278, 281, 284, 286, 291, 324
Prostate-specific antigen, 160, 208
Prostatic intraepithelial neoplasia (PIN), 210
Proteases, 226
Protein kinase B (Akt, PKB), 117
Protein kinase C (PKC), 117
Proteolysis, 191
Proto-oncogene, 84
PTCH, 72, 266, 268
PTEN, 72, 120, 210, 219, 258, 266, 268
Pulmonary heart disease, 131
Pulmonary tuberculosis, 131
Pyridyloxobutylation adducts, 90
Pyrimidine dimer, 91
Pyrrolizidine alkaloids, 44

Q

Quitting, see smoking cessation

R

Rab11, 226
Radiation, 51-55, 141, 253
Radiotherapy, 277, 317
Radon, 36, 37, 52, 184
RAS, 91, 97, 102, 114, 117, 235, 259
RB1, 44, 72, 98, 99, 104, 105, 114, 210, 230, 267
Reactive oxygen species, 86
Recombination, 71
Recombinational repair, 91
Rehabilitation, 292
Renal cell carcinoma, 72, 261, 268
Renal pelvis cancer, 85
Replication error, 86
RET, 72, 259
Retinal haemangioblastomas, 268
Retinoblastoma, 71, 72, 98, 104, 105, 265
Retinoic acid, 153, 244, 246
Retinoids, 151, 152, 154
Rho, 122
Rubber manufacture, 34, 35
Rural areas, 40

S

Saccharin, 64, 85
Salicin, 153
Salt, 63, 64, 176, 194, 233
Sarcoma, 72, 268, 281, 284
Schistosoma haematobium, 57, 58, 228, 229
Schwannoma, 268
Secondary cancers, 48
Secondary glioblastoma, 267
Selenium, 209
Seminoma, 212
Senescence, 87
Serum pepsinogen, 177
Shade, 141
Shh, 54
Sigmoidoscopy, 164
Silica, 34
Single nucleotide polymorphisms, 324
Skin cancer, 34-37, 39, 41, 49-51, 53, 68, 69, 72, 92-94, 102, 111, 141-143, 154, 255, 268
SMAD gene family, 206
SMAD2, 199
SMAD4, 199
Small cell lung cancer, 185, 186, 281
Smoke, 232
Smokeless tobacco, 23, 25, 27
Smoking cessation, 25, 28, 75, 128, 129, 132, 133, 182, 183, 310
Smoking, see tobacco smoke
Smooth muscle tumours, 68
Snuff, 22, 233
Soil pollution, 41
Solar radiation, 37
Somatic mutation, 71
Soots, 34
Spinal ependymomas, 268
Spinal tumours, 266
Spiral CT, 185
Squalamine (NHE-3 inhibitor), 123
Squamous cell carcinoma, 53, 68, 72, 141, 142, 152, 167, 182, 185, 215, 216, 223, 230, 232
Stem cell, 240, 241, 244, 286
Steroid hormones, 191
STI-571, 246, 247, 285
STK11, 250, 251
Stomach cancer, 25, 29, 36, 42, 57, 58, 61, 63-65, 85, 94, 111, 120, 131, 175, 194, 196, 238, 274, 281, 284
Subependymal giant cell astrocytoma, 268
Subungual fibroma, 268
Sulfur dioxide (SO_2), 40, 138
Sulindac, 152
Sunburn, 142, 253
Sunlight, 51, 91, 135, 141, 253
Sunscreens, 141, 152
Surgical implants, 49
Surgical oncology, 272, 314

T

T cells, 59, 149, 242, 288, 289
Talc containing asbestiform fibres, 34
Tamoxifen, 48, 49, 151, 153, 156, 192, 218, 282, 286, 291
Taxanes, 186, 282, 283, 285, 286
TCDD, 34
Telemedicine, 276
Telomerase, 108, 206
Telomere, 108
Teniposide, 50
Testicular cancer, 60, 85, 208, 273, 281, 318
Testosterone, 85
2,3,7,8-Tetrachlorodibenzo-para-dioxin (TCDD), 34
1,1,2,2-Tetrachloroethane, 138
Tetrachloroethylene, 35
Tetraphthalic acid, 85
TGF-α, 123, 191
TGF-β, 123, 191, 259, 290
TGF βR2, 250
Thioguanine, 283
Thiotepa, 49
Thymidine kinase, 111
Thyroid cancer, 51, 52, 72, 257, 268, 273, 284
Thyroidectomy, 273
TNM staging, 191, 124
Tobacco advertising, 131
Tobacco control, 128, 306-310, 313, 323
Tobacco Free Initiative, 308
Tobacco smoke, 12, 21, 37, 91, 94, 128, 134, 140, 183, 228, 233, 248, 261, 308-310, 322
Tobacco, 22, 25, 30, 39, 41, 85, 102, 128, 182, 223, 228, 233, 248, 261, 304, 308-310, 313, 321
Tobacco-specific nitrosamines, 25
Toluene, 40
Topoisomerase, 191, 283, 285
TRAIL, 290
Transforming growth factors, see TGF-α, TGF-β
Transgenic mouse models, 113, 288
Transitional cell carcinoma of the urinary tract, 48, 228
Treosulfan, 49
Trichilemmomas, 268
Trichlorobenzene, 35
Trichloroethylene, 35, 138
Trimethylpentane, 85
TSC1, 268
TSC2, 268
Tuberous sclerosis, 268
Tumour antigens, 288-290
Tumour suppressor genes, 71, 73, 84, 86, 91, 96, 98-102, 109, 121, see also p53
TUNEL assay, 116
Turcot syndrome, 268
Tyrosinaemia, 204

U

UICC, 306
Ulcerative colitis, 273

Ulcerative colitis-associated colorectal carcinoma, 86
Ultimate carcinogen, 89
Ultraviolet radiation, 34, 37, 39, 49, 51, 54, 55, 69, 92, 94, 98, 102, 115, 139, 141, 253
UPA, 226
Uracil, 85
Urocanic acid (UCA), 54
Uterine cancer, see endometrial cancer

V

Vaccine, 149
Vaginal cancer, 49
Vascular endothelial growth factor (VEGF), 123, 191, 230. 290
Vasectomy, 209
Vegetables, 30, 46, 62, 151, 153, 175, 184, 189, 194, 198, 223, 233, 258, 307
VEGF, see vascular endothelial growth factor
VHL, 72, 263, 268
Vinblastine, 286
Vinca alkaloids, 186, 214, 219, 222, 230, 241, 281-283, 285
Vincristine, 286
Vinyl chloride, 34, 35, 94, 136, 138, 204

Vitamin A, 152, 209
Vitamin D, 209
Vitamin E, 209
Vitaxin, 123
von Hippel-Lindau disease, 72, 261, 262, 265, 268

W

Water pollution, 39, 41, 140
Western lifestyle, 76, 79, 188, 307
Wilms tumour, 71, 72, 99, 261, 263, 284
Wood dust, 34, 36, 233, 238

X

Xeroderma pigmentosum, 71, 72, 92, 100, 234
X-linked proliferative disorder, 72
XLP, 72
XPB, 92
XPC, 92
XPG, 92
X-radiation, 53